Textbook of Clinical Embryology

Textbook of Clinical Embryology

Third Edition

Vishram Singh, MBBS, MS, PhD(hc), MICPS, FASI, FIMSA

Adjunct Professor, Department of Anatomy, KMC, Mangalore
Manipal Academy of Higher Education, Manipal, Karnataka, India

Editor-in-chief, *Journal of the Anatomical Society of India*

Member, Federative International Committee
for Scientific Publications (FICSP) of IFAA, Geneva

Former Professor and Head, Department of Anatomy
Santosh Medical College
Member, Academic Council and Core Committee, PhD Course
Santosh University, Ghaziabad, NCR, Delhi

Project Editor, BI Churchill Livingstone, New Delhi

Examiner in National and International Universities
Member, Editorial Board
Indian Journal of Otology; Journal of Anatomy and Cell Biology; and
National Journal of Clinical Anatomy

Ex-Vice President, Anatomical Society of India
Medicolegal Advisor, ICPS, India
Consulting Editor, ABI, North Carolina, USA
Associate Editor, Acta Medica International
Member, COPE Council (England & Wales)
Member, British Association of Clinical Anatomists (BACA)

Formerly at: GSVM Medical College, Kanpur
King George's Medical College, Lucknow
Al-Arab Medical University, Benghazi (Libya)
All India Institute of Medical Sciences, New Delhi

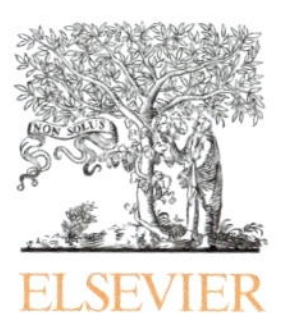

ELSEVIER

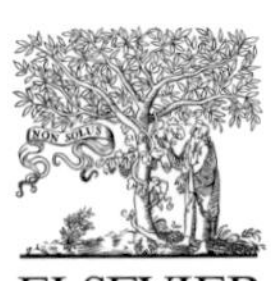

ELSEVIER

RELX India Pvt. Ltd.
Registered Office: 818, 8th Floor, Indraprakash Building, 21, Barakhamba Road, New Delhi 110 001
Corporate Office: 14th Floor, Building No. 10B, DLF Cyber City, Phase II, Gurgaon-122 002, Haryana, India

Textbook of Clinical Embryology, 3rd Edition, Vishram Singh

ISBN: 978-81-312-6396-9
eISBN: 978-81-312- 6397-6

Sr Content Strategist: Arvind Koul
Content Project Manager: Goldy Bhatnagar
Sr Cover Designer: Milind Majgaonkar
Sr Production Executive: Dhan Singh

Typeset by GW India

Printed in India by Manipal Technologies Limited, Manipal

Dedicated to

My Parents
Late Smt Ganga Devi Singh
and
Late Shri HR Singh, an ever-guiding force in my life

My Elder Sister
Late Smt Susheela Singh
for her help and cooperation during my student life

My Elder Brother
Shri Kaptan Singh
for his sacrifice for me

My Wife
Late Smt Manorama Rani Singh
for her unending support and cooperation of my pursuits

My Students
Past, and Present

Preface to the Third Edition

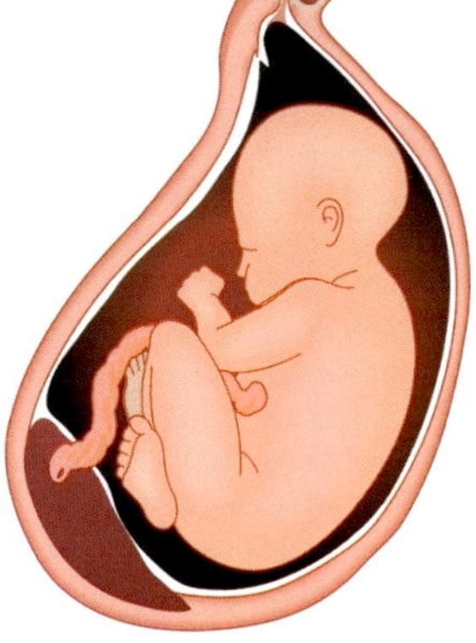

It is a matter of great pride to present before you all the third edition of *Textbook of Clinical Embryology* to view. This book is widely used not only in India but abroad also by the undergraduate and postgraduate students of anatomy, pediatrics, and obstetrics and gynecology. The popularity of this book reflects the appeal of its concept building approach and easy to understand language with clearly drawn figures. This approach has been retained in this edition as well. Based on a large number of suggestions, criticisms and comments received from the students and fellow academicians, the following major changes have been taken.

In this edition two new chapters, one on basic processes of development and molecular regulation, and another on teratology and prenatal diagnosis have been added. The chapter on medical genetics has been rewritten to include all its aspects as desired by NMC.

Further pre-embryonic and embryonic periods of development have been described on weekly basis for easy assimilation of the facts. This has led to reorganization of chapters.

In this edition new features such as addition of competencies in learning objectives new facts to remember, new line diagrams, half-tone diagrams, ultrasonographs, tables, and flowcharts have been included. In addition, at the end of each chapter the solution of clinical problems, and case studies based on text of that chapter have been discussed in detail. Most of the diagrams are completely revised and redrawn by the Author himself for easy understanding and reproducibility in the exam. The topics on fertilization, gametogenesis, extraembryonic membranes, heart and blood vessels, urogenital system, and sensory organs have been extensively revised.

In addition competencies has been added in learning objectives also.

In addition, complimentary access to online animations, chapter-wise image bank along with complete e-book is also provided.

I sincerely hope that with changes made in this edition will make this book more interesting and useful than the previous one. I would highly appreciate to receive fair comments, both good and bad, from students and teachers.

"Providing clear, simple, and uncluttered teaching material to student is a prime job of a teacher."

Vishram Singh

Preface to the First Edition

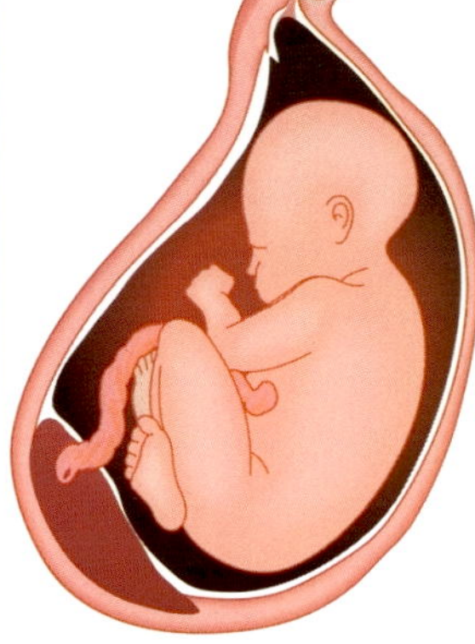

Textbook of Clinical Embryology has been carefully planned for the first year medical and dental students. It follows the revised anatomy curriculum of the Medical Council of India. Following the current trends of clinically oriented study of Anatomy, I have adopted a parallel approach of imparting basic embryological knowledge to students and simultaneously providing them its applied aspects.

To help students score high in examinations the text is written in simple language. It is arranged in easily understandable small sections. While embryological details of little clinical relevance, phylogenetic discussions, and comparative analogies have been either omitted or described in brief, all clinically important topics are described in detail. Because of increasingly significant role of molecular biology and genetics in embryology and study of birth defects, the basic molecular and genetic principles are discussed throughout the text. In addition, a separate chapter on medical genetics has been added. The tables and flowcharts given in the book summarize important and complex information into digestible knowledge capsules. Multiple choice questions have been given chapter-by-chapter at the end of the book to test the level of understanding and memory recall of the students. The numerous simple four-color illustrations and clinical photographs further assist in fast comprehension and retention of complicated information. *All the illustrations are drawn by the author himself to ensure accuracy.*

Throughout the preparation of this book one thing I have kept in mind is that thorough knowledge of embryology is required by Clinicians, especially Gynecologists, Pediatricians, and Pediatric Surgeons for physical examination, prenatal diagnostic tests, and surgical procedures. Therefore, embryological events relevant to prenatal diagnostic and surgical procedures are clinically correlated throughout the text. Further, patient-oriented problems and their embryological and genetic basis are presented at the end of each chapter for problem-based learning so that the students could use their embryological knowledge in clinical situations. Moreover, keeping in mind the relevance of embryological knowledge in day-to-day clinical practice, a separate chapter on developmental events during the entire period of gestation and their application in clinical practice is given at the end of the book.

I pay my heartfelt tribute to all the authors of various embryology books, especially *Developing Human: Clinically Oriented Embryology*, 8th edition by Keith L Moore and TVN Persaud, which I have consulted during the preparation of this book. From *Developing Human* and few other books, some photographs have been used in this book after obtaining due permission from concerned authorities (please refer to page 331 for Figure Credits).

As a teacher, I have tried my best to make the book easy to understand and interesting to read. For further improvement of this book, I would greatly welcome comments and suggestions from the readers. All these comments and suggestions can be e-mailed at indiacontact@elsevier.com and drvishramsingh@gmail.com.

'Mind perceives new ideas best only when put to test.'

Vishram Singh

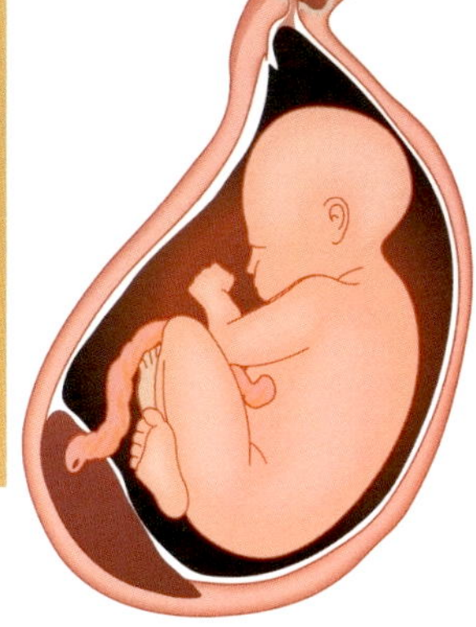

Acknowledgments

At the outset, I would like to express my gratitude to Prof. (Dr.) A. Halim, my teacher and former Prof. and Head of the Department of Anatomy, King George's Medical University, Lucknow, for creating my interest in anatomy. I learned the art of drawing simple and technically accurate line diagrams from him. May God bless him with long life.

I sincerely thank my colleagues in the Department, especially Prof. Mangala M. Pai (HOD), Prof. Latha V. Prabhu, and Dr. B. V. Murlimanju for their cooperation and appreciation of my work. I highly appreciate the help provided by Dr. Preeti Shrivastava, Associate Prof., NDMC Medical College and Hindu Rao Hospital, Delhi, for going through the proofs of this book.

I gratefully acknowledge the feedback and support of all my fellow colleagues in Anatomy throughout India, particularly:

- Prof. Punita Manik (Head of the Department), King George Medical University, Lucknow, Uttar Pradesh.
- Prof. A. Shariff (Head of the Department), AIIMS, New Delhi.
- Prof. Deepti Shastri (Dean) VMKVMC & Hospital, Salem, Tamil Nadu.
- Prof. Bipin Khade (Head of Department) Chirayu Medical College, Bhopal, Madhya Pradesh.
- Prof. T.S. Roy (Head of Department), NDMC Medical College and Hindu Rao Hospital, Delhi.
- Prof. N.C. Goel, Vice Principal and Dr. Shweta Singh, Acting Head of the Department, Hind Institute of Medical Sciences, Barabanki, Lucknow, Uttar Pradesh.
- Prof. P.K. Sharma (Head of the Department), Era Medical College, Lucknow, Uttar Pradesh.
- Prof. Poonam Kharb (Head of the Department), ITS Dental College, Ghaziabad, Uttar Pradesh.
- Prof. T.C. Singel, Zydus Medical College, Dahod, Gujarat.
- Profs Vandana Mehta (Head of the Department) and Hitendra Lohiya, Vardhman Mahavir Medical College and Safdarjang Hospital, New Delhi.
- Prof. Sneh Agrawal (Head of the Department), Lady Harding Medical College, New Delhi.
- Prof. Shashi Raheja (Head of the Department), Dr. Baba Sahib Ambedkar Medical College and Hospital, Rohini, New Delhi.
- Prof. Vanita Gupta (Head of the Department), Rama Medical College, Hapur, Uttar Pradesh.
- Profs S.L. Jethani (Medical Superintendent) and Deepa Singh (Head of the Department) and Akshya Dubey, Himalayan Institute of Medical Sciences, Jolly Grant, Dehradun, Uttarakhand.
- Prof. W.M.S. Johnson (Dean), Sree Balaji Medical College, Chennai.
- Prof. Suniti Pandey (Head of the Department), GSVM Medical College, Kanpur.
- Prof. G.M. Mahesh, Basaveshwara Medical College, Chitradurga, Karnataka.
- Prof. Sneha Guruprasad Kalthur and Dr. Prakash Babu, KMC, Manipal, MAHE, Karnataka.
- Profs C.P. Vishwanathan (Director and Emeritus Professor) and S.S. Rajasekar (Head of the Department), NRI Institute of Medical Sciences, Vishakhapatnam, Hyderabad.
- Dr. S.D. Joshi, Director Professor of Anatomy, Sri Aurobindo Medical College and P.G. Institute, Indore, Madhya Pradesh.

I would also like to express my deep sense of regards to renowned anatomists of India, especially to Prof. (Dr.) A.C. Das (my teacher), Prof. (Dr.) Inderbir Singh, Prof. (Dr.) Mahdi Hasan, Prof. (Dr.) Indra Bhargava, Prof. (Dr.) Shamer Singh, Prof. (Dr.) A.K. Datta and Dr. B.D. Chaurasia, who inspired me a lot during my student life and teaching carrier.

Lastly, I thank my daughter Dr. Rashi Singh, son Dr. Gaurav Singh and daughter-in-law Ms. Anupama Singh for helping me in the preparation of this manuscript. I gratefully acknowledge the help and cooperation received from the staff of RELX India Pvt Ltd, especially Arvind Koul (Sr. Content Strategist), Shabina Nasim (Head of Content Project Management) and Goldy Bhatnagar (Content Project Manager), in completing the project on time.

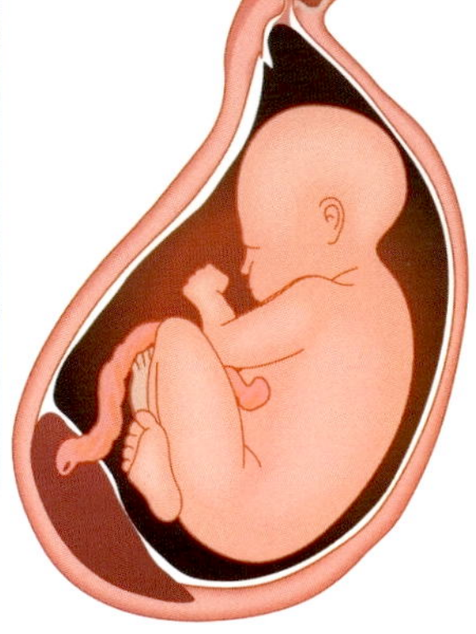

List of Animations

Contents

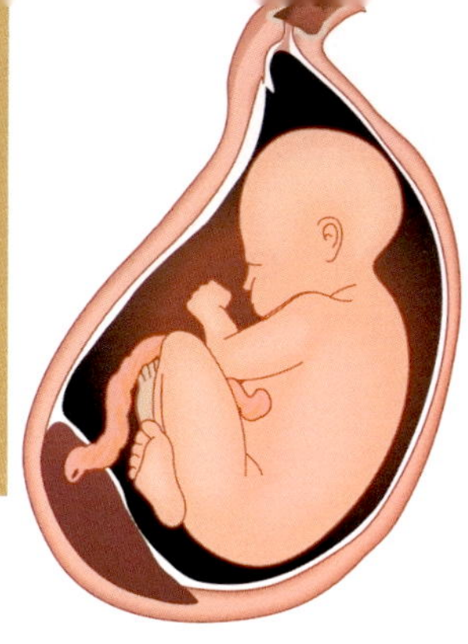

Competency Map: Embryology

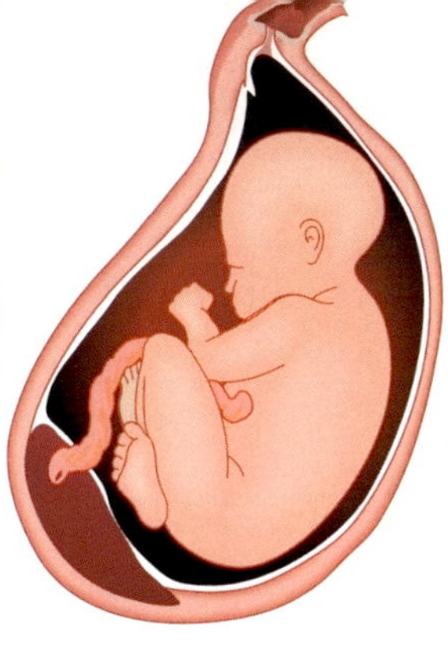

Competency code	COMPETENCY			Core (Y/N)	Chapter Nos.	Page Nos.
Topic: Introduction to Embryology						
AN 76.1	Describe the stages of human life.			Y	1	1–3
AN 76.2	Explain the terms- phylogeny, ontogeny, trimester, viability.			Y	2	12
Topic: Gametogenesis and Fertilization						
AN 77.1	Describe the uterine changes occurring during the menstrual cycle.			Y	3	25–26
AN 77.2	Describe the synchrony between the ovarian and menstrual cycles.			Y	3	28
AN 77.3	Describe spermatogenesis and oogenesis along with diagrams.			Y	4	35–37
AN 77.4	Describe the stages and consequences of fertilisation.			Y	5	45–49
AN 77.5	Enumerate and describe the anatomical principles underlying contraception.			Y	5	56
AN 77.6	Describe teratogenic influences; fertility and sterility, surrogate motherhood, social significance of "sex-ratio".			N	5	49 All topics have not been dealt in this book.
Topic: Second Week of Development						
AN 78.1	Describe cleavage and formation of blastocyst.			Y	5	50–51
AN 78.2	Describe the development of trophoblast.			Y	5 6	51 58–59
AN 78.3	Describe the process of implantation and common abnormal sites of implantation.			Y	5	53–54
AN 78.4	Describe the formation of extra-embryonic mesoderm and coelom, bilaminar disc and prochordal plate.			Y	6 6	58–61 60–62
AN 78.5	Describe in brief abortion; decidual reaction, pregnancy test.			Y	6, 5	58, 56

Continued

Competency code	COMPETENCY			Core (Y/N)	Chapter Nos.	Page Nos.
Topic: 3rd to 8th Week of Development						
AN 79.1	Describe the formation and fate of the primitive streak.	K	KH	Y	7	64–66
AN 79.2	Describe formation and fate of notochord.	K	KH	Y	7	66–68
AN 79.3	Describe the process of neurulation.	K	KH	Y	7	68–69
AN 79.4	Describe the development of somites and intra-embryonic coelom.	K	KH	Y	7, 21	69–72, 226
AN 79.5	Explain embryological basis of congenital malformations, nucleus pulposus, sacrococcygeal teratomas, neural tube defects.	K	KH	N	9 7, 12	83–84 74, 126–127
AN 79.6	Describe the diagnosis of pregnancy in first trimester and role of teratogens, alpha-fetoprotein.	K	KH	N	8	82
Topic: Fetal Membranes						
AN 80.1	Describe formation, functions and fate of-chorion: amnion; yolk sac; allantois and decidua.			Y	10	92–95
AN 80.2	Describe formation and structure of umbilical cord.			Y	10	107–108
AN 80.3	Describe formation of placenta, its physiological functions, foetomaternal circulation and placental barrier.			Y	10	96–106
AN 80.4	Describe embryological basis of twinning in monozygotic and dizygotic twins.			Y	10	108–110
AN 80.5	Describe role of placental hormones in uterine growth and parturition.			Y	10	104
AN 80.6	Explain embryological basis of estimation of fetal age.			N	30	364
AN 80.7	Describe various types of umbilical cord attachments.			N	10	106–107
Topic: Prenatal Diagnosis						
AN 81.1	Describe various methods of prenatal diagnosis.			Y	9	88–89
AN 81.2	Describe indications, process and disadvantages of amniocentesis.			Y	9	89
AN 81.3	Describe indications, process and disadvantages of chorion villus biopsy.			Y	9	89

Competency code	COMPETENCY			Core (Y/N)	Chapter Nos.	Page Nos.
AN 13.8	Describe development of upper limb.			N	12	134–136
AN 20.10	Describe basic concept of development of lower limb.			N	12	136–138
AN 25.2	Describe development of pleura, lungs, and heart.			Y	20, 22	216–224, 236–251
AN 25.5	Describe developmental basis of congenital anomalies, transposition of great vessels, dextrocardia, patent ductus arteriosus and coarctation of aorta.			Y	22	258
AN 25.3	Describe fetal circulation and changes occurring at birth.			Y	23	269–270
AN 25.4	Describe embryological basis of tracheo-esophageal fistula.			Y	20	218–219
AN 25.4	Describe embryological basis of: atrial septal defect, ventricular septal defect.			Y	22	243, 247
AN 25.6	Mention development of aortic arch arteries.			N	23	253–259
AN 25.6	Mention development of SVC, IVC and coronary sinus.			N	23	264–269
AN 39.1	Describe the embryological basis of nerve supply of extrinsic and intrinsic muscles of tongue.			Y	15	161–164
AN 43.4	Describe the development and developmental basis of congenital anomalies of face, palate, tongue, branchial apparatus, pituitary gland, thyroid gland and eye.			Y	14, 15, 16, 27, 28	148–158, 161–166, 169–177, 323–326, 328–335
AN 52.4	Describe the development of anterior abdominal wall.			N	9	115
AN 52.5	Describe the development and congenital anomalies of Diaphragm.			Y	21	226–231
AN 52.6	Describe the development and congenital anomalies of: Foregut, Midgut and Hindgut.			Y	18	188–204
AN 52.7	Describe the development of Urinary system.			Y	24	275–288
AN 52.8	Describe the development of male and female reproductive system.			Y	25	290–308
AN 64.2	Describe the development of neural tube, spinal cord, medulla oblongata, pons, midbrain, cerebral hemisphere and cerebellum.			Y	26	310–320
AN 64.3	Describe various types of open neural tube defects with its embryological basis.			N	26	322

Continued

Competency code	COMPETENCY			Core (Y/N)	Chapter Nos.	Page Nos.
Topic: Chromosomes						
AN 73.1	Describe the structure of chromosomes with classification.			Y	29	345–346
AN 73.2	Describe technique of karyotyping with its applications.			Y	29	346–347
AN 73.3	Describe the Lyon's hypothesis.			Y	29	347
Topic: Patterns of Inheritance						
AN 74.1	Describe the various modes of inheritance with examples.			Y	29	354–355
AN 74.2	Draw pedigree charts for the various types of inheritance and give examples of diseases of each mode of inheritance.			Y	29	356–358
AN 74.3	Describe multifactorial inheritance with examples.			Y	29	359
AN 74.4	Describe the genetic basis and clinical features of Achondroplasia, Cystic Fibrosis, Vitamin D resistant rickets, Haemophilia, Duchene's muscular dystrophy and Sickle cell anaemia.			N	29	359–361 All examples have not been dealt in this book.
Topic: Principle of Genetics, Chromosomal Aberrations and Clinical Genetics						
AN 75.1	Describe the structural and numerical chromosomal aberrations.			Y	29	347–350
AN 75.2	Explain the terms mosaics and chimeras with example.			N	29	353–354
AN 75.3	Describe the genetic basis and clinical features of Prader Willi syndrome, Edward syndrome and Patau syndrome.			N	29	351
AN 75.4	Describe genetic basis of variation: polymorphism and mutation.			Y	29	353–354
AN 75.5	Describe the principles of genetic counselling.			Y	29	359

1 Introduction and History of Embryology

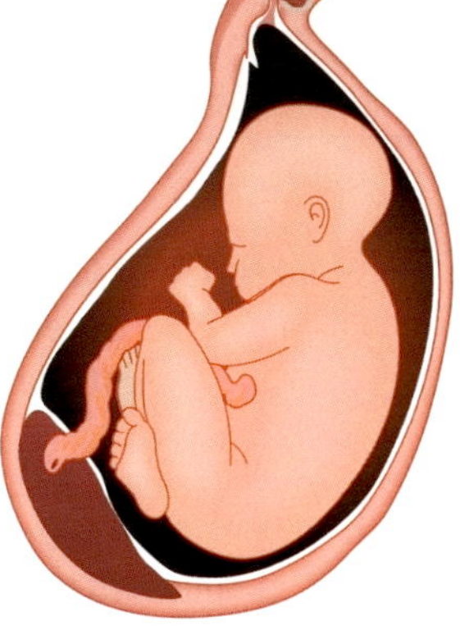

LEARNING OBJECTIVES

After studying this chapter, the student should be able to:

- Define embryology and tell how it differs from developmental anatomy.
- Divide prenatal development into preembryonic, embryonic, and fetal periods.
- Enumerate five periods of postnatal development.
- Describe the stages of human life. AN 76.1
- Write short notes on: (a) viability, and (b) trimesters. AN 76.2

OVERVIEW AN 76.1

Embryology is the science that deals with the development and growth of an individual before birth. It begins with fertilization of an oocyte (ovum) by a sperm and culminates with the birth of the baby at term. The entire period of development from fertilization to birth is termed **prenatal development**. The period of prenatal development is also called **gestation period/pregnancy**. (Pregnancy is described in detail in Chapter 30, p. 363.)

The development of an individual continues even after birth up to the age of 25 years. This period of development is termed **postnatal development**.

N.B. The term ***pregnancy*** used by clinicians refers to state of female carrying an unborn baby (products of conception) inside her uterus (Latin: *Pregnancy*, which means carrying products of conception). It consists of 38 weeks duration extending from fertilization to birth.

PRENATAL DEVELOPMENT

The prenatal development is a fascinating and awesome event. It begins with a single cell – the zygote (fertilized ovum) – and culminates after 9 months (38 weeks or 266 days) with a complex organism – the **newborn** – made of billions of cells. This involves a process called **morphogenesis**, which includes **cell division, transformation** or **specialization, migration**, and even programmed cell death (**apoptosis**).

During morphogenesis, genetic or environmental factors may affect the normal development of the baby and may cause *congenital anomalies*.

Thus, embryology helps us in understanding not only the rationale of structure and functions of each body system but also the factors responsible for causing congenital anomalies. The appreciation of these factors may assist the clinicians in preventing and treating such anomalies.

Periods of Prenatal Development

They are classified into two types:

A. **According to clinicians**

The prenatal development or pregnancy lasts for about 40 weeks. It is calculated from the first day of last menstrual cycle till birth.

The whole period of pregnancy is divided into three parts, each lasting for about 3 months and called trimesters.

- **First trimester** (week 1–week 12)
- **Second trimester** (week 13–week 28)
- **Third trimester** (week 29–week 40)

These are described in detail in Chapter 30, p. 366.

B. **According to embryologists**

The prenatal development is divided into three periods: (a) preembryonic period, (b) embryonic period, and (c) fetal period.

1. **Preembryonic period:** It extends from conception (fertilization) to the end of the 2nd week of intrauterine life (IUL).
2. **Embryonic period:** It extends from beginning of the 3rd week to the end of 8th week of IUL.
3. **Fetal period:** It extends from beginning of the 9th week to birth of the baby.

Table 1.1 Morphological events occurring during preembryonic, embryonic, and fetal periods of prenatal development

Period	Morphological Events
1. Preembryonic period (from fertilization to 2nd week)	• Formation of zygote • Initiation of cleavage • Implantation • Formation of bilaminar germ disc
2. Embryonic period (from 3rd week to 8th week)	• Formation of three germ layers • Organogenesis • Folding of embryo • Formation of miniature human • Differentiation of germ layers into specific body organs
3. Fetal period (from 9th week to birth)	Growth and specialization of the body structures

The periods of prenatal development and events occurring during these periods are shown in Table 1.1.

N.B. Clinically, the **prenatal development** is divided into two periods: (a) embryonic period and (b) fetal period.

(a) **Embryonic period:** It extends from fertilization to the end of the 8th week and the developing organism is called an **embryo**.

(b) **Fetal period:** It extends from beginning of the 9th week (3rd month) until the birth.

POSTNATAL DEVELOPMENT

The development of an individual from birth to about 25 years is called postnatal development.

Viability

It refers to the capability of fetus to survive outside the uterus.

The general age of fetal viability is 24 weeks of gestation. This means that babies born after 24 weeks of gestation can live, grow, and develop.

Periods of Postnatal Development

The postnatal development is divided into the following five periods:

1. Infancy (from birth to 1 year of age)
2. Childhood (from 2 to 12 years of age)
3. Puberty (from 13 to 16 years of age)
4. Adolescence (from 17 to 18 years of age)
5. Adulthood (from 19 to 25 years of age)

Infancy

The infancy period ranges from birth to 1 year of age and the newborn during this period is termed **infant.** The first 4 weeks of this period are very critical for the survival of the **newborn** because the transition from intrauterine to the extrauterine existence requires many changes, especially in the cardiovascular and respiratory systems. During this period there is a rapid growth of the body. This period is called **neonatal period** and the newborn during this period is termed **neonate.** If a newborn survives first few hours after birth, his/her chances of survival are usually good. The care of the baby during the neonatal period is termed **neonatology**.

N.B. The term **perinatal period** used by clinicians extends from 28th week of pregnancy to the end of 6th day after birth.

Childhood

The period of childhood extends from beginning of the 2nd year to the age of 12 years. The care of children during this period is exciting because of the constancy of change in their growth and development. Children do not stay the same during this period. As the child grows, the rate of growth slows down; however, just before puberty the growth accelerates. This is called **prepubertal growth spurt**. The medical subject dealing with the care of children in health and disease is termed **pediatrics**.

Puberty (*Latin*: Pubertas, Which Means Development of Sex Characteristics)

The puberty period ranges from 12 to 15 years in females and 13 to 16 years in males. During this period there is a very rapid physical growth and development of secondary sexual characters, and the capability of sexual reproduction is attained. The growth during puberty is dependent on the interaction of growth hormone (insulin-like growth factor 1 [IGF-1]) and sex steroids.

Adolescence

The adolescence period ranges from 17 to 18 years. This period is characterized by rapid physical growth and sexual maturation. The gonads begin to secrete testosterone and estrogen. During this period the ability to reproduce is achieved.

Adulthood (*Latin*: Adultas, Which Means Grown Up)

The adulthood period ranges from 19 to 25 years. During this period, full growth and development of body organs including ossification of bones is virtually completed.

Stages of Human Life

The stages of life refer to different phases of life through which all individuals pass in a normal lifetime. These are:

1. **Prenatal development:** from fertilization to birth
2. **Infancy:** from birth to 1 year of age
3. **Childhood:** from 2 to 12 years of age
4. **Puberty:** from 13 to 16 years of age
5. **Adolescence:** from 17 to 18 years of age
6. **Adulthood:** from 19 to 25 years of age
7. **Middle age:** from 40 to 59 years of age
8. **Old age:** from 60 years to death.

SUBDIVISIONS OF EMBRYOLOGY

1. General Embryology

It deals with the development of an individual during first 8 weeks after fertilization (i.e., it deals with preembryonic and embryonic periods). During this period a single cell called zygote (fertilized ovum) is converted into a form that externally resembles the features of a miniature human and all organs and systems are formed.

2. Systemic Embryology

It deals with the functional maturation of various organs and systems of body that are formed during the embryonic period.

3. Descriptive Embryology

It deals with the structure of different organs at various stages of development.

4. Comparative Embryology

It deals with the study of embryos in various species of animals.

5. Experimental Embryology

It deals with the results obtained from experiments of living embryos/fetuses of the lower animals.

6. Chemical Embryology

It deals with the biochemical aspect of the prenatal development.

7. Teratology

It is a branch of embryology that is concerned with the congenital anomalies or birth defects, i.e., it deals with abnormal embryonic and fetal development. Teratology is described in detail in Chapter 9, p. 83.

RECENT ADVANCES IN EMBRYOLOGY

1. **Prenatal diagnosis:** It is the detection of congenital abnormalities in an unborn child. Some of the techniques used for this purpose are as follows:
   (a) Amniocentesis
   (b) Chorionic villous sampling
   (c) Ultrasonography
   (d) Fetoscopy
   (e) Fetal blood sampling
   (f) Maternal serum screening
   (g) MRI
   For details, see p. 88.
2. **In vitro fertilization:** In vitro fertilization (IVF) of human ova and then their transfer in the uterus has now become a standard procedure throughout the world to solve the problems of infertility. On July 25, 1978, Louise Joy Brown, the first test tube baby, was born to Lesley Brown.
3. **Gene therapy:** It deals with the replacement of a deficient gene product or correction of an abnormal gene. It can be done in vitro or in vivo.
4. **Cloning:** The advancement in molecular biology has led to many sophisticated techniques that are now widely used in research laboratories for genetic regulation of morphogenesis. Now the researchers have started understanding how, when, and where selected genes are activated and expressed in the embryo during development. For example:
   (a) Now cloning is possible. The first mammal clone, **Dolly** the sheep, was cloned in 1997 (Fig. 1.1) by using the technique of somatic cell nuclear transfer.
   (b) The interest in *human cloning* has generated a considerable debate because of social, moral, ethical, and legal implications.
   (c) More recently, the cloning of a human embryo has been reported.
5. **Stem cell therapy:** *Stem cells* are cells found in multicellular organisms. These cells have the ability to

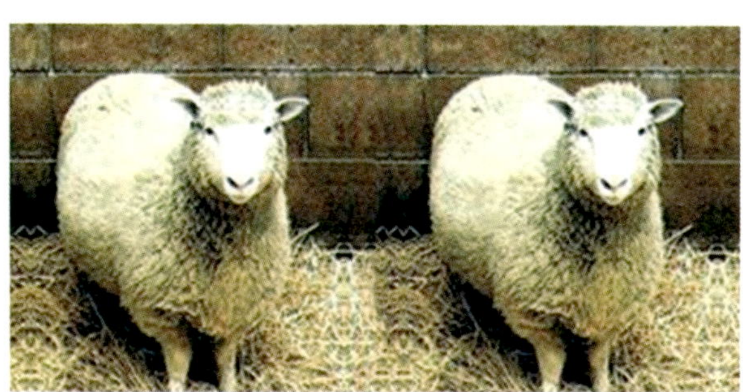

Fig. 1.1 Dolly, the first cloned sheep.

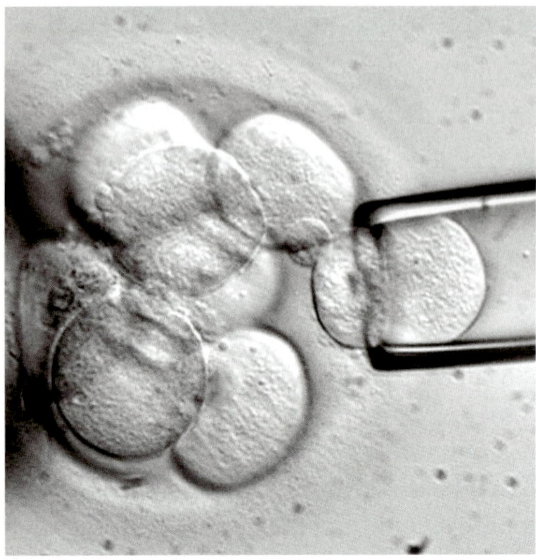

Fig. 1.2 Embryonic stem cells.

renew themselves and differentiate into a diverse range of specialized cell types. There are two broad types of mammalian stem cells:

(a) *Embryonic stem cells (ESCs)*, which are isolated from the inner cell mass of the blastocysts (Fig. 1.2). These are pluripotent, i.e., they have the ability to form different cell types.

(b) *Adult stem cells*, which are found in adult tissues, e.g., bone marrow. These cells are restricted in their ability to form different cell types and therefore are *multipotent*, not pluripotent.

The adult stem cells can be reprogrammed back into embryonic-like pluripotent cells. Such stem cells are called **induced pluripotent stem cells (iPSCs)**.

N.B. The isolation and programmed culture of human embryonic stem cells hold a great potential for the treatment of degenerative, malignant, and genetic diseases. (The embryonic stem cells are pluripotent. They are capable of self-renewal and are able to differentiate into specialized cell types.)

PURPOSE OF STUDYING EMBRYOLOGY (UTILITY AND SCOPE OF EMBRYOLOGY IN MEDICINE)

A thorough knowledge of embryology is important for the following reasons.

1. **It explains the positions and relations of various organs and neurovascular structures in adult gross anatomy.**
2. **It helps to understand the cause of development of various congenital anomalies** such as tracheoesophageal fistula, polycystic kidney, and subhepatic cecum.

   The knowledge of various factors causing congenital anomalies (such as use of alcohol, smoking, drugs, viral infections, and teratogens) can be useful in preventing their occurrence by rendering advice and adopting preventive measures.
3. Some aspects of general embryology such as gametogenesis, fertilization, and implantation are of great importance to understand the cause of **infertility and its management**. It also helps in **family planning**.
4. It forms the basis of concept of growth, repair, and regeneration of tissues, and **understanding of the development of various embryonic tumors**.
5. *In utero surgery* is nowadays possible to treat certain congenital anomalies, namely, *congenital diaphragmatic hernias* and *repair of spina bifida*, only due to in-depth study of embryology.
6. **It provides the basis for medical termination of pregnancy** in various congenital diseases, which are incompatible with life.
7. **It provides insight for use of molecular biology for genetic regulation of human development.**

HISTORY OF EMBRYOLOGY

The following text provides only a brief account of history of embryology as a mark of respect to some legends who have a significant contribution in the field of embryology.

> **"If I have seen further, it is by standing on the shoulders of the earlier giants."**
>
> *–Sir Isaac Newton*

1. **Ancient Egyptians** (3000 BCE) knew about the methods of incubation of eggs of the birds. They also believed that Aten, the Sun god, is the creator of germ in woman and seed in man and gives life to the baby in the body of mother.
2. The ***Garbha Upanishad***, an ancient scripture of Hindus (written in around 1416 BCE), describes following ideas about embryo:
   (a) Embryo comes into existence from conjugation of blood and semen during the period favorable for conception after sexual intercourse.
   (b) Developmental stages of an embryo are as follows:

• 1-day-old embryo	Formation of Kallada
• After 7 nights	Formation of vesicle
• After 1 month	Formation of spherical mass
• After 2 months	Formation of head
• After 3 months	Formation of limbs

3. **Hippocrates** (460–377 BCE) (Fig. 1.3) gave the following advice to understand the development of the embryo: Take 20 or more eggs and let them be

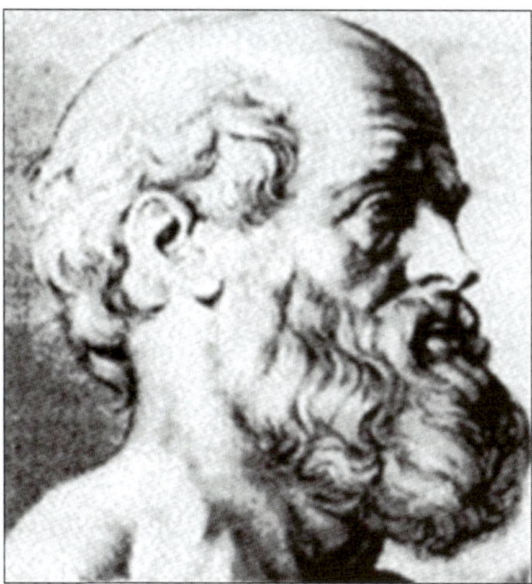

Fig. 1.3 Hippocrates (460–377 BCE).

incubated by two or more hens. Then from the second day to the day of hatching, remove one egg every day, break it, and examine it. You will exactly see how the embryo develops. This development of chick embryo can be similar to that of man.

4. **Aristotle** (384–322 BCE) (Fig. 1.4) wrote a treatise on embryology in which he described the development of the chick and other embryos. Aristotle is regarded as the *Founder of Embryology*. According to him, an embryo develops from a formless mass, which he described as a fully concocted seed with a nutritive soul and all body parts. The mass arose from menstrual blood after activation by semen.
5. **Claudius Galen** (CE 130–201) (Fig. 1.5) wrote a book on the formation of the fetus in which he described the development and nutrition of fetuses. He also described structures that are now called **allantois**, **amnion**, and **placenta**.

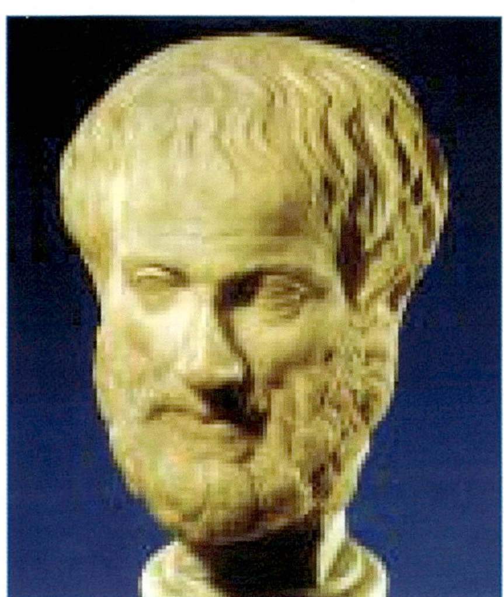

Fig. 1.4 Aristotle (384–322 BCE).

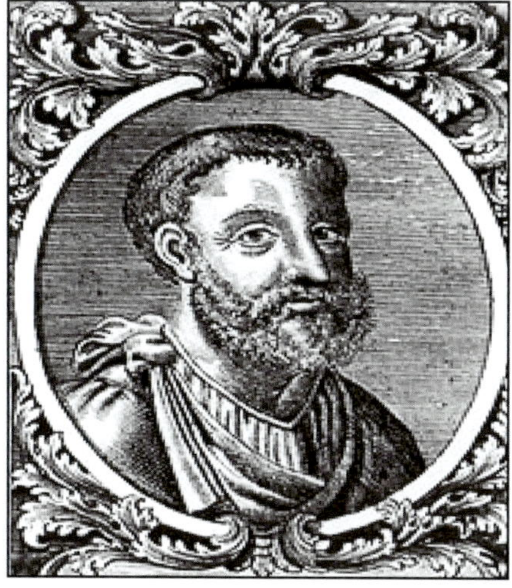

Fig. 1.5 Claudius Galen (CE 130–201).

6. **Samuel-el-Yehudi** (2nd century CE) described six stages in the formation of embryo from a "formless, rolled-up thing" to a "child whose months have been completed."
7. ***Quran*** (7th century CE), the holy book of the Muslims, describes that the human beings are produced from a mixture of secretions from the male and female. It also mentions that the human being is created from *nafla* (small drop). It also states that the resulting organism settles in the womb like a seed 6 days after its beginning. The early embryo resembles a leech and later it resembles a "chewed substance."
8. **Leonardo da Vinci** (1452–1519) (Fig. 1.6) made accurate drawings of dissections of uterus of pregnant women containing fetuses (Fig. 1.7).

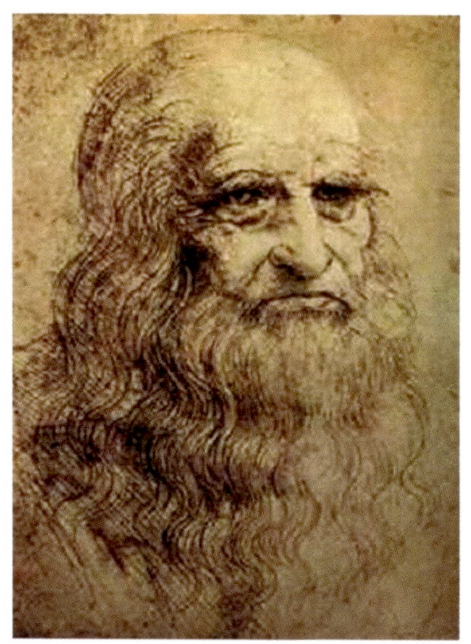

Fig. 1.6 Leonardo da Vinci (1452–1519).

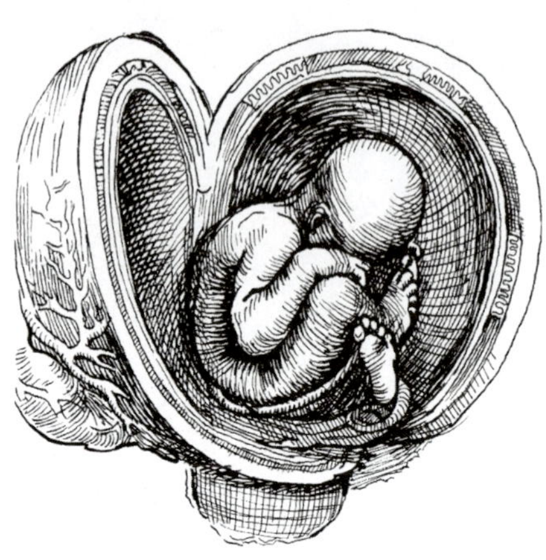

Fig. 1.7 Reproduction in Leonardo da Vinci's drawing made in the 15th century CE to show a fetus in the uterus. Modified from figure published in Publication *The Developing Human: Clinically Oriented Embryology*, 8th edition by Keith L. Moore and T.V.N. Persaud, ISBN: 9781416037064, page 9, Fig. 1.4, Copyright Elsevier, 2008.

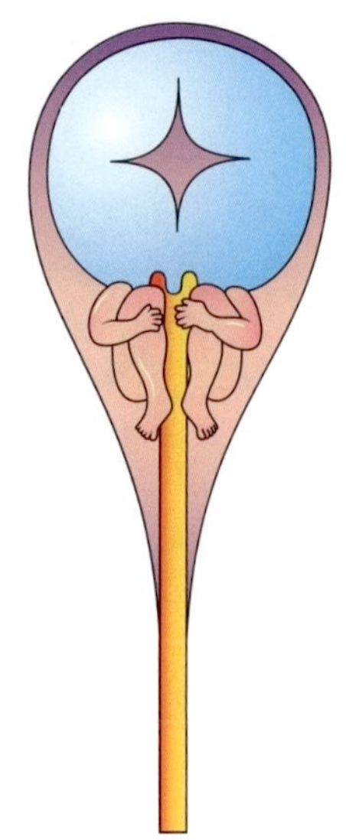

Fig. 1.8 Seventeenth century drawing of a sperm by Hartsoeker. Modified from figure published in Publication *The Developing Human: Clinically Oriented Embryology*, 8th edition by Keith L. Moore and T.V.N. Persaud, ISBN: 9781416037064, page 10, Fig. 1.6, Copyright Elsevier, 2008.

9. **William Harvey** (1578–1657) believed that male seeds or sperms after entering the womb or uterus get metamorphosed into an egg-like substance that gives rise to an embryo.
10. **Regnier de Graaf** was the first to observe vesicular ovarian follicles in 1672 with the help of simple microscopes, which are still called *Graafian follicles*.
11. **Johan Ham van Arnheim** and **Anton van Leeuwenhoek** were the first to observe a human sperm. They thought that sperms contain a miniature preformed human being that gets enlarged when sperm is deposited in the female genital tract.

    Other embryologists at this time thought that the oocyte contained a miniature human being that enlarged when it was stimulated by a sperm (Fig. 1.8).
12. **Caspar Friedrich Wolff** (1759) proposed the *layer concept*, i.e., zygote produces layers from which the embryo develops. His ideas formed the basis of the *theory of epigenesis*, which states that the development results from growth and differentiation of specialized cells. The mesonephros and mesonephric duct are called Wolffian body and Wolffian duct, respectively, after his name.
13. **Lazaro Spallanzani** (1775) said that both oocyte and sperm are necessary for initiating the development of an individual.
14. **Heinrich Christian Pander** discovered the *three germ layers* in 1817.
15. **Etienne Saint Hilaire** and **Isidore Saint Hilaire** made the significant studies of abnormal development in 1818, initiating what we now know as the *science of teratology*.
16. **Karl Ernst von Baer** (Fig. 1.9) described the *oocyte* in the ovarian follicle of a dog in 1827. He also noted cleaving zygote in uterine tube and blastocysts in the uterus. His study provided new knowledge about the origin of tissues and organs from three germ layers of the embryo, which formulated two embryological concepts: (a) *corresponding stages of embryonic development* and (b) *that general*

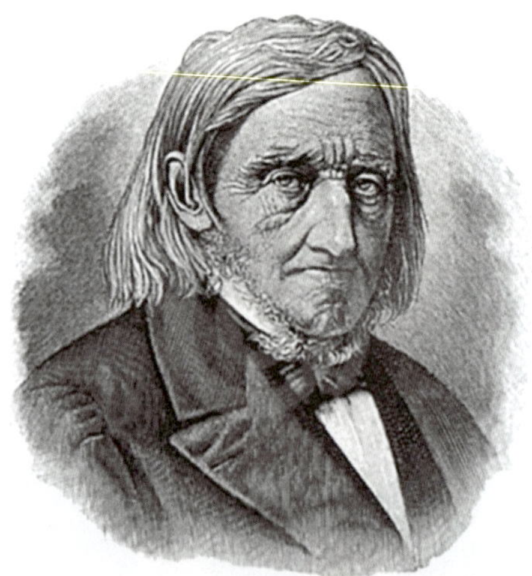

Fig. 1.9 Karl Ernst von Baer.

characteristics precede specific ones. For his significant and far-reaching contributions, he is regarded as the *Father of Modern Embryology*.

17. **Hans Spemann** (1869–1941) discovered the phenomenon of *primary induction*, i.e., how one tissue determines the fate of another. He was awarded Nobel Prize in 1935.
18. **Patrick Steptoe** and **Robert G. Edwards** (Fig. 1.10) pioneered the development of the technique of *in vitro fertilization*. Louise Brown is the first *test tube baby* born in 1978.
19. **James Till** (1931–) (Fig. 1.11) along with **Ernest McCulloch** discovered stem cells in 1960. Since the discovery of stem cells by James Till, the hope for treatment of terminal diseases has become enormous.
20. **Ian Wilmut** (1944–), an English embryologist (Fig. 1.12), is best known for leading a team that cloned a mammal from an adult somatic cell in 1996 – a Finnish Dorset lamb named Dolly (Fig. 1.1). The cloning is a cell, cell product, or organism that is genetically identical to the unit or individual from which it was derived. Clones are duplicates of each other resembling in anatomy and physiology.

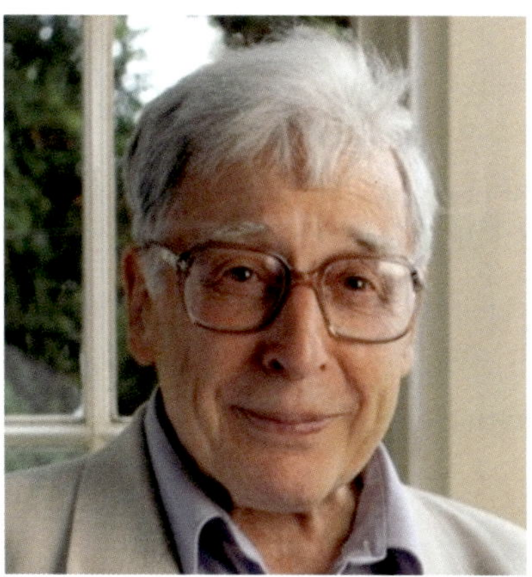

Fig. 1.10 Patrick Steptoe.

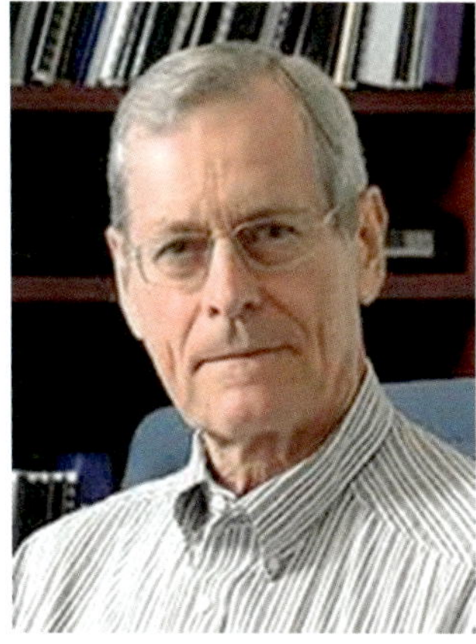

Fig. 1.11 James Till.

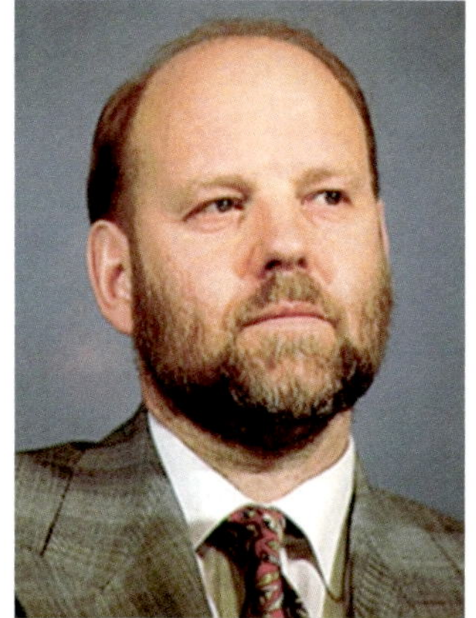

Fig. 1.12 Ian Wilmut.

EMBRYOLOGICAL TERMS

Most of the terms used in embryology are of *Latin* (L.) or *Greek* (Gr.) origin. The following text lists only those terms that are commonly used.

1. **Oocyte** (L. *Ovum* = egg): Female germ cells or sex cells produced by ovaries. **Mature oocyte** is called **secondary oocyte**.
2. **Sperm** (Gr. *Sperma* = seed): Male germ cells produced by testes.
3. **Zygote:** Cell formed by union of a sperm and secondary oocyte (ovum). The zygote is the earliest stage of embryo (i.e., the beginning of the new human being).
4. **Conceptus:** Product of conception, i.e., embryo along with its extraembryonic membranes.
5. **Cleavage:** Series of mitotic divisions of the zygote to form early embryonic cells – the *blastomeres*.
6. **Morula** (L. *Morus* = mulberry): Solid ball of 12–32 cells (blastomeres) formed 3–4 days after fertilization, just at the time when embryo enters the uterus.
7. **Blastocyst** (Gr. *Blastos* = bud, *Kystis* = capsule): It forms from late morula stage. It consists of two parts: an outer layer of small, slightly flattened cells called *trophoblasts* and inner cell mass (*embryoblast*) consisting of a group of larger polyhedral cells.

   The cavity of blastocyst (**blastocele**) separates the trophoblast from the inner cell mass except for a small area where they are in contact (embryonic pole). The embryoblast forms embryo, whereas trophoblast forms placenta.
8. **Implantation:** Attachment and subsequent embedding of blastocyst into uterine endometrium, where it develops during gestation.

9. **Gastrulation:** Formation of three germ layers (ectoderm, mesoderm, and endoderm) in the embryo.
10. **Neurulation** (Gr. *Neuron* = nerve): The process by which neural plate forms the **neural tube**. The embryo at this stage is called *neurula*.
11. **Embryo** (Gr. *Embryon*): Developing human from conception to 8th week in uterus. This period is called embryonic period (or period of organogenesis). By the end of this period, **primordia of all the major structures** of the body are formed.
12. **Primordium** (L. *Primus* = first + *Ordior* = to begin): Beginning or first discernible indication of an organ or structure.
13. **Fetus** (L. *Unborn* = offspring): Developing human from 9th week to birth.
14. **Abortion** (L. *Aboriri* = to miscarry): Expulsion of a conceptus (embryo or fetus) before it is viable, i.e., capable of living outside the uterus.
15. **Gestation** (L. *Gestation* = bearing and carrying in the womb): The process of development of embryo in the uterus from fertilization of the ovum until delivery (the period of normal pregnancy).
16. **Gestational age:** The gestational age of embryo/fetus is **calculated from presumed first day of the last normal menstrual period**. The oocyte is not fertilized until approximately 14 days (2 weeks after the preceding menstruation); hence, the **fertilization age of an embryo or fetus is 14 days less than the gestation age.**
17. **Sexual reproduction:** It involves the fusion of male and female gametes to produce an offspring.

GOLDEN FACTS TO REMEMBER

- **Founder of embryology** — Aristotle (384–322 BCE)
- **Father of modern embryology** — Karl Ernst von Baer
- **First individuals to observe human sperm** — Johan Ham van Arnheim and Anton van Leeuwenhoek
- **Carnegie collection of embryos is now in** — National Museum of Health and Medicine in the Armed Forces Institute of Pathology in Washington DC
- **First test tube baby** — Louise Brown (born in 1978)
- **First mammal cloned** — Dolly, the female domestic sheep (July 5, 1996 to February 14, 2003)
- **Inventor of first mammal cloning** — Ian Wilmut (1944)
- **Most famous Siamese twins** — Chang and Eng Bunker (born in 1811 in Siam [Thailand])
- **Stem cells were discovered in** — 1960 by James Till
- **Longest period of prenatal development** — Fetal period
- **Earliest period of extrauterine life** — Infancy (first year after birth)
- **Fertilization age** — Gestational age − 14 days

CLINICAL PROBLEM SOLVING

PROBLEMS

1. How do the terms **zygote** and **conceptus** differ?
2. The division of **prenatal development** differs among anatomists and clinicians. How?
3. **What are stem cells?** Which diseases are likely to be benefited by the stem cells?

SOLUTIONS

1. The **zygote** is a diploid single cell formed after fertilization by the union of haploid male and female gametes. It is also called a **single cell embryo**.

   The term **conceptus** refers to the product of conception, i.e., embryo and associated extraembryonic membranes.
2. The **anatomists** divide prenatal development into three periods, viz. **preembryonic, embryonic,** and **fetal,** whereas **clinicians** divide it into two periods, viz. **embryonic** (from fertilization to 8th week) and **fetal** (from 9th week to birth).
3. The stem cells are undifferentiated cells, which are capable of multiplication and differentiation into all types of specialized cells in the body. The cells of embryoblast are capable of generating all the three germ layers: ectoderm, mesoderm, and endoderm. Hence, cells of embryoblast (inner cell mass) are termed **embryonic stem cells**. These can be kept in an undifferentiated state in culture medium. By using growth factors, these can be made to form different tissue cells, e.g., muscle cells, neurons, and blood cells. The diseases that are likely to be benefited by stem cells are **Parkinson disease, Alzheimer disease, spinal cord injuries, sickle cell anemia**, etc.

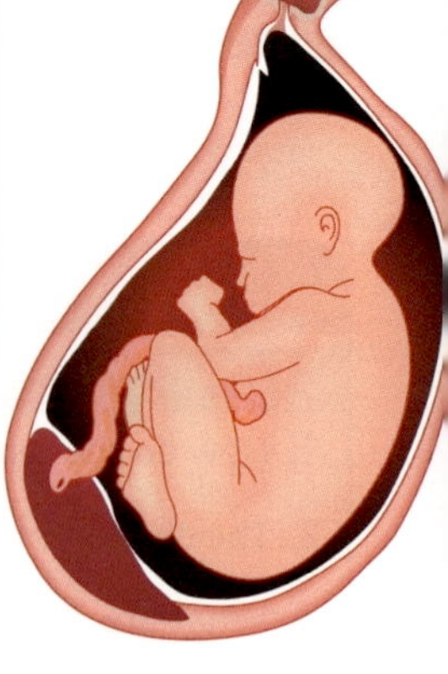

2 Basic Processes of Development and Their Molecular Regulation

LEARNING OBJECTIVES

After studying this chapter, the student should be able to:

- Give brief description of various processes of development.
- Write a short note on:
  - (a) Stem cells
  - (b) Organizer
  - (c) Ontogeny repeats phylogeny AN 76.2
- Describe in brief:
  - (a) Gene transcription
  - (b) Induction and organ formation
  - (c) Cell-to-cell signaling
  - (d) Key signaling pathways

OVERVIEW

The understanding of various processes involved in development is of immense value to analyze how a single cell embryo becomes a multicellular human, made of trillions of cells; moreover, the manner in which these cells are arranged into various tissues, organs, and organ systems. All this happen due to precise **molecular (genetic) regulation** of development.

The **genes** pass on the information necessary to make proteins, which act as **regulatory factors** in the development of various tissues and organs of the body.

A newly fertilized ovum – the **zygote** – has collection of genes called **genome** that contains all information needed to transform it from **single cell** into an **embryo** and then into an *adult*.

BASIC PROCESSES OF DEVELOPMENT

The basic processes of development are **growth, differentiation**, and **metabolism**.

1. **Growth** (Fig. 2.1):

   It occurs due to increase in number of cells, size of cells, and an intercellular substances. Hence, the growth is divided into *multiplicative growth*, *auxetic growth*, and *accretionary growth*, respectively (Fig. 2.1).

   a. *Multiplicative growth*: It occurs due to increase in number of cells as a result of mitotic cell division and termed as **hyperplasia**.

   b. *Auxetic growth*: It occurs due to increase in cell size rather than an increase in number of cells and termed as **hypertrophy**. It is seen in those cells which cannot multiply viz. **neurons, muscle fibers of myometrium of uterus** during pregnancy.

   c. *Accretionary growth*: It occurs due to **increase in intercellular substance** (also called matrix) secreted by a cell as in cartilage and bone. It is a gradual build up of matrix (i.e., intercellular substance), which leads to accretionary growth.

2. **Differentiation:** It refers to specialization of cells during formation of different tissues and organs, i.e., existing cells form new cell with special features by a process called **differentiation**.

   The differentiation could be invisible in the early embryonic cells but it becomes visible later on during the differentiation of various body tissues and organs.

   The undifferentiated cells are called **stem cells**.

   The stem cells need to be described a little bit.

   Stem cells (Fig. 2.2):

   The stem cells are cells which have potential to renew and differentiate themselves into different types of specialized cells, *viz.* **muscle cells, nerve cells, skin cells,** etc. The embryonic cells are pluripotent stem cells. For this reason the thousands of different types of cells which make up our body come from a single cell, the zygote.

   Based on potential of their differentiation, the embryonic stem cells are further divided into following types:

   (a) **Totipotent cells:** They can form all types of cells of embryo along with those of extraembryonic membranes, viz. placenta and umbilical cord, example, **zygote**.

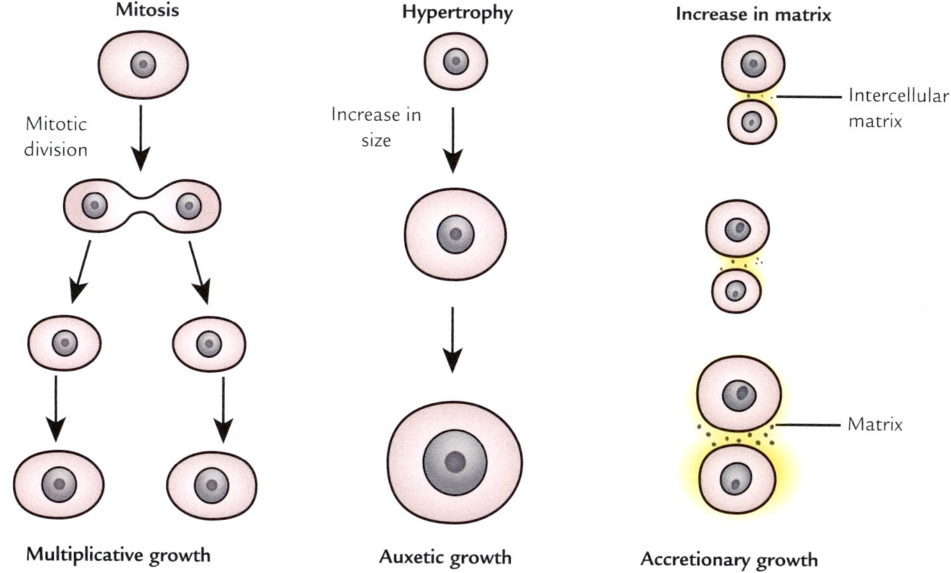

Fig. 2.1 Types of growth.

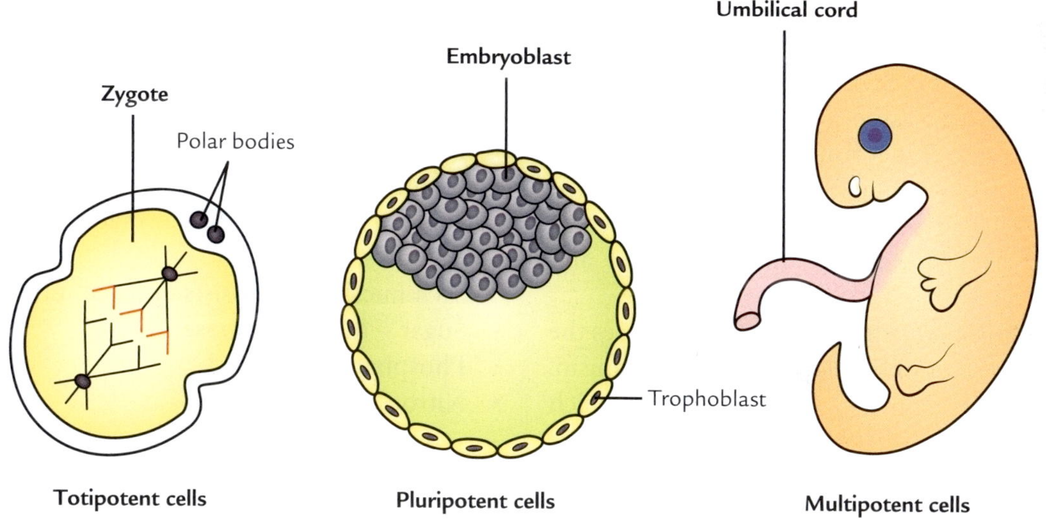

Fig. 2.2 Embryonic stem cells (ESCs).

(b) **Pluripotent cells:** They can form all types of cells of embryo but they cannot form those of extraembryonic membranes such as placenta and umbilical cord. For example, **embryoblast**.

(c) **Multipotent cells:** They can form more than one type of cells, viz. cord blood cells.

The embryonic stem cells are summarized in Flowchart 2.1.

3. **Metabolism and organizers:** The term **metabolism** in embryo refers to chemical changes in embryonic tissues or groups of cells. Some regions of developing embryo stimulate adjacent tissue to undergo morphogenetic differentiation and change their fate. This they do by liberating chemical enzymes, viz. proteins called **organizers.**

The organizers are of three types, viz. primary, secondary, and tertiary.

Primary organizer induces the adjacent region to change its fate and form the rudiment of new structure.

If this rudiment organ thus formed, also acts as an organizer, then it is called as **secondary organizer.**

If **secondary organizer**, in turn, also induces another region, then it is known as **tertiary organizer.**

For examples:

– **Primitive streak** induces formation of notochord (**primary organizer**)

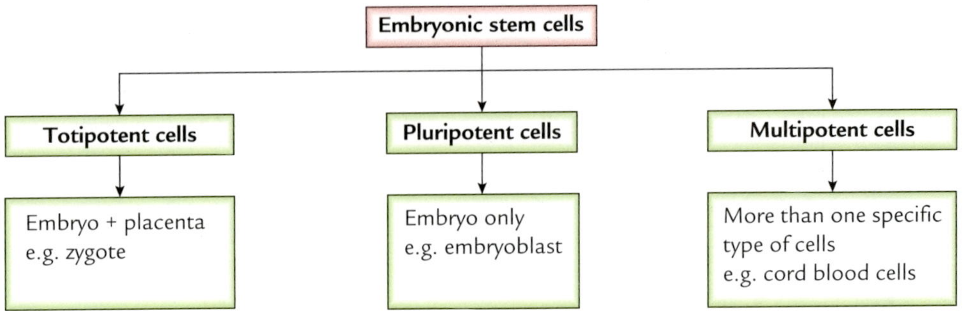

Flowchart 2.1 Types of embryonic stem cells.

- **Notochord** induces formation of neural tube **(secondary organizer)**
- **Neural tube** induces segmentation of paraxial mesoderm **(tertiary organizer)**

OTHER PROCESSES OF DEVELOPMENT

Ontogeny Repeats Phylogeny

1. **Ontogeny:** It is a branch of science which deals with complete life cycle of an organism from conception to the birth, as per blueprint hidden in its genome. The ontogeny is faithfully followed during development which involves various processes of development such as cell division, differentiation, and growth.
2. **Phylogeny:** It is a branch of science which traces the evolutionary history of development of an organism.

   It is based on a phylogenetic hypothesis which tells that all the organisms of the same phylum share a common ancestry.

   This is clearly observed during the development of certain organs, viz., development of kidney.

   The **evolutionary history of kidney** is as follows.

   Pronephros in fishes → Mesonephros in humans. Thus, as a rule during development of body organs of an organism, **ontogeny repeats phylogeny,** i.e., life cycle of an **organism repeats its ancestral history**. Thus, according to Ernst Haeckel (1866), during human development, "ontogeny repeats phylogeny".

Molecular (Genetic) Regulation and Cell Signaling

Nowadays embryology has advanced a lot from simple observational science to the one involving molecular regulation and signaling.

As we know that the development involves division, differentiation, morphogenesis, and controlled growth, all these processes occur due to proper molecular regulation and cell–cell signaling which in turn are controlled by genes.

Gene transcription:

The genes carry the blueprint of information to the cells, tissues, organs and organ systems of an organism to develop.

Structure of DNA (Fig. 2.3):

The **gene** consists of enough part of DNA strand to code for one protein.

A little description of structure of gene will make it easy to understand the above process.

The genes are located on DNA strands. The DNA molecule is made up of two strands of nucleotides, i.e., each strand of DNA is made up of a chain of nucleotides.

Each nucleotide consists of three subunits (Fig. 2.3):

- Sugar – the deoxyribose
- Phosphate group, and
- Nitrogenous base

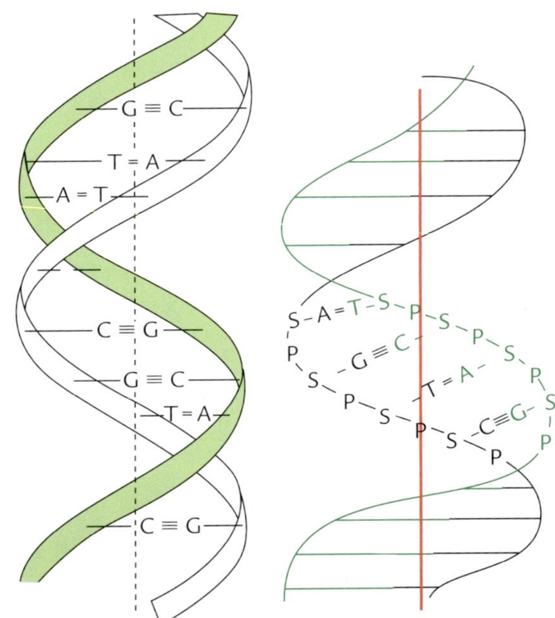

Fig. 2.3 Structure of DNA.

The phosphate sugar subunits are arranged in an alternate fashion in a DNA strand.

Each DNA strand has only one type of sugar molecule, the deoxyribose and three types of nitrogenous bases, viz.:

- **Adenine (A)**
- **Guanine (G)**
- **Thymine (T)**

The bases of two strands are held together by hydrogen bond in a specific manner, for example:

- A binds with T (A = T)
- G binds with C (G = C)
- T binds with A (T = A)
- The sequence of three nucleotides is called **codon.**
- Each gene consists of 64 such codons of structural gene (Fig. 2.4).
- Three are about 50,000 to 100,000 DNA sequences that code for RNA or protein coding sequences of structural gene.

The structural gene reveals coding sequences called **exons** and intervening noncoding sequences called **introns.**

It also possess **start and stop signals**, also called **initiator/5′** end and **termination/3′ end**, respectively, at its ends.

The presence of these signals is essential to make the gene functional (Fig. 2.4).

Exon = coding sequences
Introns = noncoding sequences

- The cells read the sequence of the gene in groups of three bases.

  There are 20,000 to 25,000 genes which code for about 100,000 proteins. That means each gene synthesizes more than one protein by a process of splicing of their introns.

  The potential number of proteins that can be synthesized is about five times more than the number of these genes.
- The **genes are involved in the synthesis of proteins,** which form the most essential components of our body such as plasma membrane, most of cytoplasm, cell organelles, intercellular substance, enzymes, hormones, antibodies, etc.

Further, most of secretory substances are proteins, although there are some nonprotein substances as well such as steroids.

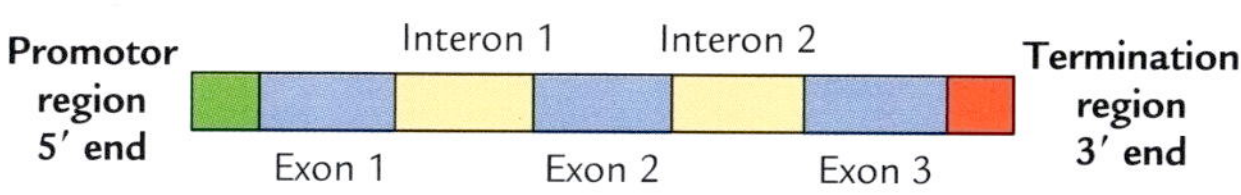

Fig. 2.4 Typical structural gene.

Factors regulating gene expression:

First transcript of nuclear gene is **pre-messenger RNA** (nRNA). As it passes out from nucleus into cytoplasm, some of its introns are removed (spliced out) and it becomes **messenger RNA** (mRNA). Thus, nRNA is longer than mRNA.

Thus, splicing process provides a provision by which the cells can produce different types of proteins from a single gene.

The effects of genes can be regulated as follows:

1. During transcription
2. During translation
3. After translation

INDUCTION AND ORGAN FORMATION

During the formation of organs (organogenesis) the cells undergo differentiation, where less specialized stem cells become more specialized cells through the expression of a set of genes.

The cell differentiation occurs as a result of cell signaling.

Induction:

The certain regions of embryo made up of group of cells cause another set of cells to change their fate. This process is called **induction.**

The group of cells or region which gives signal is called **inducer** and group of cells which change its fate is called **responder.**

The capacity of responder is called **competence** and competence requires a **competence factor.**

Examples of well-known inductions:

1. **Optic vesicle** induces the surface ectoderm to form **lens vesicle.** Here optic vesicle is inductor and surface ectoderm is **responder.**
2. Notochord induces the surface ectodermal layer of trilaminar germ disc to form neural tube.

Types of interactions between cells of two tissues, i.e., inducer and responder, are as follows:

(a) *Epithelial–mesenchymal interactions* (Fig. 2.5)
    For example:
    - Interaction between endodermal linings (epithelium) of gut and surrounding mesenchyme leads to formation of gut-derived organs, viz.:
      - Liver
      - Gallbladder
      - Pancreas
    - Interaction between endoderm (epithelium) of ureteric bud and mesenchyme of metanephric blastemal leads to formation of nephron.

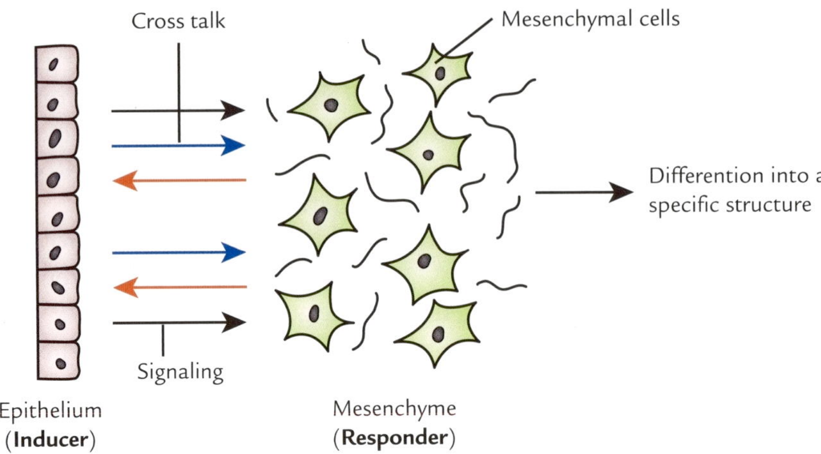

Fig. 2.5 Interaction between epithelium and mesenchyme.

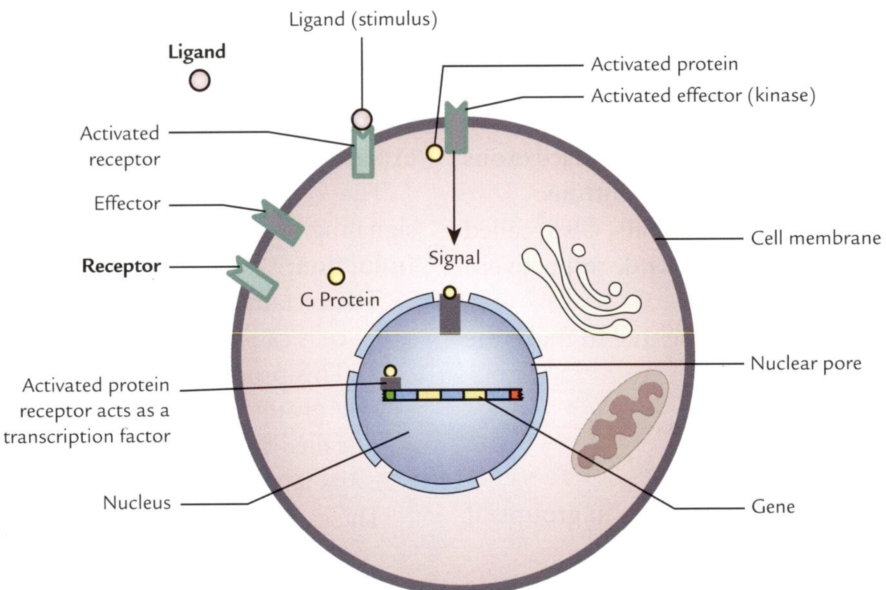

Fig. 2.6 Paracrine signaling.

– Interaction between surface ectoderm and underlying limb mesenchyme leads to the development of limbs.

(b) *Epithelial–epithelial interactions*

For example:

– Interaction between epithelium of optic cup and surface ectoderm (epithelium) leads to the formation of lens vesicle.

N.B. Although an initial signal from inducer is sufficient for responder to differentiate and change its fate but cross communication (cross-talk) is essential for differentiation of responder to continue (Fig. 2.5).

CELL-TO-CELL SIGNALING

The cell-to-cell signaling is essential for proper induction of transducer by inductor.

The signals are sent by protein molecules secreted by inducer.

Steps of cell-to-cell signaling:

There are three steps in cell-to-cell signaling:

1. Secretion of protein molecule by signaling cell
2. Transduction, i.e., binding of protein molecule to the receptor of other cell
3. Response of receptor cell

The cell-to-cell signaling occurs by two ways.

Paracrine Signaling (Fig. 2.6)

In paracrine signaling, protein molecules secreted by cells of inducer diffuse for some distance to interact with the other cells.

The protein molecule secreted by an inducer cell is called **ligand** it binds with receptor on the cell of transducer. The binding between ligand and receptor (called **ligand–receptor complex**) activates cytoplasmic protein, which in turn acts as a transcription factor.

The protein molecules (ligands) produced by inducer are in large number and called growth differentiating factors (GDFs). There are four groups of GDF3, viz.:

- Fibroblast growth factor (FGF)
- WNT
- Hedgehog
- Transforming growth factor B (TGFB)

Each group of these factors interacts with receptors of their own family.

Specific roles of various GDFs:

(a) **FGFs proteins** are produced by FGF genes
The FGFs are essential for:
 – Angiogenesis
 – Axon growth
 – Mesoderm differentiation

(b) **Hedgehog proteins** are produced by hedgehog genes. There are three hedgehog genes, viz. desert, Indian and sonic hedgehog. The sonic hedgehog (SHH) genes are used in many developmental events and may be called as **master gene** (or **morphogen**).

(c) **WNT proteins** are produced by WNT genes. There are about 15 types of WNT genes. The WNT proteins are essential for:
 - Development of limbs
 - Development of midbrain
 - Differentiation of somites
 - Differentiation of urogenital system

(d) **TGFB** is generally termed as TGFB super family because it has more than 30 family members.
It includes:
 – **Mullerian inhibiting factor (MIF)/anti-Mullerian hormone (AMH)**, which plays a significant role in sexual differentiation. The AMH gene provides instructions for making the above protein.
 – **Bone morphogenic proteins/factors (BMPs).**

 The TGFB members are responsible for:
 – Formation of extracellular matrix
 – Epithelial branching in salivary glands, lungs, and kidney
 – Bone formation
 – Regulation of cell division and cell death (apoptosis)

N.B. The other factors responsible for paracrine signaling are:
- Serotonin (5-HT)
- γ-Aminobutyric acid (GABA)
- Epinephrine
- Norepinephrine

These molecules function as important signals for embryological development, for example:

- **Serotonin (5-HT)** is essential for:
  - Proliferation and migration of cells
  - Establishing laterality, viz. gastrulation, development of heart, etc.
- **Norepinephrine** is essential for:
  - Apoptosis (programmed cell death) in interdigital spaces.

Juxtacrine Signaling

In Juxtacrine signaling, the ligands secreted by inducer do not diffuse (i.e., are not transmitted) through intercellular spaces to bind with the receptors on the other cell.

It occurs by following three ways:

(a) Protein of one cell binds directly with the receptor of other cell.
(b) Receptor of one cell binds with its ligand on the extracellular matrix secreted by another cell.
(c) Signal is directly transmitted from the cytoplasm of one cell to the cytoplasm of other cell through small conduits called gap junctions.

KEY SIGNALING PATHWAYS INVOLVED IN DEVELOPMENT

The key signaling pathways involved in development are as follows:

1. Sonic hedgehog (SHH) pathway
2. Planer cell polarity (PCP) pathway
3. Notch pathway

1. *Sonic hedgehog signaling pathway:*
   It is the key/master signaling pathway which transmits information to embryonic cells for differentiation during development.
   The different parts of embryo have different concentrations of hedgehog signaling proteins.
   – It is essential to maintain midline axis of body
   – It also plays an important role in the development of
     (a) Brain, skeleton, musculature, GIT, and lungs
     (b) In maintenance and regeneration of adult tissues by regulating adult stem cells.
2. *Convergent extension signaling pathway (planar cell polarity):*
   - The cellular signals involved in this pathway are not fully understood.

- It is found that non-canonical **WNT signaling pathway** plays an important role.

  These pathways reduce the cell-to-cell adhesion molecules to allow cells to move freely, for example:
  - During neurulation, the neural plate elongates to form neural groove between two neural folds.
  - During gastrulation, the cells move medially and embryonic axis elongates.

3. *Notch signaling pathway:*

The notch signaling pathway is highly conserved cell signaling pathway in the determination of cell fate.

There are four different types of notch receptors, viz., NOTCH1, NOTCH2, NOTCH3, and NOTCH4. The protein of notch receptor spans the cell membrane.

The ligand proteins produced by NOTCH genes bind with extracellular portions of notch receptors.

The notch signaling pathway plays an important role in the following events:
- Neuronal differentiation
- Angiogenesis
- Segmentation of somites
- Pancreatic β-cell differentiation
- Differentiation of B and T lymphocytes

CLINICAL CORRELATION

The cell-to-cell signaling is very specific. Even a subtle alteration in ligand or its receptor can alter signaling. Such alterations are caused by gene mutation and can lead to **congenital defects**.

GOLDEN FACTS TO REMEMBER

➢ **Growth factors (genes) regulating neural tube closure**	BMP (bone morphogenic proteins)
➢ **Gene**	Basic unit of heredity
➢ **Codon**	Sequence of three nucleotides in DNA or RNA strand which codes for an amino acid
➢ **Commonest type of cell-to-cell interaction**	Epithelial mesenchymal interaction
➢ **Master signaling pathway**	SHH pathway
➢ **Gene responsible for formation and maintenance of primitive streak**	Nodal gene is member of transforming growth factor β (TGF-β) family
➢ **Genetic factor responsible for spermatogenesis**	Bromodomain testes (BRDT) specific protein
➢ **Genetic factor responsible for testicular growth/ Sertoli cells**	Male-specific sex determining factor called SRY gene
➢ **Genetic factor responsible for regulation of neurulation**	WNT

CLINICAL PROBLEM SOLVING

PROBLEMS

1. **Which tissues are commonly involved in cell-to-cell interactions during embryonic development**? Give two examples.
2. **What is an organizer?** Give its types with an example.
3. What are two main types of cell signaling?

SOLUTIONS

1. The epithelial and mesenchymal tissues are commonly involved in cell-to-cell interactions during embryonic development, for example:
   (a) **Endoderm of ureteric bud** interacts with the mesenchyme of **metanephric blastema** to form nephron.
   (b) **Endoderm of gut** interacts with the **surrounding mesenchyme** to form liver and pancreas.
2. The **organizer** is a region or a group of cells in an embryo which can both induce (change in fate) and pattern (produce an organized structure) adjacent group of embryonic cells.
   The organizers are of three types:
   (a) **Primary organizer,** the first region to induce the other region to change its fate. For example, **primitive streak** induces the formation of *notochord.*
   (b) **Secondary organizer,** the one which itself is formed by primary organizer but induces another region to change its fate. For example, **notochord** induces surface ectodermal layer to form *neural tube.*
   (c) **Tertiary organizer,** the structure formed by secondary organizer but itself induces another region to change its fate. For example, **neural tube induces paraxial mesoderm to undergo segmentation.**
   The above description under points (a), (b), and (c) clearly gives examples of primary, secondary, and tertiary organizers.
3. Cell signaling are of two types:
   (a) Paracrine signaling
   (b) Juxtacrine signaling

3 Reproductive System, Ovarian Cycle, and Menstrual Cycle

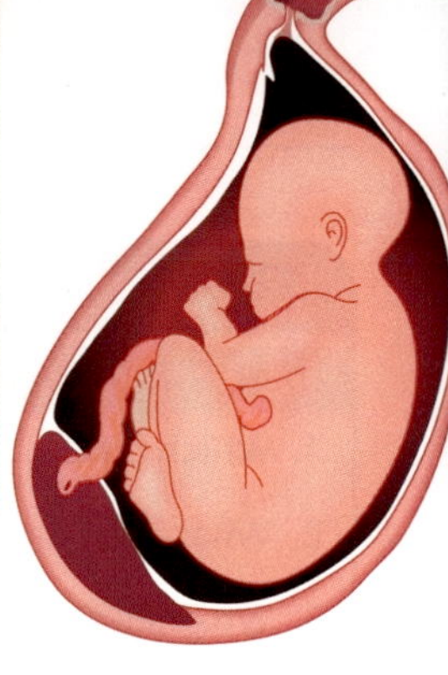

LEARNING OBJECTIVES

After studying this chapter, the student should be able to:

- Enumerate the primary and secondary reproductive organs of a male and female.
- Enumerate the components of the male and female genital tracts.
- Describe the uterine changes occuring during menstrual cycle. AN 77.1
- Describe the synchrony between menstrual and ovarian cycles in brief. AN 77.2

The reproduction is a biological process by which new offsprings are produced for continuation of species. The reproduction in human is sexual reproduction. It involves sexual intercourse between man and woman to cause fertilization, i.e., union between male and female gametes, which are produced by male and female gonads called testis and ovary, respectively. Thus reproductive system is divided into two parts: male reproductive system and female reproductive system.

MALE REPRODUCTIVE SYSTEM

OVERVIEW

The **primary reproductive organ in males** is testis. The **secondary reproductive organs in males** are scrotum, epididymis, ductus deferens, seminal vesicles, urethra, prostate gland, bulbourethral glands, and penis (Fig. 3.1). The **male genital tract** consists of vasa efferentia (efferent ductules), epididymis, vas deferens, ejaculatory duct, and urethra. The male genital tract carries sperms produced in the testis to the urethra, from where the sperms are deposited in the vagina during copulation (intercourse).

Testes

Testes are a pair of ovoid organs within the scrotum that produce **sperms** and **testosterone**. Each testis is 4–5 cm long and 2–3 cm in diameter lying within the scrotum, outside the abdominal cavity. The testis is covered by a thick, white capsule – the tunica albuginea (Fig. 3.2). The fibrous septa from the capsule extends inside substance of testis and divides it into 200–300 cone-shaped lobules. Each lobule contains 2–4 convoluted **seminiferous tubules**. The epithelial lining of the walls of these tubules contains cells in different stages of development to form *spermatozoa* through cell division. Columns of spermatogenic cells are separated by Sertoli cells. Surrounding the tubules are **interstitial cells of Leydig**, which secrete male hormone – the **testosterone**.

The seminiferous tubules start producing spermatozoa at puberty and empty their secretion (e.g., spermatozoa) into tubular network – the **rete testis**, which in turn empty into 15–20 **efferent ductules**. The efferent ductules enter into the epididymis to form the **duct of epididymis**.

N.B.

- Testes are located outside the abdominal cavity into scrotum because formation of sperms requires temperature lower than the body temperature. In scrotum the temperature is 1–3°C less than the body temperature.
- Formation of sperms continues throughout the life of men but their viability and fertilizing capacity decreases in old age.

Epididymis

Epididymis is a comma-shaped structure lying posteriorly and slightly lateral to each testis with vas deferens along its medial side. It consists of a single convoluted duct (**duct of epididymis**) formed by the union of the efferent ductules of the testis. Within the duct of epididymis, the spermatozoa mature, develop some motility, and learn a little bit of swimming. The spermatozoa show circular or even forward directional movements.

Vas Deferens

Vas deferens is a thick-walled muscular tube, about 45 cm (18 inches) long, which begins at the tail of the

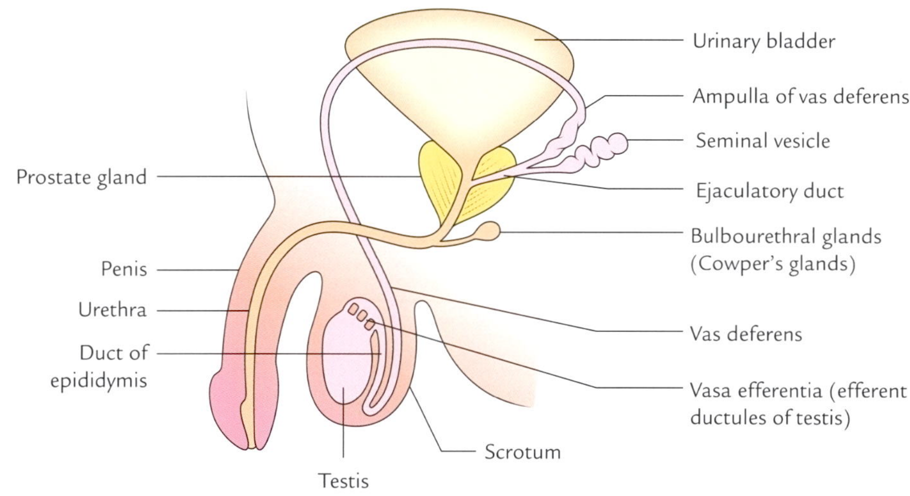

Fig. 3.1 Male reproductive system.

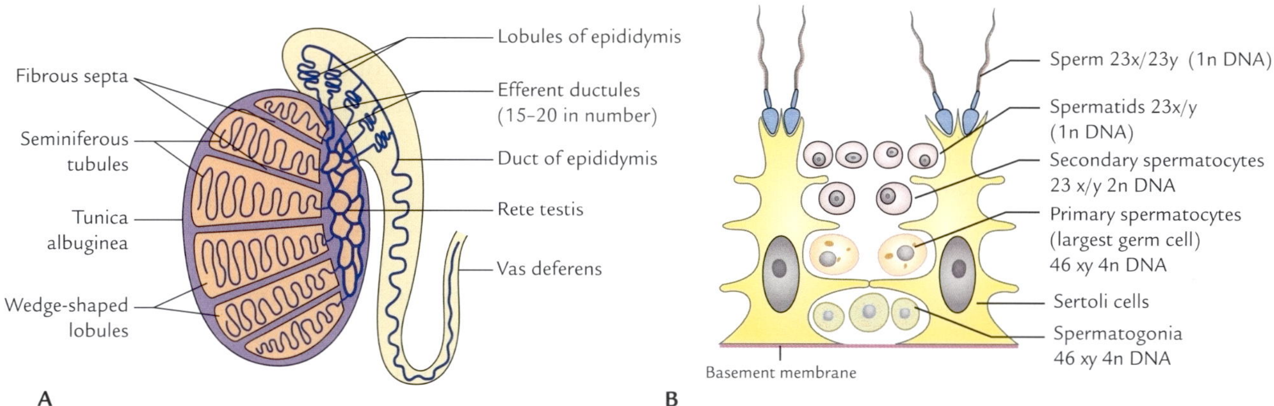

Fig. 3.2 Structure of testis. (A) Schematic vertical section of the testis showing the basic structure of testis, epididymis, and vas deferens. (B) Spermatogenic and Sertoli cells forming lining of seminiferous tubules.

epididymis as the direct continuation of the duct of the epididymis. The terminal part of each vas deferens is sacculated and is called **ampulla of vas deferens**. It serves as a **reservoir of sperm and tubular fluid**. The terminal narrow part of vas deferens joins the duct of seminal vesicle to form the **ejaculatory duct** at the base of the prostate gland. *The main function of vas deferens is to transport spermatozoa from the epididymis to ejaculatory duct.* Peristaltic contractions of smooth muscle help in propelling the semen.

Seminal Vesicles and Ejaculatory Ducts

The seminal vesicle (5 cm long) is a sacculated coiled tube adjacent to ampulla of each vas deferens. The paired seminal vesicles secrete a major portion of volume of ejaculate. These are located behind the bladder near the prostate gland. Each vesicle ends in a small duct that joins ampulla of vas deferens to form an **ejaculatory duct**. The two ejaculatory ducts are slender tubes that open into the prostatic part of the urethra. The secretion of seminal vesicles is thick and mucous like. It contains fructose that provides nutrition to sperms.

Prostate Gland

Prostate gland is a pyramidal fibromuscular gland of about the size of a chestnut. It consists of branches of tubuloalveolar glands embedded in fibromuscular stroma.

The prostate gland is situated below the urinary bladder surrounds the proximal part of the urethra and two ejaculatory ducts. It is enclosed by a thin but strong fibrous capsule. The capsule is continuous with several fibromuscular partitions. The prostatic glands secrete **prostatic fluid**, which is poured into the prostatic urethra through 10–20 ducts. The prostatic fluid contains **acid phosphatase, fibrinolysin, citric acid, amylase, prostate specific antigen,** and **prostaglandins**. The prostatic fluid forms the bulk of the semen (i.e., ejaculate).

Bulbourethral Glands (Cowper Glands)

Bulbourethral glands are two yellow, pea-sized glands located on each side of membranous urethra. These glands secrete alkaline mucus that is poured into the penile urethra just before ejaculation of the semen. The alkaline nature of these secretions protects sperms against the acidity of the urethra and vagina. The secretions of bulbourethral glands also provide lubrication during coitus.

Penis

Penis is the male erectile organ of copulation traversed by urethra. It is cylindrical in shape with a mushroom like distal end – the **glans penis**. Average size is 5.5 inches length and 4.5 inches in girth. It is used to inseminate female during sexual intercourse.

N.B. **Semen:** It is a viscid whitish fluid consisting of spermatozoa suspended in secretions of accessory glands. It is ejaculated by penis into the vagina at the time of orgasm. It consists of sperms produced by seminiferous tubules of testes and secretions of seminal vesicles, prostate gland, and bulbourethral glands. The average volume of ejaculate is 2.5–3.5 mL. Semen has a pH of 7.35–7.5, with an average sperm count of 100 million per mL. The approximate contribution by various reproductive glands is as follows:

- Prostate: 60%
- Seminal vesicles: 30%
- Testes: 5%
- Bulbourethral glands: 5%

The thin milky secretion of the prostate gland is alkaline in nature and neutralizes the acidic pH of the vagina. The movement of sperms is best at a pH of 6–6.5, whereas the vaginal pH is about 3.5–4.

The enzymes of prostatic secretion break down the coagulated proteins secreted by seminal vesicles and make the semen more liquid.

FEMALE REPRODUCTIVE ORGANS

OVERVIEW

The **primary reproductive organ in females** is ovary. The **secondary reproductive organs in females** are uterine tubes, uterus, vagina, vulva, and vestibular glands. The female genital tract consists of fallopian tube, uterus, and vagina (Fig. 3.3). The female genital tract provides the site of fertilization and site for the development of the embryo.

Ovaries

Ovaries are a pair of small ovoid organs (3 cm long × 2 cm wide × 1 cm thick) of about the size and shape of an almond. They are situated in the lateral wall of the lesser pelvis on either side of the uterus below and behind the uterine tubes. Each ovary is attached to the upper part of the uterus by the round ligament of the ovary. One end of each ovary is in contact with the fimbria of the uterine tube.

Microscopic Structure of Ovary

The outer surface of ovary is covered by a layer of cuboidal epithelium of visceral peritoneum. It is wrongly called as **germinal epithelium** as it does not contain germ cells.

The parenchyma of ovary is divided into the **thick cortex** surrounding a very **vascular medulla.** The cortex surrounding the medulla consists of high cellular connective tissue stroma mainly made up of large

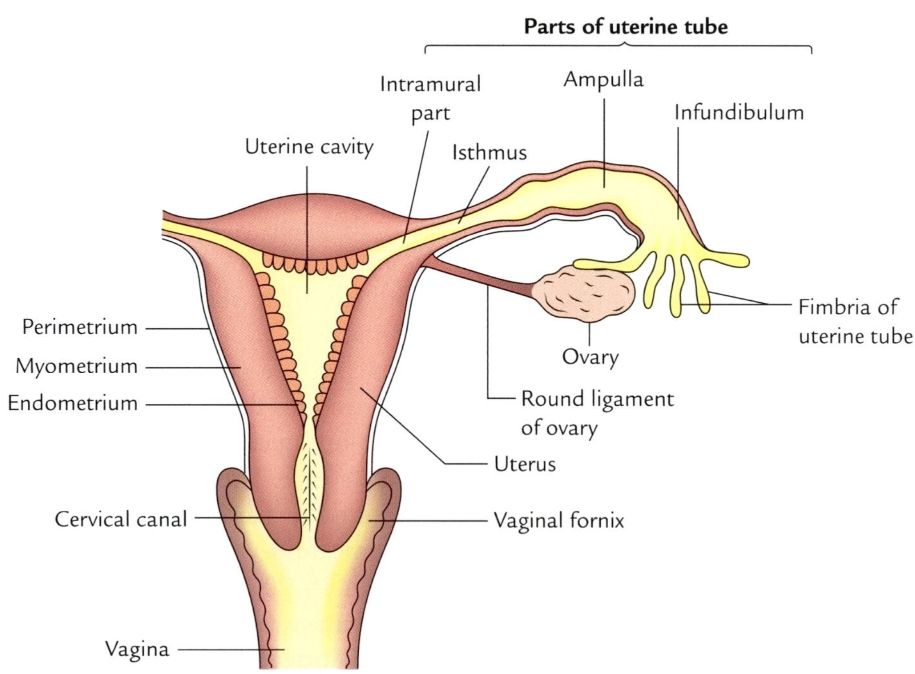

Fig. 3.3 Female reproductive system.

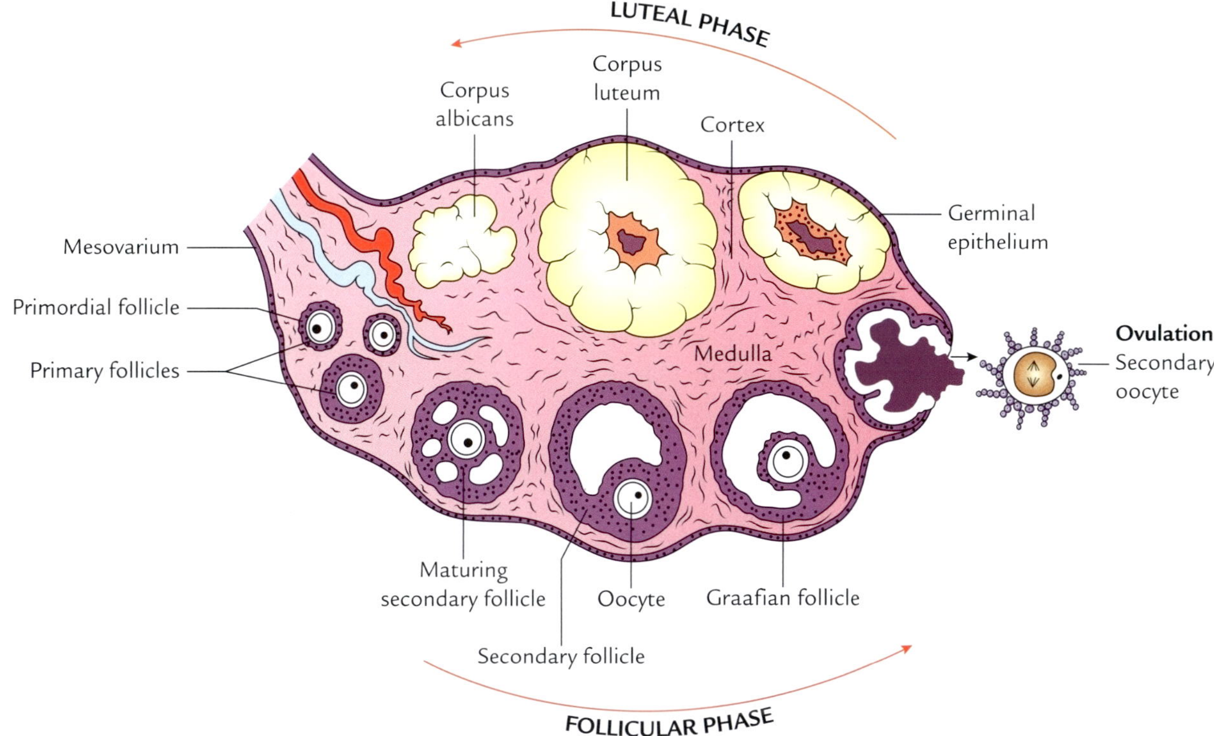

Fig. 3.4 Schematic diagram showing microscopic structure of ovary. It also shows follicular and luteal phases of ovarian cycle (i.e., various stages of development of ovarian follicles, and formation of corpus luteum and corpus albicans).

spindle-shaped fibroblasts. Before puberty, it contains numerous ***primordial follicles***. After puberty, it contains ovarian follicles in various stages of maturation and degeneration. Each follicle contains an ovum. Till puberty the ovaries remain inactive but stroma still contains immature follicles.

During child bearing age, every month one ovarian follicle matures under the influence of follicle-stimulating hormone (FSH) and ruptures to release its ovum into the peritoneal cavity. This process is called **ovulation** and recurs throughout the reproductive life of a female (**ovarian cycle**). If a woman becomes pregnant, the ovarian cycle stops temporarily.

Ovarian Cycle (Figs. 3.4 and 3.5)

During the reproductive life of a female (about 15–45 years), the ovary undergo monthly cyclic changes to release an oocyte. **Each ovarian cycle consists of 28 days.** During this cycle, follicles mature (called folliculogenesis). The folliculogenesis helps not only in the maturation of female germ cells but also in the release of a mature germ cell – the oocyte. Thus, the **ovarian cycle** is the cyclic release of ovum from the ovary.

This cycle is controlled by hormones secreted by the pituitary gland. At the onset of puberty, the pituitary gland secretes **follicle-stimulating hormone (FSH)**. Under the influence of this hormone, the primordial follicles in the ovary start growing. The growing/maturing follicles produce hormone **estrogen.** Only one follicle reaches the full development and forms

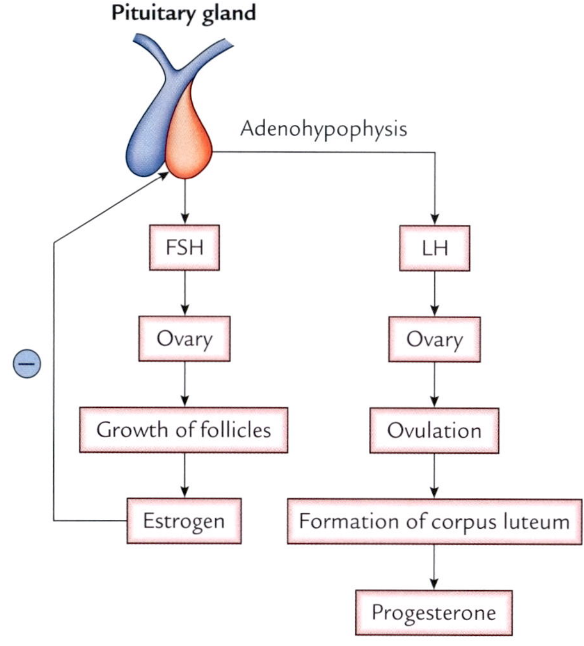

Fig. 3.5 Ovarian cycle.

Graafian follicle. Through feedback mechanism, the increased level of estrogen hormone inhibits the secretion of FSH from the anterior pituitary. The pituitary gland also secretes **luteinizing hormone** (**LH**). Under the influence of a large amount of LH, the Graafian follicle bursts and **ovulation** takes place. The ovum is released due to action of proteolytic enzymes formed by the theca externa cells that cause dissolution of capsular wall. There is plasma transudation within the follicles. As a result, follicles swell and pressure within them increases. Because of increased intrafollicular pressure and simultaneous dissolution of follicular capsular wall, follicles rupture and ovum is released (ovulation). After ovulation, the empty follicle develops into **corpus luteum**, which secretes hormone **progesterone.** The corpus luteum degenerates after 10 days if the ovum is not fertilized. The level of progesterone decreases, and again the pituitary gland secretes FSH and a new cycle starts. **Thus, the cyclic changes in the ovary comprising of development of ovarian follicles, ovulation, and formation of corpus luteum constitute the ovarian cycle.**

The **corpus luteum** persists for 2–3 months if the ovum is fertilized. By that time, placenta develops and starts secreting **progesterone** and **estrogen.** The high levels of these hormones in blood further suspend the ovarian cycle during pregnancy.

N.B. The ovarian cycles normally persist throughout the reproductive life of women except during pregnancy. The ovarian cycle terminates at menopause (at about 42–45 years of age).

Phases of the Ovarian Cycle

The ovarian cycle is divided into two phases: (a) *follicular phase* and (b) *luteal phase* (Fig. 3.10, p. 24)

1. **Follicular phase**: It corresponds to the *first half of the menstrual cycle* (Fig. 3.10, p. 24). During this phase, follicles develop and discharge only one mature oocyte. Changes in the endometrium of uterus take place due to secretion of the hormone *estrogen* produced by the developing follicles.
2. **Luteal phase**: It corresponds to the *second half of the menstrual cycle.* During this phase, the formation of the corpus luteum takes place following ovulation. Changes in uterine endometrium take place due to secretion of the hormone *progesterone.*

N.B.
- **Three important events occur during an ovarian cycle:**
  (a) Follicular development
  (b) Ovulation (release of oocyte) – the most important event
  (c) Formation of corpus luteum

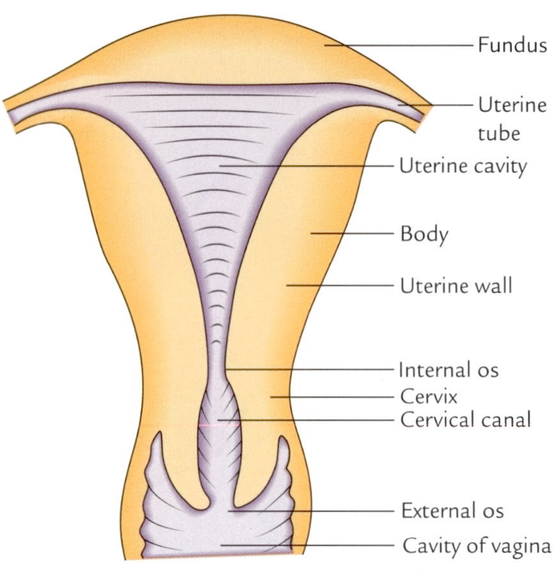

Fig. 3.6 Uterus: an internal view.

- **Output of follicular development:**
  (a) Growth and development of primary oocyte
  (b) Differentiation of follicular cells
  (c) Formation of zona pellucida
  (d) Formation of theca folliculi (viz. theca interna and theca externa)
  (e) Formation of antrum folliculi

Uterus (Fig. 3.6)

Uterus is a pear-shaped, hollow, thick-walled muscular organ present in the lesser pelvis. It is the site for implantation and development of embryo. It is about 7.5 cm long, 5 cm wide, and its walls are about 2.5 cm thick. It weighs about 30–40 g.

It has three parts: fundus, body, and cervix.

- **Fundus** is the upper dome-shaped part of the uterus above the openings of uterine tubes. It is devoid of cavity.
- **Body** is the main part of the uterus where implantation and development of fetus takes place.
- **Cervix** is the lower cylindrical part of the uterus that protrudes into the vagina.

Microscopic Structure of Body of Uterus

The uterus consists of three layers (Fig. 3.7). From superficial to deep, these are *perimetrium*, *myometrium*, and *endometrium*.

1. **Perimetrium:** It consists of peritoneum covering the uterus.
2. **Myometrium:** It is the thickest layer and consists of smooth muscle. The smooth muscle fibers are arranged in longitudinal, oblique, transverse, and circular layers. Hence, the wall of the uterus is very strong. During pregnancy, the muscle fibers undergo

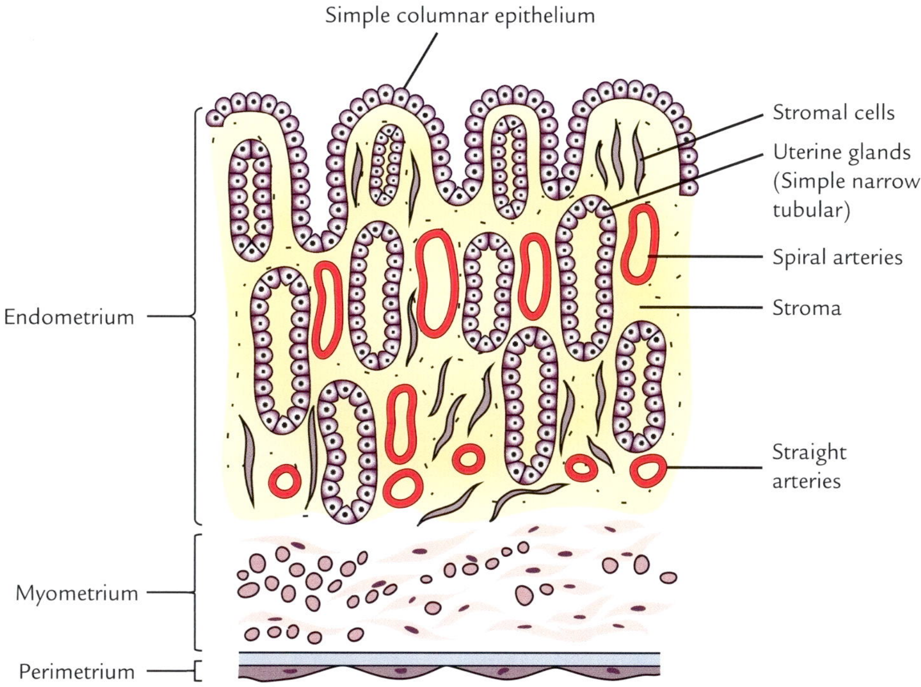

Fig. 3.7 Structure of uterine wall in the region of body uterus.

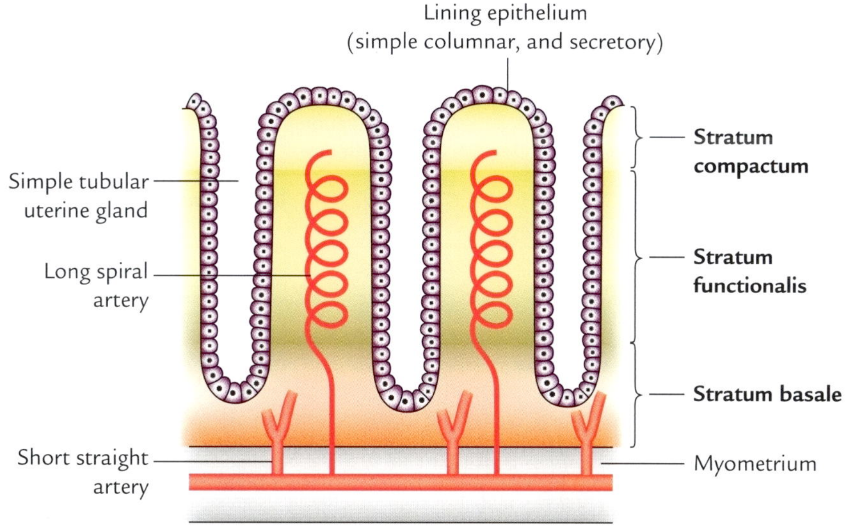

Fig. 3.8 Layers of endometrium.

hyperplasia (**hypertrophy**). This layer contains blood vessels and nerves; hence, it is also called **stratum vasculare**.

3. **Endometrium:** It is the mucous lining of the body of the uterus containing a large number of mucus-secreting glands (Fig. 3.7).

Features:

- Lined by simple columnar epithelium.
- Underlying lamina propria (connective tissue stroma) contains numerous simple tubular glands (**uterine glands**) which secrete mucous. It is highly vascular and contains number of short and long arteries (Fig. 3.8).

It is clinically divided into two parts (Fig. 3.9):

(a) **Superficial 2/3rd** or **stratum functionalis**: It undergoes cyclic monthly changes, hence termed as *stratum functionalis/stratum spongiosum.*

It is thick and edematous and supplied by long coiled endometrial arteries called **spiral arteries**. It houses upper 2/3rd of uterine glands. The stratum functionalis is highly sensitive to changes in **estrogen** and **progesterone** levels during menstrual cycle.

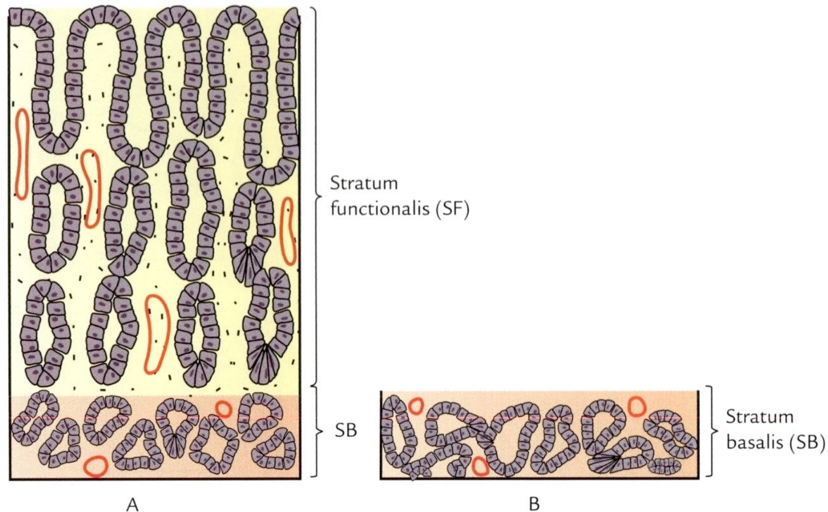

Fig. 3.9 Endometrium before and after menstruation: (A) before menstruation, (B) after menstruation (stratum functionalis is sloughed off, but stratum basalis remains intact). SF, stratum functionalis; SB, stratum basalis.

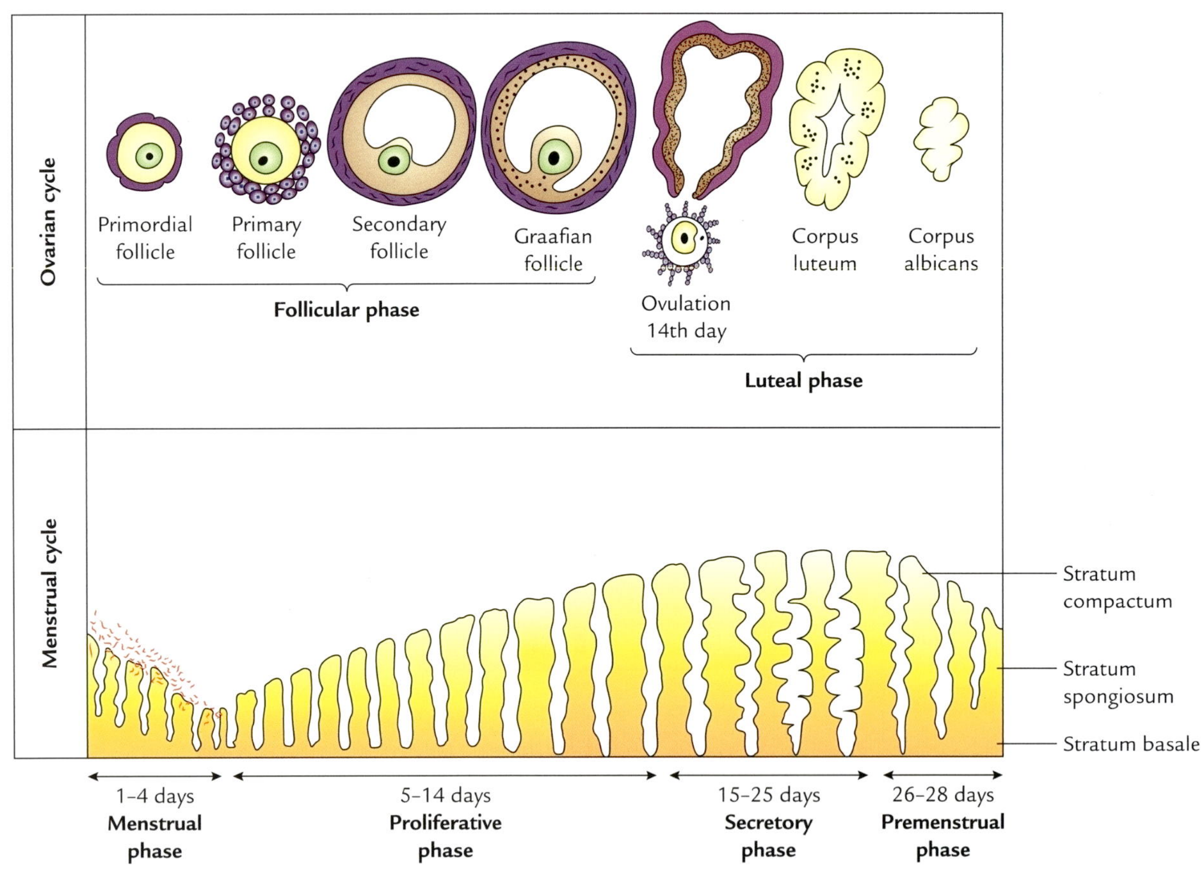

Fig. 3.10 Correlation between ovarian and menstrual cycles.

N.B. The superficial part of stratum functionalis towards the uterine lumen is thin and consists of compactly arranged stromal cells hence often termed as **stratum compactum**.

(b) **Deep 1/3rd** or **stratum basale:** It does not undergo monthly cyclic changes. It is thin and supplied by short straight arteries. It houses lower 1/3rd of uterine glands.

N.B. The **stratum functionalis** (functional layer) is sloughed off during menstruation. The basal layer remains intact, i.e., not sloughed off (Fig. 3.9).

Menstrual Cycle (Fig. 3.10) AN 77.1

During the reproductive life of a woman (from 15 to 45 years), i.e., from puberty to menopause, the uterine endometrium undergoes monthly cyclic changes called

endometrial cycle, which is commonly referred to as the **menstrual cycle** because of menstruation (flow of blood from the uterus) as a notable feature. At the age of 45 years or so the menstruation ceases and this stage is termed **menopause.** (Similar cyclic changes occur in ovaries, which constitute the ovarian cycle, see p. 21.)

Each menstrual cycle in most of the women consists of roughly 28 days. **Day 1** is the day when the menstrual flow starts. The ovulation occurs in the middle of the cycle (i.e., 14th day).

Purpose

The purpose of menstrual cycle is to prepare the endometrium for embedding of fertilized ovum (conceptus). But if the ovum is not fertilized then most of the endometrium (viz. stratum functionalis) is shed off in the form of blood flow per vaginum called **menstrual cycle.**

Uterine Changes During Menstrual Cycle

Each menstrual cycle is divided into four phases on the basis of changes that occur in the endometrium:

1. **Menstrual phase**
2. **Proliferative phase**
3. **Secretory phase**
4. **Premenstrual phase**

CLINICAL CORRELATION

1. ***Abnormal menstrual cycles:***
   (a) *Hypomenorrhea:* It is scanty blood flow during the menstrual cycle.
   (b) *Menorrhagia:* It is profuse blood flow during the menstrual cycle.
   (c) *Metrorrhagia:* It is the occurrence of bleeding between the menstrual cycles.
   (d) *Oligomenorrhea:* It is the reduced frequency of menstrual cycles.
2. ***Amenorrhea:*** It is the absence of menstruation. Amenorrhea may be of two types: primary and secondary.
   (a) *Primary amenorrhea:* It is the condition when menstrual bleeding does not occur after 16 years of age.
   (b) *Secondary amenorrhea:* It is the stoppage of menstrual cycles with normally occurring menstrual cycles before. Most common cause of amenorrhea is pregnancy.

N.B. Changes in the endometrium occur as a result of hormones (estrogen and progesterone) secreted by the ovaries (ovarian cycle), which in turn is controlled by hormones secreted by the hypothalamus and pituitary gland.

1. **Menstrual phase (menses)** (1–4 days): If the ovum is not fertilized, the corpus luteum degenerates and the level of progesterone drops down. The coiled endometrial arteries undergo spasm. The blood supply to the spongy and compact layers of the endometrium is reduced. The functional layer undergoes necrosis and sloughs off, and there is hemorrhage from the stumps of the endometrial arteries. The sloughing continues until only raw surface of the stratum basale is left.

N.B. It takes about 14 days after ovulation to breaking down the stratum functionalis of endometrium. Note that the basal layer of endometrium remains intact.

2. **Proliferative phase/follicular phase** (5–14 days): The proliferative phase coincides with the secretion of the estrogen by the maturing follicles of the ovary. Under the influence of estrogen, the remaining endometrium (stratum basale) proliferates to restore the sloughed off endometrium.
3. **Secretory phase/luteal phase** (15–25 days): The secretory phase coincides with the secretion of progesterone by the corpus luteum. The purpose of secretory phase is to make endometrium (*stratum functionalis*) thick and soft (*edematous*) for embedding of fertilized ovum. Therefore, under the influence of progesterone the endometrium undergoes the following changes during this phase:
   - Endometrium becomes soft and edematous by secretion of mucous by uterine glands.
   - Arteries become long and tortuous to supply more blood.
   - Uterine glands become elongated, dilated, and saucer shaped.

   As a result, at the end of secretory phase, endometrium becomes thick, soft, edematous, and highly vascular.
4. **Premenstrual phase** (26–28 days): If the ovum is not fertilized, the corpus luteum degenerates and blood progesterone level falls. The spiral arteries are sensitive to progesterone hormone. As a result, they undergo spasm as the progesterone level decreases. This leads to ischemic pain. The ischemic necrosis of endometrium and wall of arteries occur. As a result, blood mixed necrosed endometrium begins to slough off. This makes the beginning of menstrual phase. The teenagers (12–17 years old females) often complain of severe spasmodic pain and external spotting of blood during this phase due to spasm-like contraction of spiral arteries and ischemia of the uterine wall called **premenstrual pain.**

The features of different phases of menstrual cycle are summarized in Table 3.1.

N.B. The menstrual cycle is a continuous process, and each phase gradually passes into the next one.

Table 3.1 Features of different phases of the menstrual cycle

Phase	Features
Menstrual phase (1–4 days)	Necrosis and shedding of the functional layer of the endometrium associated with bleeding
Proliferative phase (5–14 days)	Regeneration of the functional layer of the endometrium
Secretory phase (15–25 days)	Endometrium becomes thick and soft due to increased secretory activity of endometrial glands
Premenstrual phase (26–28 days)	• Ischemia of endometrium due to reduced blood supply following spasm of tunica media of spiral arteries • Cramping or pain and external spotting of blood

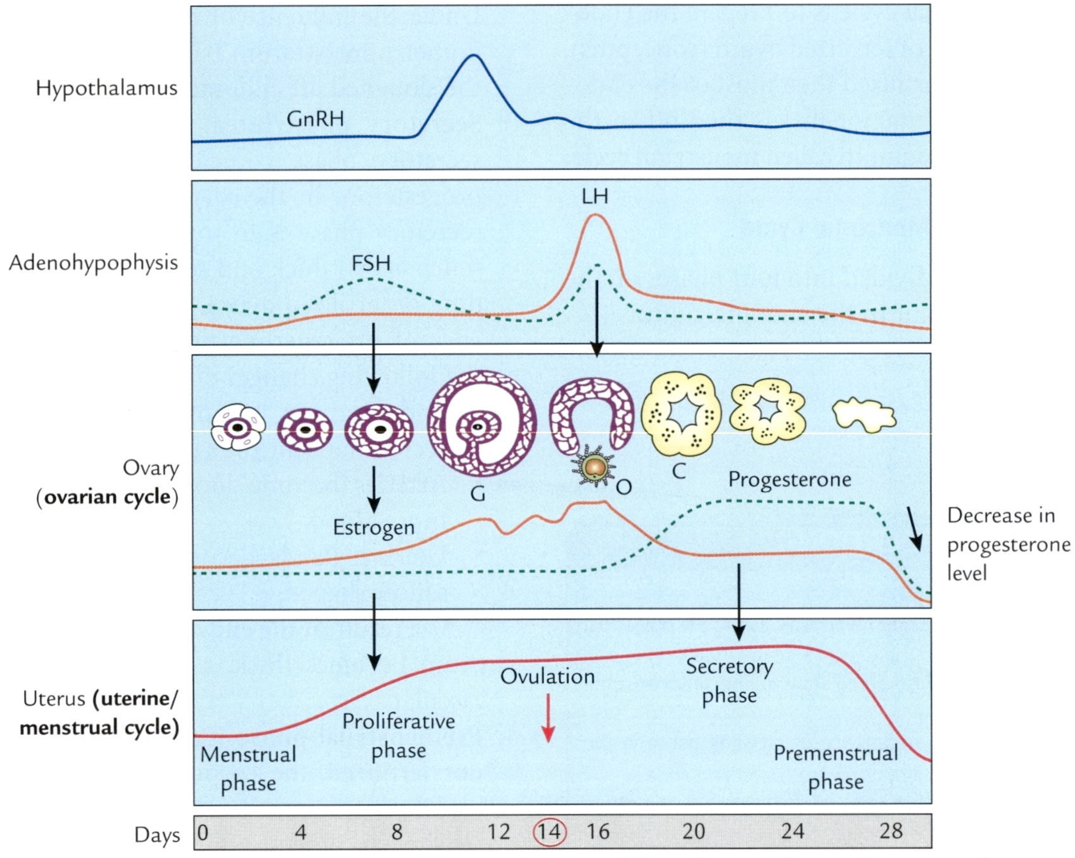

Fig. 3.11 Hormonal control of the ovarian and menstrual cycles. Note the synchrony between the two. G, Graafian follicle; C, corpus luteum; O, oocyte.

Hormonal Control of Ovarian and Menstrual Cycles (Fig. 3.11)

Both ovarian and menstrual cycles are controlled by ***the hormonal secretions of hypothalamus, adenohypophysis***, and ***ovary*** as follows (Fig. 3.11):

1. The hypothalamus secretes ***gonadotrophin-releasing hormone (GnRH)***, the key regulator of reproductive cycles.
2. The GnRH acts on the adenohypophysis, which in turn secretes FSH and LH.
3. The FSH causes maturation of one or more ovarian follicles. The ***secondary follicle*** is converted into the ***Graafian follicle.***
4. The granulosa cells of the ***secondary and Graafian follicles*** secrete ***estrogen.***
5. The estrogen stimulates the uterine endometrium to enter the ***proliferative phase*** (the level of estrogen rises to a peak just before the LH surge).
6. The LH surge stimulates ***ovulation.***
7. Following ovulation, the lutein cells of the corpus luteum secrete ***progesterone.***

8. The progesterone stimulates the uterine endometrium to enter the ***secretory phase***.

N.B. The hormones secreted by ***hypothalamus, adenohypophysis,*** **and ovary** prepare the endometrium of the uterus for implantation of the conceptus (blastocyst). If fertilization does not occur, the granulosa cells produce **inhibin**, a protein that acts on adenohypophysis and inhibits the secretion of gonadotrophins, which leads to the regression of corpus luteum. The endometrium undergoes **ischemic necrosis** due to decreased levels of progesterone and estrogen, especially progesterone secretion by the degenerating corpus luteum.

Synchrony Between Ovarian and Menstrual Cycles (Correlation Between Ovarian and Menstrual Cycles) AN 77.2

The ovarian and menstrual cycles go hand-in-hand throughout the reproductive life of women, except during pregnancy. These cycles terminate at **menopause**, usually between the ages of 45 and 55 years.

The ovarian and menstrual cycles run parallel to each other. Both these cycles are of 28-day duration.

In fact, the menstrual cycle is dependent on the ovarian cycle because the uterine endometrium undergoes cyclic changes under the influence of hormones secreted by the developing ovarian follicles and corpus luteum of the ovary.

In general, follicular phase of ovarian cycle corresponds with the first half of the menstrual cycle, whereas luteal phase of ovarian cycle corresponds with the second half of the menstrual cycle.

CLINICAL CORRELATION AN 77.5

Use of hormones in birth control (contraceptive) pills: The sex hormone estrogen with or without progesterone is used in the preparation of contraceptive pills. These hormones in contraceptive pills act on the hypothalamus and pituitary gland, resulting in **inhibition of secretion of GnRH as well as FSH and LH**, the secretion of which is essential for ovulation to occur. **The suppression of ovulation is the basis for the contraceptive pills.**

The most common variety of the contraceptive pill distributed by the government of India contains **progestin (norethisterone acetate)** 1 mg and estrogen (estradiol) 50 mg. These pills are distributed in packets, with each packet containing 28 pills. Of these 28 pills, 21 contain these hormones and 7 do not contain hormones. The woman is asked to start taking these pills 5 days after the onset of menstruation and continue without any break as long as pregnancy is not desired. Normal menstruation occurs during 7 days in which she takes pills without hormone. If the contraceptive pills are taken on a regular basis, the menstrual cycles occur regularly, each with 28 days. When she starts taking pills without hormones after 21 days, the withdrawal of hormone induces menstruation after 2 days.

GOLDEN FACTS TO REMEMBER

➢ **Total number of seminiferous tubules in each testis**	400–600
➢ **Most important function of testis**	(a) Formation of sperms (b) Production of testosterone hormone
➢ **Reproductive period of woman's life**	Period during which she can bear children (15–45 years of age)
➢ **Most important event of the ovarian cycle**	Ovulation
➢ **Menarche**	Onset of first menstruation (takes place at about 12 years of age)
➢ **Menopause**	Age at which menstruation ceases to occur (45–55 years)
➢ **Most important feature of menstrual cycle**	Monthly flow of blood per vaginum
➢ **Most important factor to initiate menstruation**	Withdrawal of progesterone and estrogen hormones
➢ **Most common cause of amenorrhea (i.e., absence of menstruation)**	Pregnancy
➢ **Most precarious time of prenatal development**	Embryonic period (3rd week to 8th week)

CLINICAL PROBLEM SOLVING

PROBLEMS

1. When an infertile (childless) couple visits a doctor, **why male fertility is evaluated first?**
2. **What are the causes of male infertility?**
3. What is the **most effective permanent method of contraception in males?**
4. In some women the cause of infertility is anovulation (i.e., cessation of ovulation). **Is it possible to induce ovulation** in these women?
5. How is ovulation assessed clinically?
6. **What is the importance of determining the time of ovulation?**
7. **Which is most precarious time of prenatal development** (i.e., period of greatest sensitivity to teratogens)? Give the embryological basis.

SOLUTIONS

1. Male fertility is evaluated first because the semen analysis is easier to perform. The average volume of semen ejaculated in the vagina during sexual intercourse is 2–6 mL (average 3.5 mL). There are usually more than 100 million sperms per mL of semen of normal males. **A man with less than 10 million sperms per mL of semen is likely to be sterile**, especially when the specimen contains immotile and abnormal sperms.
2. The common causes of male infertility are low sperm count **(oligospermia)**, poor sperm motility, abnormal sperms, and obstruction of the genital tract (e.g., vas deferens).
3. The most effective permanent method of contraception in males is **vasectomy**. This procedure involves the excision of a segment of each ductus (vas) deferens. Following vasectomy, there are no sperms in the semen or ejaculate, but the volume remains the same.

N.B. First one or two ejaculate may contain sperms.

4. In some women, ovulation does not occur due to inadequate secretion of FSH and LH. Ovulation can be induced in such women **by administrating gonadotrophins or an ovulatory agent such as clomiphene citrate**. By competing with estrogen for binding sites in the adenohypophysis, the **clomiphene citrate** suppresses the normal negative feedback loop of estrogen on the adenohypophysis. This, in turn, stimulates the release of pituitary gonadotrophins (FSH and LH) secretion, which causes maturation of several ovarian follicles and thus induces ovulation.
5. Ovulation can be assessed clinically as it is accompanied by:
   (a) A variable amount of abdominal pain in some women called *mittelschmerz* (German – mittel = mid + schmerz = pain), because ovulation results in slight bleeding in the peritoneal cavity.
   (b) A slight drop in the basal body temperature.

   In a 28-day menstrual cycle, the ovulation takes place at about the middle of the cycle, to be exact on day 14 before the start of next menstrual bleeding.

   There are many methods to find out the exact time of ovulation, but the one that is easy and commonly used is the **temperature method**. In this method, woman's body temperature is recorded every morning before she gets up and plotted on a graph. The temperature is low during menstruation, subsequently it rises, and at about the middle of the cycle it suddenly falls to rise again. The rise in temperature after sudden fall indicates that ovulation has occurred.

   Following ovulation, the basal body temperature increases by 0.3–0.5°C.

6. The importance of determining the time of ovulation is twofold:
   (a) *Rhythm method of family planning* (i.e., pregnancy is not desired): After ovulation, the ovum remains viable only for 2 days and sperms deposited in vagina remain viable only for 4 days. Therefore, fertilization can occur only if intercourse is done 4 days before ovulation to 2 days after the ovulation. Barring these 6 days, the remaining days of the menstrual cycle are regarded as **safe period**. Thus, pregnancy can be avoided if intercourse is done during safe period.
   (b) *Achievement of pregnancy* (i.e., pregnancy is desired): In case of infertility (failure to conceive), the couples are advised to have sexual intercourse during the unsafe period (i.e., 4 days before ovulation to 2 days after the ovulation), because this period is most favorable for conception.
7. The most precarious time of prenatal development for teratogenesis is during the embryonic period (i.e., from the beginning of the 3rd week to the end of the 8th week), because there is much tissue differentiation and organ formation during this period. Mostly, however, a woman does not realize that she is pregnant until it is very late. Therefore, a woman should consistently take care of herself and abstain from taking certain drugs including antibiotics (especially during 14 days before next menstruation) even if there is a remote chance that she is pregnant or might become pregnant in the near future.

4 Cell Division and Gametogenesis (Conversion of Germ Cells Into Male and Female Gametes)

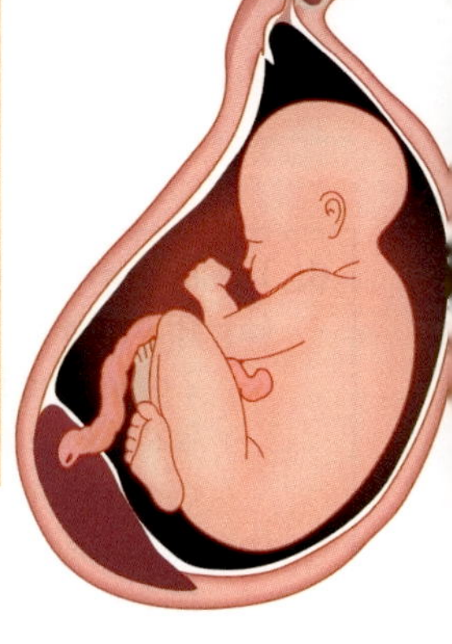

LEARNING OBJECTIVES

After studying this chapter, the student should be able to:

- Define the terms mitosis and meiosis and discuss their significance.
- List the distinguishing features between mitosis and meiosis.
- Describe spermatogenesis and oogenesis along with diagrams. AN 77.3
- Write short notes on spermiogenesis, ovulation, and corpus luteum.
- Give brief account of development of ovarian follicles and their functional significance.
- Discuss structure of male and female gametes.

OVERVIEW

The human body is made up of 60–100 trillion of cells. The body cells are broadly divided into two types: **somatic cells** and **germ cells**. The **somatic cells** undergo mitotic cell division. They are essential for growth, development, regeneration, and maintenance of various tissues of the body, whereas **germ cells** undergo meiotic cell division. They are essential for the production of gametes.

Life begins as a single cell – the zygote, formed by the union of male and female gametes. In humans, the male gametes are spermatozoa or **sperms**, which are produced by testis from puberty onward throughout life, i.e., up to death. The female gametes are **oocytes**, which are released from ovary in a cyclic fashion throughout the reproductive life of a female, i.e., from 12–45 years only.

The **gametes** are specialized cells for reproduction. Each gamete cell has a haploid (half) number of chromosomes (i.e., 23 chromosomes). Each body cell (somatic cell) has diploid (double) number of chromosomes (i.e., 46 chromosomes). The 46 chromosomes are arranged in 23 pairs. The 22 pairs of these chromosomes are called **autosomes**, whereas the 23rd pair is called **sex chromosomes**. Sex chromosomes determine the genetic sex of an individual. The sex chromosomes are of two types: X and Y. Females have two X chromosomes, whereas males have one X and one Y chromosome. Conventionally, this is expressed as a formula 44XX in females and 44XY in males.

Each **gamete** has only 23 chromosomes. In females, all oocytes are of only one type, i.e., each oocyte contains 22 autosomes and one X chromosome (22X). In males, sperms are of two types – one type contains 22 autosomes and one X chromosome (22X) and the other type contains 22 autosomes and one Y chromosome (22Y). The sperm containing X chromosomes is called **X-bearing sperm** or **gynosperm** and the sperm containing Y chromosomes is called **Y-bearing sperm** or **androsperm**.

During fertilization, if "X" chromosome combines with "X" chromosome, the **baby will be female**. On the other hand, if "X" chromosome combines with "Y" chromosome, the **baby will be male**.

CELL DIVISION

There are two types of cell divisions: *mitosis* and *meiosis*.

Mitosis

This type of cell division occurs in somatic cells. The mitotic cell division is a process in which one cell divides into two daughter cells that are genetically identical to the parent cell. Each daughter cell receives the complete complement of 46 chromosomes.

The period between the two mitotic divisions is called **interphase**. During interphase, i.e., before mitosis begins, each chromosome replicates its deoxyribonucleic acid (DNA). During this period, the chromosomes are in the form of long and thin threads (chromatin threads), which spread diffusely within the nucleus. These cannot be recognized with a light microscope (Fig. 4.1).

The various stages of mitosis are as follows (Fig. 4.2):

1. **Prophase:** In this stage, nucleolus disappears. The chromosomes become coiled.[1] They condense, shorten, and thicken. Each chromosome now consists of two parallel subunits called *chromatids*, which remain joined to each other at a narrow common region called *centromere*. However, the chromatids cannot be recognized in this stage.
2. **Prometaphase:** In this stage, the chromatids become distinguishable.

[1]Shortening of chromosomes by coiling reduces the chances of pinching off of the fragments of chromosomes.

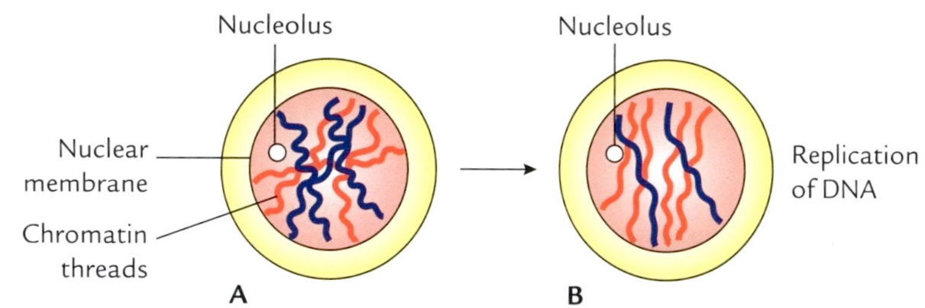

Fig. 4.1 Cell in interphase stage. (A) Early interphase. (B) Late interphase.

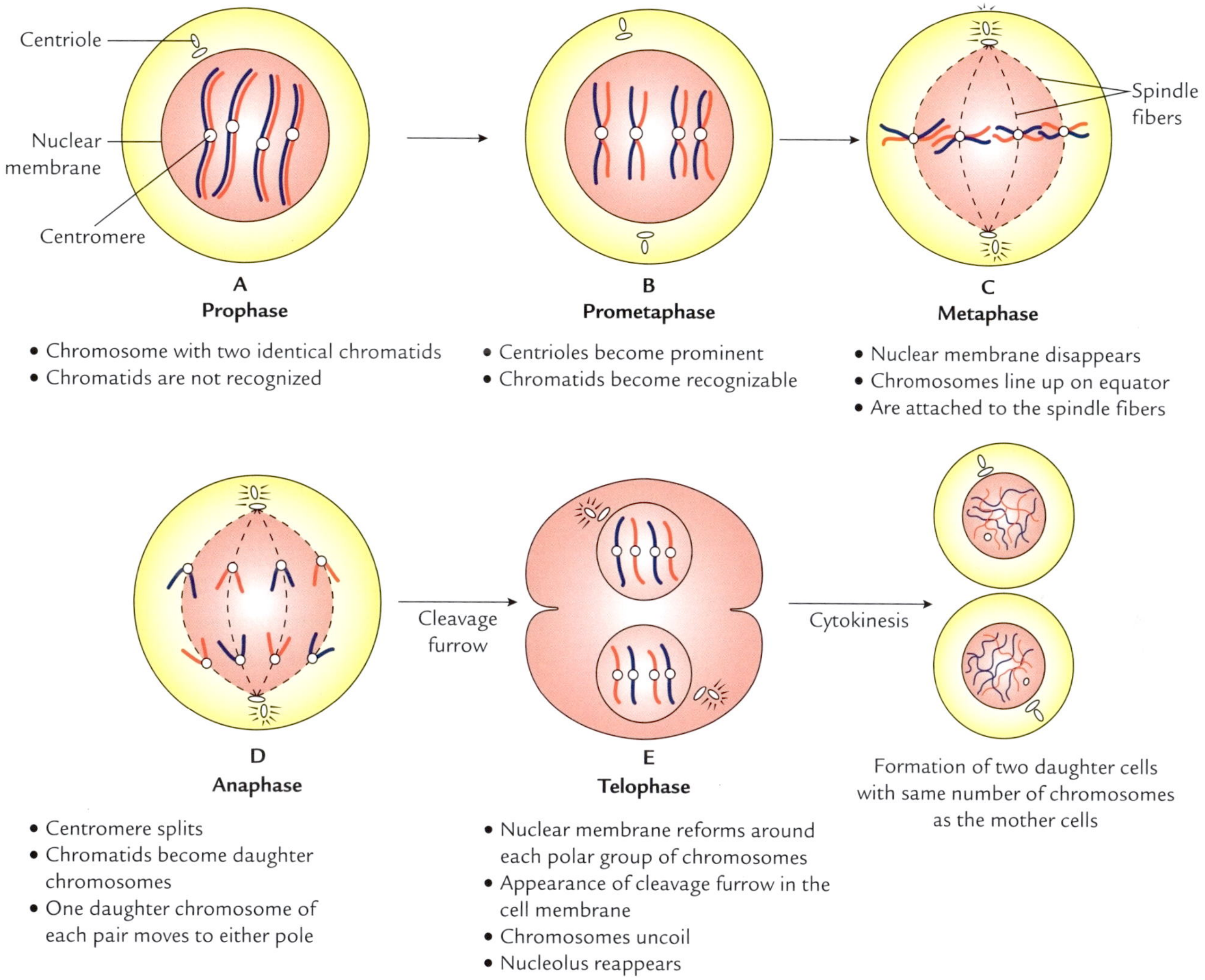

Centriole
Nuclear membrane
Centromere
Spindle fibers

A
Prophase

- Chromosome with two identical chromatids
- Chromatids are not recognized

B
Prometaphase

- Centrioles become prominent
- Chromatids become recognizable

C
Metaphase

- Nuclear membrane disappears
- Chromosomes line up on equator
- Are attached to the spindle fibers

Cleavage furrow
Cytokinesis

D
Anaphase

- Centromere splits
- Chromatids become daughter chromosomes
- One daughter chromosome of each pair moves to either pole

E
Telophase

- Nuclear membrane reforms around each polar group of chromosomes
- Appearance of cleavage furrow in the cell membrane
- Chromosomes uncoil
- Nucleolus reappears

Formation of two daughter cells with same number of chromosomes as the mother cells

Fig. 4.2 Various stages of mitosis.

3. **Metaphase:** In this stage, the nuclear membrane breaks. The double structured chromosomes (vide supra) line up in the equatorial plane of the spindle and get attached to the microtubules of the spindle extending between two centrioles, one at each pole.
4. **Anaphase:** In this stage, the centromere of each chromosome splits and the two chromatids are separated from each other. They are now called *daughter chromosomes*. The spindle fibers attached to the centromere of the chromosomes contract and pull the daughter chromosomes toward poles. Because of pull on centromere, the daughter chromosomes become V-shaped with their arms trailing as they move toward the poles.
5. **Telophase:** In this stage, the separated chromatids are migrated to the opposite poles of the spindle. The spindle fibers disappear and nuclear membrane appears around each polar group of daughter chromosomes.

The chromosomes uncoil and become less compact. The nucleolus reappears. There appears a cleavage furrow beneath the equator that deepens and separates the two daughter cells (*cytokinesis*).

> **CLINICAL CORRELATION**
>
> **Significance of mitosis**
> 1. ***Genetic stability:*** It ensures continuous succession of identical cells through generations.
> 2. ***Growth and development:*** It helps in growth and development of the body.
> 3. ***Regeneration, replacement, and repair:*** It helps in regeneration of new cells to replace the dead or damaged cells.

Meiosis (Fig. 4.3)

The meiosis is a special type of cell division that takes place only in the germ cells to produce male and female gametes. The meiosis consists of two cell divisions that take place one after the other. (a) **First meiotic division** (**meiosis I** or **reductional division**): In this division, the number of chromosomes of the daughter cells is reduced to half of the mother cell. (b) **Second meiotic division** (**meiosis II**): It is the mitotic division similar to the one described above except that there is no duplication of DNA during short interphase.

First Meiotic Division

1. **Prophase:** Prophase of the first meiotic division is very long and complicated. It is therefore subdivided into five stages.
   (a) *Leptotene:* In this stage, the chromosomes, as in mitosis, appear as slender threads. *Note*: Although each chromosome consists of two chromatids that are joined at centromere, the chromatids are not visible at this stage.
   (b) *Zygotene:* In this stage, the lengthwise pairing of homologous chromosomes begins. One of the two homologous chromosomes is from the father (**paternal chromosome**) and the other is from the mother (**maternal chromosome**). This event is called **synapsis** and each synapsing pair is called **bivalent**.
   (c) *Pachytene:* This stage is very long and may extend even for years. It is characterized by following changes:
   - The chromatids of each chromosome become visible separately. Each bivalent chromosome thus appears to have four chromatids and is called **tetrad**. Each chromatid pair is united by a **kinetochore**. There are two central chromatids and two peripheral chromatids (one from each chromosome).
   - The two central chromatids (one belonging to each chromosome) of tetrad coil over each other so that they cross at a number of points. This is called **crossing over**. Because of crossing over, the central chromatids present a cross-like configuration called **chiasmata**.

   (d) *Diplotene:* During this process, the paired homologue of tetrad starts separating. The central chromatids break at the point of crossing over and unite to the opposite chromatid. This results in exchange of genetic material between these chromatids.
   (e) *Diakinesis:* The chromosomes become more contracted and migrate toward the nuclear membrane. At the end of prophase, the nuclear membrane disappears.
2. **Metaphase:** The homologous pairs of chromosomes become arranged on the equatorial plane of the spindle.
3. **Anaphase:** In this stage, the homologous chromosomes migrate to the opposite poles of the spindle. Unlike mitosis, the chromosomes move randomly. The shorter chromosomes move earlier than the longer chromosomes.
4. **Telophase:** In this stage, the nuclear membrane is formed around the polarized group of chromosomes. The cell membrane constricts and two daughter cells are formed (**cytokinesis**). Each daughter cell thus formed contains only half the number of chromosomes (**haploid number**) with exchanged genetic material.

Second Meiotic Division

The **second meiotic division** is essentially similar to mitosis. It, however, differs from mitosis in that the DNA does not duplicate. In second meiotic division, the two daughter cells of first meiotic division form four daughter cells, each with haploid number of chromosomes.

> **CLINICAL CORRELATION**
>
> **Significance of meiosis**
> 1. ***Maintenance of normal chromosomal number:*** As the chromosome number is reduced to half during meiosis, each germ cell has *haploid number* of chromosomes. When two germ cells unite to form a *zygote*, the chromosome number is restored to normal (*diploid number of chromosomes*). Thus, because of meiosis, the chromosome number is maintained for the species.

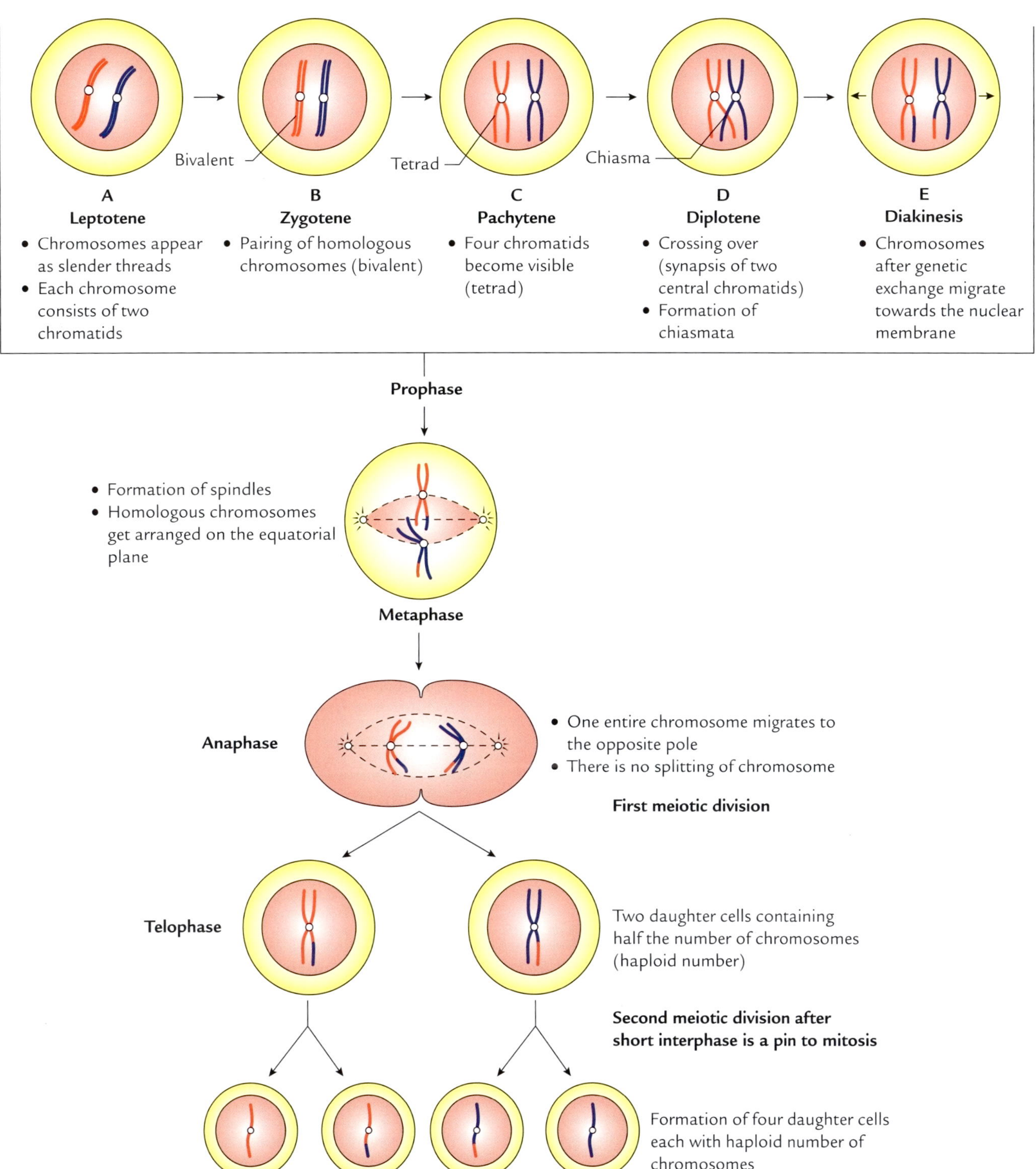

Fig. 4.3 Meiotic divisions I and II. The five stages of prophase of first meiotic division are shown by figures A, B, C, D, and E on the top.

2. ***Genetic variation:*** Because of random assortment of paternal and maternal chromosomes, and exchange of genetic material during crossing over in the meiosis, the daughter cells (i.e., gametes) have a new genetic configuration. This causes individual variations within the species, which is essential for evolution.
3. ***Hybrid vigor:*** Meiosis helps to maintain vigor in progeny through sexual reproduction.

The distinguishing features between mitosis and meiosis are given in Table 4.1.

GAMETOGENESIS

It is the process of formation of male and female gametes in an organism. Gametogenesis is a sequence of events

Table 4.1 Distinguishing features between mitosis and meiosis

Mitosis	Meiosis
Takes place in somatic cells	Takes place in germ cells
Completes in one sequence	Completes in two sequences, i.e., there are two successive divisions, namely, **meiosis I** and **meiosis II**
Crossing over of chromatids does not take place	Crossing over of chromatids takes place
Daughter cells have the same number of chromosomes as parent cells	Daughter cells have half the number of chromosomes as parent cells
Daughter cells are identical to each other and to the parent cell	Daughter cells are not identical to each other and to the parent cell
Equational division	Reductional division

involving mitotic and meiotic divisions. The gametocytes are derived from primordial germ cells (PGCs) by mitotic division.

The gametocytes undergo meiotic division to form gametes.

The PGCs develop from **epiblast** of bilaminar germ disc during the 2nd week of development. From here, first they migrate into the wall of yolk sac by week 4, then from there into developing gonad via dorsal mesentery of gut by week 5.

SPERMATOGENESIS

AN 77.3

The spermatogenesis is the process of formation of spermatozoa from spermatogonia. This process occurs in waves along the length of seminiferous tubules taking about 64 ± 4 days to complete.

The spermatogonia, which are derived from PGCs by a process called *spermatocytogenesis* (Fig. 4.4).

The PGCs are present in the wall of the seminiferous tubules of the testes.

They remain dormant in the seminiferous tubules of testes till puberty. At puberty (12–16 years), these cells undergo a series of mitotic divisions to form spermatogonia. They start forming gametes, i.e., spermatozoa, and this continues throughout the reproductive life of a male, i.e., up to old age.

The spermatogenesis can be divided into three phases:

1. **Spermatocytogenesis** (proliferation and differentiation of PGCs into spermatogonia)

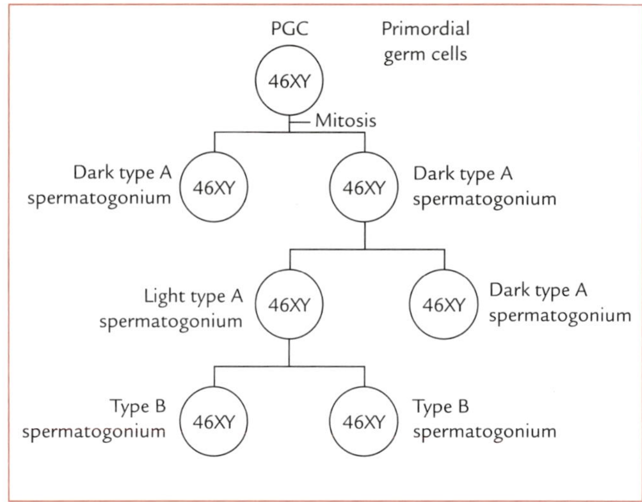

Fig. 4.4 Spermatocytogenesis.

2. **Formation of spermatids**
3. **Spermiogenesis** (transformation of spermatids into spermatozoa)

1. **Spermatocytogenesis**

   It is a process by which PGCs (stem cells) undergo repeated mitosis to replace themselves and produce a population of cells destined to become mature sperms. The PGCs divide by mitosis to form dark type A spermatogonia, which act as stem cells. Each dark type A spermatogonium undergoes mitosis to form one dark type A spermatogonium and other light type A spermatogonium. The dark type A spermatogonia are kept in reserve for repetition of the next cycle. The light type A undergoes mitotic division to form two dark type B spermatogonia.

2. **Formation of Spermatids**
   - The **type B spermatogonium** undergoes mitotic division to form two **primary spermatocytes** (largest germ cells).
   - The **primary spermatocytes** undergo **first meiotic division** (reductional division) to form two **secondary spermatocytes.** The secondary spermatocytes thus have haploid number of chromosomes.
   - Each secondary spermatocyte immediately undergoes **second meiotic division** (i.e., mitotic division without duplication of DNA) to form two **spermatids,** each with haploid number of chromosomes.
   - The spermatids are small cells of about half the size of the secondary spermatocyte and have round and darkly stained nuclei.
   - The spermatids lie close to the lumen of seminiferous tubule.

3. **Spermiogenesis**

   The spermatids are transformed into four mature spermatozoa by a process called **spermiogenesis.**

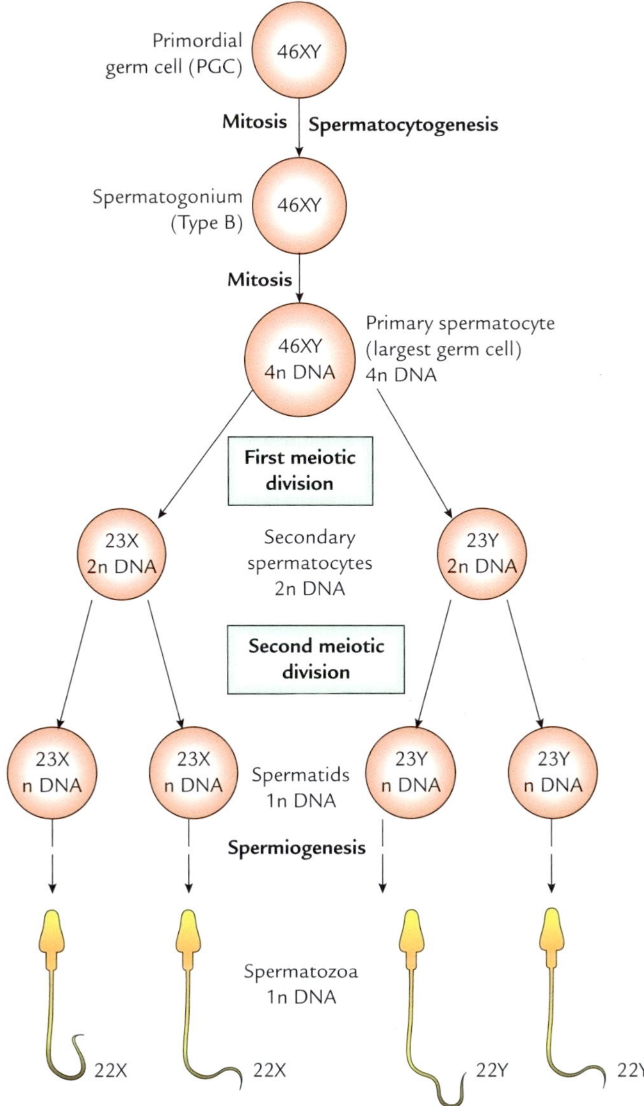

Fig. 4.5 Stages of spermatogenesis.

N.B. One primary spermatocyte forms four spermatozoa: two containing X chromosomes and two containing Y chromosomes (Fig. 4.5).

The steps of spermatogenesis are summarized in Flowchart 4.1.

To understand the process of spermiogenesis, the student must first understand the structure of spermatozoon (Fig. 4.6).

Structure of Spermatozoon (Fig. 4.6)

The spermatozoon (50 microns in length) consists of **head**, **neck**, and **tail**. The tail is further divided into three parts: **middle piece**, **principal piece**, and **end piece**. Tail forms four-fifths of the length.

Head

The head of sperm appears somewhat like a spearhead in section. It mainly consists of a **nucleus** that contains the condensed chromatin material (mostly DNA). Anterior two-thirds of the nucleus is covered by an **acrosomal cap** that contains various enzymes including **hyaluronidase** and **acrosin**.

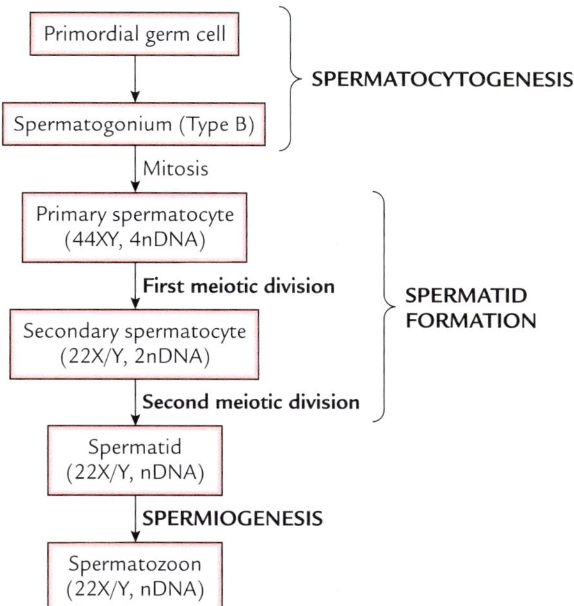

Flowchart 4.1 Stages of spermatogenesis.

Neck

The neck is narrow. It contains a funnel-shaped **basal plate** and a **centriole**. The centriole gives rise to axial filament that extends throughout the tail.

Tail

The tail consists of three parts: middle piece, principal piece, and end piece.

1. **Middle piece:** It contains the axial filament in the center, which is surrounded by spirally arranged mitochondrial sheath. At the distal end of the middle piece there is a ring-like structure through which axial filament passes. It is called *annulus* and is derived from the other centriole.
2. **Principal piece:** It is made of axial filament covered by seven outer dense fibers.
3. **End piece:** It is made of only the axial filament.

N.B.
- Structure of the axial filament is very similar to that of the cilium.
- The whole spermatozoon is covered by plasma membrane.

Figure 4.6 shows parts of the mature sperm (on the left) and sections through head, neck, middle piece, principal piece, and end piece along with their composition (on the right).

N.B. The axial filament is responsible for the movements of the spermatozoon, while mitochondria supply energy for these movements.

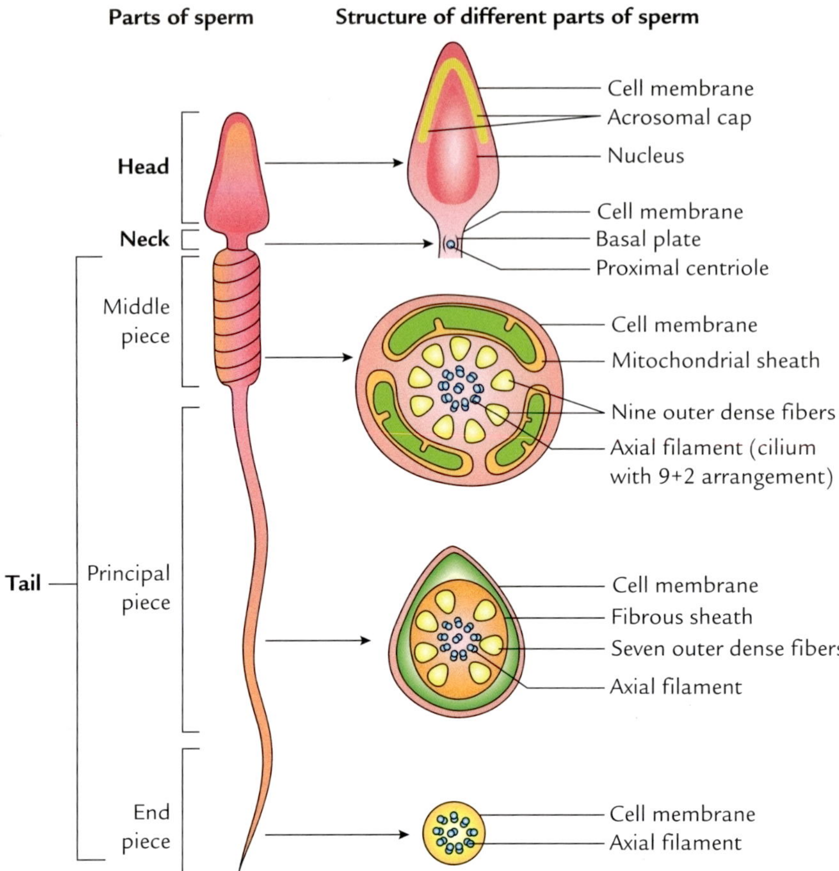

Fig. 4.6 Human sperm. The parts of mature sperm are shown on the left side, whereas the sections through the head, neck, middle piece, principal piece, and end piece along with their composition are shown on the right side.

SPERMIOGENESIS

The process by which the spermatids are transformed into mature spermatozoa is known as spermiogenesis.

Process of Spermiogenesis (Fig. 4.7)

The spermatid is more or less a circular cell containing a nucleus, Golgi apparatus, centrosome, and mitochondria. The spermatid is transformed into the spermatozoon as follows:

1. Nuclear material (chromatin) gets condensed and the **nucleus** moves toward one pole of the cell to form the **head of the spermatozoon.**
2. **Golgi apparatus** forms the **acrosomal cap** that covers anterior two-thirds of the nucleus.
3. **Centrosome** divides into **two centrioles.** One centriole becomes spherical and moves toward the posterior end of nucleus to occupy the neck region. It gives rise to the **axial filament.** The other centriole moves away from the first centriole and becomes ring shaped. It forms an **annulus/ring around the distal end of the middle piece** through which axial filament passes.
4. The part of the axial filament between the neck and annulus becomes surrounded by the mitochondria, and together with them forms the middle piece.
5. The remaining part of the axial filament elongates to form the principal and end pieces of tail. Most of the cytoplasm of spermatid is shed off but the cell membrane remains, which covers the entire spermatozoon.
6. Shedding off most of the cytoplasm (residual cytoplasm).

The structural components of the spermatid and the spermatozoon are compared in Table 4.2.

> **CLINICAL CORRELATION**
>
> **Abnormal sperms**
>
> The abnormality of sperms is common as compared to the oocytes. Morphologically, for clinicians, the sperm consists of two parts of head and tail.
>
> Sperm abnormalities can be categorized as follows:
>
> 1. ***Morphological abnormalities*** (Fig. 4.8):
>   (a) Head and tail of sperms may be abnormal (i.e., two heads, two tails)

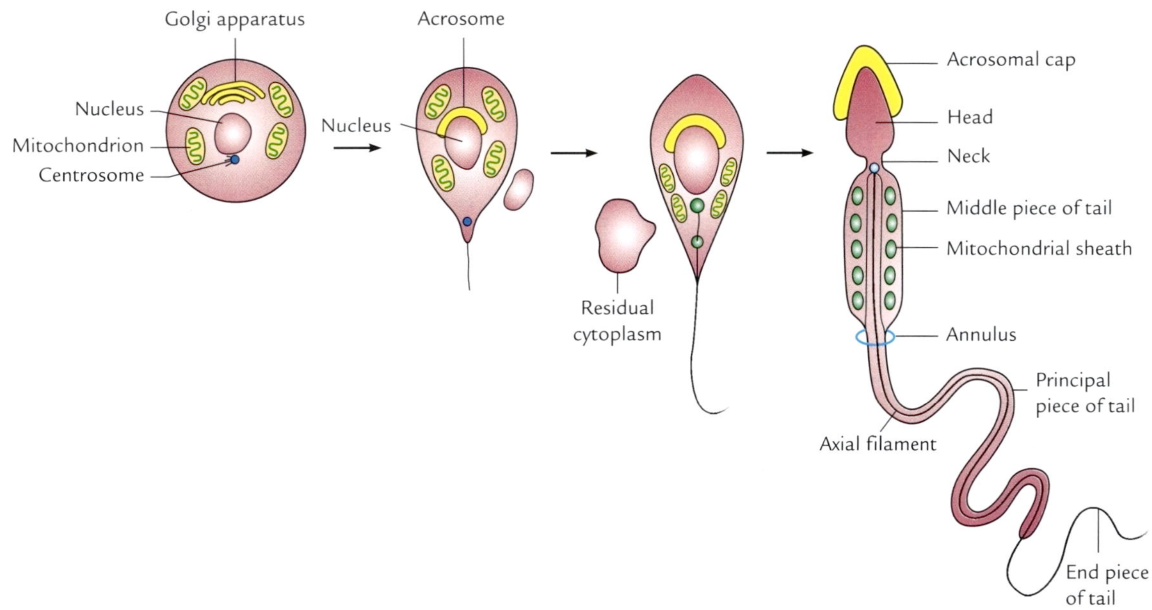

Fig. 4.7 Process of spermiogenesis.

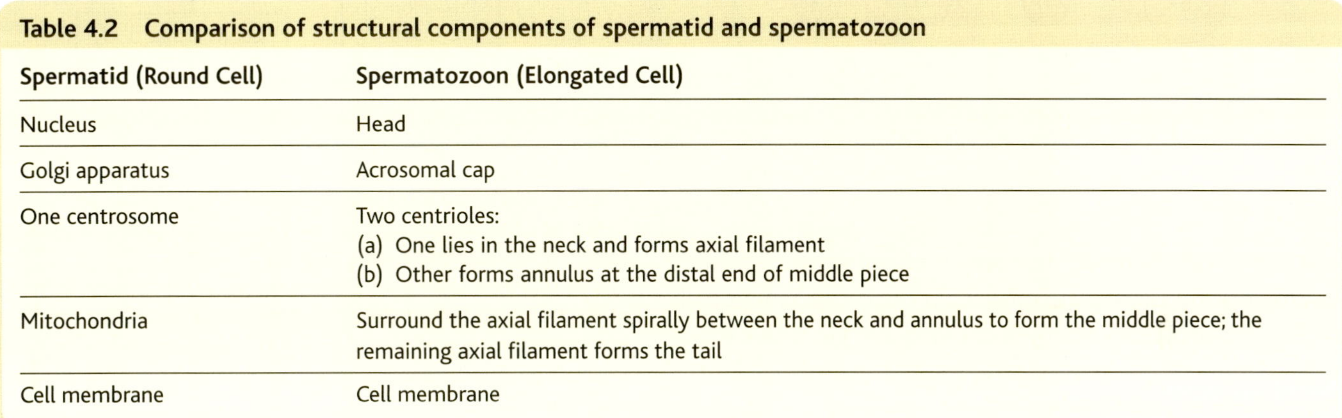

Table 4.2 Comparison of structural components of spermatid and spermatozoon

Spermatid (Round Cell)	Spermatozoon (Elongated Cell)
Nucleus	Head
Golgi apparatus	Acrosomal cap
One centrosome	Two centrioles: (a) One lies in the neck and forms axial filament (b) Other forms annulus at the distal end of middle piece
Mitochondria	Surround the axial filament spirally between the neck and annulus to form the middle piece; the remaining axial filament forms the tail
Cell membrane	Cell membrane

(b) Sperms may be giant or dwarf

(c) Sperms with double body

2. ***Immotility:*** For potential fertility, 50% sperms should be motile after 2 hours of ejaculation and some should be motile after 24 hours.
3. ***Genetic abnormalities:*** Sperm having abnormal chromosomal content (rare as compared to the oocytes).

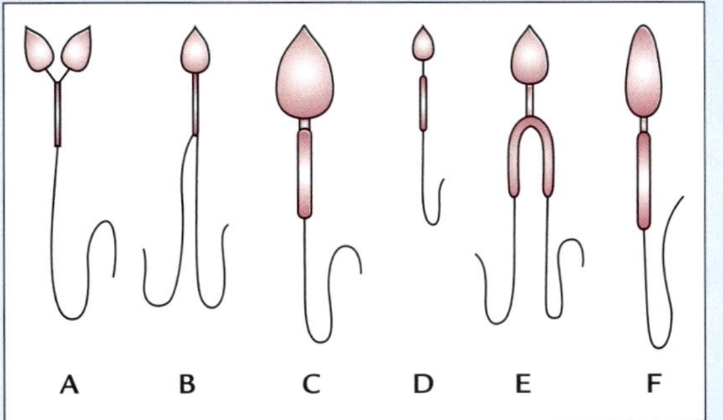

Fig. 4.8 Abnormal morphology of sperms: (A) double head; (B) double tail; (C) giant; (D) dwarf; (E) double body; (F) long head.

OOGENESIS (FIG. 4.9)

The **oogenesis** is a sequence of events (involving mitotic and meiotic divisions) by which oogonia are transformed into secondary/mature oocytes. This process begins before birth and completes by puberty.

The PGCs within ovary divide by mitosis to form a large number of oogonia.

Each **oogonium** then enlarges to form a **primary oocyte**. The primary oocyte enters the prophase of **first meiotic division** before birth. However, this division is arrested till puberty due to the presence of an oocyte maturation inhibitor (**OMI**) factor secreted by the follicular cells surrounding the oocyte. The first meiotic division **gets** completed only when primary oocytes start maturing and are getting prepared for ovulation.

At puberty, in each ovarian cycle, 5–50 primary oocytes resume their first meiotic division, which is completed just before the ovulation, forming two daughter

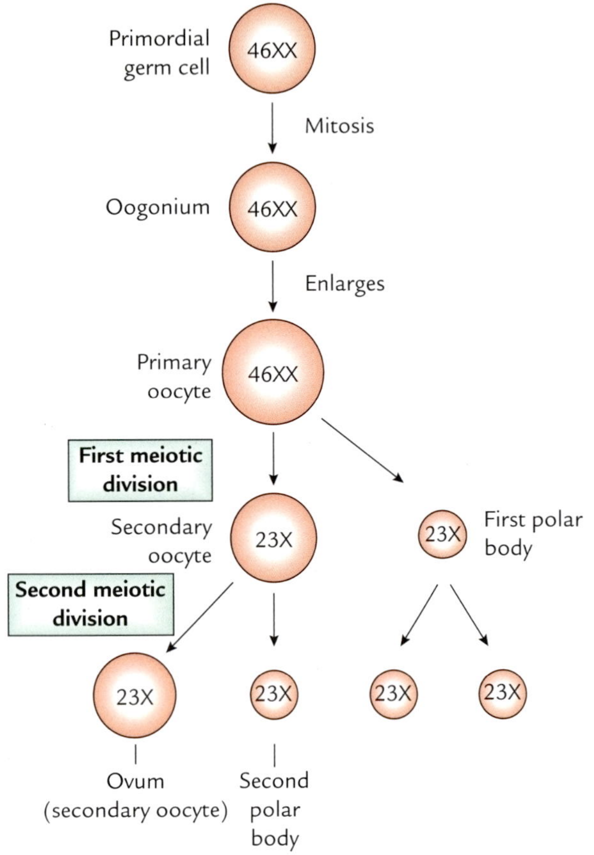

Fig. 4.9 Oogenesis.

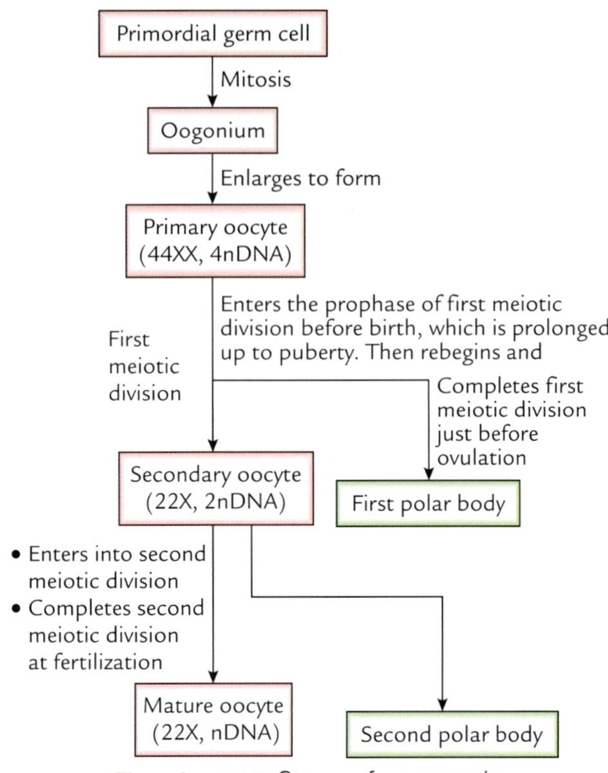

Flowchart 4.2 Steps of oogenesis.

cells each with haploid number of chromosomes. The first meiotic division is unequal; all of the cytoplasm goes to one daughter cell forming **secondary oocyte**, while the other daughter cell hardly receives any cytoplasm and forms the **first polar body**.

The secondary oocyte enters into the second meiotic division at the time of ovulation, but this division is completed only after the fertilization. The second meiotic division is also unequal and only one daughter cell receives most of the cytoplasm and forms the ovum, while the other daughter cell receives a very small amount of cytoplasm and forms the **second polar body**.

Thus, one primary oocyte forms only one ovum with 22 autosomes and one X chromosome; and three polar bodies each with 22 autosomes and one X chromosome are formed.

- Before 3rd month of intrauterine life (IUL), the PGCs undergo mitosis to form oogonia.
- Before 7th month of IUL, the oogonia continue to divide mitotically and enlarge to form primary oocytes.
- *From 7th month of IUL till birth, primary oocytes complete prophase of first meiotic division and get arrested at diplotene stage of first meiotic division by OMI.*
- From birth to puberty, primary oocyte remains in diplotene stage of first meiotic division.

N.B.

- **Oogonia** enlarge to form **primary oocytes** in late fetal period.
- In the first meiotic division, primary oocyte completes at puberty just before ovulation to form secondary oocyte.
- The secondary oocyte enters into second meiotic division immediately after ovulation. At the time of ovulation, secondary oocyte is in metaphase stage of second meiotic division, which continues till fertilization. The secondary oocyte completes its meiotic division only when it is fertilized.
- At birth, the ovary contains about two million germ cells. Thereafter, most germ cells degenerate and, by puberty, when ovulation begins only about 40,000 oocytes are left in the ovary. Out of which only 400–500 ovulate.

The steps of oogenesis are summarized in Fig. 4.9 and Flowchart 4.2.

The differences between spermatogenesis and oogenesis are given in Table 4.3.

The differences between the male and female gametes are given in Table 4.4.

Oogenesis is accompanied by development and growth of the follicles.

FURTHER DETAILS

Development of Ovarian Follicles

The development of ovarian follicles is essential for growth and maturation of female gametes and ovulation.

The ovarian follicles are complexes formed by primary oocyte and surrounding stromal cells of an ovary.

Table 4.3 Differences between spermatogenesis and oogenesis

Spermatogenesis (Process of Formation of Male Gametes)	Oogenesis (Process of Formation of Female Gametes)
Occurs in testes	*Occurs in ovaries*
• Primary spermatocytes form after birth at puberty • Starts at puberty	• Primary oocyte forms before birth • Starts before birth (10th week) and stops from birth to puberty (i.e., for about 12 years) and then restarts at puberty (i.e., 12 years of age)
• Production of sperms occur throughout life from puberty to old age	• Production of ova (one per month) occurs only during reproductive life from puberty (12 years) to menopause (45 years)
One primary spermatocyte forms four sperms (i.e., four male gametes)[a]	One primary oocyte forms only one mature oocyte (i.e., one gamete)*
It is not accompanied by development and growth of any such structures as follicles	It is accompanied by development and growth of follicles
Hardly contains any cytoplasm	Contains good amount of cytoplasm to provide nutrition to the embryo

*One primary spermatocyte forms four sperms and each sperm hardly contains any cytoplasm, because it survives only for 2–4 days and does not need to provide nutrition to the conceptus, and hence does not need a stored nutrition. On the other hand, one primary oocyte forms only one mature oocyte/ovum to retain maximum cytoplasm because fertilized ovum (conceptus) takes 4 days to become blastocyst. During this period, it derives its nutrition from stored food in the ovum. The polar bodies are formed merely to get rid of unwanted number of chromosomes in the female gamete and hardly contain any cytoplasm.

Stages of Development

The various stages of development of ovarian follicles are: (1) *primordial follicle*, (2) *primary follicle*, (3) *secondary follicle*, and (4) *Graafian follicle* (Fig. 4.10).

1. **Primordial follicle:** The oogonium gets covered by a single layer of flat epithelial cells – the **follicular cells** (which are derived from stromal cells of ovary) – to form the **primordial follicle**. The oogonium within the follicle contains single large nucleus with prominent eccentric nucleolus.
2. **Primary follicle:** The flattened follicular cells become columnar and form the **primary follicle**. The follicular cells proliferate to form several layers. The follicular cells are now called **granulosa cells** (also called membrana granulosa). The primary oocyte and its granulosa cells secrete a glycoprotein substance that forms a thick homogeneous membrane between the granulosa cells and the primary oocyte. This membrane is termed **zona pellucida**. The granulosa cells rest on the **basement membrane** that separates these cells from the surrounding stromal cells. This is called **multilaminar (maturing) primary follicle.**
3. **Secondary follicle:** Small fluid-filled cavities appear between the follicular cells. These cavities fuse together to form a large cavity – **the antral cavity/antrum** – and the follicle is termed **secondary (vesicular) follicle.**
4. **Graafian follicle:** The antrum gradually increases in size and pushes the oocyte toward one side of the follicle. The granulosa cells that surround the oocyte are called **cumulus oophoricus (or cumulus ovaricus)** and those that attach the oocyte to the wall of the follicle are called **discus proligerus.**

As the follicle expands, the stromal cells surrounding the granulosa cells become condensed to form a covering called **theca interna** (theca = covering). Outside the theca interna, some fibrous tissues get condensed to form another covering of the follicle called **theca externa.** The ovarian follicle is now fully matured and is termed Graafian follicle.

Table 4.4 Differences between male and female gametes

Features	Sperm (Male Gamete)	Secondary Oocyte (Female Gamete)
Size	Very small, about 2 μm in width	Very large, about 120 μm in diameter
Length	More (60 μm)	Less
Motility	Highly motile	Immotile
Amount of cytoplasm	Absent/very little cytoplasm	Large amount of cytoplasm to provide nutrition to conceptus
Types	Two types: (a) X-bearing sperms (22 + X) and (b) Y-bearing sperms (22 + Y)	Only one type (22 + X)

N.B.

- All ovarian follicles (primordial, primary, and secondary) contain primary oocytes (44XX). The primary oocyte completes first meiotic division to form secondary oocyte (22X) and first polar body in Graafian follicle just before ovulation.
- The cells of theca interna later secrete estrogen hormone and together they form the **thecal gland.**

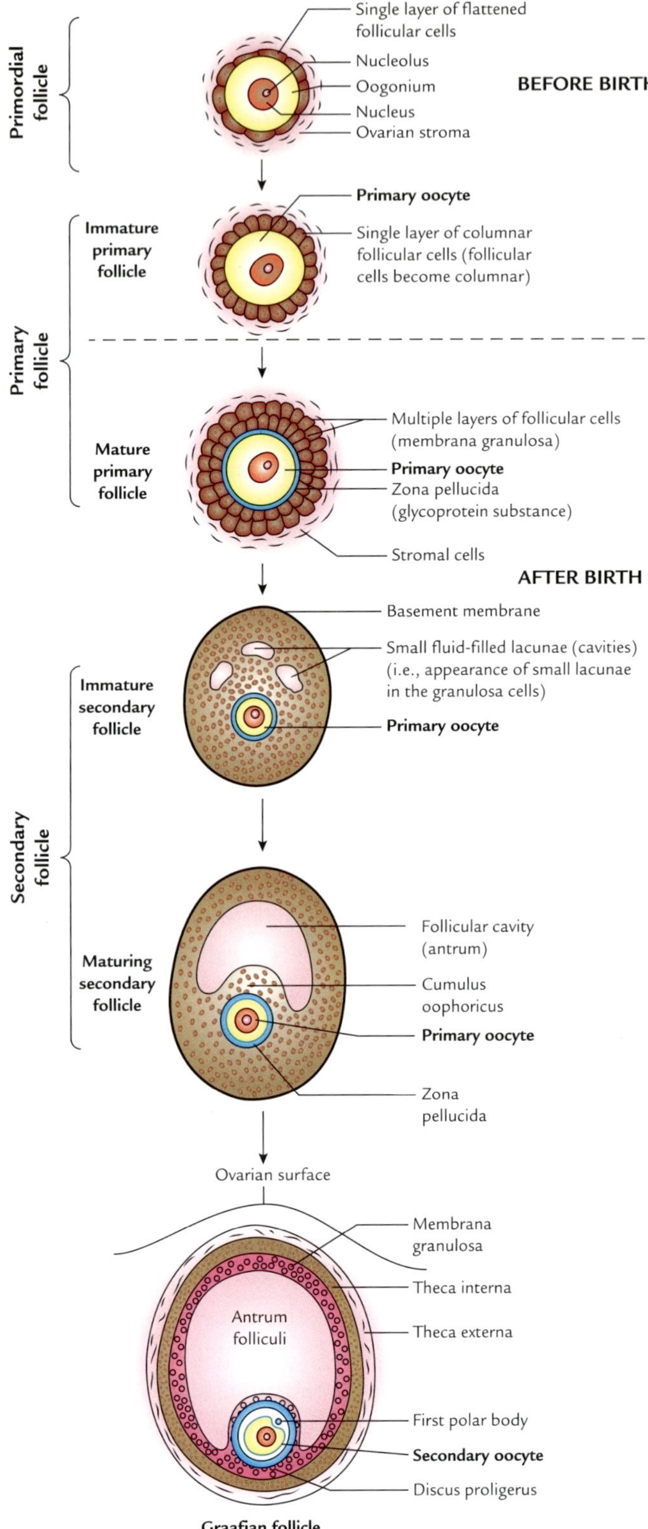

Fig. 4.10 Development of ovarian follicles.

Ovulation (Fig. 4.11)

It is a process of shedding off an ovum from the ovary.

Around 14th day in a 28-day menstrual cycle (to be very specific on 14th day before the onset of next menstrual cycle), the Graafian follicle, under the influence of follicle-stimulating hormone (FSH) and luteinizing hormone (LH), enlarges and becomes so big that it not only reaches the surface of the ovary but also forms a bulge on the surface of ovary. The theca and stroma on this side of follicle become very thin. A small avascular area (**stigma**) appears in the most convex superficial position of the follicle and, at the same time, the cells of cumulus oophoricus become loosened due to the accumulation of intercellular fluid.

Ultimately, under the surge of LH, the primary oocyte resumes the first meiotic division to form **secondary oocyte**. The second meiotic division also begins but arrested in metaphase. The follicle ruptures, and the ovum is released from the cortex of the ovary (**ovulation**). ***At the time of ovulation, the secondary oocyte is in metaphase stage of second meiotic division, which continues till fertilization.***

Final factors responsible for ovulation:

1. *High concentration of LH* increases **collagenase activity** (activity of proteolytic enzymes), which digests collagen fibers in and around the Graafian follicle.
2. *Increased prostaglandin levels* in response to LH surge causes **contraction** of smooth *muscle fibers* around the Graafian follicle.
3. *Increased fluid pressure* within follicular cavity.
4. *Enzymatic digestion* of follicular wall.

CLINICAL CORRELATION

Determination of time of ovulation

It can be done by various methods:

1. *Calender method:* Ovulation occurs 14th day before the onset of next menstrual cycle ± 1 day.
2. *Measurement of body temperature during midcycle:* It decreases (0.3–0.5°C) just before the ovulation and increases 0.3–0.5°C just after the ovulation.
3. *Estimation of hormones (FSH and LH) by Elisa strips:* There is an increase in LH and decrease in FSH at the time of ovulation.
4. *Ultrasonography:* The process of ovulation can be detected by ultrasonography.
5. *Mittelschmerz:* It is one-sided lower abdominal pain often associated with vaginal spotting.

Structure of the Female Gamete (Secondary Oocyte; Fig. 4.12)

1. It is a **very large cell** and measures more than 100 microns in diameter.
2. Its nucleus is not visible because nuclear membrane dissolves for second meiotic division. Spindle and chromosomes attached to it in the equatorial plane (metaphase stage) are seen.

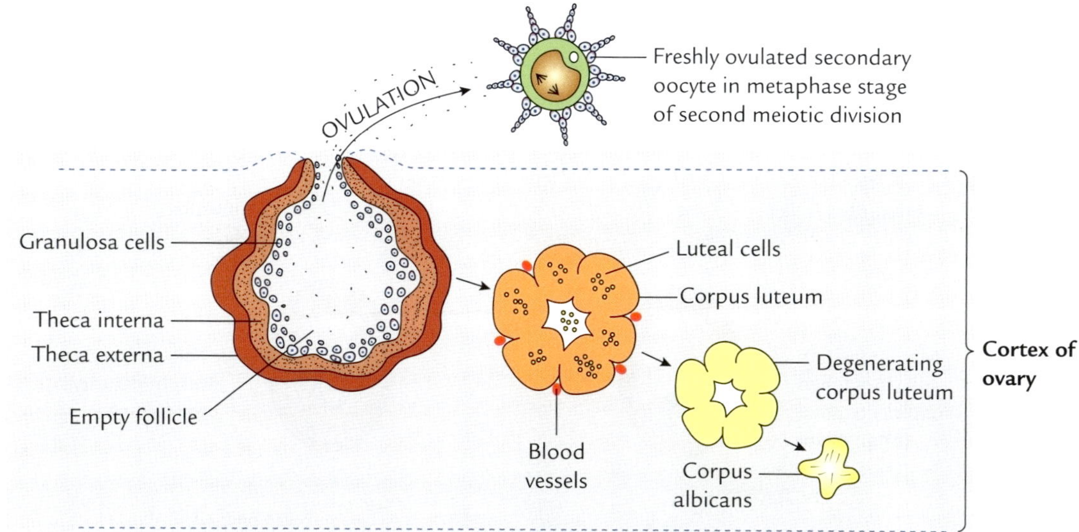

Fig. 4.11 Ovulation and formation of corpus luteum.

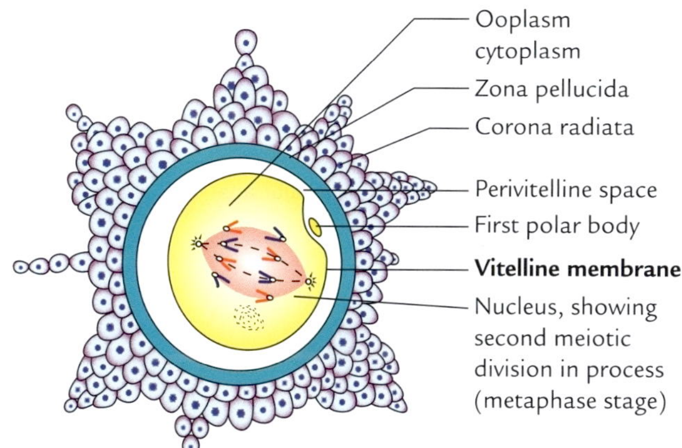

Fig. 4.12 Structure of female gamete – the ovum (secondary oocyte).

3. It is surrounded by the zona pellucida, which in turn is surrounded by cells of corona radiata.
4. A distinct space is present between the cell membrane called ***vitelline membrane*** and zona pellucida. It is termed ***perivitelline space.***
5. It contains first polar body.

N.B. The students must be aware that following terms are liberally used for female gametes by various authors, viz.
(a) Secondary oocyte
(b) Mature oocyte
(c) Ovum
(d) Oocyte

Corpus Luteum

After ovulation, the wall of the empty follicle (consisting of granulosa cells and cells of theca interna) collapses (crumbled and folded) and gets transformed into a kind of endocrine gland called as **corpus luteum.** Under the influence of LH (secreted by the pituitary gland), the follicular cells enlarge and become polyhedral. The yellowish pigment develops in these cells of corpus luteum, which are now called **lutein/luteal cells.** These cells secrete **progesterone** and some **estrogen.** Under the influence of progesterone together with some estrogen, the uterine endometrium enters into secretory phase in preparation for the implantation of embryo.

Types of corpus luteum

The corpus luteum is of two types:

(a) **Corpus luteum of pregnancy**

If fertilization occurs, the corpus luteum persists for 3–4 months under the influence of HCG secreted by the trophoblast of embedded blastocyst in the endometrium. This is called the ***corpus luteum of pregnancy.*** Progesterone secreted by the corpus luteum maintains the pregnancy for initial 3–4 months and thereafter the pregnancy is maintained by progesterone secreted by ***placenta.***

(b) **Corpus luteum of menstruation**

If fertilization does not occur, the corpus luteum lasts only for 10–14 days. Thereafter it degenerates and is gradually transformed into a mass of fibrous tissue called **corpus albicans** (white body). This is called the **corpus luteum of menstruation.**

Fate of Ovarian Follicles (Fig. 4.13)

In each ovarian cycle, a number of ovarian follicles begin to develop but only one reaches maturity. The fate of ovarian follicles is as follows:

1. The one that reaches maturity, ruptures and sheds off a secondary oocyte. The wall of empty follicle collapses to form corpus luteum (vide supra).

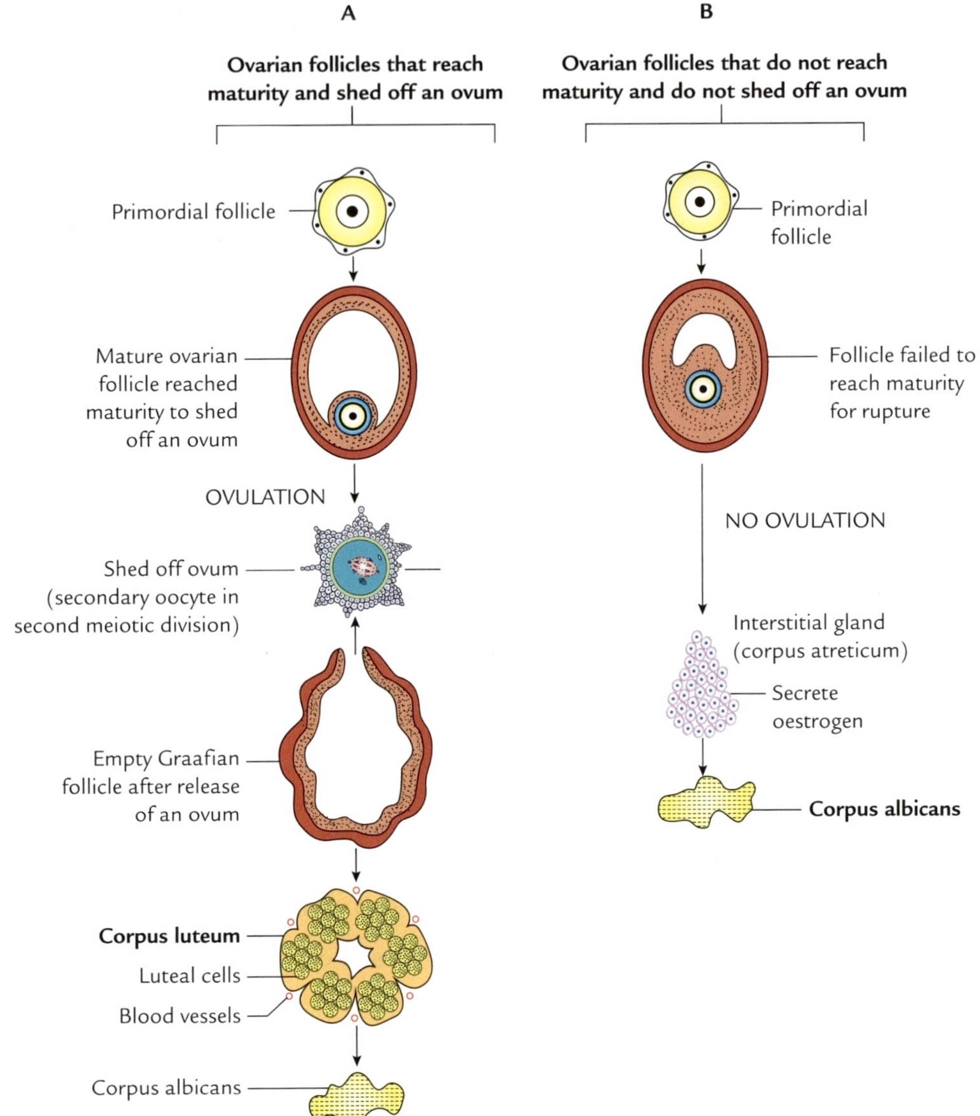

Fig. 4.13 Fate of ovarian follicles. (A) Fate of mature follicles (Graafian follicle), which rupture and shed off secondary oocytes. (B) Fate of those follicles that do not reach maturity to shed off ova.

2. The follicles that fail to reach maturity, undergo degeneration. The oocyte and granulosa cells of each follicle disappear. However, the cells of theca interna proliferate to form **interstitial gland** (**corpora atretica**). These glands secrete estrogen for some period of time and then degenerate to form a mass of fibrous tissue similar to the **corpus albicans**.

CLINICAL CORRELATION

Abnormal oocytes (female gametes)

The occurrence of abnormal oocytes is rare as compared to sperms. However, the following types of abnormalities of oocytes may occur:

1. ***Oocytes may be binucleated or trinucleated.*** Although such oocytes may give rise to twins or triplets, but they usually degenerate before reaching the maturity.
2. ***Oocytes with abnormal chromosomal contents*** may occur due to nondisjunction of chromosomes in meiosis I or meiosis II. The abnormal oocyte instead of having 23 chromosomes may contain 24 chromosomes or 22 chromosomes.

N.B. If oocyte with 24 chromosomes is fertilized by a normal sperm (23 chromosomes), a zygote with 47 chromosomes is produced (i.e., trisomy). The **trisomy** 21 or **Down syndrome** is most common type of trisomy. Similarly, if an ovum with 22 chromosomes is fertilized by a normal sperm (23 chromosomes), a zygote with 45 chromosomes will be produced (i.e., **monosomy**), e.g., **Turner syndrome** (45, X0). For details see Chapter 29.

GOLDEN FACTS TO REMEMBER

Largest germ cells in the seminiferous tubules	Primary spermatocytes
Duration of reproductive life of a female	About 30 years (i.e., 15–45 years)
Secondary oocyte completes its second meiotic division	Just after fertilization
Usual period of viability of sperm after ejaculation	48 hours (but may survive up to 4 days in female genital tract)
Usual period of viability of an unfertilized ovum	24 hours (but may survive up to 2 days)
Number of spermatozoa formed from one primary spermatocyte	4
Number of ova (female gametes) formed from one primary oocyte	1
A person is likely to be sterile if number of healthy sperms per mL is less than	10 million
Number of ovarian follicles that undergo ovulation during entire reproductive life of a woman (i.e., 12–42 years)	400–500
Number of ovarian follicles present at puberty	40,000
Number of primary oocytes that get matured and complete their first meiotic division before ovulation	5–30
Total period required for the process of spermatogenesis	60–75 days (about 2$\frac{1}{2}$ months)
State of ovum (secondary oocyte) at the time of ovulation	Metaphase stage of second meiotic division
Time required by an oogonium to develop into mature oocyte	More than 12 years; 2 months and 14 days

CLINICAL PROBLEM SOLVING

PROBLEMS

1. **During evaluation of male fertility an analysis of semen is made.** Why?
2. **Is it possible to have a baby of desired sex?**
3. **What is the safe period of the menstrual cycle?** Give the embryological/anatomical basis.
4. **Give the embryological basis of high incidence of chromosomal abnormalities in the offsprings of women who marry late.**
5. **Can the offsprings of men who marry late be affected?**

SOLUTIONS

1. The analysis of semen is done (a) to count the number of sperm per mL of semen, (b) to see morphological abnormalities of sperms, and (c) to see motility of sperm. Knowledge of these facts is essential to clinicians because a man with less than 10 million sperms per mL of semen is likely to be sterile, especially when specimen contains immotile and abnormal sperms.
2. Yes, it is possible to have a baby of desired sex nowadays.

   Sperms are of two types: **X-bearing sperms (gynosperms)** and **Y-bearing sperms (androsperms)**. When an ovum (X) is fertilized by a Y-bearing sperm, the offspring will be a **baby boy**, and if an ovum (X) is fertilized by an X-bearing sperm, the offspring will be a **baby girl**. Various **in vitro techniques** are now used to separate X and Y sperms using the following criteria:
   (a) Difference in swimming abilities of X- and Y-bearing sperms.
   (b) Different speeds of migration of sperms. The Y-bearing sperms move faster than X-bearing sperms.
   (c) Difference in the appearance of X- and Y-bearing sperms. The Y-bearing sperms are long and thin, whereas X-bearing sperms are short and thick.
   (d) Difference in DNA content of X- and Y-bearing sperms. The DNA content is 2.8% more in X-bearing sperm than that in Y-bearing sperm.

N.B. Thus, the use of a selected sperm sample in artificial insemination may produce a baby of desired sex.

   There is also a claim that a couple can choose the sex of their child, if they can manage the following things:
   (a) If the sexual intercourse is done on day of ovulation, i.e., 14th day (counted backward from the first day of the next menstrual cycle) ± 1 day.
   (b) If the sexual intercourse is done after female takes an alkaline douche.
   (c) If the frequency of sexual intercourse is reduced as much as possible.
3. The ovulation occurs on the 14th day of the menstrual cycle before the start of the next menstruation with variation of ± 1 day. The 14th day is counted backward from the last day of the menstrual cycle. The viability of sperm is not more than 2–3 days and viability of ovum is only 24 hours. Keeping all these factors in mind, if coitus (intercourse) is avoided for 1 week between 11th and 17th day the pregnancy can be avoided. Barring this week, the rest of the period of the menstrual cycle is termed **safe period.**
4. The commonest cause of abnormal chromosome number in a gamete is the nondisjunction during meiosis I or II.

   Prolonged dormancy of primary oocytes may be the reason for the high incidence of chromosomal abnormalities in offsprings of older women. Remember that primary oocytes are formed by the 5th month of intrauterine life. **The primary oocyte enters the prophase of first meiotic division before birth, but this division is arrested till puberty. At puberty, the primary oocyte reassumes first meiotic division, which is completed just before ovulation.**

   The secondary oocyte enters the second meiotic division at the time of ovulation, but gets arrested in metaphase stage and completed only if it is fertilized. Trisomy 21 (Down syndrome) is the most common chromosomal abnormality in offsprings born to women older than 35 years.
5. Yes. An increased incidence of achondroplasia (a congenital skeletal anomaly due to disturbance of endochondral ossification at the epiphyseal plate, particularly of long bones during fetal life) is associated with paternal age. Achondroplasia is the common cause of **dwarfism** (shortness of stature).

5 First Week of Development: Fertilization, Cleavage, Blastocyst Formation, and Implantation

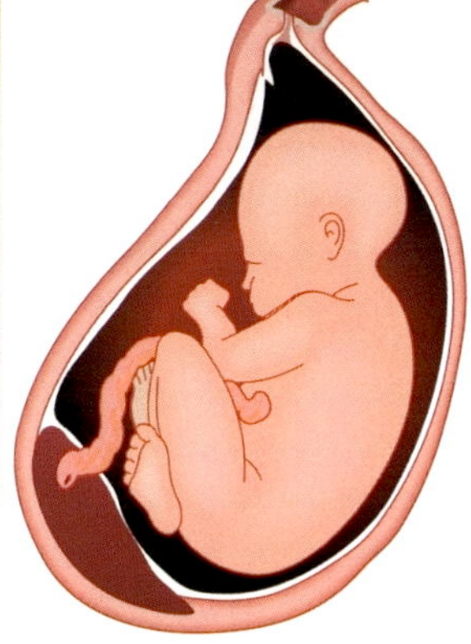

LEARNING OBJECTIVES

After studying this chapter, the student should be able to:

- Describe the stages and consequences of fertilization. AN 77.4
- Give the commonest site of fertilization and implantation.
- Enumerate:
  (a) Oocyte barrier
  (b) Components of secondary oocyte
- Describe the cleavage and formation of blastocyst. AN 78.1
- Write short notes on (a) capacitation of sperms and (b) morula.
- Describe the sterility, fertility, and surrogate mother. AN 77.6
- Describe the process of implantation and discuss the common abnormal sites of implantation. AN 78.3
- Enumerate and describe the anatomical principles underlying contraception. AN 77.5

OVERVIEW

The **fertilization** is the union of haploid male and female gametes to form diploid **zygote**–a single cell embryo.

The zygote undergoes a series of mitotic division called **cleavage** to form **blastocyst**. The blastocyst gets **implanted** into the uterine endometrium to develop into **full term fetus along with placenta**. The placenta secrete a hormone called human chorionic gonadotrophin (HCG), which forms the basis of pregnancy test.

In about 30%–40% cases spontaneous expulsion of embryo called **abortion** occurs due to severe genetic abnormalities.

FERTILIZATION AN 77.4

Fertilization is the process of fusion of male and female gametes (pronuclei) to form a **zygote**. It takes place within 24 hours of ovulation in the most dilated part of the uterine tube – the **ampulla**. The results of fertilization are (a) **determination of genetic sex of embryo**, (b) **restoration of diploid number of chromosomes,** and (c) **initiation of cleavage.** Fertilization is essential for propagation of species and their evolution.

For a proper understanding, fertilization is described under the following headings: **approximation of gametes, fusion of gametes**, and **results of fertilization.**

Approximation of Gametes (Fig. 5.1)

(a) Migration of Sperms

During coitus (sexual intercourse), a male ejaculates about one teaspoonful of semen containing 200–300 million sperms into the female's vagina. This high number is needed because of the high rate of sperm mortality in the female genital tract. Only 200–300 sperms survive

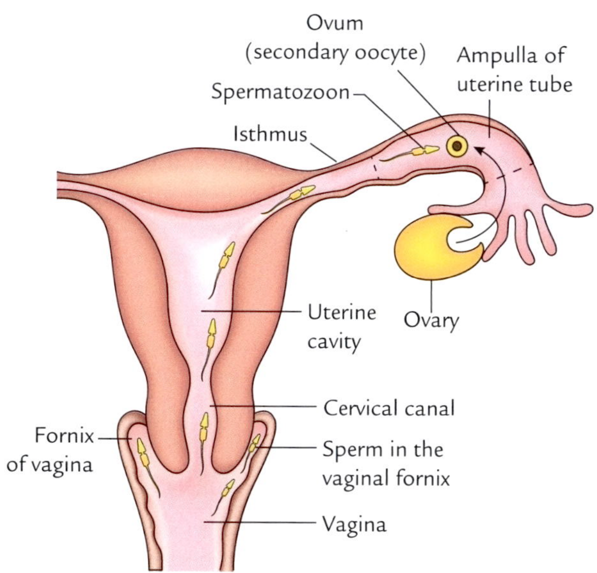

Fig. 5.1 Approximation of male and female gametes.

(i.e., only hundreds out of millions) and reach to contact the female gamete – the secondary oocyte in the uterine tube.

The journey of sperms from the vagina to the ampulla of uterine tube is promoted by prostaglandins present in the semen. The prostaglandins cause powerful contraction of uterine muscle, which is substantiated by oxytocin released by neurohypophysis. Uterine contractions create a negative pressure in the uterine cavity. Consequently, the sperms are sucked in from the vagina into the uterine cavity. The movement of sperms from the cervix to the isthmus of the uterine tube occurs primarily by their own propulsive action, i.e., whip-cord like movements of their own tail and to some extent, the movement is also assisted by fluid currents created by uterine cilia. It takes about 2–7 hours for the sperms to reach from the cervix to the ampulla of the uterine tube.

Note that only 1% of sperms deposited in vagina enter into uterine cervix. Out of this, only 300–500 sperms reach the uterine tube at the time of fertilization.

(b) Transport of an Oocyte (Fig. 5.1)

Just before the ovulation the fimbriated end of the fallopian tube becomes closely applied to the surface of the ovary, and its finger-like fimbriae start moving back and forth (**sweeping action**) over the ovarian surface. As the secondary oocyte is discharged on the surface of ovary, the sweeping action of fimbriae and fluid currents produced by cilia of the mucous lining of fimbria sweeps the ovum (secondary oocyte) into the infundibulum of the uterine tube as soon as it is discharged from the ovarian follicle.

From infundibulum, the oocyte passes to the ampulla of the tube mainly by the peristaltic movements of the tubal wall and movements of cilia.

The sperms again become motile due to **chemoattractants** produced by cumulus cells surrounding the oocyte and swim to the ampulla for fertilization. The majority of sperms die within 24 hours.

Other Details

Viability of gametes. The female gametes (mature oocytes) generally remain viable for 24 hours after ovulation. They are usually fertilized 12 hours after ovulation.

The male gametes (sperms) generally remain viable for 48 hours in the female genital tract.

N.B. According to some authorities, female and male gametes may survive up to 2 and 4 days, respectively.

Fertilization barriers. Before fertilization, the female gamete is protected by three barriers. From superficial to deep, these are:

1. **First barrier**, which is formed by **corona radiata** which is made up of 2–3 layers of follicular (granulosa) cells ovarian follicle surrounding a developing oocyte.
2. **Second barrier**, which is formed by **zona pellucida** (made of glycoproteins, ZP1, ZP2, and ZP3). It is a thick membrane of glycoprotein surrounding oocyte deep to corona radiata.
3. **Third barrier**, which is formed by **vitelline membrane** of oocyte itself. It is a structure made of protein fibers surrounding plasma membrane of oocyte.

The zona pellucida needs to be described in detail.

Zona pellucida. The zona pellucida is a **thick transparent membrane of 3 glycoproteins** (ZP1, ZP2, and ZP3) surrounding the ovum. It is an extracellular matrix formed by secretions from oocyte and zona granulosa cells.

Functions of zona pellucida

1. Protects oocytes and early embryos (viz. zygote, morula) during development.
2. Allows diffusion of uterine secretion (witch's milk) for nourishment of blastomeres.
3. Regulates interaction between oocyte and sperms around it during fertilization.
4. The ZP3 protein of zona pellucida binds with the receptor on membrane surrounding sperm heads and evokes *acrosomal reaction*.
5. On penetration by sperm it undergoes zonal reaction and becomes impermeable to other sperm to prevent polyspermy.
6. Prevents ectopic implantation of blastocyst.

The trophoblast has a strong tendency to stick with the endothelium to which it comes in contact with. The zona pellucida prevents the sticking of the trophoblast with the endothelium during the journey of fertilized oocyte from ampullary region of the uterine tube to the uterine cavity. **The most important function of zona pellucida is to prevent implantation of the blastocyst at sites other than the normal, thus preventing *ectopic pregnancy*.**

Therefore, the sperm must be able to disintegrate and pass through these barriers. Sperms get this ability to pass through these barriers by two processes: (a) **capacitation** and (b) **acrosome** reaction.

Capacitation

The capacitation is the final step of maturation of sperms, which make them competent to fertilize an oocyte. The capacitation occurs after ejaculation of sperms into the female genital tract; it lasts for about 7–10 hours. During capacitation, the glycoprotein coat and seminal plasma proteins covering the plasma membrane of sperm in the acrosomal region are removed by chemicals secreted by uterus. Now sperms' tails start to beat more vigorously. Only capacitated sperm undergoes acrosome reaction and fertilizes the ovum.

Acrosome Reaction

Acrosome reaction occurs when capacitated sperm comes in contact with the zona pellucida (i.e., acrosome reaction is induced by zona proteins). This reaction leads to release of enzymes, such as **hyaluronidase** and **acrosin,** from acrosomal cap. The antigenic coating of the sperm initiates an immunological reaction between the **oocyte's fertilizin** and the **sperm's antifertilizin**.

CLINICAL CORRELATION

Significance of capacitation: Capacitation of sperms is a prerequisite for fertilization.

It is now confirmed by experiments that the freshly ejaculated sperms are infertile and must be in the female genital tract for at least 7 hours before they can fertilize a secondary oocyte.

During in vitro fertilization, the capacitation of sperms is induced artificially by treating the ejaculate with a solution consisting of gamma-globulin, free serum, follicular fluid, dextran, serum dialysate, and adrenal gland extract.

Stages of Fertilization (Fig. 5.2) AN 77.4

To fertilize the ovum (secondary oocyte), the sperm has to break three barriers (may be called **fertilization barriers**) which surround and protect it.

The sequence of events taking place during fertilization is as follows:

1. **Penetration of corona radiata:** About 300–400 capacitated sperms come in contact with corona radiata. They liberate hyaluronidase enzymes, which digest the chemical substance binding the cells of corona radiata. Now the sperm freely penetrates the corona radiata to reach the zone pellucida through the movements of its tail.
2. **Penetration of zona pellucida:** When the head of sperm comes in contact with glycoproteins of zona pellucida, an **acrosome reaction** occurs. The acrosome releases digestive enzymes (**acrosin and pepsin-like substances**), which cause lysis of the zona pellucida and plasma membrane around the head of the sperm. This allows the sperm to penetrate through the zona pellucida and reach into the perivitelline space. Once the sperm penetrates the zona pellucida, a change in the properties of zona pellucida (**zona reaction**) occurs that makes it impermeable to other sperms to prevent polyspermy.
3. **Penetration of vitelline membrane:** When the plasma membranes of sperm head come in contact with the plasma membrane of oocyte (called vitelline membrane), the latter breaks down at the site of fusion. This allows the head of the sperm to enter into the cytoplasm of the oocyte leaving behind the discarded body and tail of sperm on the oocyte surface. As soon as the head and neck of sperm enters the oocyte, a **calcium wave** appears in the cytoplasm of oocyte that makes oocyte membrane impermeable to other sperms.

N.B. **Polyspermy** is prevented by integrin peptides of vitelline membrane and zona reaction of zona pellucida by not allowing the entry to more than one sperms (vide supra).

4. **Formation of female pronucleus:** The penetration of oocyte by the sperm activates the oocyte to complete its second meiotic division. Thus, two cells are produced: one cell containing all the cytoplasm is called **mature oocyte** and the second cell containing hardly any cytoplasm is called second polar body.

   The maternal chromosomes (22 + X) of mature oocyte condense and arrange themselves in a vesicular pattern to form the **female pronucleus.**
5. **Formation of male pronucleus:** The sperms move forward to come in close contact with the female pronucleus. Its nucleus becomes swollen and forms the male pronucleus. Morphologically, the male and female pronuclei are indistinguishable. Each chromosome in male and female pronuclei is made of only one chromatid. The pronuclei (both haploid) grow and replicate their DNA, i.e., change from haploid (n) to diploid ($2n$). Now each chromosome in male and female pronuclei consists of two chromatids. The oocyte containing two haploid nuclei is called **ootid.**
6. **Formation of zygote:** The male and female pronuclei lose their cell membrane and chromosomes of two nuclei (23 in each) mix together to form diploid (i.e., 46 chromosomes). The ootid becomes a zygote. The chromosomes in zygote become arranged on a cleavage spindle in preparation for cleavage of

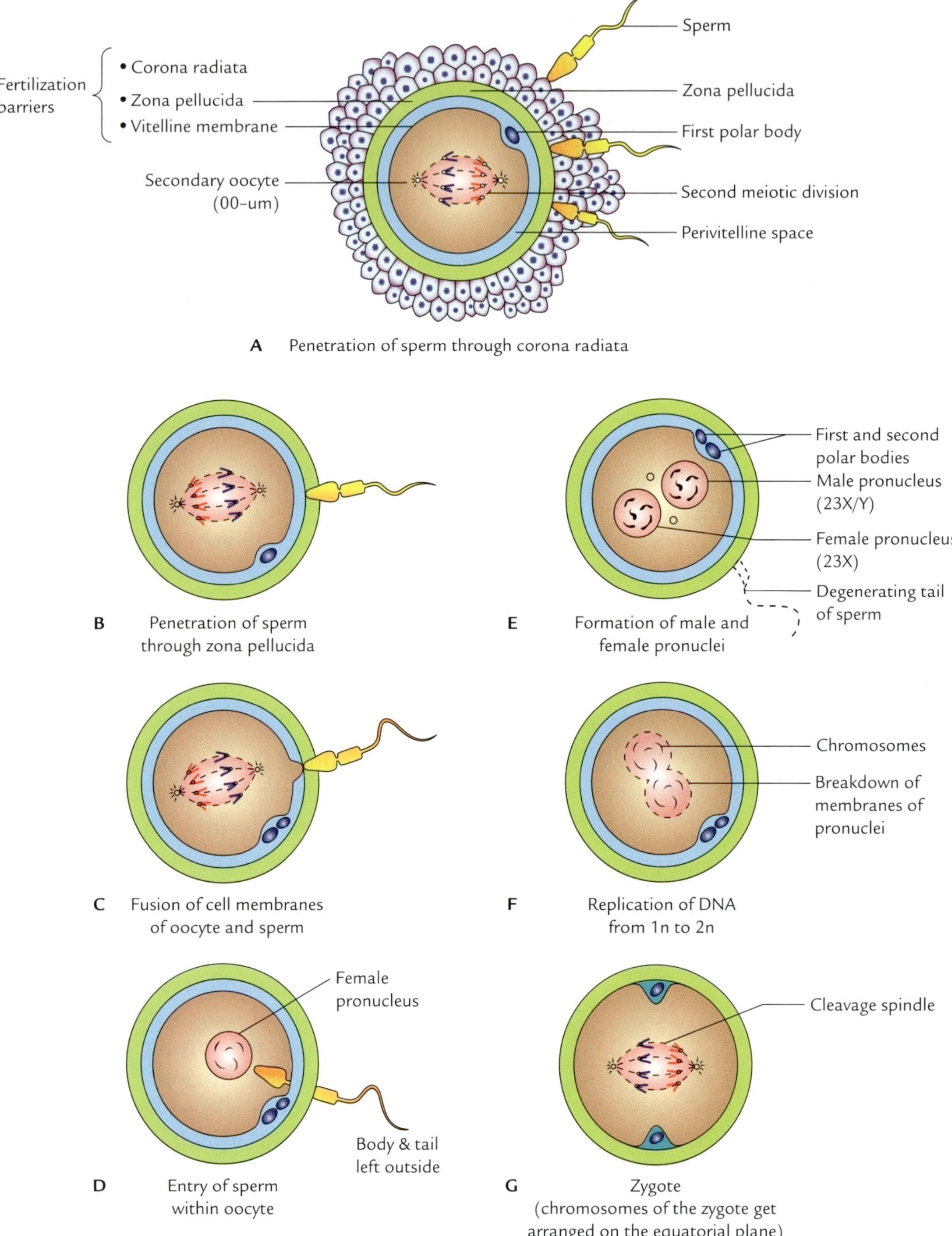

Fig. 5.2 Steps/phases of fertilization and formation of the zygote.

zygote. The chromosomes split longitudinally at the centriole and sister chromatids move to the opposite poles, providing each cell of the zygote with a normal diploid number of chromosomes and DNA. As the sister chromatids move to the opposite poles, a furrow appears on the surface of the cell and two cells are formed.

Results of Fertilization

AN 77.4

The main results of fertilization are as follows:

1. **Completion of second meiotic division of the female gamete:** As soon as the sperm enters into the secondary oocyte, the latter completes its second meiotic division and extrudes the second polar body into the **perivitelline space.**

2. **Restoration of diploid number of chromosomes:** The male and female pronuclei (both haploid) fuse with each other to restore normal diploid number of chromosomes.
3. **Determination of chromosomal sex of the new individual:** The oocytes are only of one type, i.e., they contain only "X" chromosomes, whereas the sperms are of two types: (a) "Y"-bearing sperms (**androsperms**) and (b) "X"-bearing sperms (**gynosperms**). If an oocyte (X) is fertilized by a Y-bearing sperm, the result will be a **male baby**, and if an oocyte is fertilized by an X-bearing sperm, the result will be a **female baby**. *Therefore, it is the father who is responsible for determination of the sex of the baby, and not the mother.*
4. **Initiation of cleavage:** Fertilization stimulates the zygote to undergo a series of rapid mitotic divisions. This is called **cleavage**.
5. **Variation of human species**: It occurs due to mingling of maternal and paternal chromosomal complements of two different species. For examples, if the ovum of one species (e.g., tiger) is fertilized by the sperm of other species (e.g., lion), the baby born will be called **liger**. Similarly, if the ovum of a female donkey is fertilized by the sperm of a horse, the baby born will be called **mule**.

N.B. During fertilization only head of sperm enters into oocyte and its body and tail are left outside on the surface of zona pellucida; hence, child does not have any mitochondrial DNA from father because mitochondria are present around the body of sperm. Therefore, all the mitochondrial DNA in child comes only from mother. Thus, one can say genetically children are closer to mother than father.

CLINICAL CORRELATION

- **Sterility and infertility:** AN 77.6 The **sterility** is inability to produce a biological child while infertility is **inability** to conceive after a certain period.
- **In vitro fertilization (IVF):** The *in vitro fertilization* is a process by which ovum is fertilized outside the human body. IVF is now a common procedure used in various laboratories to help couples for whom normal pregnancy is not possible due to tubal occlusion, disorders of ovulation, etc.

Steps of IVF: The following techniques are used in a sequential manner for IVF and embryo transfer (Fig. 5.3).

1. *Stimulation of ovary:* The follicular growth in the ovary is stimulated by administration of gonadotrophins/clomiphene citrate.
2. *Retrieval of oocytes:* Several mature oocytes are collected by needle aspiration from ovarian follicles by laparoscopy or with the assistance of ultrasound visualization.
3. *Collection of sperms:* The ejaculate is collected by masturbation, and the sperms are separated from the seminal fluid and capacitated artificially by exposure to ionic solution (see Clinical Correlation on p. 47).

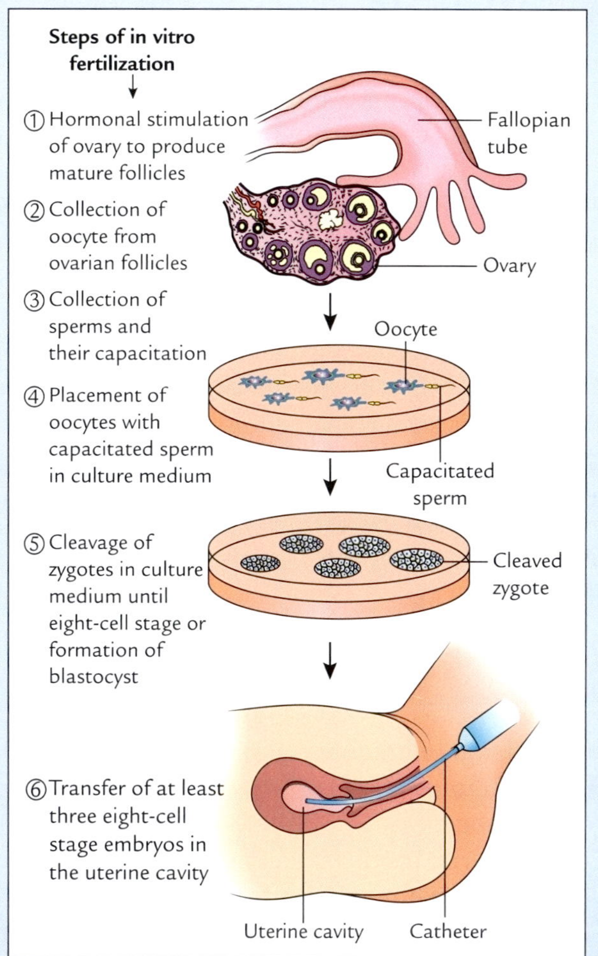

Fig. 5.3 Various steps of in vitro fertilization and embryo transfer.

4. *Fertilization:* The oocytes are placed in the culture medium and capacitated sperms are added immediately (i.e., oocytes and sperms are cultured together).
5. *Culture of embryo:* The cleavage is allowed to proceed in vitro till the 8-cell stage of the embryo or sometimes up to the stage of blastocyst formation.
6. *Embryo transfer:* At least three *8-cell stage embryos* are transferred into the uterus to develop to full-term fetus. At least three embryos are placed in the uterus because of the low success rate of implantation. The remaining embryos are frozen for further use in case the first attempt of IVF fails to cause pregnancy.

The in vitro pregnancy is supported at least for two weeks by **progesterone**.

N.B. IVF of oocytes and transfer of cleaving zygotes into the uterus have provided an opportunity for many women who are sterile due to tubal occlusion.

- **Surrogate mothers:** AN 77.6 Some women have normal ovaries and produce mature oocytes but are unable to become pregnant due to agenesis of the uterus or hysterectomy. In such cases, IVF may be performed and the embryos are transferred to another woman's uterus (after pretreatment with progesterone) for development and delivery.

Unusual Modes of Fertilization and Cleavage

- **Superfecundation and superfetation**

  The superfecundation is the fertilization of two or more oocytes during the same menstrual cycle (within a day or two) by sperms from separate acts of coitus. In this condition, the fetuses are of the same age. (**Heteropaternal superfecundation** may occur when two oocytes are fertilized by two different males.)

  The **superfetation** is the fertilization of a second oocyte of different menstrual cycle during pregnancy. This gives rise to fetuses of different ages.

N.B. Under normal conditions, the ovulation ceases during pregnancy, but sometimes an aberrant ovulation may take place during pregnancy, and if an ovum is fertilized at a subsequent period, then it leads to multiple births with newborns of different ages.

- **Multiple births**

  The occurrence of multiple births has increased in many countries. This is due to more exposure of females for fertility therapies, viz. (a) induction of ovulation by administering *gonadotrophins* and (b) *in vitro fertilization* (IVF).
- **Parthenogenesis**

  The term parthenogenesis refers to reproduction of an ovum without fertilization. It is seen in number of vertebral species such as fish, etc. However, occasionally, in human beings the oocyte gets activated without sperm penetration and starts multiplication but there is no record of any viable birth so far.

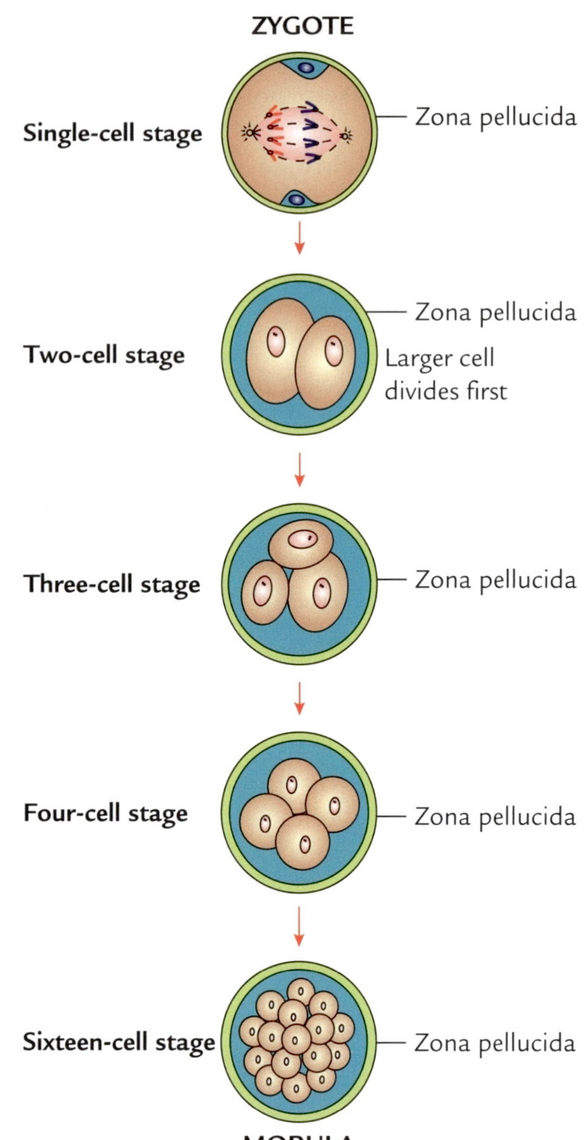

Fig. 5.4 Cleavage of zygote (i.e., series of mitotic divisions of the zygote).

CLEAVAGE AND BLASTOCYST FORMATION (BEGINNING OF DEVELOPMENT OF A NEW OFFSPRING)

The life of new individual (embryogenesis) begins after fertilization by a process called cleavage of zygote. This leads to the development of a blastocyst – a primordium of early embryo. The cleavage of zygote occurs due to metabolic activation of the oocyte during fertilization by the sperm.

Cleavage (Fig. 5.4) AN 78.1

The cleavage consists of repeated mitotic divisions of the zygote into smaller units. This results in a rapid increase in the number of cells. These cells are called **blastomeres**, which become smaller with each successive cleavage division. The division of zygote starts just after fertilization and continues as the zygote passes along the uterine tube. During cleavage, the zygote is surrounded by a thick zona pellucida.

The zygote divides to form two cells of which one is smaller than the other (**two-cell stage of embryo**). The larger cell divides first giving rise to **three-cell stage.** The smaller cell divides next and the embryo consists of four cells that divide to form eight cells. The eight cells further divide to form 16 cells.

A **16-cell stage embryo** resembles a mulberry fruit and is termed **morula.** In **morula**, the **blastomeres** are very small and contain very little cytoplasm to survive.

Blastocyst Formation (Fig. 5.5) AN 78.1, AN 78.2

The morula enters into the uterine cavity about 4 days after fertilization. The endometrial fluid penetrates the zona pellucida and enters into the intercellular spaces of the morula. Gradually, the intercellular

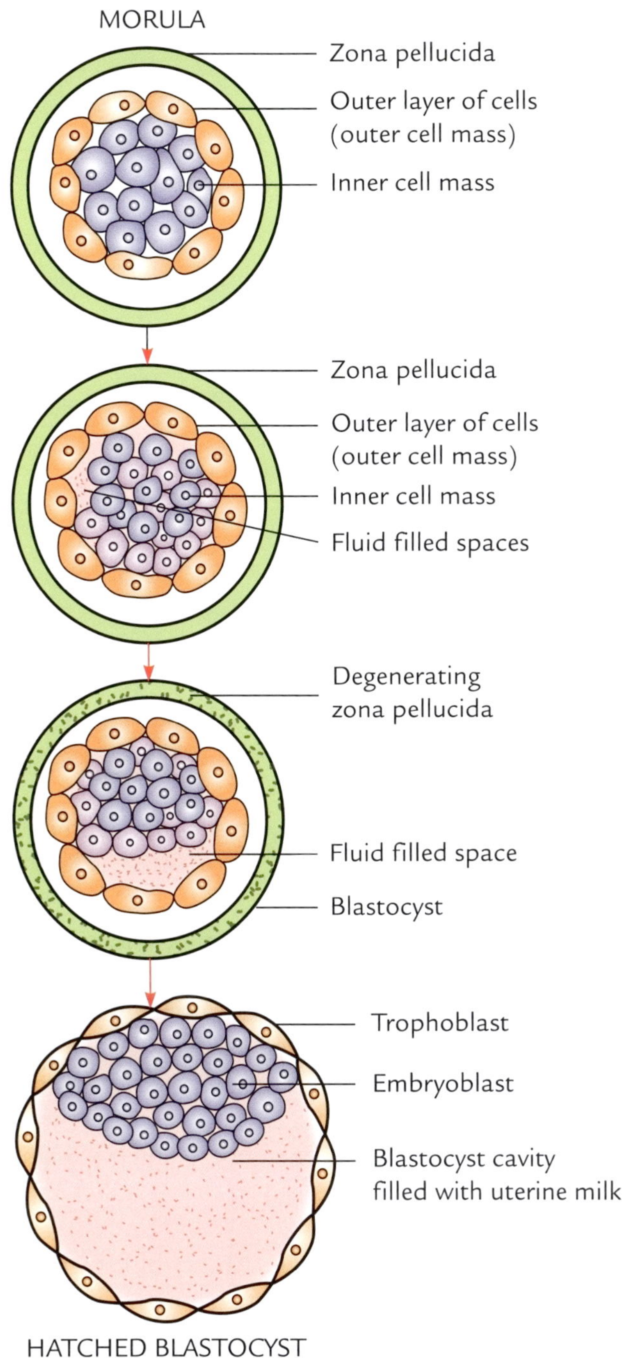

Fig. 5.5 Formation of blastocyst.

spaces coalesce to form a single large cavity called blastocyst cavity. At this stage, the embryo is called blastocyst. The blastocele is filled with fluid rich in nutrients, which is secreted by the endometrium of the uterus. This fluid is also termed **uterine milk**.

The cells now get arranged into two groups: (a) a group of cells in the center of morula is called **inner cell mass (embryoblast)** and (b) cells at the periphery of morula are called outer cell mass (**trophoblast**).

As the cavity enlarges, the outer cells forming the trophoblast become flattened (Gk. *Trophe* = nutrition). The inner cell mass called **embryoblast** becomes compact and is attached to the trophoblast at one pole – the **embryonic pole**.

Hatching of Blastocyst

As the blastocyst increases in size, the zona pellucida gradually disintegrates and disappears. The shedding of zona pellucida leads to **hatching of blastocyst**. Now blastocyst is ready to attach on endometrium at its embryonic pole.

Fate of blastocyst:

(a) **Embryoblast** gives rise to embryo.
(b) **Trophoblast** gives rise to placenta, which provides nutrition to the embryo.
(c) **Blastocele** forms yolk sac.

Timing of Various Stages of Cleavage Development of Blastocyst and Implantation

These are (Fig. 5.6)**:**

Day 1 – Zygote in fallopian tube
Day 2 – 4-Cell stage in fallopian tube
Day 3 – 8-Cell stage in fallopian tube
Day 4 – 16-Cell stage (morula) in uterine cavity
Day 5 – Blastocyst in uterine cavity
Day 6 – Hatching of blastocyst in uterine cavity
Day 7 – Beginning of implantation

CLINICAL CORRELATION

Hydatidiform vesicular mole (Fig. 5.7): This clinical condition occurs due to abnormal development of trophoblastic cells following fertilization of an empty oocyte (absent/inactive pronucleus) by a sperm (**monospermic mole**) or due to fertilization of an empty oocyte by two sperms (**dispermic mole**). This leads to the death of the embryo. As a result, the chorionic villi fail to complete their development and undergo degenerative changes. These degenerating villi form cystic swellings called hydatidiform moles, which resemble a bunch of grapes. Moles secrete higher level of human chorionic gonadotrophins (HCG), causing early signs and symptoms of pregnancy.

Hydatidiform mole is also called **molar pregnancy**.

Clinical features of hydatidiform mole:

- Preeclampsia during the first trimester
- Elevated levels of HCG (>100,000 mIU/mL)
- Enlarged uterus and dark brown to bright red vaginal bleeding
- Hydatidiform mole resembles a **bunch of grapes**
- Presence of vesicles in urine
- No fetal movements
- No fetal heart sounds
- Ultrasound reveals **snowstorm appearance** of the uterine cavity

Continued

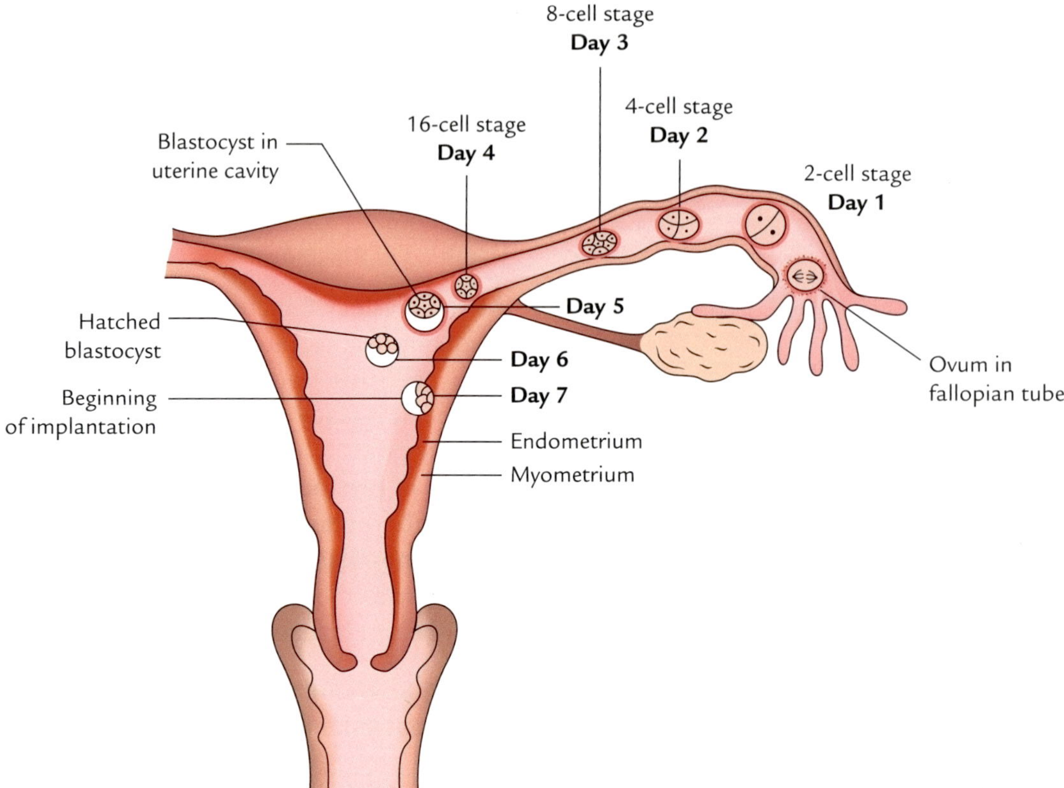

Fig. 5.6 Events during first week of development. (Timing of fertilization, various stages of cleavage, development of blastocyst and beginning of implantation.)

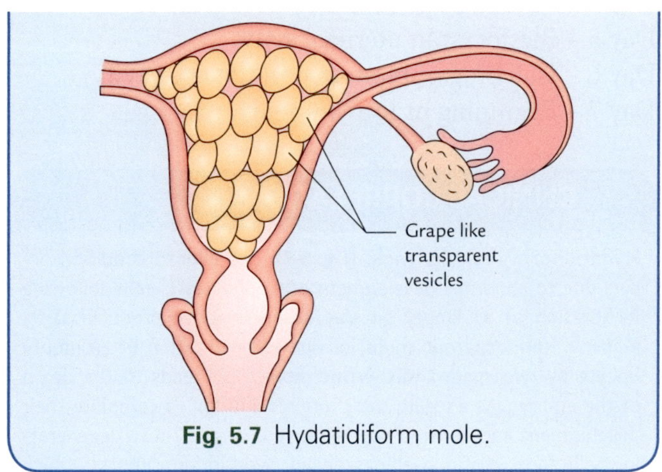

Fig. 5.7 Hydatidiform mole.

N.B.

- Around 3%–5% of hydatidiform moles undergo malignant change forming **choriocarcinoma**.
- There are **two types of hydatidiform moles**: (a) **complete type** in which there is no existence of embryo at all and (b) **partial type** in which part of the embryo is seen.
- Majority of hydatidiform moles are monospermic, i.e., an empty oocyte having no female pronucleus is fertilized by a single sperm.

IMPLANTATION

The implantation is a process by which the moving blastocyst is first attached to the epithelial lining of endometrium and then gets embedded into the uterine endometrium. The embryo remains attached with endometrium till birth.

The implantation occurs in the upper part of the posterior wall of uterine cavity.

The blastocyst surrounded by zona pellucida enters into the uterine cavity on day 5.

The blastocyst enlarges, the zona pellucida disintegrates, and blastocyst is released on day 6, called **hatching of blastocyst.**

Now sticky polar *trophoblast* adheres/binds with the epithelial lining of uterine endometrium, on day 7.

The trophoblast secretes *proteolytic enzymes*, which erodes uterine epithelium to create passage for blastocyst into the uterine endometrium of secretory phase.

N.B. Further embedding takes place in 2nd week of development, but brief account is given here for better understanding of students.

The blastocyst burrows deeper and deeper in the endometrium until it completely disappears from the surface.

The polar trophoblast forms finger-like projections called villi, which gets intimately associated with maternal tissue (decidua basalis) to form placenta.

The penetration defect in the uterine endometrium is closed by *fibrin plug* made up of blood clot and cellular debris. The implantation is described in detail in Chapter 6.

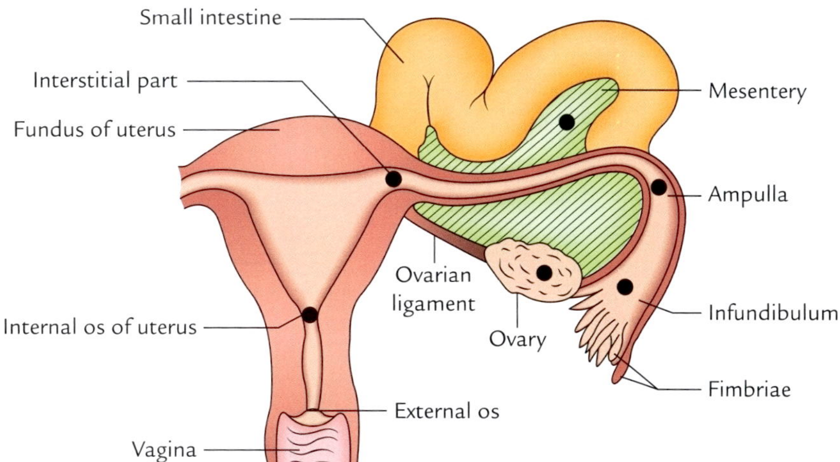

Fig. 5.8 Abnormal sites of implantation.

Normal Site of Implantation

Normally, the blastocyst is implanted in the upper part of the posterior wall of the uterine cavity. The implanted conceptus produces a small swelling on the surface of endometrium.

Abnormal Sites of Implantation AN 78.3

These may be within the uterus or outside the uterus (Fig. 5.8).

1. **Abnormal sites of implantation within the uterus:** In the lower uterine segment near the *internal os*. It leads to the development of **placenta previa**.
2. **Abnormal sites of implantation outside the uterus.** It is termed as **ectopic pregnancy**.
   (a) **In the uterine tube** (*tubal implantation*)*:* Here it may take place in the (a) ampulla, (b) infundibulum, or (c) interstitial part, in order of frequency.
   (b) **In the abdominal cavity** (*abdominal implantation*)*:* Here it implants most frequently in the peritoneal lining of the rectouterine pouch (pouch of Douglas), but may implant at any place covered by peritoneum, e.g., mesentery.
   (c) **In the ovary** (*ovarian implantation*)*:* Fertilization and implantation may occur while ovum is still within the ovary.

CLINICAL CORRELATION

1. **Placenta previa (abnormal uterine implantation**; Fig. 5.9): Normally, the blastocyst is implanted on the upper part of the posterior wall of the uterine cavity and the developed placenta is attached to the *upper uterine segment* (upper two-thirds of the body). Occasionally, the blastocyst is implanted in the lower part of uterine cavity near the internal os and then the developed placenta is attached to the *lower uterine segment* (lower one-third of the body of uterus). It is termed **placenta previa**.
   The various degrees of placenta previa are as follows (Fig. 5.9):
   (a) ***First degree:*** The attachment of the placenta does not extend up to the internal os.
   (b) ***Second degree:*** The attachment of the placenta extends up to the internal os but does not cover it.
   (c) ***Third degree:*** The edge of the placenta covers the internal os but when the os dilates during child birth the placenta no longer occludes it.
   (d) ***Fourth degree:*** The placenta completely covers/bridges the internal os even when the os is fully dilated during childbirth. The placenta previa of the fourth degree is also sometimes termed *central placenta previa.*
   The placenta previa, especially the fourth degree, can cause severe bleeding after the first trimester of pregnancy or during parturition (i.e., birth of the baby).

N.B.

- The placenta previa is one of the commonest causes of antepartum bleeding. The position of placenta previa during pregnancy is determined by routine ultrasonography.
- **Ectopic pregnancy:** The implantation of the blastocyst outside the uterus is called **ectopic pregnancy** (Fig. 5.8). Depending upon the site of implantation, it can be of the following types:
  (a) ***Tubal pregnancy*** (95%): In about 95% of the cases, ectopic pregnancies occur within the uterine tube, mostly in the ampullary region (80%) and are referred to as **tubal pregnancies.**
  Complications
  (i) *Tubal abortion:* In this abortion, choriodecidual hemorrhage occurs around the conceptus, which gets detached and expelled into the tubal lumen. It is often seen in ampullary implantation.
  (ii) *Tubal rupture:* It commonly happens if implantation occurs in isthmus or interstitial part of the tube. The rupture leads to internal hemorrhage. Clinically, it presents as heavy vaginal bleeding and severe belly pain, especially on one side. The patient goes in a state of acute shock. The tubal pregnancies are terminated through medical and surgical intervention.

Continued

(b) ***Abdominal pregnancy*** (1%). If implantation occurs in:
 (i) Peritoneal lining of the rectouterine pouch (*pouch of Douglas*).
 (ii) Mesentery of the intestinal loop or the omentum.

(c) ***Ovarian pregnancy*** (3% – primary ovarian pregnancy). If implantation occurs in ovary.

N.B. Ectopic pregnancies usually do not develop normally in unfavorable locations and lead to death of the embryo and severe hemorrhage in the mother during the 2nd month of pregnancy. Rarely does an extrauterine embryo develop to full term.

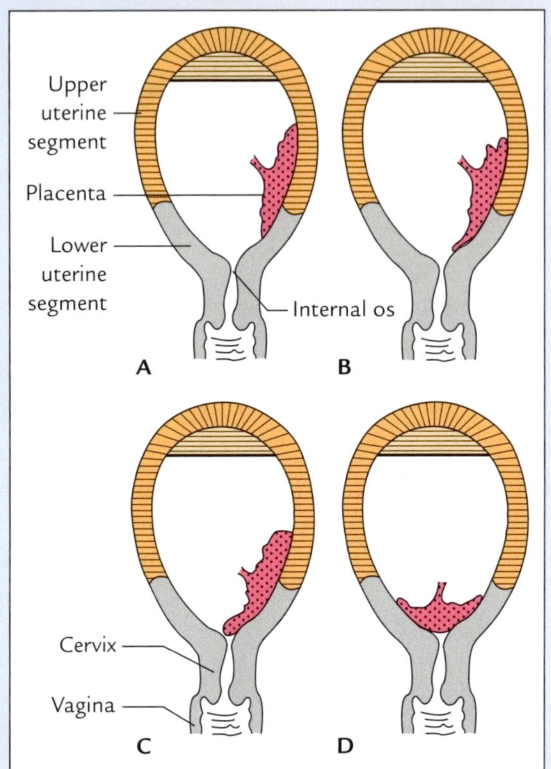

Fig. 5.9 Types of placenta previa: (A) first degree, (B) second degree, (C) third degree, (D) fourth degree.

GESTATIONAL AGE OF DEVELOPMENTAL EVENTS IN FIRST WEEK

Developmental Event	Time of Occurrence
➢ Fertilization	Day 1 (within 24 h of ovulation)
➢ 4-cell embryo	Day 2
➢ 8-cell embryo	Day 3
➢ Morula	Day 4
➢ Blastocyst	Day 5
➢ Hatching of blastocyst	Day 6
➢ Implantation	Day 7

GOLDEN FACTS TO REMEMBER

➢ **Life span of sperm after ejaculation**	24–48 h
➢ **Life span of ovum after ovulation**	24–48 h
➢ **Number of sperms reaching the site of fertilization**	300–500
➢ **Transport time of sperms from cervix to fallopian tube**	2–7 h
➢ **Commonest site of fertilization**	Ampulla of uterine tube (the most dilated part of uterine tube)
➢ **Most important function of zona pellucida**	Prevents the implantation of blastocyst at unwanted/ abnormal sites
➢ **Fertilization barriers (oocyte barriers)**	(a) Corona radiata (b) Zona pellucida (c) Vitelline membrane
➢ **Transcription factor responsible for formation of inner cell mass and trophoblast**	Oct4 and Nanog
➢ **Unicellular embryo**	Zygote
➢ **Most of the hydatidiform moles are**	Monospermic
➢ **Time taken by ovum to reach fallopian tube from ovary**	25 min
➢ **State of ovum at the time of fertilization**	Second meiotic division in metaphase stage
➢ **Day of contact of blastocyst with endometrium**	Day 7

CLINICAL PROBLEM SOLVING

PROBLEMS

1. **Which factors are responsible for transport of sperms from vagina to uterine tube?**
2. **What are the primary causes of infertility in men and women?** Why have incidences of infertility increased in the past few decades? What are the possible reasons?
3. A woman with bilateral tubal block but proper oogenesis is not able to conceive (i.e., become pregnant). She is prepared to go to any extent to have a child. What will the clinician likely to suggest her?
4. If a person has low sperm count but wants his wife to conceive. What are the fertility options?
5. **Give the embryological basis of pregnancy testing.**
6. What is human chorionic gonadotrophin? What is its clinical significance?
7. Why does each pronucleus replicate its DNA during the growth of male and female pronuclei?
8. **Which factors prevent polyspermy?**
9. Describe the embryological/anatomical principles underlying contraception (i.e., basis of fertility control in males and females/family planning). AN 77.4

SOLUTIONS

1. The factors responsible for transport of sperms from vagina to uterine tube are:
   (a) Liquefaction of semen, by fibrinolysin in it.
   (b) Contraction of uterine muscle by semen prostaglandins and oxytocin secreted by neurohypophysis during sexual intercourse.
   (c) Aspiration of sperms by vacuum created by uterine contractions.
   (d) Propulsion of sperms by whip-like movements of their tail.
2. The term **infertility** means inability to conceive (i.e., become pregnant). Infertility occurs in about 20% of married couples. The major causes of infertility in women are **polycystic ovarian syndrome (PCOS)**, primary ovarian insufficiency (POI) and **blockage of uterine tubes**, whereas the major cause of infertility in men is low sperm count (**oligospermia**), abnormal sperm function or blockage.
3. The clinician will suggest her to go for assisted reproductive technology (ART). The IVF is given in detail on p. 49, although the success rate is low (about 20%).
4. The fertility options are:
   (a) Intrauterine insemination (IUI).
   (b) *In vitro fertilization* (IVF).
   (c) IVF with intracytoplasmic sperm injection (ICSI), i.e., transfer of sperm into cytoplasm of oocyte.
5. The pregnancy test is done by assaying HCG in maternal blood at day 8 and in maternal urine at day 10.
6. Human chorionic gonadotrophin (HCG) is a glycoprotein produced by syncytiotrophoblast, which stimulates the production of progesterone by corpus luteum. This is clinically significant because the progesterone produced by the corpus luteum is essential for maintenance of pregnancy until the 8th week. Thereafter, placenta takes over the production of the progesterone.
7. Both male and female pronuclei (both haploid) replicate their DNA so that each cell of the two-cell stage zygote has a normal amount of DNA (i.e., 2*n*).

8. The following two factors prevent polyspermy during fertilization:
   (a) **Zona reaction:** As the sperm penetrates, a change in the properties of zona pellucida occurs that makes it impermeable to other sperms.
   (b) **Vitelline block:** As the sperm enters into the oocyte, **calcium waves** appear in its cytoplasm. These calcium waves initiate the release of enzymes from the cortical granules lining the plasma membrane of the oocyte. Because of the release of cortical granules, the vitelline membrane undergoes a change. The changed vitelline membrane becomes impermeable to other sperms (i.e., works as a vitelline block).

9. The embryological and anatomical principles underlying contraception in females and males are given as follows:

In Females	In Males
• **Temporary methods** 1. *Prevention of union of sperm and oocyte:* (a) By avoiding coitus during the fertile period of the menstrual cycle (10–17 days). The remaining days of the menstrual cycle are safe. (b) By using mechanical barrier such as diaphragm/cervical cap. (c) By using spermicidal jellies/cream (not really useful). 2. *Prevention of implantation:* ***By using intrauterine contraception devices (IUCD)*** such as a copper-T. 3. *Prevention of ovulation* ***by using contraceptive pills*** *with or without suppressing normal menstrual cycle.* A ***contraceptive*** pill is a combination of progesterone analogue – ***progestin and estrogen.*** 4. *Medical termination of pregnancy* ***(MTP):*** This is done only till 12 weeks of pregnancy.	• **Temporary methods** 1. *Prevention of union of sperm and oocyte:* ***By using mechanical barrier, such as condom,*** during coitus. The discharged seminal fluid then collects in the condom and not in the vagina. 2. *Prevention of production of sperms* ***by using the contraceptive pill:*** A **male pill** has been developed and tested in clinical trials. It contains synthetic androgen that prevents both LH and FSH secretion that either stop the production of sperms (70%–90% of men) or reduce it to the level of infertility.
• **Permanent methods** ***Tubectomy:*** The fallopian tube on each side is ligated at two places and the intermediate part is removed.	• **Permanent methods** ***Vasectomy:**** The vas deferens on each side is ligated at two places and the intermediate part is removed.

*The most effective method of permanent contraception in males is vasectomy.

6

Second Week of Development: Implantation, Bilaminar Germ Disc, and Prechordal Plate

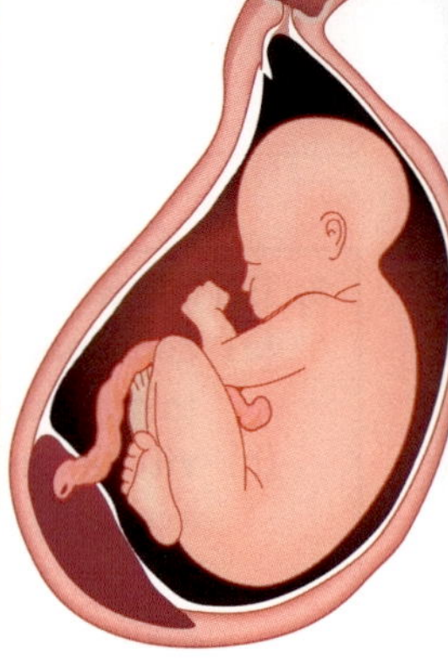

LEARNING OBJECTIVES

After studying this chapter, the student should be able to:

- Describe the development of trophoblast. AN 78.2
- Describe in brief the formation of bilaminar germ disc. AN 78.4
- Describe the development of:
  (a) Extraembryonic mesoderm AN 78.4
  (b) Extraembryonic coelom/chorionic cavity AN 78.4
  (c) Secondary yolk sac
  (d) Prechordal plate AN 78.4
- Give reasons why second week of development is termed as **week of 2's.**

OVERVIEW

During second week of development the embryo gets embedded into the endometrium of posterior wall of uterus and remains associated with it till birth. Further embryoblast is converted into flat **bilaminar germ disc**. This is followed by the formation of amniotic sac, yolk sac, and chorionic cavity.

The bilaminar germ disc and associated amniotic sac and yolk sac remain suspended in the large chorionic cavity by the connecting stalk (Fig. 6.4). The comfort and nutrition to embryo is supplied first by uterine endometrium and then by fetomaternal circulation.

IMPLANTATION (FIG. 6.1)

The blastocyst consists of an **inner cell mass, blastocyst cavity and outer cell layer or trophoblast**. The polar **trophoblast** is an area of trophoblast overlying the inner cell mass.

- At the end of first week, i.e., **on day 7**, the **polar trophoblast** of the blastocyst being sticky in nature gets attached to the columnar epithelium of endometrium of posterior uterine wall.

The uterine endometrium is partly eroded by the proteolytic enzymes secreted by the polar trophoblast and blastocyst gets partly embedded.

- **On day 8**, the trophoblast differentiates into two layers: an **inner cytotrophoblast** and **outer syncytiotrophoblast.**
- **On days 9–10**, the syncytiotrophoblast divides mitotically very fast to grow rapidly. In the process its cells lose their adjacent cell membranes to form a multinucleated protoplasmic mass called syncytiotrophoblast.
  - Syncytiotrophoblast secretes more proteolytic enzymes and further invades deep into the endometrium. As a result, blastocyst goes deeper and deeper until it gets completely imbedded. Now it lies deeper and completely disappears from surface.

Note that at the time of embedding the uterine endometrium is in its secretory phase. As the blastocyst is embedded, the endometrium surrounding it undergoes **decidual reaction**. It is characterized by following changes:

- Increase in intercellular substance and its vascularity.
- Stromal cells enlarge and become filled with glycogen and lipid, and become **decidual cells**.
- Endometrial glands become elongated and tortuous and looks *saucer-shaped* in section.
- Long endometrial arteries elongate and become more tortuous.
- Several small lacunar spaces appear in the syncytiotrophoblast which fuse with each other to form **large lacunar spaces**.
- **On days 11–12**, lacunar spaces enlarge further and communicate with each other.
  - The cords of syncytiotrophoblast between the lacunae are called **trabeculae**.
  - The syncytiotrophoblast erodes maternal vessels. As a result, lacunar spaces get filled with maternal blood. Further, the trophoblast forms finger-like

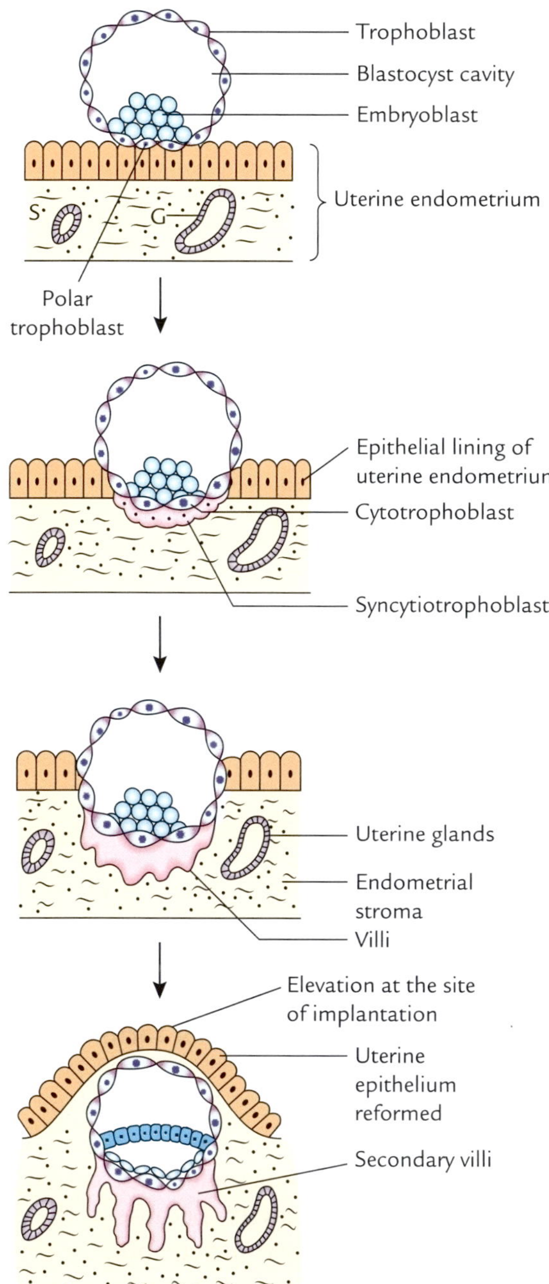

Fig. 6.1 Steps of implantation.

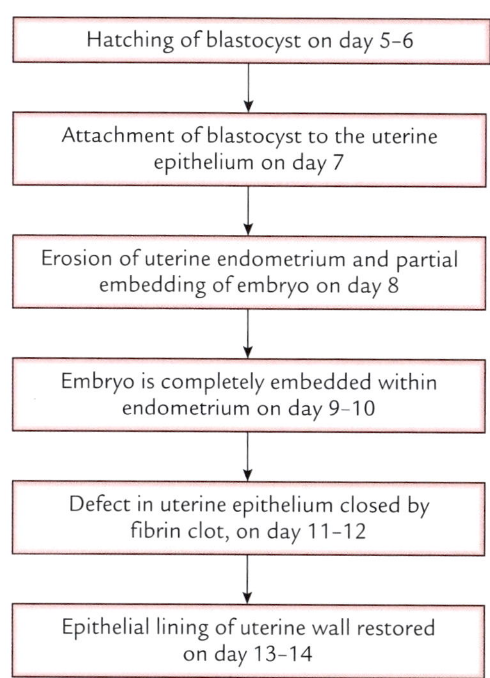
Hatching of blastocyst on day 5–6

Attachment of blastocyst to the uterine epithelium on day 7

Erosion of uterine endometrium and partial embedding of embryo on day 8

Embryo is completely embedded within endometrium on day 9–10

Defect in uterine epithelium closed by fibrin clot, on day 11–12

Epithelial lining of uterine wall restored on day 13–14

Flowchart 6.1 Showing implantation of blastocyst.

projections into columns (trabeculae) of syncytiotrophoblast, called **villi.**

The somatopleuric mesoderm invades the center of each villus with **fetal blood vessels**, thus establishing **fetomaternal circulation.**

Now the "fetal" blood vessels are separated from maternal blood only by some fetal tissue called *placental barrier*.

- **On days 11–12,** the epithelial defect on endometrial surface caused during the process of implantation is closed by **fibrin plug** made up of blood clot and cell debris.
- **On days 13–14,** the defect is completely epithelialized, and surface of uterine epithelium becomes smooth but still remains slightly elevated. The process of implantation is summarized in Flowchart 6.1.

FORMATION OF BILAMINAR GERM DISC (FIG. 6.2)

As we already know that the blastocyst is a spherical structure consisting of an outer layer of flattened cells called **trophoblast** and an inner mass of cells at one pole (embryonic pole) called **inner cell mass** or **embryoblast**. It also contains a cavity between inner cell mass and trophoblast called **blastocyst cavity.**

On day 8, the cells of embryoblast differentiate into two germ layers:

1. ***Hypoblast***, a layer of small **cuboidal cells** adjacent to the blastocyst cavity. It is also called primitive endoderm.
2. ***Epiblast***, a layer of high **columnar cells** toward the embryonic pole.

The **embryo is now disc shaped** and made up of two germ layers, **epiblast** and **hypoblast**, hence it is termed **bilaminar germ disc**.

Further Development

- **Formation of amniotic cavity** (Fig. 6.2):

  As the bilaminar germ disc forms, a small cavity appears within the epiblast called **amniotic cavity.** Soon it enlarges and gets filled with amniotic fluid.

  The floor of this cavity is formed by epiblast while its roof is formed by amniogenic cells.

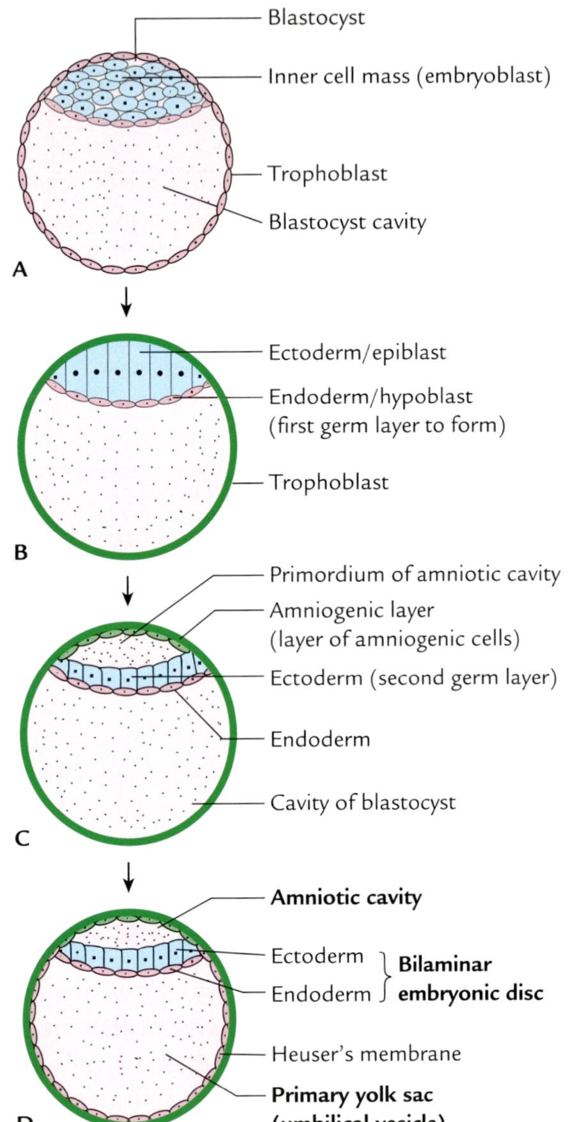

Fig. 6.2 Formation of bilaminar embryonic disc. Also note the formation of amniotic cavity and primary yolk sac. The layer of trophoblast is shown by a thick single green layer in lower three figures for the sake of simplicity.

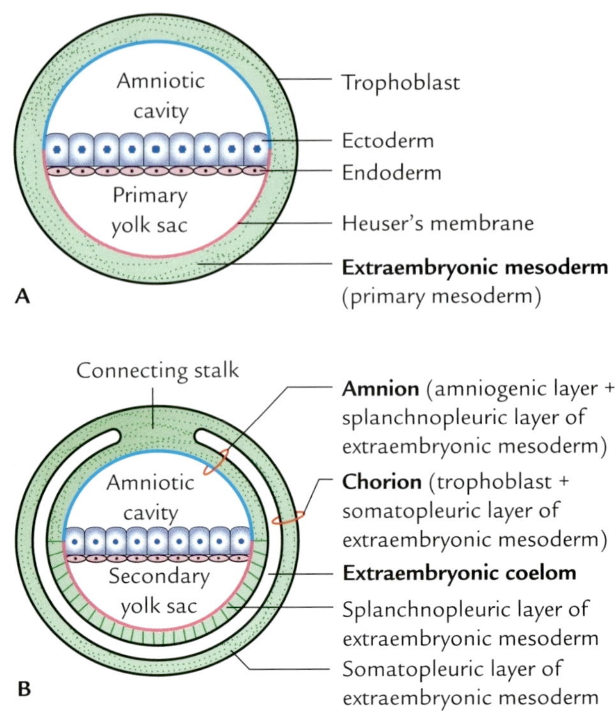

Fig. 6.3 Formation of extraembryonic mesoderm (A) and extraembryonic coelom and connecting stalk (B).

- **Formation of primary yolk sac:**
  On day 9, at the embryonic pole, the cells of hypoblast proliferates to form flattened cells, which migrates and lines the inner surface of trophoblast surrounding the blastocyst cavity and forms the **Heuser's membrane**. Now the blastocyst cavity is called as **primary yolk sac.**
- **Formation of extraembryonic mesoderm, extraembryonic coelom, and connecting stalk** (Fig. 6.3):
  - The cells of trophoblast give rise to a mass of cells that separate the amniotic cavity and primary yolk sac from the trophoblast. This cell mass is termed **extraembryonic mesoderm.** (According to some authorities, **extraembryonic mesoderm** is derived from the cells lining the primary yolk sac.) The extraembryonic mesoderm is also termed **primary mesoderm.**
  - The **term extraembryonic mesoderm is so coined because this mesoderm lies outside the embryonic disc** and **does not form any tissues of the embryo itself.**
  - A number of small cavities appear in the extraembryonic mesoderm that later coalesce together to form **extraembryonic coelom/extraembryonic cavity or chorionic cavity.** Because of the development of **extraembryonic coelom,** the primary yolk sac becomes smaller and is now termed **secondary yolk sac.**
  - The extraembryonic coelom does not extend into that part of extraembryonic mesoderm where it connects the embryonic disc with the part of trophoblast. This part of extraembryonic mesoderm forms the **connecting stalk.** With the development of blood vessels the connecting stalk becomes umbilical cord.
  - Because of the formation of extraembryonic coelom, the extraembryonic mesoderm splits into two layers:
    - The part lining the trophoblast is called **somatopleuric layer of extraembryonic mesoderm** or **parietal layer** of the extraembryonic mesoderm.

- The part lining the yolk sac is called **splanchnopleuric layer of extraembryonic mesoderm** or **visceral layer** of extraembryonic mesoderm.

- **Formation of chorion and amnion:**

The development of extraembryonic coelom leads to the formation of two membranes: (i) chorion and (ii) amnion.

- ***Chorion:*** It consists of somatopleuric layer of extraembryonic mesoderm and trophoblast covering it.
- ***Amnion:*** It consists of roof of amniogenic layer consisting of amniogenic cells and splanchnopleuric layer of extraembryonic mesoderm covering it.

CHORIONIC CAVITY/GESTATIONAL SAC (FIG. 6.4)

The **chorionic cavity** is a large fluid-filled cavity surrounding the embryo, i.e. it is a space which completely surrounds primary yolk sac, bilaminar germ disc and amniotic sac except where bilaminar germ disc is attached to the cytotrophoblast by a connecting stalk.

The embryo (bilaminar germ disc) along with amniotic sac and yolk sac (secondary yolk) is suspended in the large chorionic cavity by a connecting stalk (Fig. 6.4).

CLINICAL CORRELATION

The gestational sac can be seen by endovaginal ultrasound in pregnant woman at about 3–5 weeks of gestation. When the mean sac diameter is 2–3 mm. It serves as a first sign of early pregnancy.

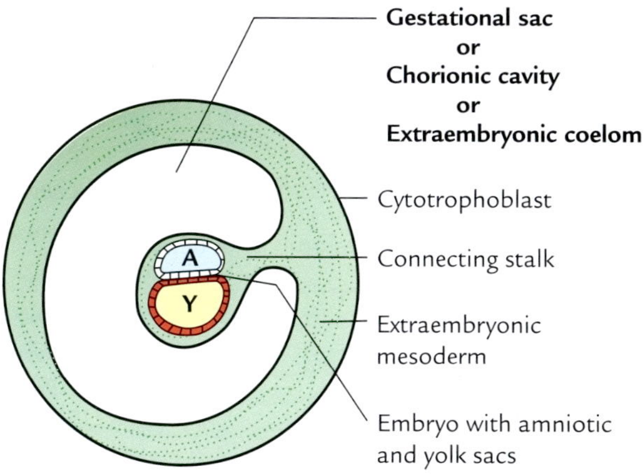

Fig. 6.4 Gestational sac (also called chorionic cavity. Y, yolk sac; A, amniotic sac.

FORMATION OF PRECHORDAL PLATE (FIG. 6.5)

At one end of the embryonic disc, a rounded area becomes thicker than the rest of the bilaminar germ disc. This rounded area is termed **prechordal plate.**

- In the region of prechordal plate, the cuboidal endodermal cells become columnar.
- With the development of prechordal plate, the cranial and caudal ends of the embryo are determined. The end at which the prechordal plate appears is called **cranial (head) end** and the other end is termed **caudal (tail) end.**

The prechordal plate also determines the *central axis of the embryo and acts as an organizer of head region.*

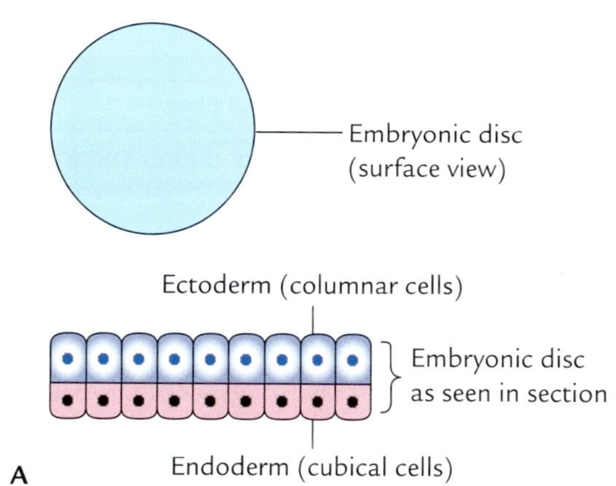

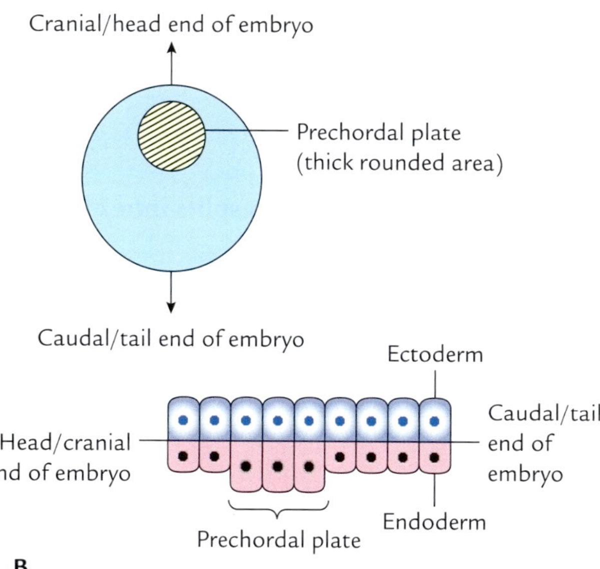

Fig. 6.5 Formation of prechordal plate. (A) **Bilaminar embryonic disk:** surface view (above) and as seen in section along the long axis of embryonic disc (below). (B) **Prechordal plate:** surface view (above) and as seen in section along the long axis of bilaminar embryonic disc (below).

These developmental events are given in Flowchart 6.2.

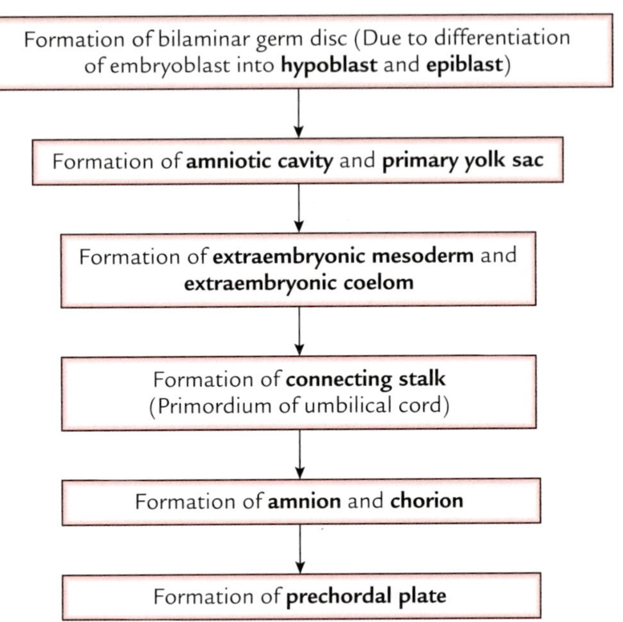

Flowchart 6.2 Developmental events during second week of preembryonic development.

KEY DEVELOPMENTAL EVENTS DURING SECOND WEEK OF PREEMBRYONIC DEVELOPMENT

The major developmental events in second week occur in pairs, hence second week of development is known as **week of 2's**. They can be easily remembered by a **mnemonic** as follows.

Mnemonic: week of 2's.

- **Embryoblast differentiates into 2 layers:**
  - Epiblast
  - Hypoblast
- **Formation of 2 cavities:**
  - Amnionic cavity
  - Yolk sac cavity
- **Extraembryonic mesoderm splits into 2 layers:**
  - Somatopleuric layer
  - Splanchnopleuric layer
- **Trophoblast differentiates into 2 layers:**
  - Cytotrophoblast
  - Syncytiotrophoblast
- **Formation of 2 chorioamniotic membranes:**
  - Amnion
  - Chorion
- **Formation of 2 types of villi:**
  - Primary villi
  - Secondary villi

GESTATIONAL AGE OF KEY DEVELOPMENTAL EVENTS

Developmental Event	Time of Occurrence
Formation of bilaminar germ disc	Day 8
Formation of amniotic cavity	Day 8
Differentiation of trophoblast into two layers, viz. cytotrophoblast and syncytiotrophoblasts	Day 8
Formation of primary yolk sac	Day 9
Complete implantation of blastocyst	Day 12
Establishment of fetomaternal circulation	Days 11–12
Formation of secondary yolk sac	Days 13–14
Formation of prechordal plate	Day 14

GOLDEN FACTS TO REMEMBER

Most characteristic feature during second week of development	Formation of bilaminar germ disc
First organ to develop for hemopoiesis	Yolk sac
Decidua	Uterine endometrium of secretory phase
Decidual reaction	Thickening of functional layer of uterine endometrium
Defect in uterine endometrium caused by implantation is closed by	Fibrin plug made up of blood clot and cell debris
Gestational sac	Extraembryonic coelom
First germ layer to develop	Endoderm

CLINICAL PROBLEM SOLVING

PROBLEMS

1. **Give the embryological basis of pregnancy testing.**
2. **What is human chorionic gonadotrophin?** What is its clinical significance?
3. What is **decidual reaction**? Give its clinical significance.
4. **Even during pregnancy sometimes menstrual cycle occurs. Why**?
5. What is the **significance of prechordal plate**?
6. What is **embryotroph**?

SOLUTIONS

1. The pregnancy test is done by assaying human chorionic gonadotrophin (HCG) in maternal blood on day 8 and in maternal urine on day 10. Because it is secreted by syncytiotrophoblast by then.
2. Human chorionic gonadotrophin is a glycoprotein produced by syncytiotrophoblast, which stimulates the production of **progesterone** by corpus luteum. This is clinically significant because the progesterone produced by the corpus luteum is essential for maintenance of pregnancy until the 8th week. Thereafter, placenta takes over the production of the progesterone.
3. It is a change which occurs in the functional layer of uterine endometrium surrounding the implanted blastocyst under the influence of increased level of hormone progesterone. These are:
   - Stromal cells are enlarged and contain glycogen and lipid to become **decidual cells.**
   - Increase in intercellular substance
   - Endometrium becomes edematous
   - Increase in the tortuosity of endometrial glands and spiral arteries.

   The decidual reaction plays a central role in the maintenance of pregnancy. **The process of decidual reaction is the most critical event that occurs in uterine endometrium during pregnancy.**
4. After pregnancy, **fetomaternal circulation** get established in the later part of second week of development. The lacunar spaces become filled with blood and fetal capillaries enter into core of villi.

   Occasional bleeding may occur through defect in the endometrium at the site of implantation due to increased maternal blood flow in the lacunar spaces.
5. The significance of prechordal plate:
   (a) Establishes craniocaudal axis of an embryo
   (b) Acts as organizer of head region (patterning of cranial neural tube)
   (c) Gives rise to the endodermal layer of oropharyngeal membrane.
   (d) Rupture of this membrane establishes opening of mouth.
6. It is a nutrient material composed mainly of secretion from uterine glands and substances in uterine blood. It contains proteins and amino acid which nourishes embryo prior to formation of placenta.

7 Third Week of Embryonic Development: Gastrulation, Primitive Streak, Notochord, Neural Tube, Intraembryonic Mesoderm, and Somites

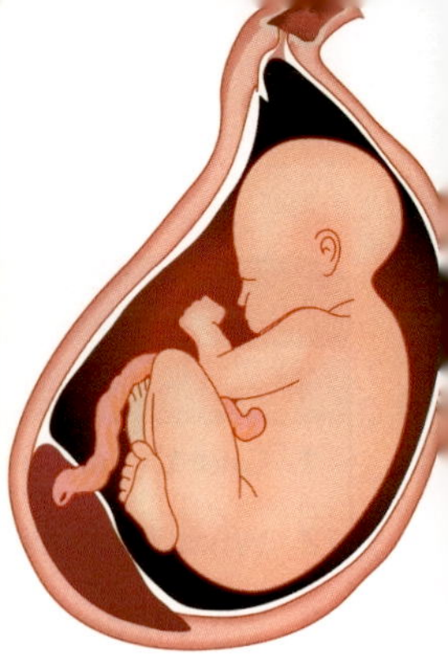

LEARNING OBJECTIVES

After studying this chapter, the student should be able to:

- Describe the formation and fate of primitive streak. AN 79.1
- Describe the formation and fate of notochord. AN 79.2
- Describe the process of neurulation. AN 79.3
- Describe the development of somites and intraembryonic development. AN 79.4
- Write short notes on intraembryonic mesoderm, septum transversum, and intraembryonic coelom.
- Discuss in brief the subdivisions of intraembryonic mesoderm.
- Describe briefly the formation, subdivisions, and fate of somites.

OVERVIEW

The knowledge of **gastrulation, primitive streak, notochord, and neurulation/neural tube formation** is of utmost importance for students to understand various congenital anomalies such as **teratomas, neural tube defects**, and **gastroschisis**. Proper knowledge of intraembryonic mesoderm helps in understanding the development of somites, urogenital and cardiovascular systems, and body cavities (pericardial, pleural, and peritoneal cavities).

GASTRULATION

The gastrulation refers to the **formation of three germ layers**, viz. **ectoderm** (surface layer), **mesoderm** (middle layer), and **endoderm** (deepest layer) from **pluripotent epiblast**, during the third week of development.

The bilaminar germ disc is converted into trilaminar germ disc through the formation of primitive streak.

PRIMITIVE STREAK (FIG. 7.1)

Appearance of primitive streak is the first sign of gastrulation. It appears as a **linear thick band on the dorsal surface of bilaminar embryonic disc at its caudal end in the midline.** It is formed due to proliferation and migration of cells of epiblast in the midline. The cells forming primitive streak are **pluripotent**, i.e., they have the ability to form all types of adult cells.

- Primitive streak **becomes visible on the dorsal surface of embryonic disc on day 15*** of embryonic development.
- The cranial end of the primitive streak presents a round elevated area called **primitive node.** A small depression appears in this node called **primitive pit**. Concurrently, a narrow groove appears in the midline of primitive streak called **primitive groove**. The primitive groove is continuous cranially with the primitive pit.

Formation of Three Germ Layers

All the three primary germ layers are derived from epiblast as follows (Fig. 7.2):

- Cells of epiblast migrate toward the primitive streak. As they reach in the region of the primitive streak, they become flask shaped, detach themselves from the epiblast, and slip beneath it.
- The detached flask-shaped cells of epiblast move inward (invaginate) toward the hypoblast. Some of these cells replace the hypoblast cells to form the **endoderm** and others come to lie between the

*__Mnemonic:__ Number of days on which primitive streak appears, correspond to the number of letters in term "PRIMITIVE STREAK."

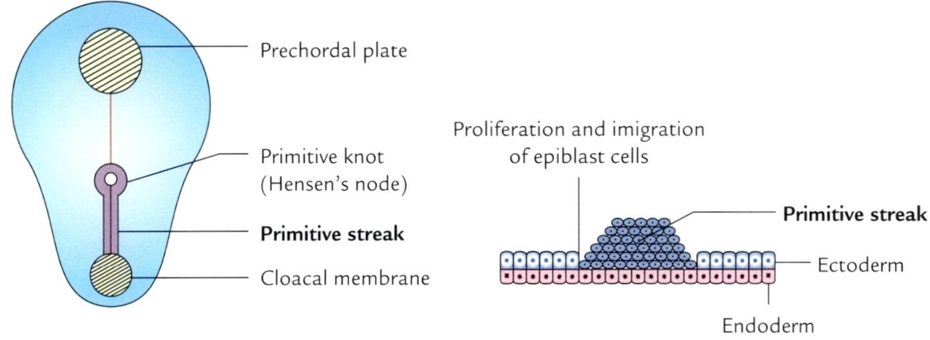

Fig. 7.1 Formation of primitive streak (surface view. The figure on the right side is the transverse section of embryo showing primitive streak.

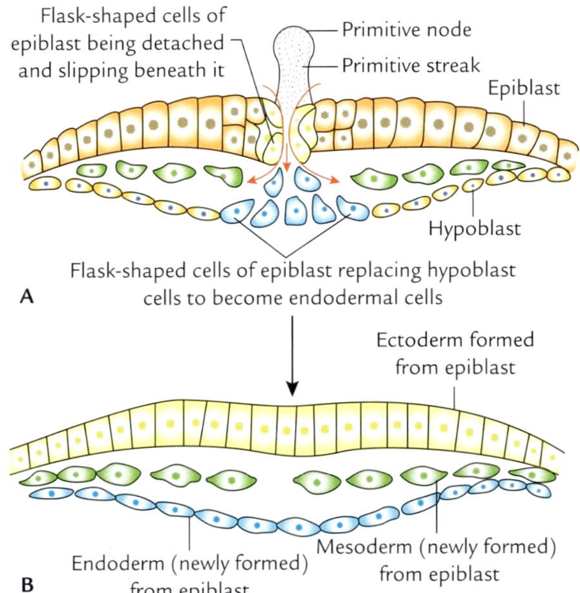

Fig. 7.2 Formation of the three germ layers (according to new concept).

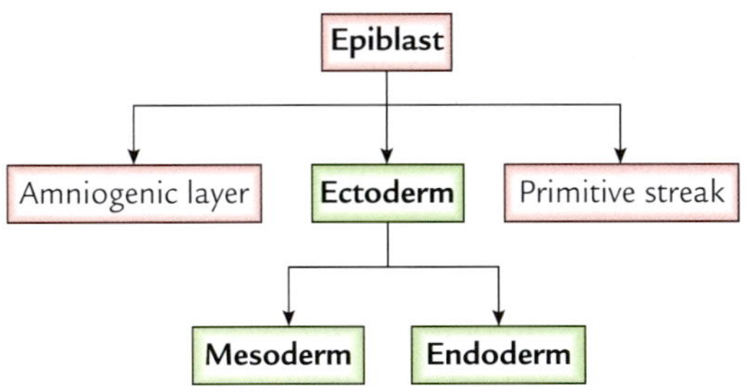

Flowchart 7.1 Formation of the three germ layers from epiblast.

epiblast and the newly formed endoderm to form the **mesoderm**. The remaining cells of the epiblast now form the **ectoderm** (Flowchart 7.1).

Derivatives of three germ layers: In general, ectoderm gives rise to nervous system, mesoderm gives rise to musculoskeletal system, and endoderm gives rise to inner lining of gastrointestinal, respiratory, and urinary tracts. For details see p. 76, Chapter 8.

Classical Concept of Formation of Three Germ Layers

Here the bilaminar germ disc is considered to be made of a superficial layer of **ectoderm** and deep layer of **endoderm**. The **primitive streak** is formed due to proliferation and migration of cells of ectoderm in the midline on the dorsal surface of embryonic disc.

Formation of Intraembryonic Mesoderm

The cells from bottom of primitive groove spread between ectoderm and endoderm to form the **intraembryonic mesoderm, the 3rd germ layer.**

Mode of spread of intraembryonic mesoderm (Fig. 7.3): The intraembryonic mesoderm spreads in cranial, caudal, and lateral directions into all parts of the embryonic disc except in the following three regions:

- ***Region of prechordal plate,*** where the ectoderm and endoderm are in firm contact with each other and later form the **buccopharyngeal membrane.**
- ***Region of cloacal membrane*** (*circular area at the caudal end of the disc*), where the ectoderm and endoderm are in an intimate contact with each other.
- ***Region of notochord:*** Midline between the prechordal plate and primitive knot; this area is occupied by the notochord.

N.B.

- Anterior to the prechordal plate, the intraembryonic mesoderm of two sides is continuous with each other. The mesoderm in this area forms **septum transversum**.
- As the embryonic disc enlarges and elongates, the connecting stalk becomes smaller and comes to lie at the caudal end of the embryo.
- At the caudal end of the embryo, the intraembryonic mesoderm passes beyond the embryonic disc and becomes continuous with the mesoderm of the connecting stalk made up of extraembryonic mesoderm.

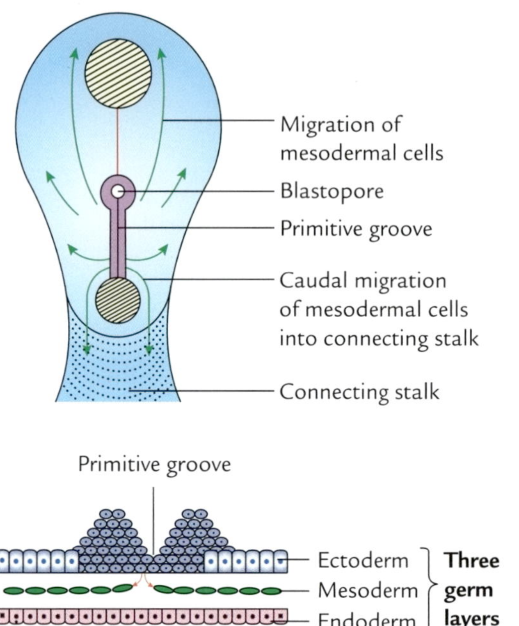

Fig. 7.3 Formation of primitive streak and intraembryonic mesoderm.

Functions of Primitive Streak AN 79.1

- Gives rise to intraembryonic mesoderm (third layer of embryonic disc)
- Formation of septum transversum
- Formation of notochord
- Determines the future craniocaudal axis of the embryo
- Demarcates the embryo into left and right halves.

Fate of Primitive Streak AN 79.1

The primitive streak actively forms intraembryonic mesoderm by ingression of its cells up to the end of the 3rd week of intrauterine life (IUL). Thereafter, it regresses craniocaudally and completely disappears by the end of the 4th week.

CLINICAL CORRELATION

Sacrococcygeal teratoma (Fig. 7.4) AN 79.5

Normally, the primitive streak undergoes degenerative changes and disappears completely by the end of the 4th week of IUL (vide supra). However, if the remnants of the primitive streak persist after the 4th week, the totipotent (pluripotent) cells of the primitive streak give rise to a large **precoccygeal tumor** called **sacrococcygeal teratoma.** Its large size may cause an obstructed labor or even death of the baby.

Sacrococcygeal teratoma is the most common tumor in newborns, occurring in 1:37,000 pregnancies. It occurs more commonly in female babies. The tumor usually becomes malignant during infancy, and therefore must be removed before 6 months of age.

It is situated at the base of coccyx (tail bone). The excessive blood flow through tumor often lead to heart failure (called hydrops). It is easily diagnosed by ultrasonography and babies are often delivered by caesarian section (Fig. 7.4).

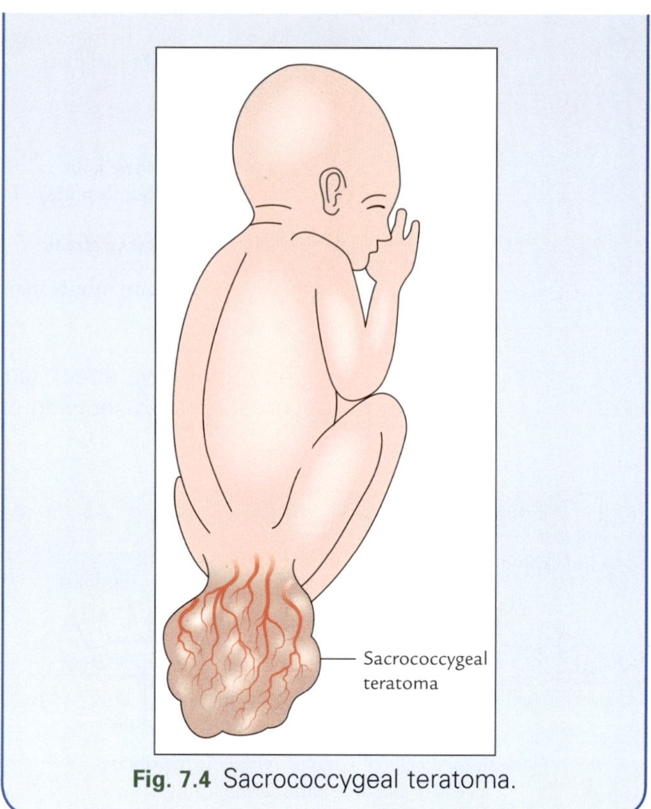

Fig. 7.4 Sacrococcygeal teratoma.

NOTOCHORD

Notochord is a midline cord of cells that develops in the region between the *primitive streak* and the *prechordal plate of embryonic disc.* It develops from the primitive knot (Hensen's node) of the primitive streak (Fig. 7.5).

Development of Notochord

Understanding of development of notochord is essential because it forms the central axis of the embryonic disc and induces the formation of neural tube.

The notochord develops from the primitive knot. The various stages of development of notochord are as follows (Figs 7.6 and 7.7):

1. Cells of **primitive knot** of the primitive streak proliferate to form *prenotochordal cells* that move inward (i.e., invaginate) to produce a central depression called **blastopore.**

   From the bottom of the blastopore, the *prenotochordal cells* of the primitive knot migrate forward in the midline between the ectoderm and the endoderm of the bilaminar embryonic disc to form a solid cord of cells called **notochordal process** or **head process.** Remember that the notochordal process lies between ectoderm and endoderm. Hence, the **ectoderm forms the floor of amniotic cavity and endoderm forms the roof of the yolk sac.**

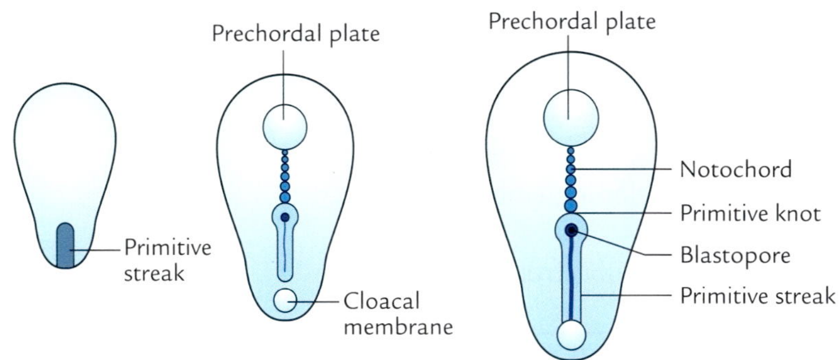

Fig. 7.5 Dorsal view of the embryonic disc showing the development of notochord.

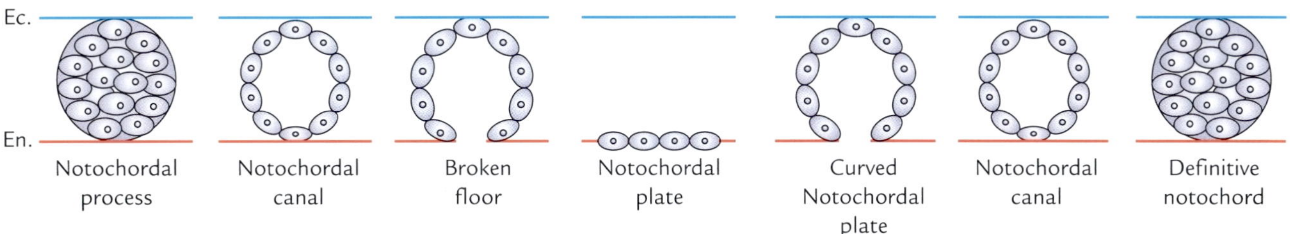

Fig. 7.6 Stages of development of notochord as seen in horizontal section. Ec, ectoderm; En, endoderm.

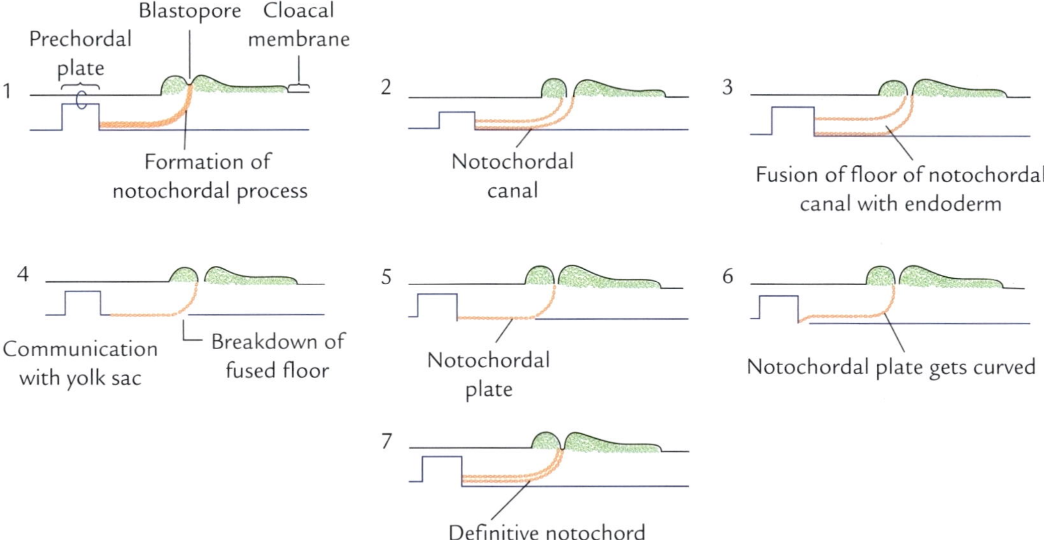

Fig. 7.7 Stages of development of notochord as seen in longitudinal section.

2. The notochord increases in length by extending caudally as the primitive streak recedes caudally and regresses.

   The notochordal process gets canalized to form **notochordal canal**. The notochordal canal is continuous with the blastopore.
3. The floor of notochordal canal fuses with the endoderm.
4. Later both the fused parts (wall of notochordal canal and part of endoderm) breakdown. The notochordal canal now communicates above with the amniotic cavity and below with the yolk sac. At this stage, the amniotic cavity and the yolk sac are in communication with each other.
5. Gradually, the walls of the canal become flattened to form a flattened plate called **notochordal plate.**
6. The notochordal plate gets curved to form a canal.
7. The proliferation of cells of the tube converts it into a solid cord of cells to form **definitive notochord.** The endoderm is restored, and now the notochord is completely separated from the endoderm.

N.B. The proximal part of the *notochordal canal* persists temporarily as **neurenteric canal** and forms a transitory communication between the **amniotic cavity** and the **yolk sac** (umbilical vesicle).

Functions of Notochord

AN 79.2

1. It forms the central axis of the developing embryo (embryonic disc).
2. It induces the formation of neural tube from the overlying ectoderm.
3. It provides central column around which vertebral bodies and intervertebral discs develop.

Fate of Notochord

AN 79.2

1. Notochord is present in all the animals belonging to phylum Chordata.
2. In human beings, notochord appears only in embryo. In later life, it disappears but its remnants are seen in the form of **nucleus pulposus** of the intervertebral discs and **apical ligament of dens** of second cervical vertebra.

CLINICAL CORRELATION

Chordoma: This is a rare tumor that arises from the remnants of notochord. It is formed either in the cranial region or in the sacral region. In the cranial region, it is seen at the base of the cranium and has a tendency to spread into the nasopharynx. It commonly occurs in men late in life, i.e., over 50 years of age. About 30% of these tumors are malignant.

NEURULATION/FORMATION OF THE NEURAL TUBE (FIG. 7.8)

AN 79.3

The process of formation of neural tube is called **neurulation.** The neural tube is formed from the ectoderm overlying the notochord as under:

1. The notochord induces the overlying ectoderm to differentiate into specialized cells called **neuroectodermal cells.**
2. The neuroectodermal cells proliferate to form a thick plate called **neural plate.** The neural plate extends in midline from prechordal plate to the primitive knot.
3. The margins of the neural plate get elevated (**neural folds**) as paraxial mesoderm proliferates on either side of the notochord. This leads to the formation of **neural** groove flanked by **neural** folds. The neural groove becomes deeper and neural folds move toward midline to fuse with each other to form a cylindrical **neural** tube. The fusion of neural folds (i.e., **closure of neural tube**) begins in the middle and gradually extends in cranial and caudal directions. Before the completion of fusion, the neural tube communicates with the **amniotic sac** via two openings, namely, **cranial neuropore** and **caudal neuropore.** The amniotic fluid circulates in the neural tube through these neuropores.

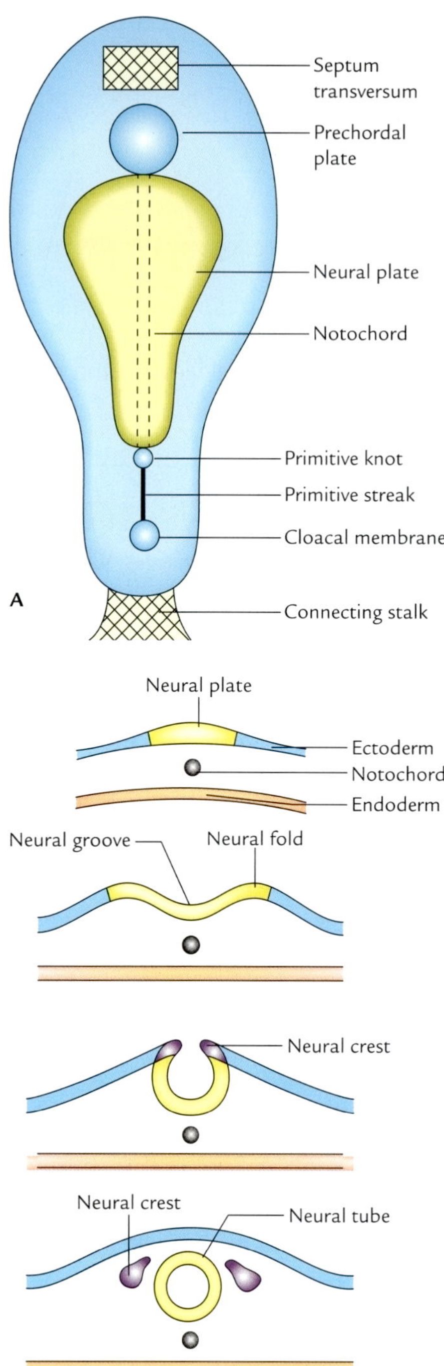

Fig. 7.8 Formation of neural tube. (A) Neural plate as seen on the dorsal surface of the pear-shaped embryonic disc. (B) Horizontal sections of embryo showing various stages of development of neural tube.

During the closure of the neural groove, the cells at the tips of neural folds (**neural crests**) do not take part in the formation of neural tube. When the surface ectoderm is restored, they form bilateral masses dorsolateral to the neural tube, deep to surface ectoderm.

The anterior neuropore closes on day 25 (at 20 somite stage), whereas caudal neuropore closes on day 27 (at 25 somite stage).

The neural tube forms central nervous system while neural crest cells form peripheral nervous system.

The cranial part of neural tube enlarges and forms the brain, whereas the caudal part of neural tube remains tubular and forms the spinal cord. **Further development of the brain and spinal cord and derivatives of neural crests is described in detail in Chapter 26.**

N.B. The formation of neural tube is induced by notochord.

INTRAEMBRYONIC MESODERM AN 79.4

Intraembryonic mesoderm is the middle layer of trilaminar embryonic disc. It is derived from primitive streak. It lies between ectoderm and endoderm except at the following three sites:

(a) Prechordal plate
(b) Notochord
(c) Cloacal membrane.

It lies on either side of the notochord. The intraembryonic mesoderm of two sides meet in front of Prechordal plate to form *cardiogenic plate* (for details see p. 235).

Subdivisions of Intraembryonic Mesoderm

The **intraembryonic mesoderm** on either side of neural tube divides into three longitudinal columns. From the medial to lateral side, these are **paraxial mesoderm**, **intermediate mesoderm**, and **lateral plate mesoderm** (Fig. 7.9).

1. **Paraxial mesoderm:** The mesoderm lateral to neural tube condenses to form the paraxial mesoderm.
2. **Intermediate mesoderm:** The mesoderm in between the paraxial mesoderm and lateral plate mesoderm is termed intermediate mesoderm. It is not only intermediate in position but also intermediate in thickness as compared to paraxial and lateral plate mesoderms.
3. **Lateral plate mesoderm:** The mesoderm in the lateral part of embryonic disc remains thin and forms lateral plate mesoderm.

Fate of Paraxial, Intermediate, and Lateral Plate Mesoderms

Paraxial Mesoderm

The paraxial mesoderm undergoes segmentation to form **somatomeres** and **somites.**

Development of somatomeres

The paraxial mesoderm is a thick, longitudinal column of mesodermal cells that lies on each side of the notochord and the developing neural tube.

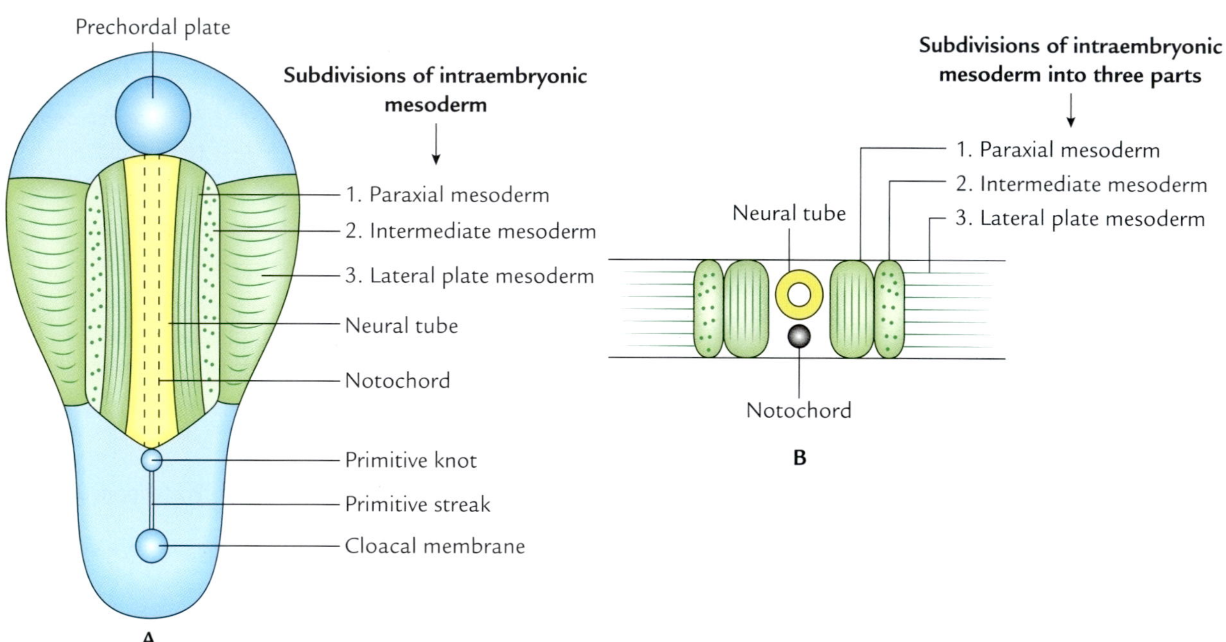

Fig. 7.9 Subdivisions of intraembryonic mesoderm. (A) As seen in embryonic disc. (B) As seen in the horizontal section of the embryonic disc.

It undergoes segmentation and gets organized into segments known as **somatomeres. They are loose masses of paraxial mesoderm.** The somatomeres are formed in the craniocaudal sequence towards the end of 3rd gestational week.

The **first pair of somatomeres** appears in cephalic region of the embryo and the formation proceeds craniocaudally. Each somatomere consists of mesodermal cells arranged in concentric whorls around the center of the unit.

Somatomeres 1–7, which are located from cephalic to otic vesicle, do not condense to form somites but contribute to mesoderm of the head and neck region, which forms all the striated muscles in this region.

The remaining somatomeres located caudal to otic vesicle condense to form well-defined cubical blocks called **somites.**

Development of somites (Gr. Soma = body) (Figs 7.10 and 7.11)

These are cubical blocks of paraxial mesoderm located caudal to otic vesicle on each side of developing neural tube. The somites first appear in the future occipital region of the embryo. The first pair forms on day 20 at a short distance caudal to the otic vesicle/placode. Subsequent pairs form in craniocaudal sequence. Thus, cranial somites are oldest and caudal somites are youngest.

About 38 pairs of somites appear between days 20 and 30 of development (**somite period of human development**). By the end of the 5th week, about 42 days, 44 pairs of somites are formed in the human embryo. Out of these, 4 are occipital, 8 are cervical, 12 are thoracic, 5 are lumbar, 5 are sacral, and from 8 to 10 are coccygeal. The somites form visible surface elevations on either side of the midline.

The first pair of somites appears in the occipital region on day 20 (vide supra) and subsequently approximately three pairs of somites are added each day until the end of the 5th week. Thus, while the somites are forming, the number of somites provides a good index of the age of the embryo (Table 7.1).

Correlation between somites and spinal nerves

As discussed earlier, somites begin to form at the cranial end of the paraxial mesoderm and continue to do so caudally. In craniocaudal direction, they are termed **occipital, cervical, thoracic, lumbar,** and **coccygeal somites.** Caudal to the occipital region, the number of somites corresponds to the number of spinal nerves in the region. Thus, there are 8 cervical, 12 thoracic, 5 lumbar, and 5 sacral somites corresponding to same number of spinal nerves in these regions. The number of coccygeal somites, however, exceeds the number of coccygeal nerves, but the extracoccygeal somites degenerate.

Structure and fate of somites (Fig. 7.12)

- Each somite is triangular in shape with a small slit-like cavity in its center.

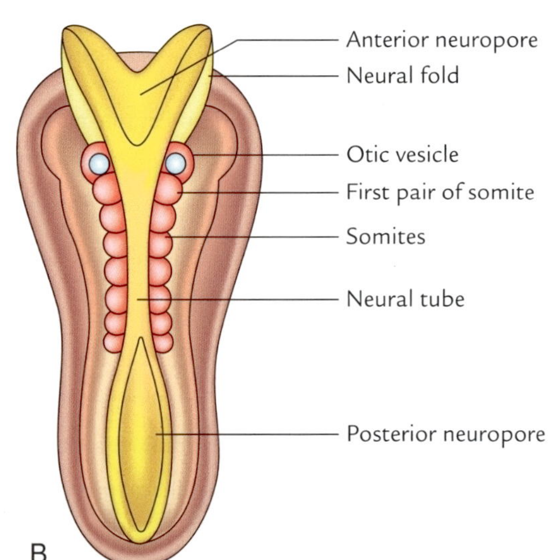

Fig. 7.10 Formation of somites. Dorsal view of a 22 days old embryo. (A) Actual specimen. (B) Idealized figure. Neural folds are fused opposite somites to form neural tube. The neural tube is in open communication with amniotic cavity through anterior and posterior neuropores. The somites are visible on each side of the neural tube.

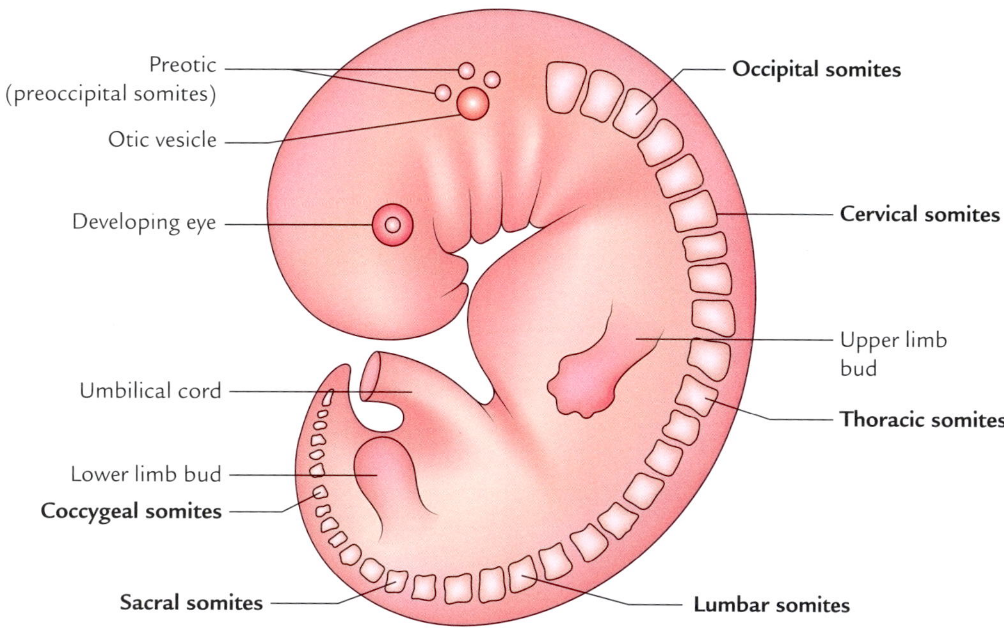

Fig. 7.11 Lateral view of a 30-days-old embryo. A total of 38–39 pairs of somites are visible: 4 occipital, 8 cervical, 12 thoracic, 5 lumbar, 5 sacral, and 4–5 coccygeal.

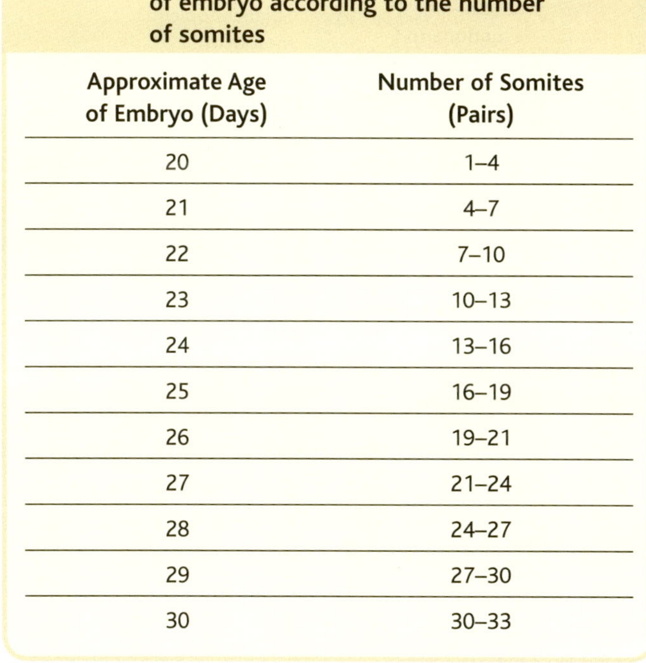

Table 7.1 Estimation of the approximate age of embryo according to the number of somites

Approximate Age of Embryo (Days)	Number of Somites (Pairs)
20	1–4
21	4–7
22	7–10
23	10–13
24	13–16
25	16–19
26	19–21
27	21–24
28	24–27
29	27–30
30	30–33

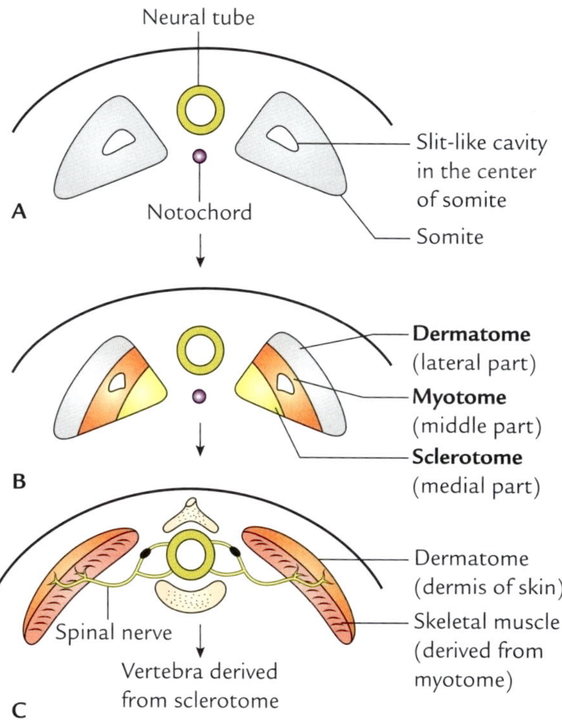

Fig. 7.12 Subdivisions of somites.

- Each somite is divided into three parts: medial, middle, and lateral.
  - The **medial part** is called **sclerotome**, which forms vertebrae and ribs.
  - The **middle part** is called **myotome**, which forms skeletal muscles.
  - The **lateral part** is called **dermatome**, which forms the dermis of the skin.

Intermediate Mesoderm

The intermediate mesoderm forms most of the genitourinary system, e.g., **kidneys, testes, ovaries,** etc.

Lateral Plate Mesoderm

The lateral plate mesoderm forms **body wall** and **body cavities**. Initially, it is involved in the formation of intraembryonic coelom.

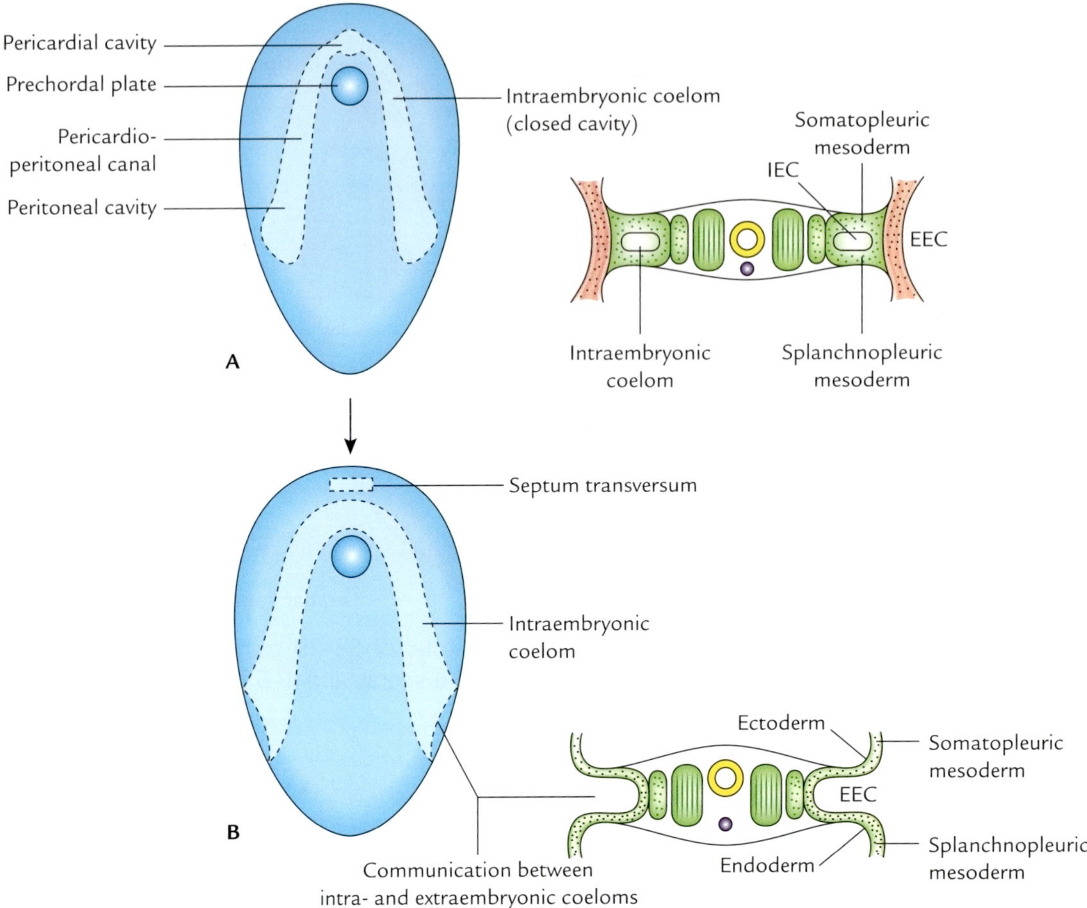

Fig. 7.13 Intraembryonic coelom (surface view on the left and transverse view on the right). (A) Early stage. Note that it is a closed cavity. (B) Late stage. Note that it is communicated with extraembryonic coelom. IEC, intraembryonic coelom; EEC, extraembryonic coelom.

Formation of intraembryonic coelom (Fig. 7.13)

The lateral plate of mesoderm of two sides is continuous with each other anterior to the prechordal plate (primitive buccopharyngeal membrane).

A large number of small cavities appear on each side of the lateral plate mesoderm and mesoderm anterior to the prechordal plate. All these cavities coalesce (fuse) together to form a single large horseshoe-shaped cavity called **intraembryonic coelom.**

Subdivisions of intraembryonic coelom

During the 2nd month, the intraembryonic coelom is divided into three parts:

- Part anterior to the prechordal plate called **pericardial cavity.**
- Right and left limbs of the intraembryonic coelom called **peritoneal cavities.**
- Canals through which pericardial cavity communicates with the peritoneal cavities are termed **pericardioperitoneal canals.**

N.B. Initially, the horseshoe-shaped intraembryonic coelom is a closed cavity, but soon it establishes communication with the extraembryonic coelom (Fig. 7.13).

Formation of somatopleuric and splanchnopleuric layers of mesoderm

As a result of formation of intraembryonic coelom, the lateral plate mesoderm is divided into two layers: somatopleuric mesoderm and splanchnopleuric mesoderm:

1. *Somatopleuric (parietal) layer* lies in contact with the ectoderm.
2. *Splanchnopleuric (visceral) layer* **lies in contact with the endoderm.**

The **somatopleuric mesoderm** contributes to the development of the body wall, whereas splanchnopleuric mesoderm contributes to the development of walls of the viscera (e.g., viscera of gastrointestinal and respiratory tracts).

- The intraembryonic mesoderm lying anterior to the pericardial cavity is called **septum transversum,** which contributes to the development of **liver** and **diaphragm.**

Table 7.2 Derivatives of intraembryonic mesoderm (paraxial, intermediate, and lateral plate mesoderm)

Paraxial Mesoderm	Intermediate Mesoderm	Lateral Plate Mesoderm
• Striated muscles of head and neck region • Axial skeleton • Muscles of trunk • Muscles of limbs	• Connective tissue of gonads • Metanephric blastema • Smooth muscle and connective tissues of reproductive system • Most of genitourinary system	• Diaphragm • Pericardial cavity • Peritoneal cavity • Body wall • Wall of gastrointestinal and respiratory tracts

- The epicardium of heart develops from **splanchnopleuric mesoderm** lying in front of the prechordal plate.

The derivatives of paraxial mesoderm, intermediate mesoderm, and lateral plate mesoderm are summarized in Table 7.2.

TIMING OF KEY DEVELOPMENTAL EVENTS

Developmental Event	Time of Occurrence
➢ Primitive streak	Day 15 (**Mnemonic**: 15 letters in term "primitive streak")
➢ Notochord	Day 17
➢ Intraembryonic mesoderm	Day 19
➢ Neural tube	Day 21
➢ First pair of somite	Day 20
➢ Primitive heart tube	Day 21

GOLDEN FACTS TO REMEMBER

➢ **First sign of gastrulation**	Appearance of primitive streak
➢ **Primitive streak appears on**	15th day of embryonic development
➢ **Most common tumor in the newborns**	Sacrococcygeal teratoma
➢ **Mother of intraembryonic mesoderm**	Primitive streak
➢ **First pair of somites appears at the end of**	3rd week
➢ **Most of the axial skeleton is derived from**	Somites
➢ **Oldest somites**	Occipital somites
➢ **Youngest somites**	Coccygeal somites
➢ **Genes responsible for orderly sequencing of somites**	Notch signaling genes
➢ **Teratoma**	Tumor arising from the remnant of primitive streak
➢ **Chordoma**	Tumor arising from the remnant of notochord
➢ **Remnants of notochord in adults**	(a) Nucleus pulposus (b) Apical ligament of dens
➢ **Swimming pool of embryo**	Amniotic cavity
➢ **Neurulation**	Process of formation of neural tube

CLINICAL PROBLEM SOLVING

PROBLEMS

1. **What do you understand by the term teratomas? Give the embryological basis.**
2. The **teratomas are located either as midline structures or as the paramedian structures of the body. Why? Give the embryological basis.**
3. An ultrasound done in 3rd trimester of pregnancy reveals a **large vascular mass tumor near the sacral region of female fetus. What is the possible diagnosis?**
4. **Enumerate the midline structures in the embryonic disc.**

SOLUTIONS

1. The **teratomas are congenital tumors** that arise from pluripotent embryonic cells of remnants of the primitive streak. These tumors commonly contain tissues derived from all the three germ layers such as hair tissues, neural tissues, etc. (derivatives of ectoderm); intestinal and respiratory epithelium (derivatives of endoderm); and muscle, connective tissue, fat, cartilage, and bone (derivatives of mesoderm). Consequently, the **teratoma consists of a heterogeneous mass of tissues.**
2. The **teratoma arises from remnants of pluripotent cells of primitive streak – a midline structure in the embryo.** In the embryonic life, these cells lie in the midline beneath the coelomic epithelium in association with the hindgut. Normally, these cells migrate to the gonadal ridges forming ovaries and testes. Therefore, teratomas commonly arise in gonads (i.e., testes and ovaries), which are located in the paramedian regions of the body, but may also arise in the midline structures of the body, i.e., in mediastinum, presacral, and coccygeal regions.

N.B. The most common site of teratoma is ovary.

3. This mass represents **sacrococcygeal teratoma**, a tumor which arises from remnants of primitive streak in the coccygeal region.

   It is a germs cell tumor, hence it contains different types of body tissues derived from ectoderm, mesoderm, and endoderm, such as hair – ectodermal in origin, muscle – mesodermal in origin, bone – mesodermal in origin, and teeth – both ectodermal and mesodermal in origin.
4. In craniocaudal order these are:
   1. Septum transversum
   2. Pericardial sac
   3. Buccopharyngeal membrane
   4. Neural plate and notochord
   5. Primitive node
   6. Primitive streak
   7. Cloacal membrane

8 Fourth to Eighth Weeks of Embryonic Development: Organogenesis and Folding of Embryo

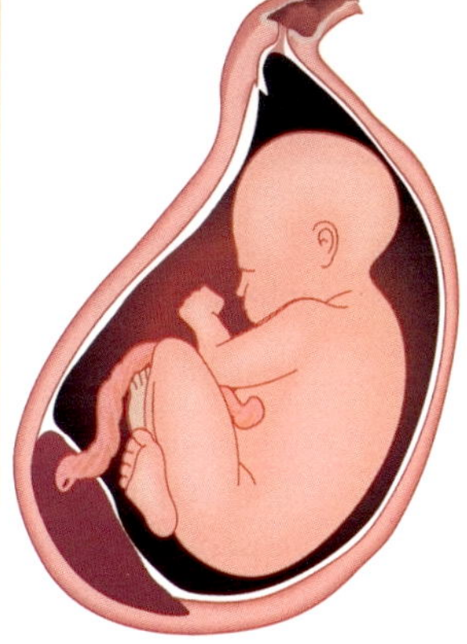

LEARNING OBJECTIVES

After studying this chapter, the student should be able to:

- Enumerate the structures derived from three primary germ layers.
- Enumerate the structures as seen in transverse and mid-sagittal sections of embryo during 4th week before folding.
- Give brief description of connecting stalk during 5th week of intrauterine life.
- Enumerate the salient external features of 8th-week-old embryo.
- Enumerate the major effects of folding of embryo.

OVERVIEW

This period of development (i.e., from 4th to 8th weeks) is the actual **period of organogenesis.**

Three primary germ layers, which were formed during 3rd week of development, undergo differentiation to form various tissues and organs of the body during 4th to 8th weeks.

As a result of formation of various organs and folding of the trilaminar germ disc, the embryo acquires a **"miniature human form."**

THREE GERM LAYERS (FIG. 8.1)

The three germ layers are formed during 3rd week of development from the epiblast of bilaminar germ disc. From superficial to deep, these are (Fig. 8.1):

1. Ectoderm
2. Mesoderm
3. Endoderm

All the tissues and organs of the body are derived from these three layers.

In general, the ***ectoderm*** gives rise to the nervous system and lining of the surface of the body.

The ***mesoderm*** gives rise to the musculoskeletal, cardiovascular, reproductive, and urinary systems of the body.

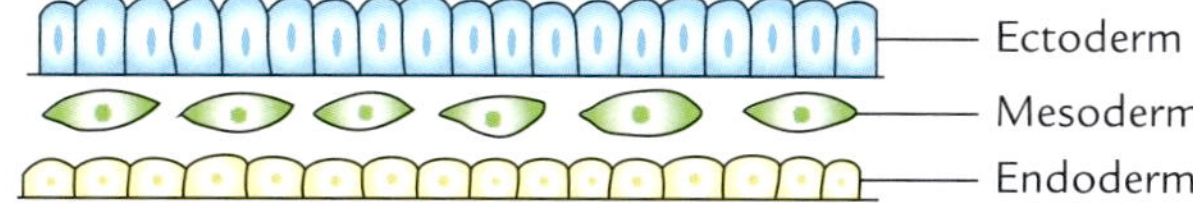

Fig 8.1 Three primary germ layers.

The ***endoderm*** forms the lining of gastrointestinal and respiratory tracts and their derivatives.

The structures derived from these three primitive germ layers are given in detail in Table 8.1.

FOLDING OF EMBRYO

As a result of rapid embryonic growth and development of various organs, especially the **neural tube and somites,** the circular trilaminar embryonic disc undergoes folding both in median and horizontal plane to form a more cylindrical embryo, establishing the **miniature form of human body** (Fig. 8.2).

Disposition of Structure Before Folding

Before folding, the disposition of structures in germinal disc is as follows:

1. *As seen in midsagittal section between amniotic cavity above and yolk sac below*

   In craniocaudal order, these are (Fig. 8.3):
   - Septum transversum
   - Pericardial cavity/sac
   - Buccopharyngeal membrane
   - Neural tube, notochord, primitive streak
   - Cloacal membrane
2. *As seen in transverse section*

   These are (Fig. 8.4):
   - Amniotic cavity
   - Ectoderm
   - Neural tube
   - Endoderm
   - Yolk sac

Table 8.1 Structures (tissues and organs) derived from three germ layers

Ectoderm	Mesoderm	Endoderm
• Central nervous system • Peripheral nervous system • Sensory epithelium of nose, eye, and ear • Derivatives of neural crest cells (see p. 310) • Pituitary gland • Epidermis of skin and its appendages, viz. hair, nails • Enamel of teeth • Lining of all orifices on the surface, viz. – Oral cavity – Nasal cavity – External auditory meatuses • Subcutaneous glands – Sweat glands – Sebaceous glands • Mammary glands	• Muscles, viz. skeletal, smooth, and cardiac • Heart, blood vessels, lymph vessels • Connective tissues • Bones and cartilages • Kidneys and ureters • Spleen • Gonads – Testes – Ovaries • Uterus and vagina • Serous membranes – Pleura – Pericardium – Peritoneum – Synovial membrane	• Epithelium lining of: – GIT – Respiratory tract – Biliary tract • Glands – Thyroid – Parathyroid – Thymus • Epithelial lining of: – Pharyngotympanic tube – Tympanic cavity – Mastoid antrum • Epithelial lining of: – Urinary bladder – Urethra • Epithelial lining of tonsils

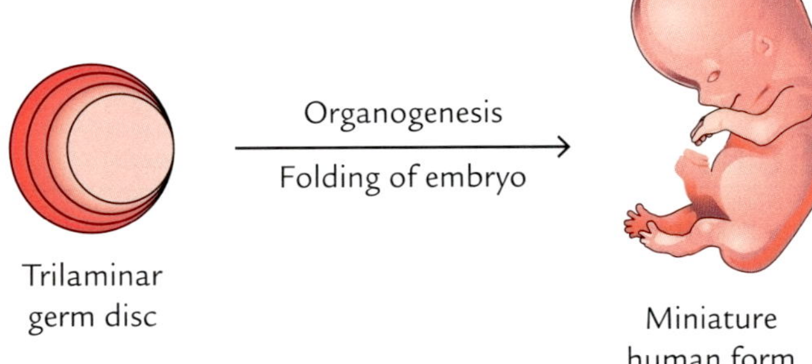

Fig 8.2 Formation of miniature human.

Processes of Folding

As discussed earlier, the folding of an embryonic disc is a significant event in the establishment of the miniature form of the human body. As a result of folding, the flat embryonic disc becomes somewhat cylindrical embryo.

The folding occurs in both median and horizontal planes due to rapid growth of the embryo.

Folding of Embryo in the Median Plane/Craniocaudal Folding (Fig. 8.3)

The craniocaudal folding, i.e., folding in median plane, occurs due to growth of neural tube in length.

The folding of embryo in the median plane occurs as follows (Fig. 8.3):

- There is a progressive increase in the length of embryo (embryonic disc), but its head and tail ends remain relatively close together. Consequently, the embryonic disc bends ventrally producing a dorsal convexity and bulges upward into the **amniotic cavity**.
- With further increase in the length of embryonic disc, the head and tail ends also get folded on itself to form **head fold** and **tail fold**, respectively. As a result of the formation of head and tail folds, the head and tail ends of embryo move ventrally.

a. **Head fold**

The head fold is formed at the end of 3rd week, due to rapid growth of the cranial portion of neural tube (future forebrain) and relative stiffness of notochord. The forebrain grows cranial beyond the oropharyngeal membrane.

As a result, the following changes take place:

- **Septum transversum**, which was lying cranial to **buccopharyngeal membrane**, now comes to lie ventral to it.
- Septum transversum, which was lying in front of pericardial cavity, now lies behind the pericardial cavity.
- Heart tube, which was lying below the pericardial cavity, now lies above the **pericardial cavity.**

b. **Tail fold**

The tail fold is formed due to rapid growth and elongation of caudal portion of neural tube (future spinal cord) and relative stiffness of primitive streak.

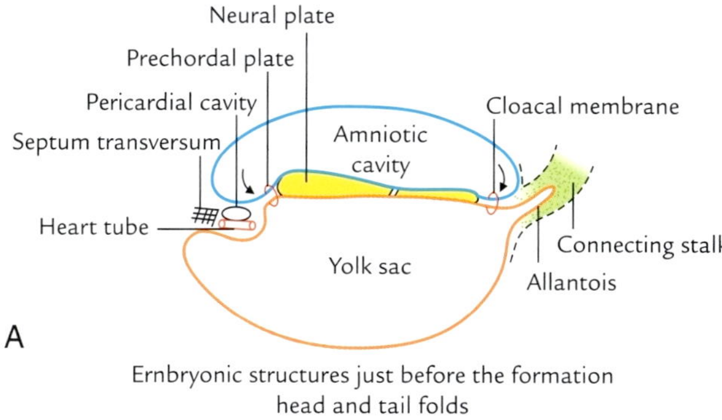

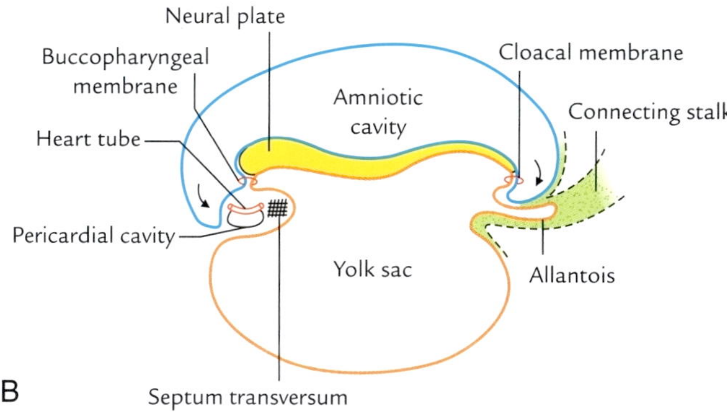

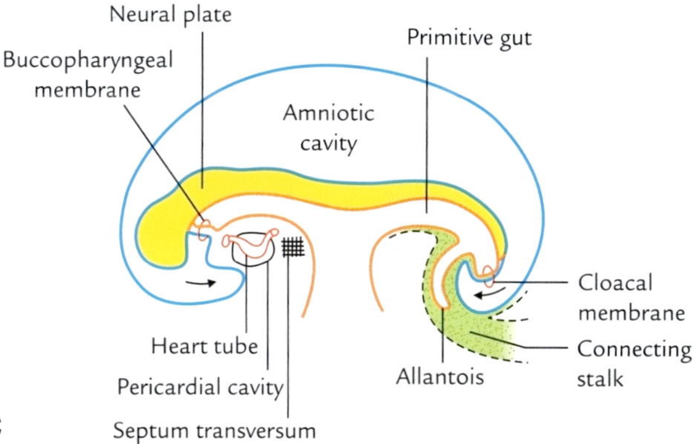

Fig 8.3 Arrangement of structures of embryo before and after the folding (formation of head and tail folds) as seen in median longitudinal sections. (A) Embryonic disc with its important components. (B) Embryonic disc after formation of head fold. Note that the heart tube comes to lie on the roof of the pericardial cavity, and septum transversum becomes caudal to the pericardial cavity. (C) Note the changed relations between septum transversum, pericardial cavity, heart tube, and cloacal membrane.

As a result, the following changes take place:

- Tail region grows beyond the cloacal membrane which eventually comes to lie ventrally.
- Dorsolateral part of yolk sac gets trapped within the tail fold to form hindgut. Its terminal portion gets dilated to form cloaca.
- The cloaca is now separated from amniotic cavity by the cloacal membrane.
- Connecting stalk now gets attached on the ventral aspect of embryo in the umbilical region. The connecting stalk is the site of continuation of:
  - Amnio ectodermal reflexion
  - Intraembryonic and extraembryonic coelom

Folding of Embryo in the Horizontal Plane/Lateral Folding (Fig. 8.4)

The lateral folding of embryo in the horizontal plane occurs due to rapid growth of somites on either side of spinal cord.

- Superficial layer of ectoderm thickens in the middle to form neural plate, which in turn forms neural tube to lie in midline below the ectoderm.
- The margins of ectoderm roll upward to become continuous above with the wall of the amniotic cavity. The margins of endoderm roll downward to become continuous with the wall of yolk sac.
- The middle layer of intraembryonic mesoderm in the middle holds the two tubes (amniotic cavity above and yolk sac below) together.
- **The folding of sides of the embryo forms right and left lateral folds. The lateral folds move medially toward midline and fuse to each other to form the anterior abdominal wall. However, in the center of the anterior abdominal wall a somewhat circular aperture remains, which represents the future umbilicus.** This also makes embryo cylindrical.
- With the formation of lateral folds in embryo, communication between midgut and yolk sac narrows to form the **vitellointestinal duct** (**omphaloenteric duct**).
- As the embryo folds on itself, the amniotic cavity expands enormously and completely surrounds the embryo. Now the embryo floats freely in the amniotic fluid within amniotic cavity, which serves as a *swimming pool* for the *embryo*.
- Because of enormous expansion of amniotic cavity, the extraembryonic coelom gets almost completely obliterated and the amnion forms the covering of the umbilical cord.

EFFECTS OF FOLDING OF EMBRYO (FIG. 8.5)

1. Because of the formation of folds on all sides, the flat embryonic disc becomes cylindrical, leaving an opening on the ventral aspect called **umbilical ring**.

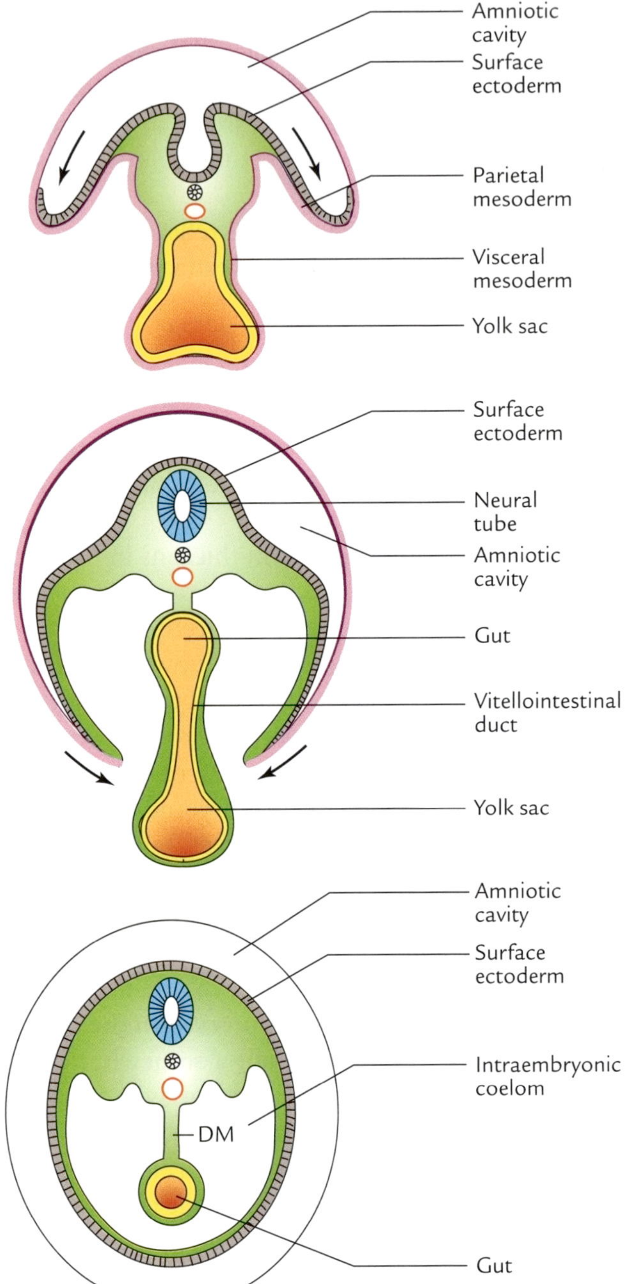

Fig 8.4 Lateral folding of embryo as seen in transverse section of embryos at various stages of development. DM, dorsal mesentery.

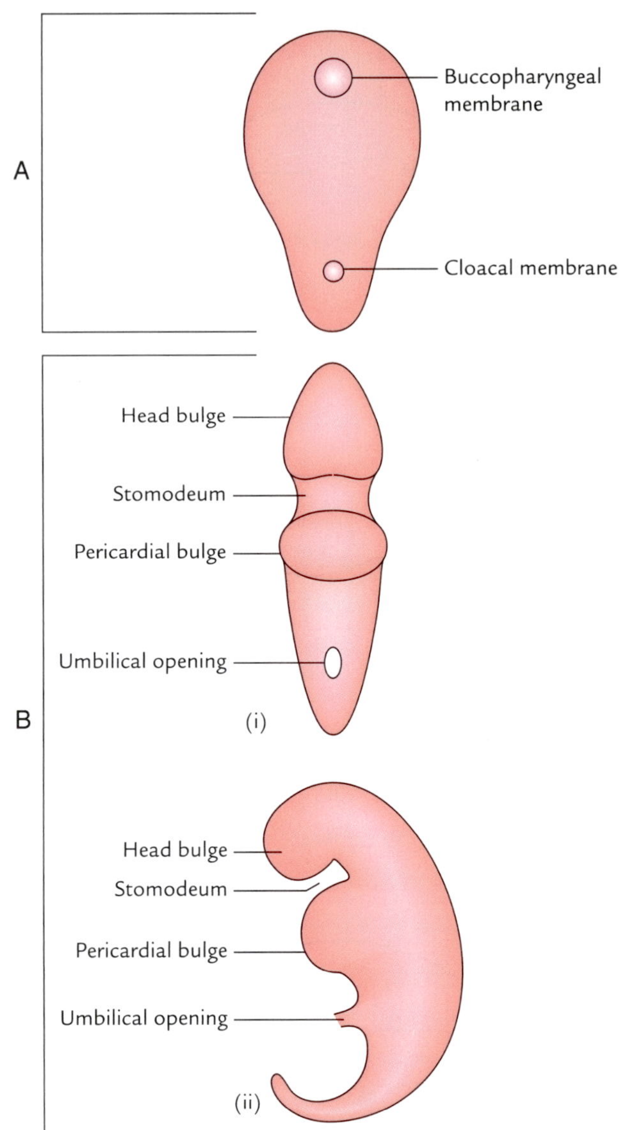

Fig 8.5 Folding of the embryo. (A) Embryonic disc before folding. (B) Embryo after folding: (i) frontal view and (ii) lateral view.

2. The ectoderm forms the outer covering of the embryo.
3. The embryo becomes completely surrounded by the amniotic cavity.
4. The part of yolk sac gets incorporated in the embryo to form the **primitive gut**.
5. The cranial end of primitive gut is now separated from **stomodeum** by **buccopharyngeal membrane**, and the caudal end of primitive gut is separated from **proctodeum** by the **cloacal membrane**.
6. The connecting stalk (future umbilical cord) now becomes attached to the ventral aspect of embryo around the umbilical opening.
7. The allantois now gets connected to the terminal part of the hindgut.
8. The head containing brain now forms the cranial-most part of the embryo.
9. The **septum transversum** and **pericardial cavity** now lie on the ventral aspect of the cranial end of the embryo, with heart tube lying dorsal to the pericardial cavity.
10. The septum transversum now lies caudal to the primitive heart tube and pericardial cavity.
11. A depression is formed between head bulge and pericardial bulge (Fig. 8.5). This depression is

called **stomodeum** and is separated from the cranial end of foregut by the buccopharyngeal membrane.

12. **Two halves of the peritoneal cavity now fuse to form a single peritoneal cavity.**

The arrangement of structures of embryo before and after the folding (formation of head and tail folds) is shown in Fig. 8.7 and summarized in Table 8.2.

N.B. All the major organ systems begin to develop during the embryonic period. By the end of this period, i.e., during the 8th week, the human embryo has a **distinct human appearance**.

FORMATION OF EARLY UMBILICAL CORD AND PRIMITIVE GUT

Primordium of Umbilical Cord

The primordium of umbilical cord is formed by connecting stalk.

The expansion of amniotic cavity leads to folding with ventral shifting of amnio-ectodermal junction and formation of umbilical ring which surround *connecting stalk.*

Structures present within connecting stalk in 5th week are (Fig. 8.6):

1. Extraembryonic mesoderm
2. Vitellointestinal duct
3. Remnants of yolk sac
4. Allantois (It gets partly incorporated into the embryo.)

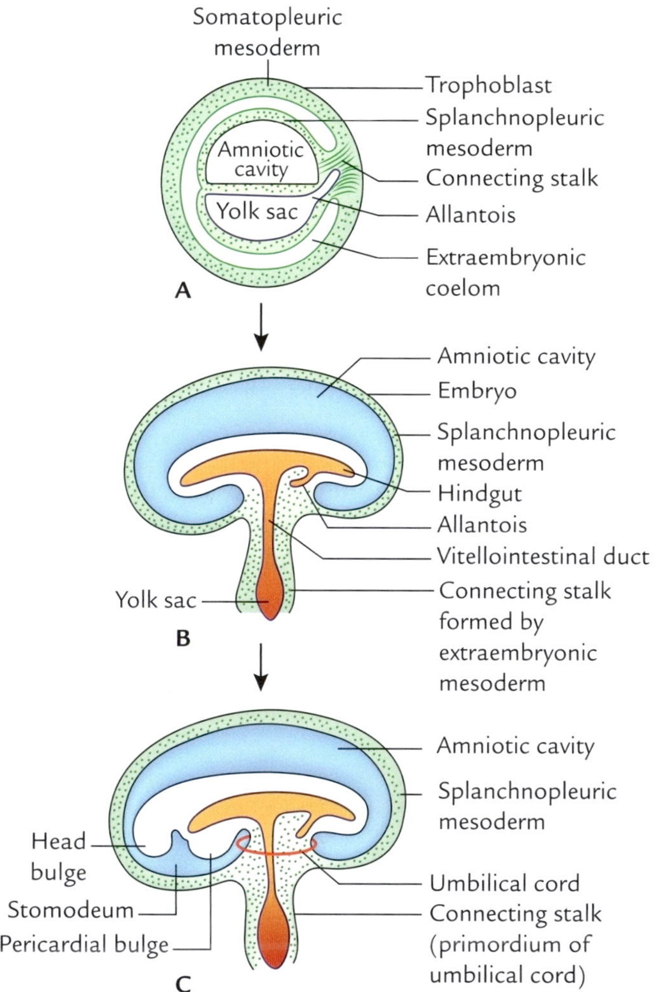

Fig 8.6 Folding of the embryo and formation of the **umbilical cord**.

Table 8.2 Arrangement of important structures of embryo before and after the folding in craniocaudal direction

Before Folding of Embryo	After Folding of Embryo
Septum transversum lies cranial to the pericardial cavity and heart tube	Septum transversum lies caudal to the pericardial cavity and heart tube
Heart tube lies below the pericardial cavity	Heart tube lies above the pericardial cavity (i.e., heart tube jumps from the floor of the pericardial cavity to its roof)
Prechordal plate	Prechordal plate forms buccopharyngeal membrane/oral membrane
Cranial part of the neural plate lies above and behind the primitive buccopharyngeal membrane	Cranial part of the neural plate lies above and in front of buccopharyngeal membrane/oral membrane and forms the cranialmost structure of the embryo
Yolk sac lies below the embryo	Most of yolk sac is taken up with the embryo to form primitive gut
Connecting stalk is attached at the caudal aspect of the embryo	Connecting stalk is attached on the ventral aspect of the embryo
Allantois is directed caudally	Allantois is directed ventrally

A small diverticulum arises from the caudal part of the yolk sac and grows into the connecting stalk attached to the caudal end of the embryo called allantois (allantoic diverticulum).

FORMATION OF PRIMITIVE GUT (FIG. 8.7)

Because of the formation of head and tail folds, the part of yolk sac becomes enclosed within the embryo to form a long tubular structure called **primitive gut**. The primitive gut forms most of the gastrointestinal tract.

- The primitive gut is divided into three parts: **foregut**, **midgut**, and **hindgut**. The midgut is in wide communication with the yolk sac through a wide channel – the primordium of **vitellointestinal duct (yolk stalk)**.

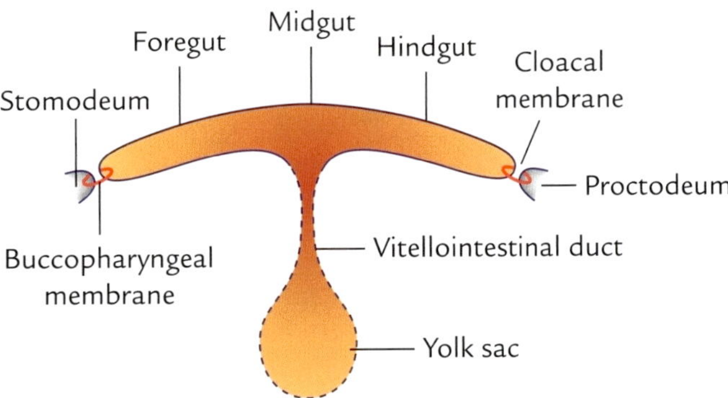

Fig 8.7 Folding of the embryo and formation of **primitive gut**.

SALIENT FEATURES OF ORGANOGENES DURING 4TH TO 8TH WEEKS OF DEVELOPMENT

The salient features of organogenes during 4th to 8th weeks of development are given below in tabular form:

Week	Development of tissues and organs
Fourth week (days 22–23)	1. Complete formation of neural tube by closure of anterior and posterior neuropores. 2. Differentiation of cranial part of neural tube into the brain vesicles. 3. Four to 12 somites. 4. Formation of optic vesicles and optic placodes. 5. Appearance of upper and lower limb buds. 6. Formation of three pairs of pharyngeal arches.
Fifth week	1. Enlargement of cranial part of neural tube. 2. Fine swellings around primitive mouth, viz. frontonasal, maxillary, and mandibular. 3. Appearance of cervical sinus. 4. Upper limb buds become paddle shaped. 5. Lower limb buds appear flipper like.
Sixth week	1. Appearance of nasal processes. 2. Buccopharyngeal membrane ruptures. 3. Appearance of auricular hillocks around 1st pharyngeal cleft. 4. Development of brain vesicles.
Seventh week	1. Appearance of notches between digital rays in the primordia of hands and feet. 2. Formation of umbilical hernia. 3. Appearance of ossification centers in limb bones.
Eighth week (Fig. 8.8)	1. Development of face. 2. Development of eyes with closed eyelids. 3. Auricles have acquired more or less final shape. 4. Head is proportionately large. 5. Limbs and digits are more or less well defined. 6. Hands and feet move ventrally. 7. Tail disappears. 8. Differentiation of external genitalia. 9. Coordinated limb movements start occurring.

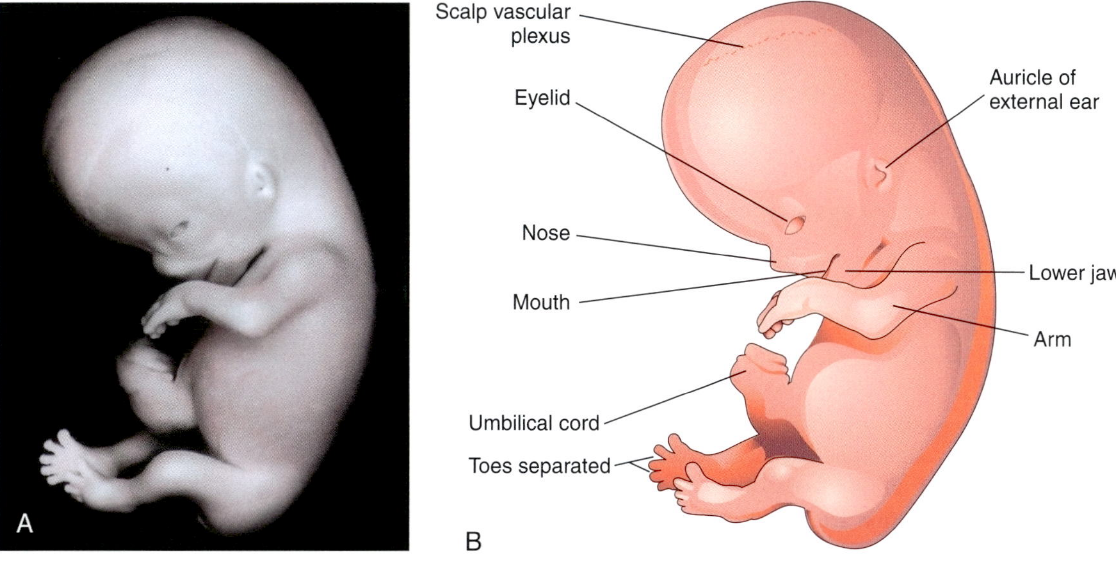

Fig 8.8 Lateral view of an embryo at the end of 8th week (56 days). (A) Actual but not labelled. (B) Idealized and labelled. (*Source:* From Nishimura H, Semba H, Tanimura T, Tanaka O: Prenatal development of the human with special reference to craniofacial structures: an atlas, Washington, DC, 1977, National Institutes of Health.)

GESTATIONAL AGE OF KEY DEVELOPMENTAL EVENTS

Developmental Event	Time of Occurrence
➢ Pharyngeal arches	Day 24
➢ Upper limb buds	Days 26–27
➢ Lower limb buds	Day 28
➢ Optic pits and lens placodes	Day 28
➢ Appearance and facial swellings around stomodeum	Day 30
➢ Auricular hillocks around first pharyngeal cleft	Days 29–35

GOLDEN FACTS TO REMEMBER

➢ **Most important features of embryonic period (3rd to 8th weeks of development)**	Organogenesis
➢ **Swimming pool of embryo**	Amniotic cavity
➢ **Buccopharyngeal membrane ruptures**	During 6th week
➢ **Cloacal membrane ruptures**	During 7th week
➢ **Gestation period when embryo is seen in miniature human form**	End of 8th week

CLINICAL PROBLEM SOLVING

PROBLEMS

1. **Why 3rd to 8th week of embryonic development is very important for the normal development of the baby and the most sensitive period for teratogens?**
2. Give the embryological basis of **agenesis**, **aplasia**, and **atresia**.
3. **What is the origin of neural crest cells? Discuss their migration.**
4. **Enumerate the organs and structures that maintain contact with the external world.**

SOLUTIONS

1. The period of pregnancy from 3rd to 8th week of gestation is critical because it is this period during which cell populations responsible for organ formation are established and primordia of various organs are being formed.

   Early in the 3rd week of embryonic development, three primary germ layers responsible for organogenesis begin to form. Later in the 3rd week, the differentiation of central nervous system begins, and over the next 5 weeks, the primordia for major organ systems are established.

   Thus, in **3rd to 8th week of pregnancy the cells are rapidly proliferating and critical cell–cell signals are occurring.** These phenomena are extremely sensitive to disruption by teratogens. Therefore, **if during this period, the developing baby is exposed to teratogens it will suffer from various types of birth defects (congenital malformations).**

2. • ***Agenesis*** is complete failure of organ to develop due to absence of primordial tissue made up precursor cells.
   • ***Aplasia*** is failure of organ to develop after the initial development (rudimentary development).
   • ***Atresia*** is a condition in which duct or orifice in the body is closed. *Atresia* differs from stenosis in the sense that *atresia* is complete closure while *stenosis* is partial closure, i.e., narrowing.

3. The **neural crest cells** arise from the junction between neural plate and surface ectoderm, i.e., **from edges of neural folds.** The key proteins responsible for their formation are **bone morphogenetic protein-5 (BMP-5).**

   In cranial region they migrate before the closure of neural folds, whereas in caudal region they migrate after the closure of neural folds. **The neural crest cells are multipotent stem cells and migrate to various sites in embryo to form number of cell types,** viz. peripheral nervous system, melanocytes, glial cells, neuroendocrine cells, cardiac septa, etc., and **organs,** viz. craniofacial cartilages and bones.

   One third of birth defects occur in the region of head and face such as **cleft lip** and **cleft palate**, etc.

4. These are:
   (a) Central nervous system (CNS)
   (b) Peripheral nervous system (PNS)
   (c) Sensory epithelium of **nose** (olfactory epithelium), eye (retina), and ear (receptors of ear).

9 Teratology/Birth Defects, Prenatal Diagnosis, and Fetal Therapy

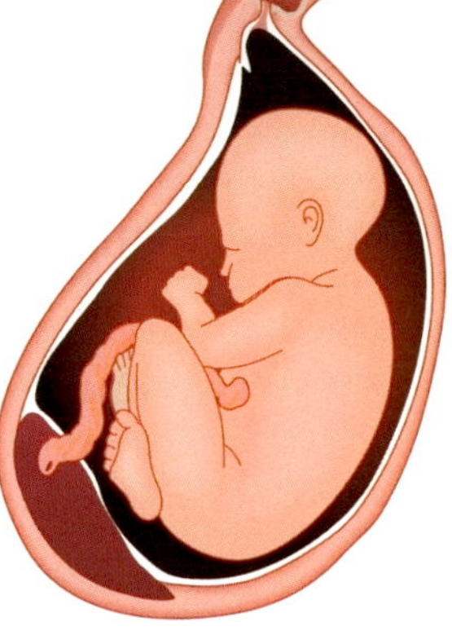

LEARNING OBJECTIVES

After studying this chapter, the students should be able to:

- Give the brief account of environmental factors responsible for birth defects.
- Describe the role of teratogens and alfa-fetoprotein during pregnancy. AN 79.6
- Write short notes on: (a) teratogenesis, (b) teratogens, (c) types of birth defects, and (d) principles of teratogenesis.
- Enumerate the genetic factors responsible for birth defects.
- Describe the various methods used for prenatal diagnosis of birth defects. AN 81.1
- Describe the indications, process, and disadvantages of chorionic villus biopsy. AN 81.3

OVERVIEW

Teratology is the study of abnormalities caused during developments. It is very often thought to be same as birth defects but it is not. The range of teratology is much broader than that of birth defects because it includes anomalies occurring during non-birth stages also.

The **birth defects/congenital malformations** are structural defects present at the time of birth.

The agents or factors responsible for causing various anomalies are termed **teratogens**.

The most common birth defects are:

(a) Congenital heart defects
(b) Cleft lip/cleft palate
(c) Neural tube defects
(d) Down syndrome
(e) Blood disorders (viz. thalassemia, sickle cell disease)

TERATOLOGY/BIRTH DEFECTS

It is the study of congenital abnormalities including the causes, mechanisms and patterns of abnormal development. The study of birth defects or congenital anomalies is essential because they are responsible for more than 20% of intrauterine deaths and are observed in about 2.5% live born babies.

Types of Birth Defects

The birth defects occur prenatally and may be identified before birth. There are four types of birth defects: **malformations, disruptions, deformations,** and **dysplasias.**

(a) ***Malformations:*** These are structural defects in the body due to abnormal embryonic or fetal development, viz. *cleft lip* and *cleft palate.*
(b) ***Disruptions:*** These result in morphological alternations of otherwise normal developing structures due to disruption of processes caused by factors such as *vascular anomalies, anoxia, teratogens, amniotic bands,* viz. *missing digits or limbs.*
(c) ***Deformations:*** These are abnormalities of shape of a part of body caused by mechanical forces. They usually involve musculoskeletal system, viz. **clubfoot** caused by compression in amniotic cavity.
(d) ***Dysplasias:*** These are abnormal organizations of cells (i.e., dyshistogenesis) due to the presence of abnormal cells. It may occur at microscopic level, viz. **hip dysplasia** where socket of hip, i.e., acetabulum, fails to develop properly.

Frequency of Congenital Anomalies Affecting Various Systems

1. Musculoskeletal system: 30%
2. Integumentary system: 20%
3. Central nervous system (CNS): 14%
4. Gastrointestinal system: 9%
5. Genitourinary system: 9%
6. Respiratory system: 2%

Causes of Birth Defects

The various causes of birth defects are:

1. **Environmental factors: 15%**
   - *Infection* during pregnancy
   - *Drug exposure* during pregnancy
   - *Exposure to various chemical agents* during pregnancy
   - *Exposure to ionizing radiation* during pregnancy
2. **Genetic or hereditary factors: 30%**
   - Chromosomal anomalies
   - Gene mutation
3. **Multifactoral factors, i.e. combination of genetic and environmental factors (55%):** It has been found that 15% birth defects are caused by environmental factors, 30% by genetic factors, and remaining 55% are caused by the combination of genetic and environmental factors (also called multifactorial inheritance [Fig. 9.1]).

N.B. The **major birth defects** are structural changes in one or more parts of the body. These are *anophthalmos, anotia/microtia, cleft lip* and *cleft palate, esophageal atresia, gastroschisis, muscle dystrophy, omphalocele, anencephaly, neural tube defects,* upper and lower limb defects (viz. *Amelia* and *meromelia*), *cardiac defects, Down syndrome, anophthalmia/microphthalmia, diaphragmatic hernia.*

A. ENVIRONMENTAL FACTORS

The environmental factors or agents that cause malformation in an embryo are called **teratogens.**

The process of by which congenital malformations are produced by a teratogens in an embryo is called **teratogenesis.** The induction of malformation by teratogens is called **teratogenicity.**

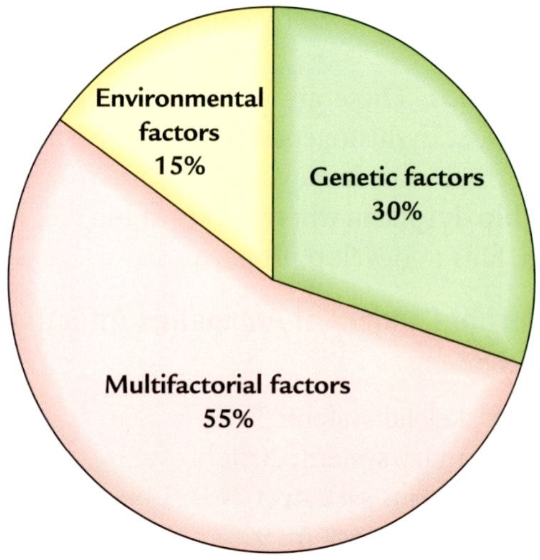

Fig. 9.1 Percentage of birth defects caused by various factors.

Classification of Teratogens

AN 76.6

1. **Infective agents:** German measles or rubella, cytomegalovirus (CMV), toxoplasmosis herpes simplex virus, varicella virus (chickenpox), HIV.
2. **Chemical agents:** Organic mercury, lead, potassium iodide, etc.
3. **Drugs:**
   (a) *Pharmacological drugs*
   - Thalidomide
   - Anticonvulsants, viz. phenytoin

   (b) *Social drugs*
   - Alcohol
   - Cocaine
   - Tobacco smoking
4. **Irradiation:**
   - X-rays
   - Atomic explosions
5. Other factors
   - *Hormones*, viz. androgenic hormones, diethylstilbestrol, maternal diabetes, oral contraceptives, *in vitro fertilization*, maternal obesity, nutritional deficiencies, viz. folic acid, iodine, hypoxia, hypothermia, etc.

Principles of Teratogenicity

There are 3 principles of teratogenicity:

- ***Genetic susceptibility*** (i.e., genotype of an embryo)
- ***Developmental stage/period of development,*** which is susceptible to teratogen
- **Dose of drug or chemical**

The details are as under:

1. The *genetic susceptibility* refers to increased chance of developing congenital anomalies due to the presence of one or more gene mutations and/or a family history of increase risk of developing disease.
2. *Developmental stage/period* susceptible to teratogens to cause birth defects. The susceptibility of embryo to teratogens depends on its stage of development (Fig. 9.2).

   During ***first two weeks***, teratogens usually damage all or most of the cells leading to death and abortion of embryo but if they damage few cells, the embryo recovers and develops without congenital anomalies.

   Between ***3rd to 8th weeks*** (i.e., ***period of organogenesis***) is the most sensitive period of development for teratogens to cause congenital anomalies.

   The ***9th to 38th weeks*** is the period of functional maturity, hence least sensitive to teratogenesis.

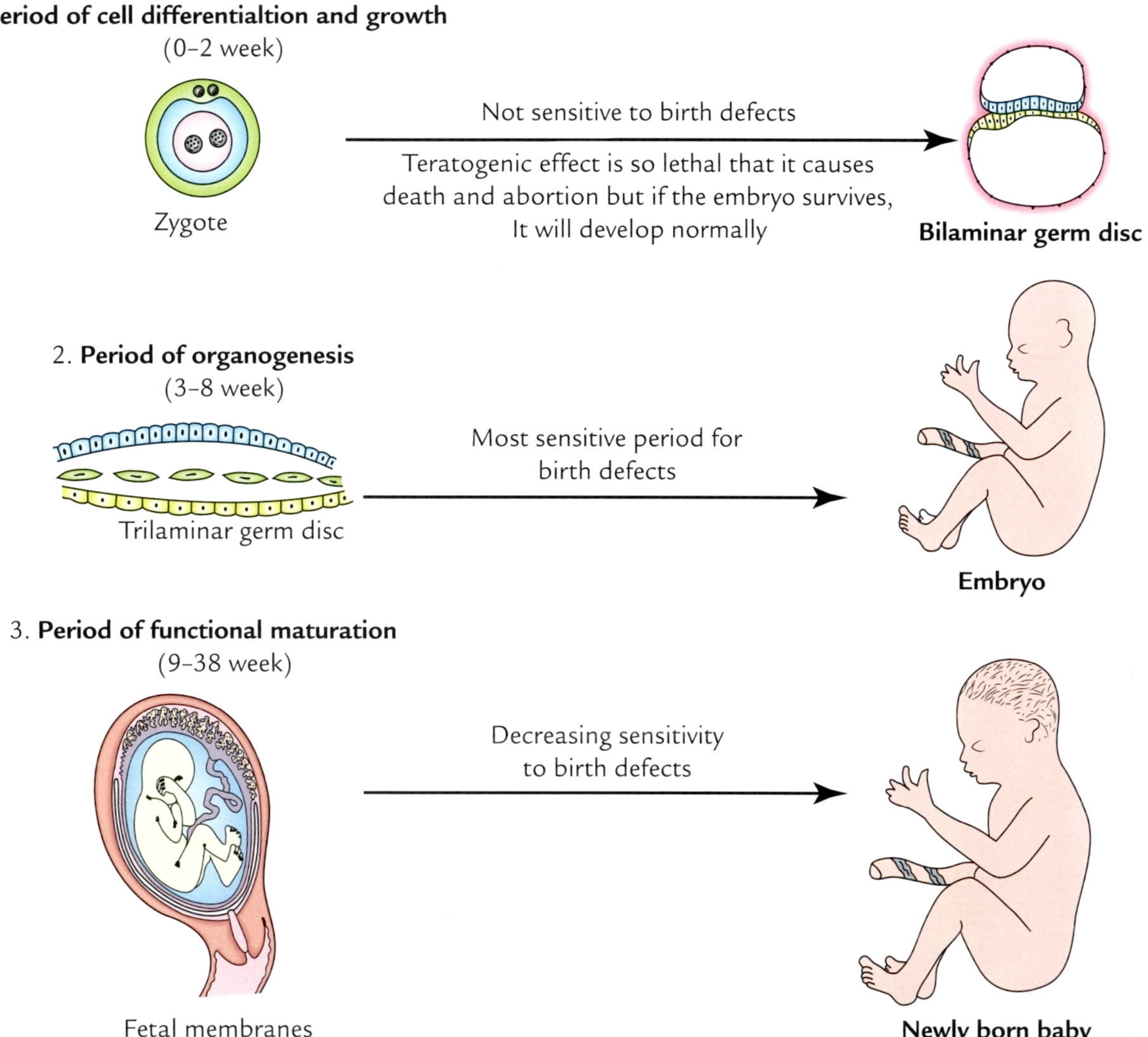

Fig. 9.2 Period of susceptibility to teratogens causing birth defects.

N.B. The clinicians must know the periods of susceptibility to teratogens during pregnancy.

3. ***Doses of drugs or chemicals:*** The high doses of teratogens usually are more deleterious than the low doses, but the amount of dose differs according to developmental stage. One should always remember that a dose may be lethal but not teratogenic; on the other hand, dose may not be lethal but teratogenic.

N.B. These factors determine which genes are turned on and off, thereby influencing the way an embryo develops and its tissues and organs function.

1. Infectious agents

(a) ***German measles (or rubella):*** If pregnant women get affected by German measles (also called rubella) in early stages of gestation, their offsprings may suffer from congenital anomalies. The type of abnormality depends on the stage of embryonic development, at the time of infection during pregnancy. For example:
   - *Cataract:* If infection occurs during 8th week of pregnancy.
   - *Glaucoma:* If infection occurs during 8th week of pregnancy.
   - *Heart defects:* If infection occurs during 5th to 10th weeks.
   - *Hearing loss:* If infected during 9th week.
   - *Teeth abnormalities:* If infected during 6th to 9th weeks.

(b) ***Cytomegalovirus (CMV):*** The developing embryo gets infected by mother only if she is suffering from infection by CMV/by this virus from mother only even if she is asymptomatic.

The various malformations produced include *microcephaly, visual impairment, intellectual disability*, etc.

N.B. Other viral infections such as **herpes simplex virus** and **varicella virus** can also cause congenital abnormalities.

(c) ***Toxoplasmosis:*** It is a disease caused by protozoon parasite – the *Toxoplasma gondii*, one of the world's most common parasites. It usually occurs by eating undercooked contaminated food. It is transmitted to embryo from mother during pregnancy.

Diseases caused by toxoplasmosis include **hydrocephalus, cerebral calcifications, mental retardation,** and **microphthalmos.**

(d) ***Congenital syphilis:*** It is a bacterial infection which usually occurs and spreads by sexual contact. This infection is very rare these days. However, if occurs it will definitely cause congenital deafness and mental retardation.

2. Radiation

It is now well established that radiation is mutagenic agent which causes **mutation of genes in germ cells** and subsequent congenital anomalies.

It is observed that offsprings of mothers who are treated with high doses of X-rays during pregnancy suffer from congenital anomalies such as **microcephaly, skull defects, spina bifida, cleft palate,** etc.

3. Chemical agents

(a) ***Organic mercury:*** The organic mercury poisoning of mothers can cause congenital anomaly of brain affecting motor skills.

(b) ***Lead:*** The lead poisoning in pregnant mother can affect *hemopoietic, gastrointestinal, and urinary system of the developing fetus.*

Lead-based paint and its dust are common sources of exposure to lead poisoning.

(c) ***Potassium iodide:*** It is seen that if potassium iodides are used by pregnant women, the iodine readily crosses placenta and often causes teratogenic effects such as *congenital goiter* and *hypothyroidism*. Therefore, throughout the pregnancy, the number of doses of potassium iodide should be kept to a minimum.

4. Drugs

(a) ***Pharmacological drugs***

(i) *Thalidomide:* It is an antinauseant and sleeping pill and if taken by pregnant women in early pregnancy causes *Amelia* and *meromelia*, i.e., total or partial absence of limbs respectively.

N.B. Thalidomide is used even now as an immunomodulatory agent in the treatment of *AIDS* and other immunological disorder such as *leprosy*.

(ii) *Isotretinoin (Accutane):* It is a class of medications called retinoids – analogues/polymers of *vitamin A*. They regulate epithelial growth rate and often used for the treatment of *cystic acne* or severe *recalcitrant nodular acne*, which may become suppurative or hemorrhagic.

(iii) *Aminopterin:* It is a 4-amino derivative of folic acid. It is an antineoplastic drug with immunosuppressive properties and often used in chemotherapy. It is an antagonist of folic acid, hence if given in higher doses it will cause abortion or congenital anomalies like anencephaly, meningocele, hydrocephalus, and cleft lip/cleft palate.

(iv) *Anticonvulsant drugs* (viz. phenytoin and trimethadione): The trimethadione if taken by pregnant woman it may cause major malformations such as *heart defects, facial defects,* and *microcephaly*. These defects together produce a syndrome called **fetal hydantoin syndrome**.

Similarly, **trimethadione** will cause trimethadione syndrome characterized by malformed ears, cleft palate, cardiac defects, and urogenital and skeletal anomalies.

(v) *Other drugs* such as **triazolam** (a variety of benzodiazepines used for better sleep), warfarin (an anticoagulant drug), and clomiphene (an ovulatory stimulant) should not be given to pregnant women.

(b) ***Illicit drugs, alcohol, and cigarette smoking:*** The *alcohol* intake during social gathering is a main problem in today's society.

The consumption of alcohol during pregnancy causes ***fetal alcohol syndrome*** characterized by:

- Short palpebral fissures
- Hypoplasia of maxilla
- Altered joint mobility, and
- Ventricular septal defects (VSDs)

(c) ***Hormones:*** Unnecessary use of hormones such as **progestins** and **diethylstilbestrol** in pregnant woman used to avoid abortion should also be avoided, as these hormones may cause androgenic activities and cancer vagina, respectively.

A small list of some of the drugs which are absolutely contraindicated or to be avoided at the best is given in Table 9.1.

Table 9.1 List of drugs that should not be given to pregnant women at all or to be avoided at best

Drugs Absolutely Contraindicated in Pregnancy	Drugs with Definitive Evidence of Risk to Fetus
• Thalidomide – *an antinausea drug* • Methotrexate, busulfan, chlorambucil – *anticancerous drugs*	• Tetracycline • Doxycycline • Streptomycin • Amikacin • Tobramycin } *Antibiotics*
• Phenytoin (Dilantin) • Trimethadione • Antiepileptic drugs	• Phenobarbital (a barbiturate) – *a sedative*
• Triazolam (benzodiazepine) – *a hypnotic drug*	• Valproic acid – *an antiepileptic drug*
• Warfarin – *an anticoagulant drug*	• Diazepam – *an antianxiety drug*
• Clomiphene – *an ovulatory stimulant*	• Alprazolam – *an antianxiety drug*

5. Maternal factors

(a) ***Diabetes mellitus:*** Pregnant mothers with uncontrolled ***diabetes mellitus***, particularly during embryogenesis/organogenesis, are three or four times more prone to produce birth defects in their offsprings such as holoprosencephaly and sirenomelia (caudal dysgenesis).

(b) ***Nutritional deficiencies:*** The nutritional deficiencies in mothers during pregnancy are associated with certain birth defects. For example:
- *Folic acid deficiency* leads to *neutral tube defects.*
- *Iodine deficiency* may cause *endemic cretinism.*

(c) ***Obesity:*** Recently, it is found that women with obesity are associated with twofold increased risk of *neural tube defects* in their offsprings.

(d) ***Hypoxia:*** The hypoxia in mothers is often associated with low birth weight babies.

6. Mechanical factors

Certain birth defects such as clubfoot, congenital dislocation of hip, intrauterine amputations, etc. may occur due to **malformed uterus, oligohydramnios**, and **amniotic bands** formed due to rupture of amnion during early pregnancy.

B. GENETIC FACTORS (CHROMOSOMAL ABNORMALITIES AND GENE MUTATION)

The genetic factors are responsible for 30% birth defects. **The chromosomal abnormalities** account for 20% of major birth defects, whereas **gene mutations** account for another 10%.

1. Birth Defects Caused by Chromosomal Abnormalities

Numerical Abnormalities

(a) ***Due to numerical abnormalities involving autosomes:*** These occur due to the presence of an extra chromosome. For examples:

(i) ***Trisomy 21 or Down syndrome (47 XY 21):***
- Occurs due to nondisjunction of chromosomes during meiosis.
- Frequency increases with advance maternal age.
- Affected baby has **oblique palpebral fissure, epicanthus,** and **transverse crease in hand (Simian crease**). For details see p. 349, Chapter 29.

(ii) ***Trisomy 18 or Edward syndrome (47 XY 18):*** Affected baby presents microcephaly, drooping eye lids, **rocker bottom feet** (i.e., convex plantar aspects), **low set ears**, etc.). Also see p. 350, Chapter 29.

(iii) ***Trisomy 13 or Patau syndrome (47 XY 13):*** Affected baby presents **cleft lip** and **cleft palate, microphthalmia, mental retardation**, etc. Also see p. 350, Chapter 29.

(b) ***Due to numerical abnormalities involving sex chromosomes:*** These occur due to abnormal sex chromosomal complement. For examples:

(i) ***Klinefelter syndrome (47 XXY):*** Affected baby is male and presents the following features: **testicular atrophy, gynecomastia, long limbs,** etc. For details see p. 350, Chapter 29.

(ii) ***Turner syndrome (45 XO):*** Affected baby presents gonadal dysgenesis, webbed neck, shield-like chest, pin-point nipples. For details see p. 350, Chapter 29.

(iii) ***Triple X syndrome/super female (47 XXX):*** The affected female baby shows **delayed motor skills, delayed speech and learning abilities, and scanty menses.**

Structural Abnormalities

The structural abnormalities occur due to breakage of one or more chromosomes. The congenital abnormalities depend on what happens to broken pieces. For examples:

(a) **Cri-du-chat syndrome (Cat's cry syndrome)**
- Occurs due to deletion of short arm of chromosome 5 which is lost.
- Affected baby presents a cat-like cry, microcephaly, and heart defects.

(b) **Prader–Willi syndrome (Paternal 15q)**
- Occurs due to microdeletion of long arm of chromosome 15 derived from father (i.e., microdeletion of paternal chromosome called paternal imprinting).
- Affected child present short stature, pot-belly, small hands, and feet. For details see p. 351.

(c) **Angleman syndrome (Maternal 15q)**
- Occurs due to microdeletion of long arm of chromosome 15 derived from mother (i.e., microdeletion of maternal chromosome)
- Affected child is prone to unprovoked long periods of laughter, mental retardation and unable to speak. For details see p. 351.

(d) **Down syndrome due to Robertsonian translocation (Functional trisomy 21)**

In this, short arms of two acrocentric chromosomes 14 and 21 are deleted and lost but their long arms join together to form a long 21 chromosome, which functions as two 21 chromosomes, thus causing functional trisomy 21 leading to Down syndrome. For details see p. 348.

2. Birth Defects Caused by Gene Mutations

Many congenital malformations both structural and functional are caused by inheritance of single gene mutation. The examples are as follows:

- *Structural malformation*, viz. **Marfan syndrome** due to autosomal dominant inheritance.
- *Functional malformations*, viz. *phenylketonuria*, *homocystinuria*, and *galactosemia* due to autosomal recessive inheritance.

For details see Chapter 29.

C. BIRTH DEFECTS CAUSED BY MULTIFACTORIAL INHERITANCE

These are:
- **Talipes**
- **Congenital heart defects**
- **Neural tube defects**
- **Cleft lip and cleft palate**
- **Congenital hip dysplasia/dislocation**

In such cases, environmental factors interact with genotype to produce phenotype.

N.B. Multifactorial disorders are more common than single gene and chromosomal disorders. The preventive measures rely on avoidance of environment factors, which can be explained by genetic counseling. Also see p. 358, Chapter 29.

PRENATAL DIAGNOSIS AN 81.1

It is done to detect various congenital anomalies of fetus during pregnancy.

The various methods of prenatal diagnosis are:
1. Ultrasonography
2. Maternal serum screening
3. Amniocentesis
4. Chorionic villus sampling
5. Fetoscopy
6. Magnetic resonance imaging (MRI)
7. Cordocentesis/percutaneous umbilical cord blood sampling (PUCBS)

1. Ultrasonography

It is a noninvasive and safe technique to be used during pregnancy. It is mostly used to assess the age and fetal growth during intrauterine life.

The **birth defects** that can be detected by ultrasound are:
- Neural tube defects, viz. ***anencephaly and spina bifida***
- Abdominal wall defects, viz. ***omphalocele***
- Heart defects, viz. ***interventricular septal defect***
- Facial defects, viz. ***cleft lip and cleft palate***

In addition, ultrasound is also used to screen for **Down syndrome** and some other chromosomal anomalies, viz. Klinefelter syndrome, by using soft tissue markers (Fig. 9.3) such as:

(a) **Nuchal translucency** (also called **nuchal test**)

(b) **Nasal bone shadow**

The nuchal test involves measuring the thickness of translucent space on the back of neck of fetus as fluid accumulates here, in Down syndrome and heart defects. The nasal bone is either absent or small in such cases.

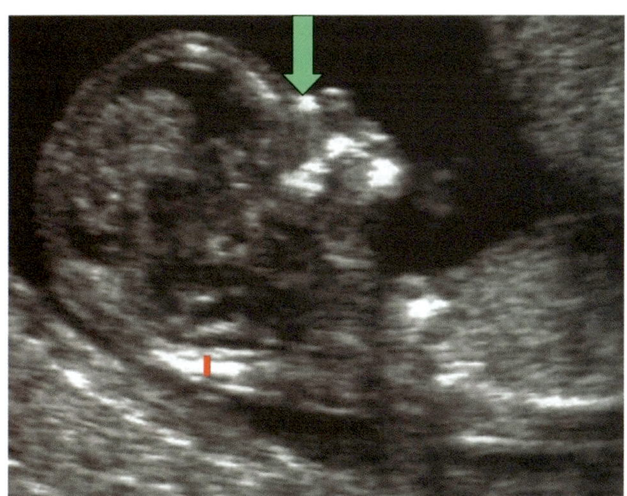

Fig. 9.3 Soft tissue markers in Down syndrome. Green arrow shows nasal bone shadow while red line shows nuchal translucency. (*Source: Journal of Crash Course:* Obstetrics and Gynaecology: Prenatal Diagnosis; 2009, Elsevier.)

N.B. This test must be performed during weeks 11–14 of pregnancy, especially in pregnant women of age 35 years and above. If the thickness of translucency is more and nasal bone shadow is absent, maternal serum screening test is done. *The risk is assessed by combining three things: translucency test, report of maternal serum screening, and mother's age.*

2. Maternal Serum Screening (Triple Screening Test in Pregnancy)

It is a noninvasive technique done during second trimester (i.e., 4th–6th month of pregnancy).

It is done to search for three biochemical markers of fetus. For example:

(a) *Serum* **α-fetoprotein levels:** They are:
  (i) Increase in neural tube defects, etc.
  (ii) Lowered in monosomies and trisomies.

(b) *Human chorionic gonadotropins (HCG) levels:* They are decreased in monosomies, viz. Turner syndrome and trisomies, viz. Down syndrome.

(c) *Estriol and inhibin A:* It promotes growth of the uterus and prepares female body for delivery. Estriol level starts increasing during 8th week of pregnancy. The concentrations of **HCG** and **inhibin A** are raised, with low **estriol** levels in Down syndrome.

3. Amniocentesis

It is an invasive technique and done between weeks 14–15 of pregnancy.

In this procedure, a needle is passed through the anterior abdominal wall of mother (i.e., transabdominally) into the amniotic sac of fetus under ultrasound guidance (Fig. 9.4).

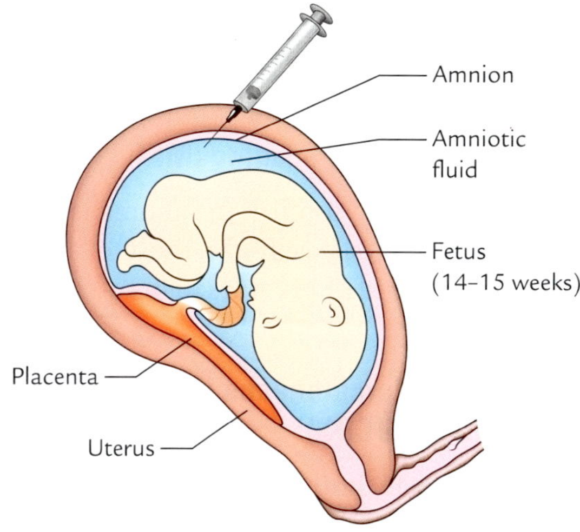

Fig. 9.4 Amniocentesis: Removal of amniotic fluid from amniotic cavity.

About 20–30 mL of amniotic fluid is withdrawn to preform the following tests:

(a) **To analyze the level of α-fetoprotein**

(b) **To perform karyotyping of fetal cells.** Note that fetal cells (epithelial cells from fetal skin) float in the amniotic fluid.

4. Chorionic Villus Biopsy/Sampling (CVS) AN 81.3

Indications for Chorionic Villus Sampling

It is done in pregnant women who have increased risk (risk >1:150) of fetal chromosomal or genetic abnormalities found during antenatal screening.

It is an **invasive technique** done after 10 weeks of pregnancy.

Process

By this technique, about 5–30 mg of villus tissue is aspirated by needle through transabdominal or transvaginal route from the placenta.

- It is done much before amniocentesis.
- **The villus tissue is used for karyotyping to detect various chromosomal anomalies, inborn errors of metabolism and X-linked disorders.**

Disadvantages

It has high risk of abortion.

5. Fetoscopy

It is an invasive procedure. In this procedure, a small incision (3–4 mm) is made in the abdominal wall and an endoscope (fiberoptic lighting instrument) is inserted through the abdominal and uterus to observe the various congenital anomalies directly. Usually, it provides a surgical access.

6. Magnetic Resonance Imaging (MRI)

It is sometimes done to confirm the anomalies detected by ultrasonography, especially for those of brain and spinal cord, because MRI provides high soft tissue contrast and resolution.

7. Cordocentesis/Percutaneous Umbilical Cord Blood Sampling (PUCBS)

- It is an **invasive technique** and done not earlier than 17 weeks of pregnancy.
- By this technique, blood sample is withdrawn from umbilical vein through an ultrasound-guided needle and examined for chromosomal anomalies.

It is done to detect blood-associated conditions, viz. fetal anemia. It is usually done when diagnosis is not made by other prenatal tests.

N.B. This test carries a significant risk, hence it should be done only when other tests are inconclusive and in pregnancies with high risk for genetic disorders.

FETAL THERAPY

With the recent advances in the medical field, now the fetal therapy is possible. These are as follows:

1. **Fetal transfusion**

   Now blood transfusion is given to anemic fetuses by inserting a needle in umbilical vein of umbilical cord, under ultrasound guidance. Fetal anemia occurs in conditions like *erythroblastosis fetalis.*

2. **Fetal medical treatment**

   Now fetal treatment of conditions like cardiac arrhythmias compromised thyroid function, etc. is possible. The drugs are given to mother which reaches fetus by crossing placental barrier or can be administered directly to fetus by intramuscular injection in gluteal region or through umbilical vein.

   Now good medical centers have a separate branch of medicine called **maternal fetal medicine** (**MFM**) to manage health concerns of mother and fetus.

3. **Fetal surgery**

   The surgery in fetus is now possible to treat conditions like *congenital diaphragmatic hernia, spina bifida defects*, and *placing shunts* to remove fluid from organs and cavities.

   In ex-utero surgery, the uterus is opened, and fetus is operated directly. This procedure allows to ensure proper establishment of fetal airway before completion of delivery and clamping of umbilical cord.

4. **Stem cell transplantation and gene therapy**

   Now *in utero* stem cell transplantation is possible because fetus does not develop immunocompetence before 18 weeks of gestation. The hemopoietic stem cells have great potential in this regard for treating immunodeficiency and hematological disorders.

GOLDEN FACTS TO REMEMBER

➢ Most lethal period of gestation to teratogens	First two weeks
➢ Most susceptible period of gestation for birth defects (i.e. teratogenesis)	Third to 8th weeks of gestation, i.e., period of organogenesis
➢ Syndrome	A group of anomalies occurring together which have a specific common cause
➢ Most common type of birth defects	Congenital heart defects
➢ Gestation period for development of immunocompetence	After 18 weeks of gestation, i.e., after $4^1/_2$ months/ 2nd trimester
➢ Most common method used to diagnose prenatal birth defects	Ultrasonography

CLINICAL PROBLEM SOLVING

PROBLEMS

1. What are the **factors which put the woman at higher risk in pregnancy?**
2. Name the factors that influence the effect of teratogens.
3. Which vitamin is recommended to married females of child-bearing age as a supplement?
4. Which drugs are safe to take during pregnancy?
5. Is cigarette smoking safe during pregnancy?

SOLUTIONS

1. These are:
   - **Advanced maternal age,** 35 years and above.
   - **Previous history, genetic problems,** viz. Down syndrome, etc.
   - **Poorly controlled diabetes mellitus.**
   - **Abnormal ultrasound findings,** viz. thick nuchal translucency and small nasal bone.
2. These are:
   - Genetic susceptibility, viz. genotype of mother and embryo.
   - Period of gestation/developmental stage.
   - Dose and duration of exposure to teratogen.
3. Folic acid, 400 μg daily to prevent neural tube defects.
4. These are:
   Penicillin including amoxicillin, ampicillin, erythromycin, cephalosporins, etc. Similarly, local anesthetic agents, salicylates (aspirin) in low doses are also safe.
5. Cigarette smoking is not safe during pregnancy because it may lead to **preterm birth, low birth weight** and **defects of lip** etc. The smoking during pregnancy also increases the risk of sudden infant death syndrome (SIDS).

10 Extraembryonic Membranes, Placenta, Umbilical Cord, and Multiple Pregnancy

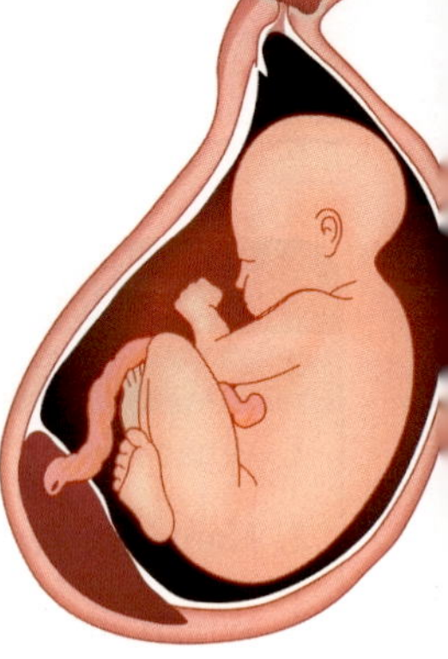

LEARNING OBJECTIVES

After studying this chapter, the student should be able to:

- Define extraembryonic membranes and give brief account of each of them.
- Write short notes on (a) amnion (b) chorion, (c) yolk sac, (d) allantois and (e) decidua. AN 80.1
- Enumerate the functions and fate of amnion, chorion, yolk sac, allantois, and decidua. AN 80.1
- Describe the development of placenta in detail and give its main functions. AN 80.3
- Write short notes on (a) fetomaternal circulation and (b) placental barrier. AN 80.3
- Describe the umbilical cord in brief and give its functions. AN 80.2
- Describe the various types of umbilical cord attachments. AN 80.7
- Give the embryological basis of (a) placenta previa, (b) cord prolapse, and (c) oligohydramnios.
- Describe the embryological basis of twining in monozygotic and dizygotic twins. AN 80.4

EXTRAEMBRYONIC MEMBRANES

OVERVIEW

The **extraembryonic/fetal membranes** are membranous structures that develop from zygote but do not form any part of the embryo proper. In other words, while many intraembryonic events form tissues and organs of the embryo, a number of extraembryonic structures develop as well. These are called **extraembryonic membranes**, namely, **amnion**, **chorion**, **yolk sac**, **allantois**, **placenta**, and **umbilical cord** (Figs 10.1 and 10.2).

The extraembryonic membranes appear parallel to embryo and help in its development. They are responsible for protection, respiration, excretion, and nutrition of embryo and fetus. At birth, placenta, umbilical cord, and other extraembryonic membranes are separated from the fetus and expelled from uterus as an **afterbirth**. The knowledge of extraembryonic membranes is essential to perform prenatal diagnostic procedures, such as amniocentesis and chorionic villous biopsy.

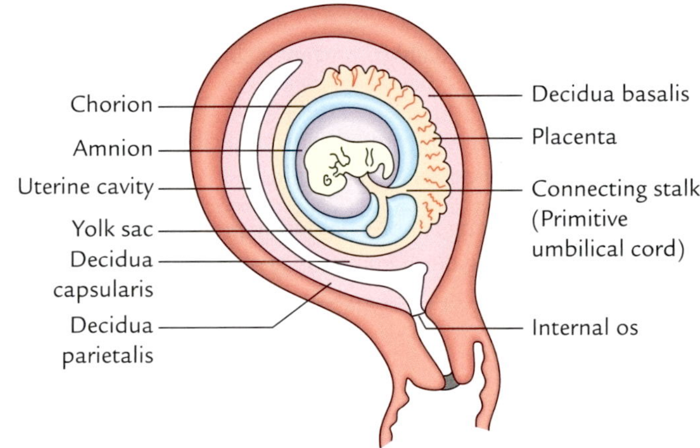

Fig. 10.1 Extraembryonic membranes.

N.B. In reptiles, birds, and mammals there are **four extraembryonic membranes** viz.: (a) amnion, (b) chorion, (c) yolk sac, and (d) allantois. But in placental mammals, two more extraembryonic membranes form viz. *placenta* and *umbilical* cord, which connect the embryo to the mother's uterus.

Amnion (Fig. 10.2) AN 78.4, AN 80.1

- Amnion is a thin extraembryonic membrane that loosely envelops the embryo forming an amniotic sac that is filled with the **amniotic fluid**.
- The amniotic sac is lined by ectodermal cells of inner cell mass and amniogenic cells of trophoblast. Note: Amniogenic cells line the roof and lateral walls of the amniotic sac and do not cover its floor.
- As the amniotic sac enlarges during the late embryonic period (at about 8 weeks) due to collection of more amniotic fluid within it, the amnion gradually surrounds the whole embryo and ensheathes the developing umbilical cord.
- The amniotic cavity grows at the expense of extraembryonic coelom, which gets obliterated and fusion occurs between amnion and chorion (Fig. 10.2D).

As a result, amniotic sac or bag of waters is surrounded by double-layered thin membrane consisting of amnion and chorion.

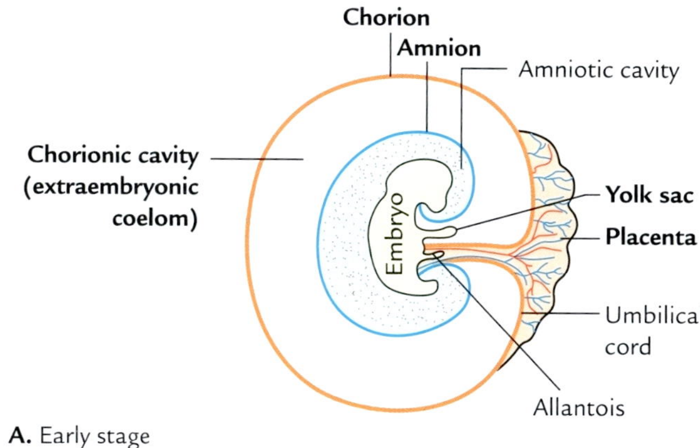

A. Early stage

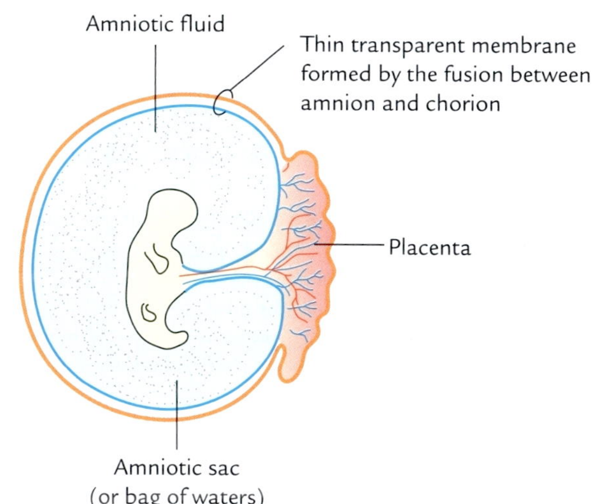

B. Later stage

Fig. 10.2 Formation of amnion and chorion.

Amniotic Fluid

Amniotic fluid is a clear, watery fluid containing salt, sugar, urea, and proteins. It is derived from

A. amniotic cells by filtration or secretion,
B. fetal urine when kidneys start functioning,
C. secretion of lung cells, and
D. secretion by placenta.

Constituents of Amniotic Fluid

The amniotic fluid contains

1. metabolites and hormones (HCG, HPL);
2. cells that are sloughed off from fetal lungs, placenta, and amniotic sac (all these cells have same genetic composition);
3. fetal urine.

Functions of the Amniotic Fluid

As a buoyant medium, the amniotic fluid performs following functions for the embryo and the subsequent fetus:

1. It permits symmetrical development and growth.
2. It provides a water-cushion to protect the developing embryo and fetus from jolts that the mother may receive.
3. It helps to maintain a consistent pressure and temperature.
4. It allows free fetal movements – an important prerequisite for musculoskeletal development and blood flow.
5. It forms hydrostatic bag (**bag of waters**) that helps in dilatation of the cervix at the beginning of the labor (childbirth).

N.B. The addition of fetal urine and swallowing of amniotic fluid by the fetus maintains the quantity of the amniotic fluid to the optimum.

Chorion (Fig. 10.2)

- It is a highly specialized extraembryonic membrane that participates in the formation of the placenta.
- It is formed by the somatopleuric layer of extraembryonic mesoderm and trophoblast. Numerous small finger-like projections arise from its surface called **villi**.
- On the side of decidua capsularis, the chorion villi regress/disappear, leaving a smooth surface called **chorion laeve** (**smooth chorion**).
- On the side of decidua basalis, the chorion villi further develop and grow in the decidua basalis to contribute the fetal portion of the placenta. It is called **chorion frondosum (leafy chorion)**. For details see p. 97.

CLINICAL CORRELATION

1. **Amniocentesis** (see Fig. 9.4): AN 81.2 It is a procedure by which the amniotic fluid is aspirated from the amniotic cavity for diagnostic purposes. It is usually done at 14th or 15th week of pregnancy, when the amniotic sac contains 175–225 mL of amniotic fluid. It is done (a) to examine the chromosomes in cells of amniotic fluid for detection of genetic diseases such as Down syndrome, (b) to detect defective enzyme involved in the formation of myelin sheath in *Tay–Sachs* disease by biochemical techniques, and (c) to detect neural tube defects.

Continued

The **sex of a fetus** can also be detected by chromosomal studies. Because fetal urine is added to the amniotic fluid, it can be used to study fetal enzymes and fetal hormones. The presence of **high levels of α-fetoproteinin** amniotic fluid indicates neural tube defects. Also see Chapter 9, p. 89.

2. **Oligohydramnios:** It is a clinical condition in which the volume of amniotic fluid in the amniotic cavity is less than normal. The normal amount of fluid at full term is 700–1000 mL. If this volume becomes 400 mL or less, it is termed oligohydramnios. It occurs due to placental insufficiency with reduced placental blood flow, agenesis of kidneys, and loss of amniotic fluid due to preterm rupture of amnion.
3. **Polyhydramnios:** The excessive accumulation of amniotic fluid (e.g., 2000 mL or more) in the amniotic cavity leads to a clinical condition called *polyhydramnios*. It occurs due to esophageal atresia or defects of central nervous system (CNS) because of which the fetus is unable to swallow the amniotic fluid and consequently the fluid is not absorbed in the gastrointestinal tract (GIT) of the fetus.
4. **Amniotic bands:** Occasionally, the **inner layer of amniotic sac (or bag of water)**, the amnion, peals away from sac and encircles around the part of baby body, viz. digits and limbs and causes congenital anomalies such as **amputations and constrictions of digits.**
5. **Normally rupture of membranes of amniotic sac** (i.e., amnion and chorion) occur just before the onset of labor but if it occurs before 37 weeks, it is termed **preterm rupture of membrane** (PROM). The exact causes of PROM are unknown. But the risk factors include sever polyhydramnios, smoking, etc.

Yolk Sac AN 80.1

The yolk sac is an endodermal sac lying ventral to the embryo (bilaminar embryonic disc) (Fig. 10.3). In humans it hardly contains any nutritive yolk inside it. **It is the first element seen within gestational sac during ultrasonography on weeks 5–7.**

Development of Yolk Sac

The yolk sac develops from the cavity of blastocyst (blastocele) and passes through following three stages of development.

1. **Primary yolk sac:** The cavity of blastocyst is converted into **primary yolk sac** when it is **lined by flattened cells** derived from endoderm of embryoblast (or according to some from trophoblast). This lining formed of flattened cells is called Heuser membrane. It is attached to the undersurface of the embryonic disc. The primary yolk sac is formed at the end of the second week.
2. **Secondary yolk sac:** With the appearance of extraembryonic coelom, the primary yolk sac becomes smaller and is termed secondary yolk sac. **The cells lining the yolk sac becomes cuboidal.**
3. **Tertiary yolk sac or definitive yolk sac:** It is a remnant of the secondary yolk sac. As embryo folds, it takes up most of the yolk sac inside the body of the embryo to form primitive gut. The **portion of yolk sac not taken up inside the body of the embryo** is termed **tertiary/definitive yolk sac.** It communicates with the midgut via *vitellointestinal duct.*

N.B. Yolk sac is also called umbilical vesicle.

Functions of Yolk Sac

1. **Hemopoiesis:** It produces blood for the embryo until the liver is formed during the 6th week.
2. **Formation of primitive gut:** Its dorsal portion forms the *primitive gut.*
3. **Houses primordial germ cells after being formed by epiblast:** The primordial germ cells form from the wall of the yolk sac and migrate to the developing gonads during the 4th week, where they form primitive germ cells (*spermatogonia or oogonia*).
4. **Formation of allantois:** A small diverticulum that arises from the caudal part of the yolk sac.

CLINICAL CORRELATION

Meckel's diverticulum: The stalk of the yolk sac (vitellointestinal duct) usually detaches itself from the midgut by the 6th week and the yolk sac gradually shrinks as the pregnancy advances. But sometimes it persists as Meckel's diverticulum (for details see p. 198).

Allantois (Allantoenteric Diverticulum) AN 80.1

Allantois is a small diverticulum that arises from the caudal wall of the yolk sac on day 16 and extends into the connecting stalk (also see p. 77).

After the folding of embryo, the allantois is connected with the dilated terminal part of the hindgut called **cloaca.**

Functions of Allantois

1. It is vascularized by allantoic vessels that later become **fetal umbilical arteries and vein.**
2. In adults, it is represented by **median umbilical ligament.**
3. It also contributes a bit to the formation of urinary bladder (viz. apex of urinary bladder).

N.B. In lower animals, the allantois acts as a reservoir of urine. In humans, it is a vestigial structure.

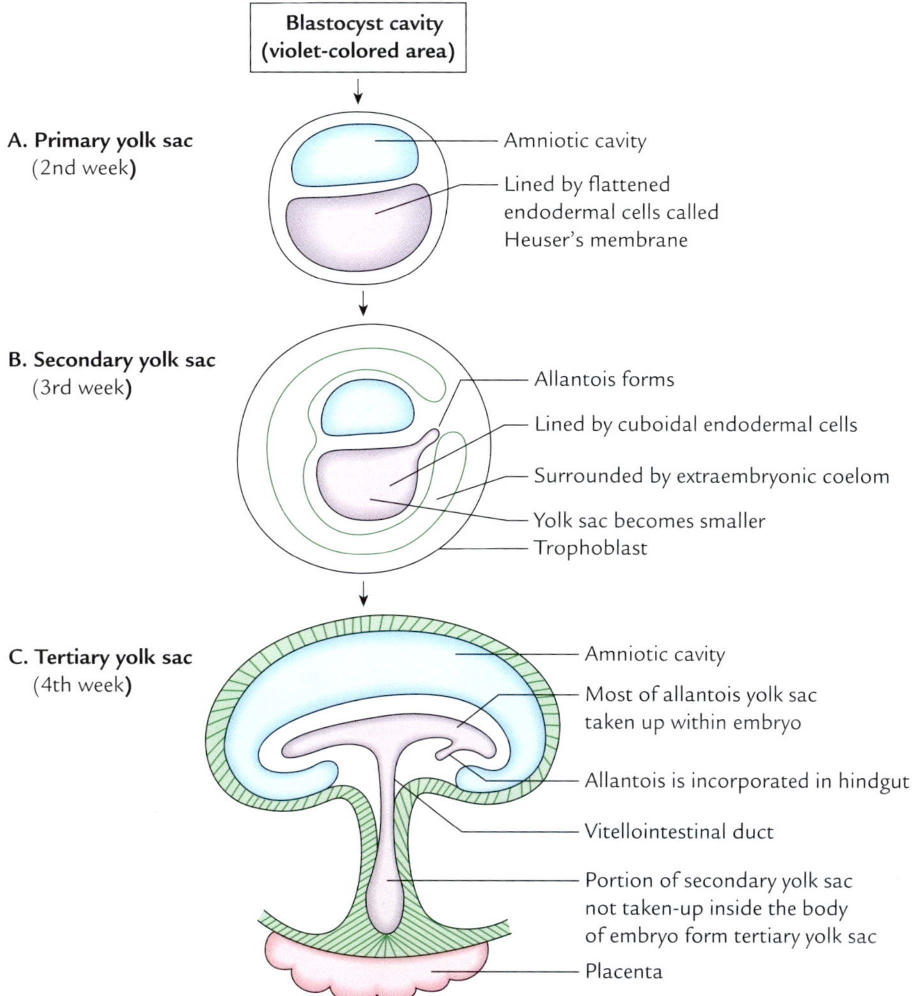

Fig. 10.3 Stages of development of yolk sac. (A) **Primary yolk sac** (lined by Heuser membrane made of flattened cells derived from endoderm). (B) **Secondary yolk sac** (becomes smaller due to the formation of extraembryonic coelom and cells lining it becomes cuboidal). (C) **Tertiary yolk sac** (part of secondary yolk sac which is not taken up inside the embryonic disc).

CLINICAL CORRELATION

Urachal cyst, sinus, or fistula: The extraembryonic portion of allantois degenerates during the 2nd month of intrauterine life.

The part of intraembryonic portion gets incorporated into apex of urinary bladder and the remaining part involutes to form a thick urinary tube called **urachus**. After birth, the urachus becomes a fibrous cord called **median umbilical ligament**, which extends from apex of urinary bladder to the umbilicus. The failure of urachus to obliterate/fibrose leads to the formation of **urachal cyst**, **sinus**, or **fistula** (for details see p. 284).

IMPLANTATION AND DECIDUA AN 80.1

For proper understanding of the development of placenta, the students should first understand implantation and decidua.

Implantation (see Fig. 6.1) AN 78.3

Implantation is a process by which the blastocyst is embedded within the endometrium of the uterus. The intimate contact of fetal and maternal tissues occurs by implantation of the blastocyst.

N.B.

- **Types of implantation**
- *Interstitial implantation:* In this type, the blastocyst is embedded in the endometrium of the uterine wall, e.g., humans.
- *Eccentric implantation:* In this type, the blastocyst is embedded in the uterine crypts, e.g., rats.
- *Central implantation:* In this type, the blastocyst is implanted in the uterine cavity, e.g., cows.

Decidua (Gravid Endometrium) AN 78.5

The decidua is a modified uterine endometrium during pregnancy. It is so called because it separates/sheds off after birth (in Latin, *decidua* = *falling off*).

Decidual reaction

The uterine endometrium is changed into decidua under the influence of progesterone and hCG. This process of formation of decidua is called **decidualization** and changes that occur in endometrium together form **decidual reaction.**

Features of decidual reaction:

- Stromal cells become enlarged and get filled with glycogen and lipid. Now they are called as **decidual cells.**
- Intercellular substance increases, as a result endometrium becomes **edematous.**
- Endometrial arteries become more tortuous.
- Endometrial glands become enlarged and tortuous, and their saw-toothed appearance increases.

Thus, the functional layer of endometrium around gestational sac becomes thick, soft, highly vascular, and rich in nutrients. It is now called as **decidua.**

The decidua provides protection and nutrition to embryo.

> **CLINICAL CORRELATION**
>
> The decidual reaction can be seen by ultrasonography as a thick layer of endometrium around the gestational sac as early as 4–5 weeks of pregnancy.
>
> A thin decidua of less than 2 mm around gestational sac is one of the features of **anembryonic pregnancy**.

N.B.

- As the blastocyst is implanted, the syncytiotrophoblast of conceptus starts secreting human chorionic gonadotropin (HCG) hormone, which intensifies the changes that has occurred in the endometrium during secretory phase.
- The molecular mechanism of implantation involves synchronization between the invading blastocyst and receptive endometrium (i.e., implantation occurs due to mutual interaction between the cells of trophoblast and endometrium).

Parts/subdivisions of decidua

The decidua is divided into three parts (Fig. 10.4), according to its relationship to the conceptus.

1. **Decidua basalis:** It is that part of decidua which lies deep to the embryo (developing blastocyst). It is *decidua basalis* which forms maternal part of placenta.
2. **Decidua capsularis:** It is that part of decidua which forms a capsule around the embryo and separates it from the uterine cavity.
3. **Decidua parietalis:** Rest of the decidua (excluding decidua basalis and decidua capsularis) is termed *decidua parietalis*.

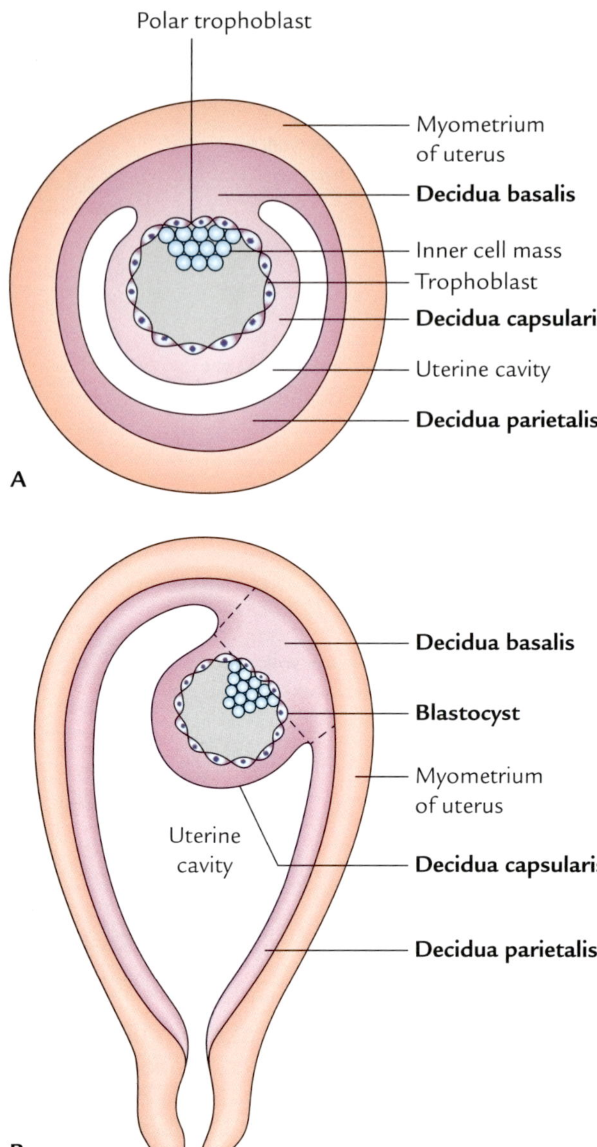

Fig. 10.4 Parts (subdivisions) of decidua. (A) As seen in the horizontal section of uterus. (B) As seen in the coronal section of uterus.

PLACENTA

> **OVERVIEW**
>
> The placenta is a highly vascular compact disc-like structure (having a diameter of 15–20 cm and weighing about 500 gm) by which the fetus is attached to the mother's uterine wall through umbilical cord. It consists of two components: maternal and fetal. It is the only organ that develops from two different individuals who are genetically different, i.e., fetus and mother.
>
> The placenta provides O_2 and nutrients to fetus and removes CO_2 and metabolic waste products from fetus. The *fetal component of placenta* develops from chorion and the maternal component from the *decidua basalis.*

Development of Placenta

AN 78.2

The placenta is a **fetomaternal organ**. It consists of two components: (a) fetal component and (b) maternal component. The fetal component develops from **chorion frondosum** and the maternal component develops from **decidua basalis**.

Structural Components of Placenta

The **fetal component** consists of amnion, extraembryonic mesoderm, chorion, and chorionic villi (made of chorion and *umbilical vessels*), whereas **maternal component** consists of thin layer of *decidua basalis, decidual septae, decidual blood vessels* and *blood within placental lacunae.* By the end of 4th month decidua basalis is almost completely replaced by the fetal part of the placenta.

Stages of Development of Placenta

The various events/stages involved in the development of placenta are as follows:

1. **Formation of chorion frondosum and chorion laeve** (Fig. 10.5)
   (a) **Small finger-like projections** arise from **chorion** (trophoblast and underlying extraembryonic mesoderm) into the decidua surrounding conceptus, i.e., **decidua basalis** and **decidua capsularis.**
   (b) As the chorionic sac enlarges, the chorionic villi in relation to decidua capsularis get compressed and degenerated. As a result, this part of chorion becomes smooth and is now called **chorion laeve.**
   (c) The chorionic villi in relation to decidua basalis are not compressed and hence do not degenerate. Rather they grow extensively into the decidua basalis. This part of the chorion is called **chorion frondosum.**
2. **Formation of trabeculae and intervillous spaces** (Fig. 10.6)
   (a) The cells of trophoblast (made up of single layer of cuboidal cells) proliferate and move on its surface. These cells lose their cell membranes to form a continuous sheet of cytoplasm containing many nuclei. This sheet/layer is called **syncytiotrophoblast**. Thus, trophoblast is differentiated into two layers: (a) a deep layer called **cytotrophoblast** and (b) a superficial layer called **syncytiotrophoblast.**
   (b) The syncytiotrophoblast grows rapidly, erodes the decidua basalis, and becomes thick. The small cavities (**lacunae**) appear in thickened syncytiotrophoblast. The syncytiotrophoblast continues to erode the decidua basalis. The lacunae increase in size. They are separated from each other by portions of syncytiotrophoblast termed **trabeculae** (**villous primordia**).
   (c) As the syncytiotrophoblast further grows, it erodes the blood vessels of the decidua basalis; as a result the *blood enters into the lacunae* along with the secretions of the endometrial glands. Later the lacunae communicate with each other around the trabeculae and form the **intervillous spaces.**
3. **Development of chorionic villi** (Fig. 10.7)
   The chorionic villi are of three types, which develop in succession as follows:
   a. **Primary villi:** The cytotrophoblast forms finger-like projections that invade the trabeculae of syncytiotrophoblast in its center. These finger-like projections of cytotrophoblast surrounded

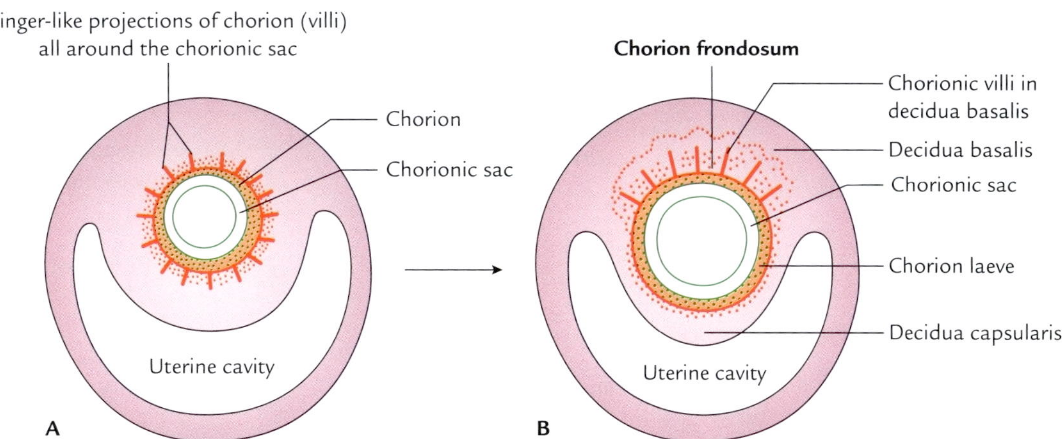

Fig. 10.5 Formation of chorion frondosum and chorion laeve. (A) Formation of villi all around the chorionic sac. (B) Regression of chorionic villi in relation to decidua capsularis.

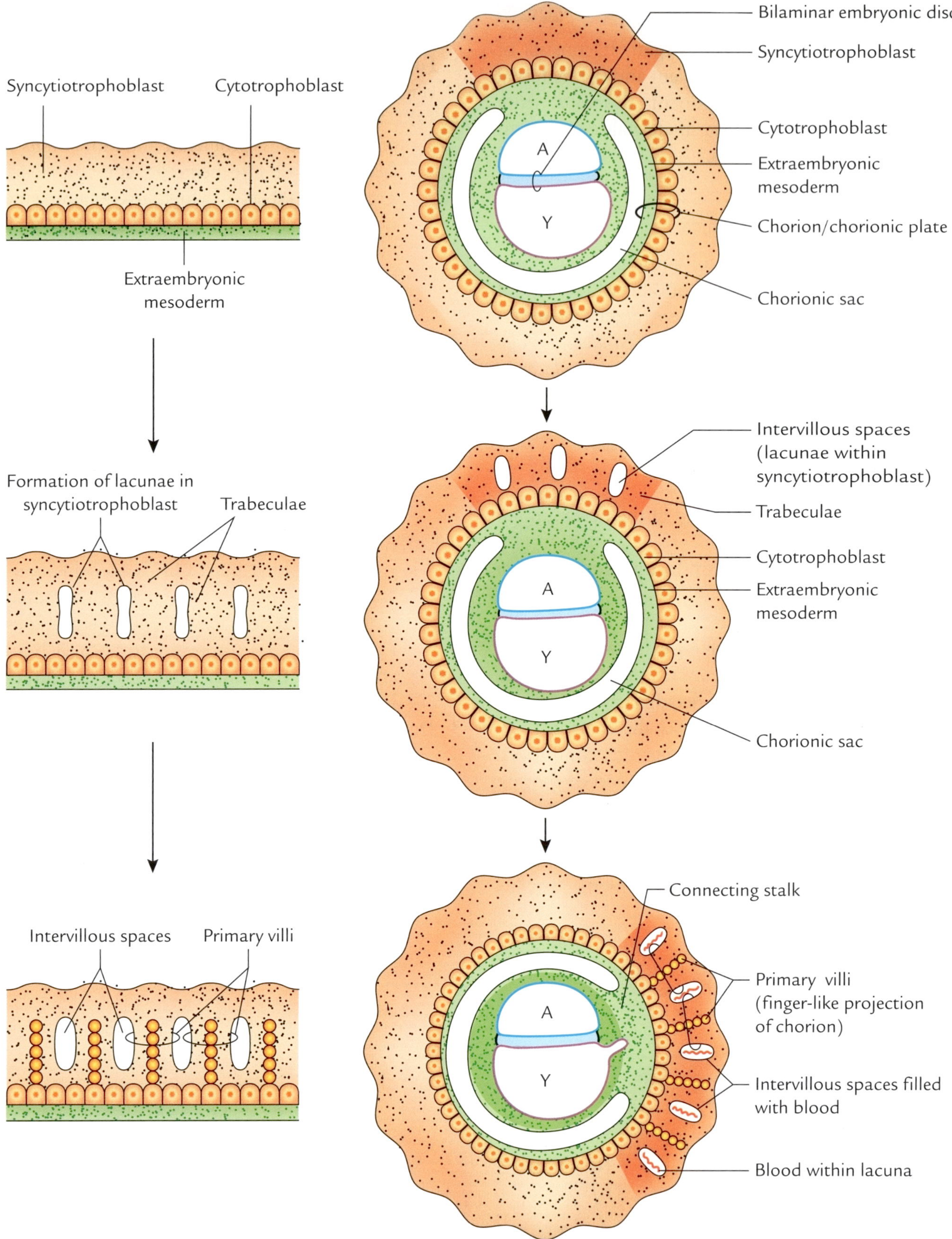

Fig. 10.6 Formation of trabeculae, primary, villi, and intervillous spaces. A, amniotic cavity; Y, yolk sac.

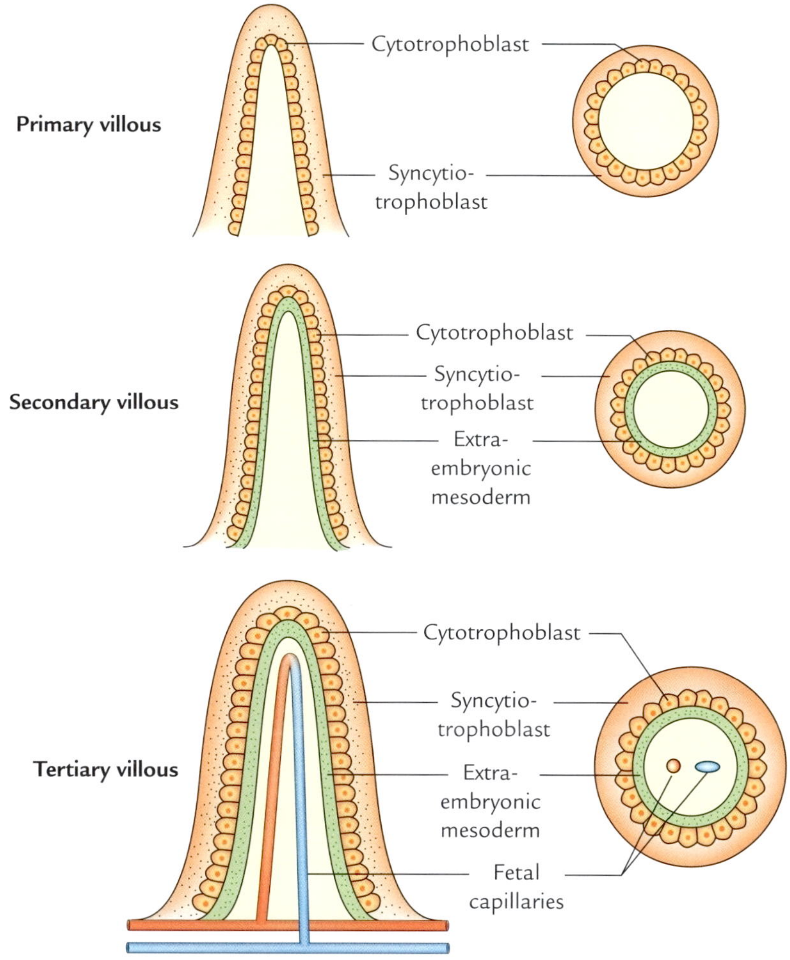

Fig. 10.7 Three stages of development of villi. Figures on the right side are the sectional views of three types of villi.

Table 10.1 Differences in composition of primary, secondary, and tertiary villi

Types of Villus	Composition
Primary villus	Core of cytotrophoblastic cells covered by a layer of syncytiotrophoblast
Secondary villus	Core of mesoderm covered by a single layer of cytotrophoblast, which in turn is covered by syncytiotrophoblast
Tertiary (definitive) villus	Fetal capillaries appear in the mesodermal core covered by layers of cytotrophoblast and syncytiotrophoblast, respectively

by a layer of syncytiotrophoblast are called the *primary villi*.

b. **Secondary villi:** The extraembryonic somatopleuric mesoderm lying deep to the cytotrophoblast now invades the center of each villus to form *secondary villi*.

c. **Tertiary villi:** The blood vessels develop and invade in the mesoderm of the secondary villi to form *tertiary villi*.

The composition of three types of villi is summarized in Table 10.1.

4. **Formation of cytotrophoblastic shell and anchoring villi**

The cells of cytotrophoblast in the apical region of each villus proliferate, pierce and pass across the layer of syncytiotrophoblast to form a continuous layer of cytotrophoblast called **cytotrophoblastic shell**. The cytotrophoblastic shell in turn is attached to decidua basalis (Fig. 10.8).

The formation of cytotrophoblastic shell divides the syncytiotrophoblast into outer and inner layers that undergo **fibrinoid degeneration**. After fibrinoid

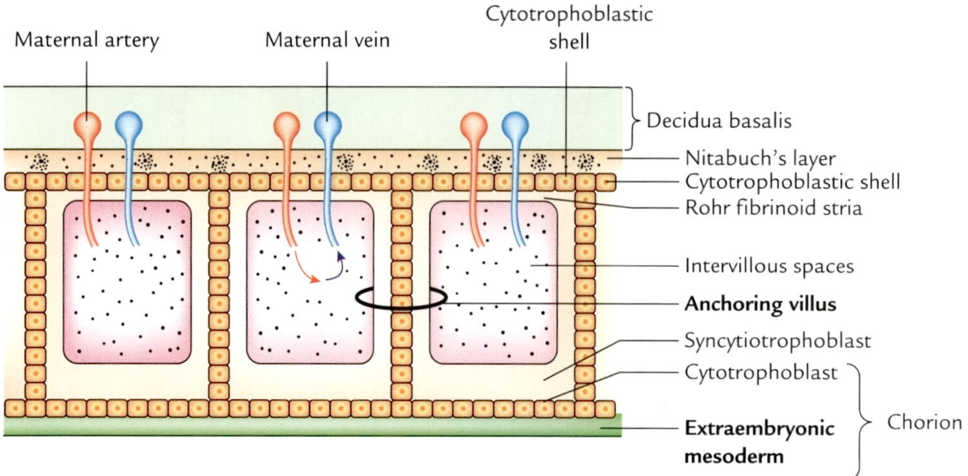

Fig. 10.8 Formation of cytotrophoblastic shell.

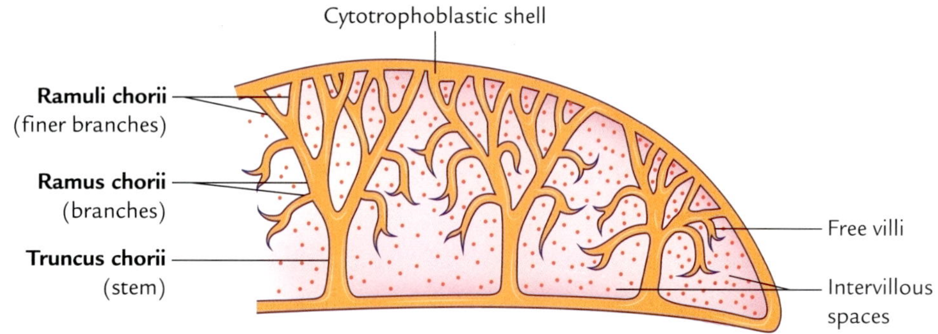

Fig. 10.9 Anchoring villi. Note each anchoring villi consists of a stem called *truncus chorii*, which divides into a number of branches called *ramus chorii*, which in turn divide into a number of finer branches called *ramuli chorii*.

degeneration, the outer layer forms **Nitabuch layer** and the inner layer forms the **Rohr fibrinoid stria.**

Both Nitabuch membrane and Rohr fibrinous stria play a major role in an immunological separation between fetal and maternal tissues to prevent rejection of fetus (fetal tissue an antigen) by the mother.

Because of the formation of cytotrophoblastic shell, the syncytiotrophoblast is completely isolated from the decidua basalis. The cytotrophoblastic shell (Fig. 10.9) fixes (anchors) all villi to the decidua. *These villi are now attached at one end to chorion (fetal side) and to the decidua basalis at the other end (maternal side)*. Because the villi are now fixed at both the ends, these are now called as ***anchoring villi*** (Fig. 10.9).

Branching Pattern of Anchoring Villi

The branching pattern of anchoring villus is as follows:

The anchoring villi give off numerous offshoots that grow and move freely into intervillous spaces filled with blood as **free villi.** This increases the surface area for absorption of nutrients.

- **Truncus chorii** are the stems of anchoring villi.
- **Ramus chorii** are direct branches from stem of anchoring villi.
- **Ramuli chorii** are the branches of ramus chorii.

The ramuli chorii are attached to the cytotrophoblastic shell (Fig. 10.9).

In addition to this, the new villi are further added from chorionic side; thus, converting the intervillous spaces into a **bag of vascular sponges.**

The chorionic villi from chorion thus maximize the fetal surface area that comes in contact with maternal blood for exchange of gases, nutrients, etc.

Lobulation of Placenta (Fig. 10.10)

After the formation of cytotrophoblastic shell and anchoring villi, a number of septa grow inward from decidua into the intervillous spaces and divide the maternal surface of placenta into (15–20) irregular

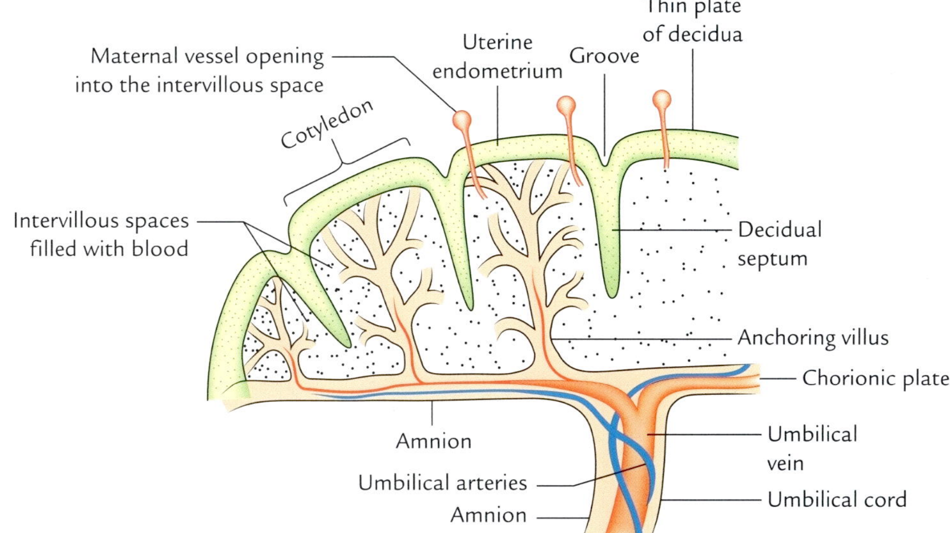

Fig. 10.10 Formation of cotyledons (lobes) of placenta. Placenta consists of 15–20 cotyledons, and each cotyledon contains 2–3 anchoring villi.

convex areas (lobes) called **cotyledons**. Each cotyledon contains 2–3 anchoring villi. As the pregnancy proceeds, the placenta also enlarges to meet the need of the fetus. At term the placenta covers nearly 30% of the internal surface of the uterus.

Full-Term Placenta

The fully formed placenta is a disc-shaped compact mass of vascular tissue.

Features (Fig. 10.11)

- Shape and size: Flat circular disc having a diameter of 15–20 cm, thick in the center (2–5 cm), and thin at periphery.
- Weight: 500–600 g
- Surfaces: Two (maternal and fetal).

Differences between maternal and fetal surfaces of placenta: These are given in Box 10.1.

> **CLINICAL CORRELATION**
>
> After birth, placenta is carefully inspected for missing cotyledons. If the cotyledons remains attached to uterine wall, after birth they may cause severe postpartum bleeding.

Placental Barrier or Placental Membrane AN 80.3

The **placental membrane** separates maternal blood from fetal blood within placenta. Thus, there is no mixing of maternal and fetal blood in the placenta.

The intervillous spaces are filled with maternal blood derived from endometrial arteries and drained by endometrial veins. The chorionic villi contain fetal blood vessels.

The **maternal blood** in the intervillous space is separated from the **fetal blood** within the fetal blood vessels present in the villi by placental membrane (also called *placental barrier*) made up of fetal tissue.

It is across this membrane that the exchange of gases, nutrients, and waste products takes place between maternal and fetal blood.

Constituents of Placental Barrier/Membrane (Fig. 10.12)

- **In early part of pregnancy**

  Until about 20 weeks of pregnancy, the placental membrane is thick and made up of five layers. From the maternal side to fetal side, these are:
  1. syncytiotrophoblast,
  2. cytotrophoblast,
  3. basement membrane of cytotrophoblast,
  4. mesoderm in the core of villus, and
  5. endothelium and basement membrane of fetal capillaries.
- **In later part of pregnancy**

  In later part of pregnancy, as the nutritional demands of fetus increases, the placental membrane becomes thin to increase the efficiency of transport of nutrients and gases across it.

Thus, in the early part of pregnancy, i.e., up to 20 weeks, the placental membrane is about 0.025 mm thick, but in the later parts of pregnancy, it remains only 0.002 mm thick.

Maternal surface
- Cobblestone appearance (i.e., presents groove and elevations)

Fetal surface
- Smooth and shinning
- Covered with transparent amniotic membrane
- Attachment of umbilical cord in center

Umbilical cord
Smooth chorion
Cotyledons
Grooves

Umbilical cord
Umbilical cord attached in the center
Amnion (transparent)
Chorionic vessels radiating under amnion

A. Maternal surface of placenta

B. Fetal surface of placenta

Fig. 10.11 Full-term placenta with umbilical cord. Real specimen showing features on its maternal surface (A) and on its fetal surface (B). (*Source:* These figures were published in Publication *The Developing Human: Clinically Oriented Embryology*, 8th edition by Keith L. Moore and T.V.N. Persaud, ISBN: 9781416037064, Fig. 7.13A and B, Copyright Elsevier, 2008.)

Box 10.1 Differences Between Maternal and Fetal Surfaces of Placenta

Maternal Surface	Fetal Surface
• Rough and irregular	• Smooth and shining
• Presents 15–20 cotyledons (round slightly bulging area separated by grooves), giving a cobblestone appearance	• Presents attachment of umbilical cord nearly in the center with chorionic vessels radiating toward periphery
• Covered by thin layer of decidua basalis	• Covered by chorionic plate which in turn is covered by amnion

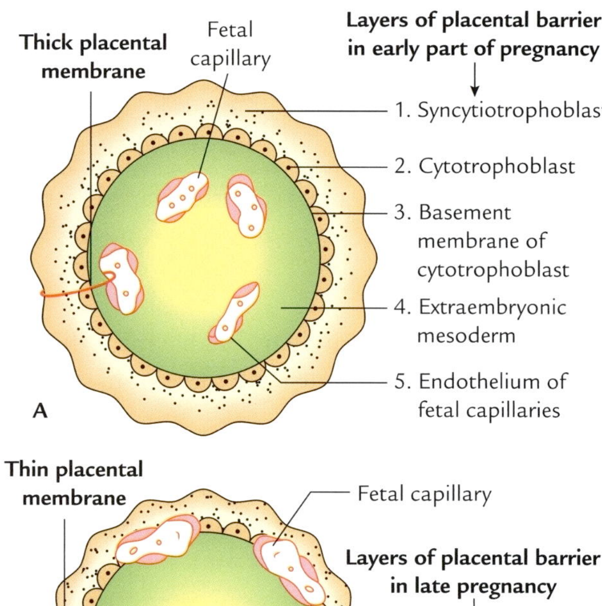

Fig. 10.12 Placental membrane (barrier). (A) In early pregnancy. (B) In late pregnancy.

N.B. However, at the end of pregnancy, the efficiency of placental membrane reduces due to deposition of fibrinoid material on the surface of the membrane.

Factors responsible for thinning of placental membrane:

1. Syncytiotrophoblast becomes thin.
2. Cytotrophoblast disappears.
3. Two basement membranes disappear.
4. Endothelial cells of fetal capillaries become thin.

Thus, after 20 weeks of pregnancy the placental membrane consists of only two layers, viz.:

1. Thin syncytiotrophoblast
2. Endothelial cells of fetal capillaries

N.B. The placental membrane/barrier measures about 14 m^2. The total surface area of placental membrane is roughly equal to the absorptive area of the GIT.

In humans, maternal blood is separated from fetal blood by chorionic tissue; hence human **placenta is termed hemochorial.**

N.B. **Phylogenic classification of placenta:** It is based on maternal and fetal tissues that come in contact. Phylogenetically, the placenta is classified into following five types.

	Type	Maternal Tissue	Fetal Tissue
1	Epitheliochorial (in pig)	Endometrial epithelium	Chorion
2	Endotheliochorial (in dog, cat, etc.)	Endothelium of blood vessel	Chorion
3	Hemoendothelial (in rabbit)	Blood in intervillous space	Endothelium of fetal blood vessel
4	Hemochorial (in human)	Blood in intervillous space	Chorion

Placental Circulation (Fig. 10.13)

The placental circulation brings maternal and fetal circulations in close relationship.

The placental blood flow increases at term and amounts to about 500 mL/min.

The circulation of blood in the placenta is of two types: maternal and fetal.

Uteroplacental Circulation

About 80–100 spiral arteries and number of veins of uterine endometrium (decidua basalis) open into the intervillous spaces. The blood enters the intervillous space through spiral arteries, and under the pressure of blood in arteries, the blood reaches right up to the chorionic plate. It then slowly passes around the branches of villi for exchange across the very thin placental membrane. Then the blood from intervillous space is drained by the veins of decidua basalis.

N.B.
- Blood circulation in the intervillous spaces begins as early as on 9th day of pregnancy.
- In fully formed placenta, the intervillous space contains 150 mL of blood, which is replaced every 15–20 seconds (i.e., three to four times per minute).

Fetoplacental Circulation AN 80.5

The fetal blood comes to placenta through two umbilical arteries. These arteries enter the chorionic plate underneath the amnion. They break up into small branches which enter the stems of chorionic villi. Each of which in turn divides into primary, secondary, and tertiary

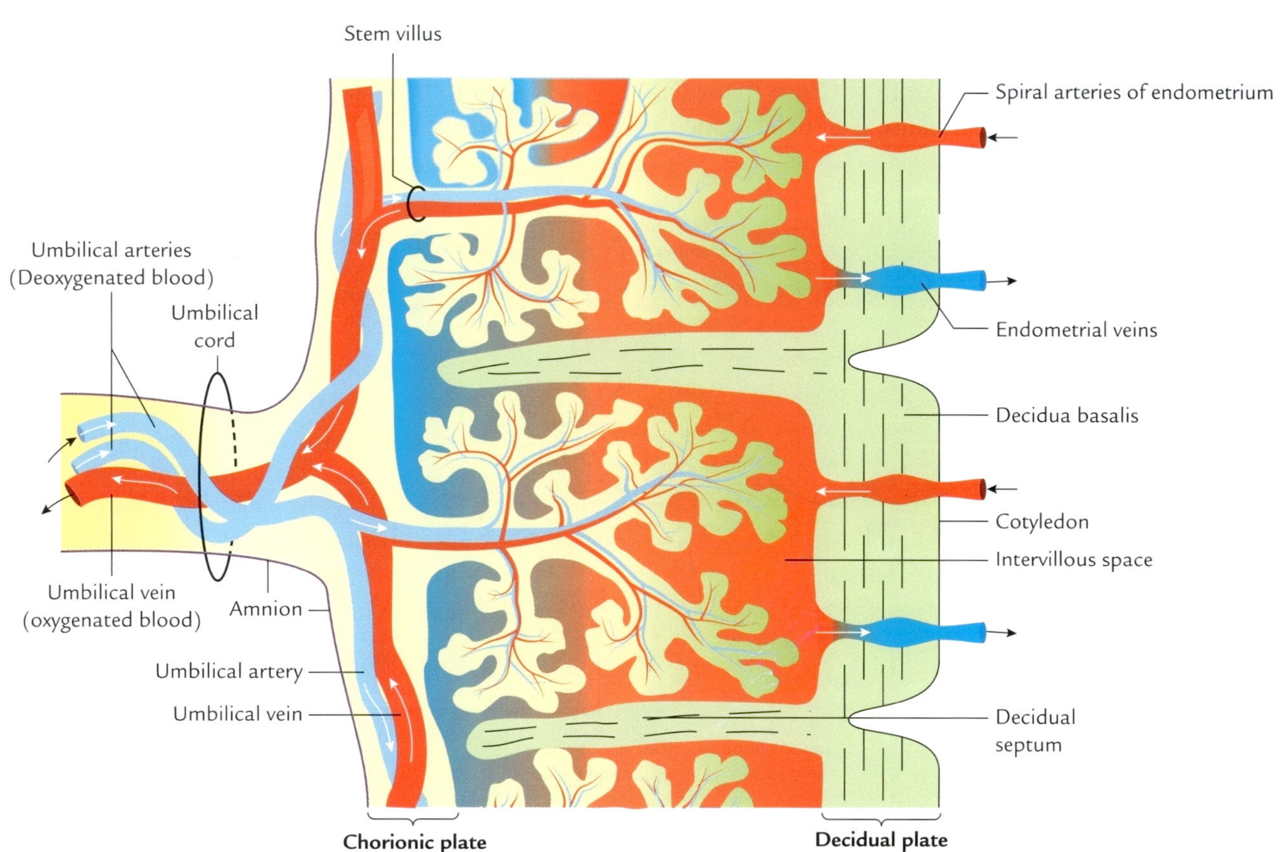

Fig. 10.13 Placental circulation.

branches corresponding to branches of stem villi. It gets oxygenated in placenta by diffusion of O_2 from maternal blood.

The veins from the chorionic villi drain into the umbilical vein that carries blood rich in O_2 and nutrients to the fetus from placenta.

Functions of Placenta

The placenta subserves the following functions (Fig. 10.14):

1. **Exchange of gases:** This involves supply of O_2 from maternal blood to fetal blood and removal of carbon dioxide (CO_2) from fetal blood to maternal blood. A full-term fetus takes about 20–30 mL of O_2 per minute from the maternal blood. Therefore, even a short interruption of O_2 supply to the fetus may prove fatal.
2. **Transport of nutrients:** Carbohydrates, fats, proteins, amino acids, vitamins, and electrolytes are transported from maternal blood to fetal blood.
3. **Excretion of waste products** of metabolism like urea, uric acid, etc. into the maternal blood.
4. **Transmission of maternal antibodies:** Maternal antibodies (IgG), α-globulins, and immunoglobulins can cross the placental barrier and pass from mother to the fetus, and thus provide passive immunity to the fetus against infections/diseases such as diphtheria, measles, and poliomyelitis but not against chicken pox and whooping cough.
5. **Barrier function:** Acts as a barrier to many bacteria and organisms. Some of these or their toxins manage to cross the barrier and may cause fetal defects such as measles, rubella, syphilis, etc. It also acts as a barrier for maternal hormones such as ACTH and TSH.
6. **Production of hormones and their role in uterine growth and parturition:** Placenta also acts as temporary endocrine gland and produces the followings hormones:
   - Progesterone
   - Estrogen
   - Human chorionic gonadotropin (HCG)
   - Human chorionic somatomammotropin (HCS)
   - Human placental lactogen (HPL)
   - Relaxin

   (a) ***Progesterone*** maintains pregnancy by supporting the lining of endometrium.

   (b) ***Estrogen***, which promotes uterine growth and development of mammary gland. It also sensitizes the myometrium by oxytocin which stimulates uterine muscles to contract to begin labor/parturition.

   (c) ***HCG***, which has an effect similar to luteinizing hormone (LH) of the pituitary gland to maintain corpus luteum.

   (d) ***Human placental lactogen (HPL)/somatomammotropin (HCS)***, which helps to feed growing baby. It has an anti-insulin effect on maternal blood causing increased plasma level of glucose and amino acids in maternal blood, and enhances utilization of glucose by the fetus.

   (e) ***Relaxin*** relaxes pelvic ligaments and widens cervix to facilitate parturition.

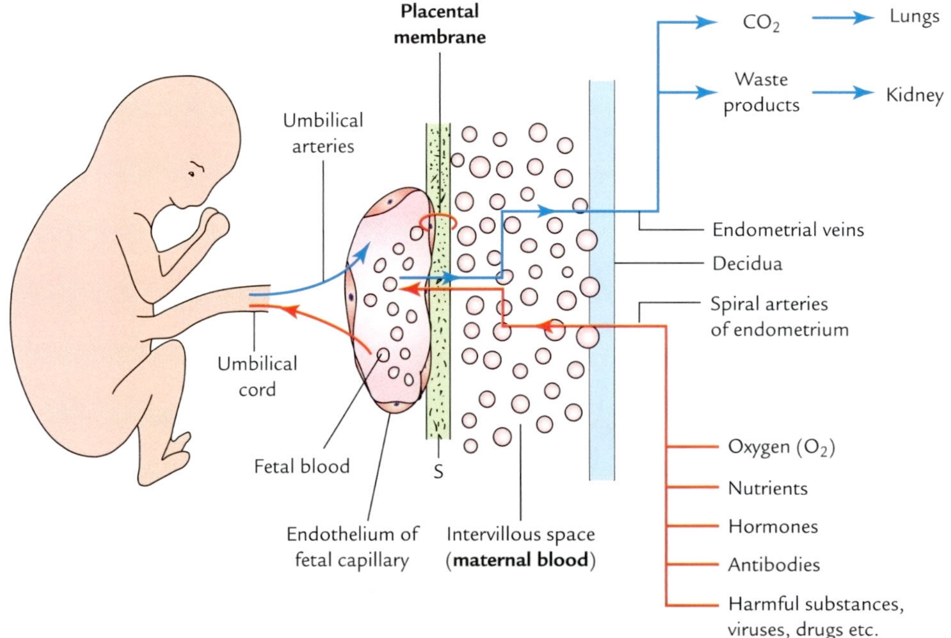

Fig. 10.14 Transport across the placental membrane. S, syncytiotrophoblast.

7. **Storage function:** It acts as a storage house for glycogen, calcium, and iron in early months of pregnancy. However, this function is taken over by liver soon.

Congenital Anomalies of the Placenta

The congenital anomalies of the placenta are grouped into three types:
(a) Anomalies due to abnormal adherence of chorionic villi to uterus.
(b) Anomalies due to abnormal shape.
(c) Anomalies due to abnormal site of attachment of umbilical cord.

A. Anomalies due to Abnormal Adherence of Chorionic Villi to Uterine Wall (Fig. 10.15)

1. **Placenta accreta**, if the chorionic villi are attached to endometrium.
2. **Placenta increta**, when chorionic villi penetrate the full thickness of myometrium.
3. **Placenta percreta**, if chorionic villi penetrate full thickness of myometrium and perimetrium (uterine serosa).

B. Anomalies due to Abnormal Shape (Fig. 10.16)

Normally, the placenta is circular and discoid/discoidal (circular disc shaped). The various anomalies of the shape of placenta are discussed as follows.
1. **Bilobed (bidiscoidal) placenta:** The placenta consists of two lobes.
2. **Multilobular placenta:** The placenta consists of more than two lobes.
3. **Diffuse placenta:** The placenta is thin and not disc shaped. It occurs when chorionic villi persist all around the blastocyst.

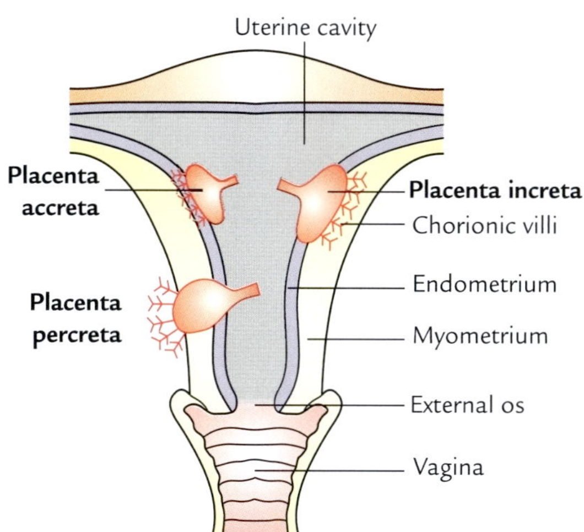

Fig. 10.15 Anomalies of placenta due to abnormal adherence of chorionic villi.

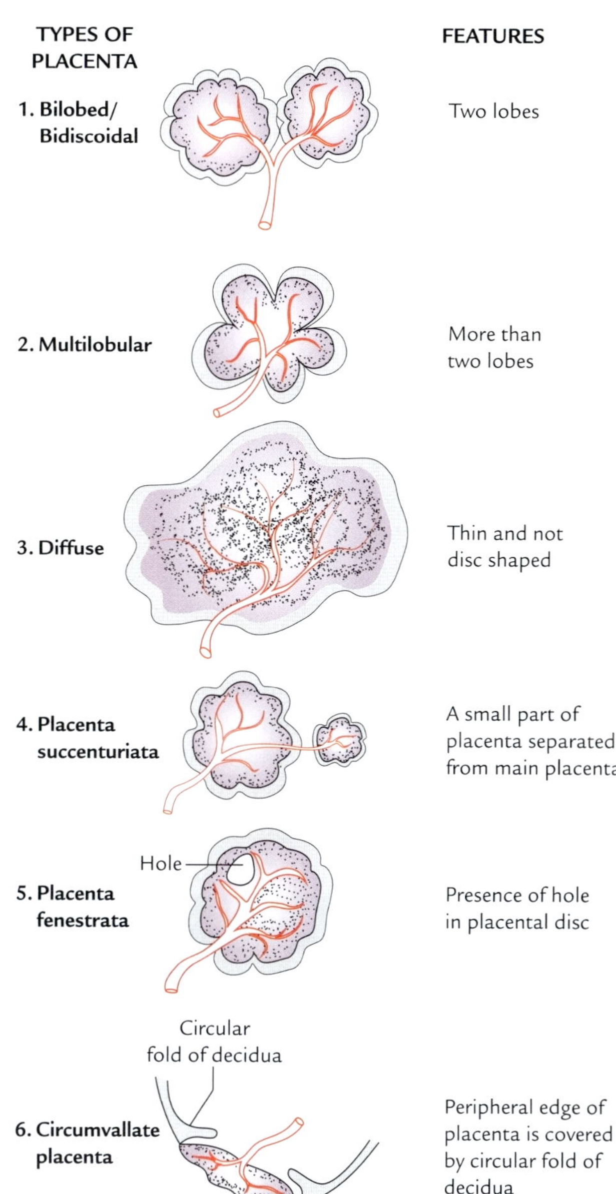

Fig. 10.16 Anomalies of placenta due to shape.

4. **Placenta succenturiata:** In this type, a small part of the placenta is separated from the main (rest) part of the placenta, but remains connected through blood vessels and placental membranes.
5. **Placenta fenestrata:** In this type, a hole is present in the placental disc.
6. **Circumvallate placenta:** In this type, the peripheral edge of the placenta is covered by a circular fold of the decidua.

C. Anomalies due to Abnormal Site of Attachment of Umbilical Cord (Fig. 10.17 C, D, and E)

Normally, the umbilical cord is attached to the center or within 3 cm from center of placenta on its fetal side.

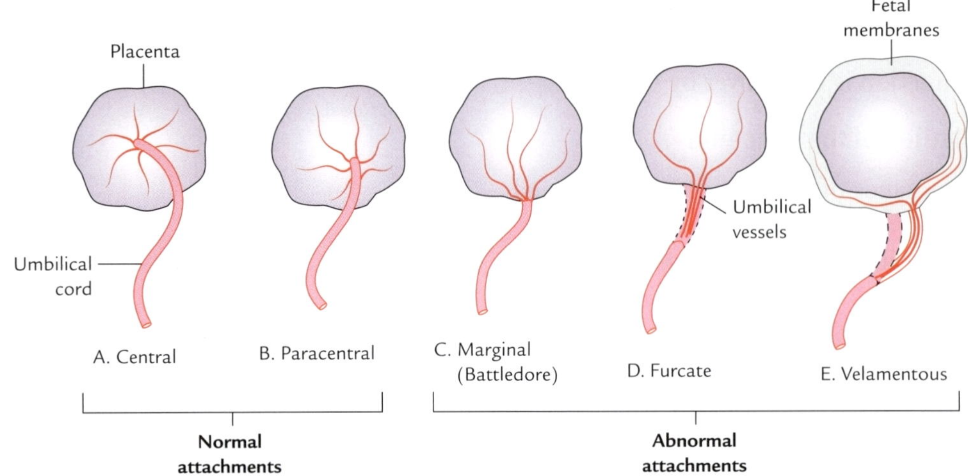

Fig. 10.17 Various types of umbilical cord attachment to placenta. Anomalies of placenta due to abnormal umbilical cord attachment are shown in Figures C, D, and E.

The various anomalies of placenta due to abnormal attachment of umbilical cord are as follows.

1. **Marginal (Battledore) placenta** (Fig. 10.17C): When the cord is attached to the margin of the placenta.
2. **Furcate placenta** (Fig. 10.17D): When blood vessels of umbilical cord divide before reaching the placenta.
3. **Velamentous placenta** (Fig. 10.17E): When the umbilical cord is attached to chorioamniotic blood vessels to proceed unprotected and ramify there before reaching the placenta.

N.B. Anomalies due to abnormal implantation of placenta in the uterine cavity, e.g., placenta previa (see p. 53).

CLINICAL CORRELATION

Erythroblastosis fetalis (hemolytic disease of the fetus) (Fig. 10.18)

If during pregnancy, the fetus is Rh +ve and mother is Rh –ve in such a case some fetal blood cells enter into maternal blood during parturition at the time of birth, and act as *antigen*. As a result, there occurs an **antigen–antibody response**, and antibodies are formed in the maternal blood. This baby will not be affected by these antibodies in the present case, but in subsequent pregnancies the maternal antibodies (against the fetal antigens) pass across the placenta into the fetus and cause breakdown of fetal red blood cells producing a clinical condition called **erythroblastosis fetalis** (or **hemolytic disease of the fetus**)

In most severe cases the baby dies in the womb due to severe anemia. However, in less severe cases, the baby is born with anemia, which can be treated with blood transfusion. Earlier the disease was called **erythroblastosis fetalis** because in some cases severe haemolysis stimulates the increased production of fetal blood cells, i.e. erythroblasts.

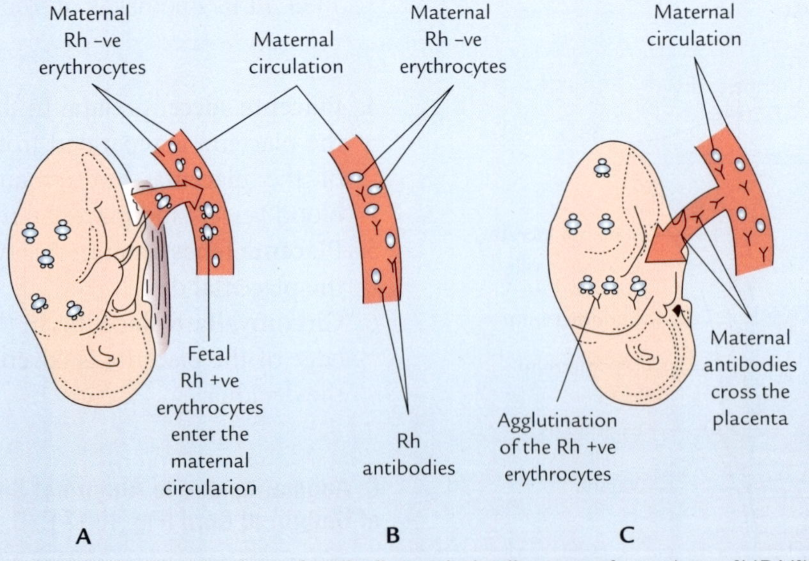

Fig. 10.18 Erythroblastosis fetalis (hemolytic disease of newborn [HDN]).

UMBILICAL CORD

AN 80.2, AN 80.7

The umbilical cord is a long (about 52 cm), twisted, cord-like structure by which fetus is attached to the mother (uterine wall via placenta). It connects umbilicus of a fetus to the center of fetal surface of the placenta, which is covered by glistening amniotic membrane (Fig. 10.19). The cord presents **false knots.** They are formed as the baby moves during pregnancy or delivery.

N.B. The umbilical cord has natural spiral twists, because the umbilical vein is longer than the umbilical arteries.

Measurements (At Full Term)

Length: 50–55 cm (about 2 feet)
Breadth: 1–2 cm

Development

The umbilical cord develops from connecting stalk (the part of extraembryonic mesoderm in which the extraembryonic coelom does not develop).

Initially, the mesodermal bar of connecting stalk is attached to the roof of amniotic cavity at one end and trophoblast at the other end (see Fig. 8.6).

Gradually, with the further development of embryo, it becomes narrower and moves to the caudal end of the embryo. Later with the formation of head and tail folds, it moves ventrally in the region of umbilicus (for details, see Fig. 8.6, p. 79). Now it connects the embryo with chorion. As the placenta develops the connecting stalk connects the fetus with the placenta.

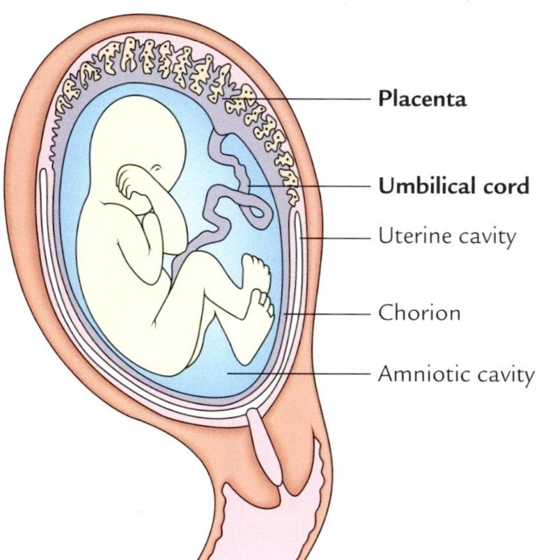

Fig. 10.19 Umbilical cord and well-developed placenta. Note amnion and chorion are fused.

The umbilical vessels develop in the connecting stalk during 3rd week of development and the extraembryonic mesoderm of connecting stalk undergoes mucoid degeneration to form a gelatinous substance called Wharton jelly. The Wharton jelly protects the umbilical vessels.

As the amniotic cavity enlarges, it obliterates the extraembryonic coelom and forms a tubular sleeve around the umbilical cord.

N.B. **Beaded appearance of umbilical cord:** The umbilical vessels are longer than the cord, and hence twisting and bending of vessels leads to beaded appearance of the umbilical cord.

Contents of Umbilical Cord (Fig. 10.20)

1. Two umbilical arteries
2. One umbilical vein (left umbilical vein)
3. Wharton jelly
4. Remains of allantoic diverticulum
5. Remains of vitellointestinal duct (remnant of yolk sac)

N.B. In early embryonic life, there are two umbilical veins. Thereafter, right vein disappears, and **left is left.**

In one out of 200 newborns, only **single umbilical artery** is present. These babies are often associated with cardiac anomalies.

Functions of Umbilical Cord

The **umbilical arteries** arising from ventral divisions of internal iliac **arteries carry deoxygenated blood from fetus to the placenta.** After oxygenation in the placenta, the **umbilical vein carries oxygenated blood from the placenta to the fetus.** Note **placenta is an organ of respiration in fetus.**

Types of Umbilical Cord Attachments to Placenta (Fig. 10.17)

These are:

1. **Central** (about 90%), when attached in the center, normal.

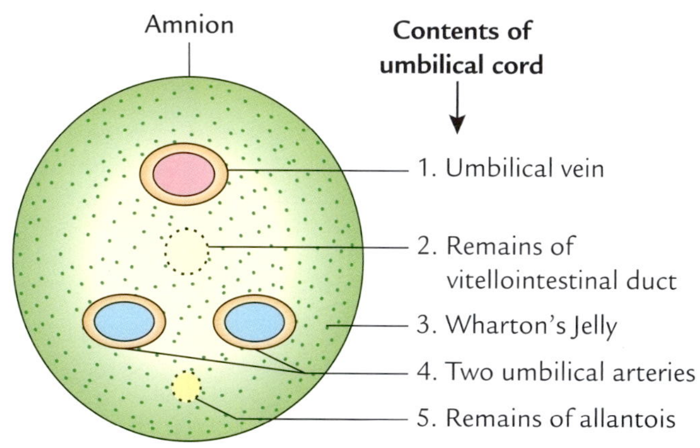

Fig. 10.20 Cross section of the umbilical cord.

2. **Eccentric/paracentral**, when attached, about 2 cm away from center of placenta, normal.
3. **Marginal (battledore)**, when attached on the margin (70%) of placenta.
4. **Furcate**, when blood vessels divide before reaching placenta.
5. **Velamentous**, when attached to chorioamniotic membranes.

CLINICAL CORRELATION

Complications of Umbilical Cord:

(a) ***Cord prolapse:*** If the cord is long, it is likely to prolapse through the uterus during parturition (childbirth), leading to a clinical condition called *cord prolapse*. In this condition, the cord is likely to be compressed between fetal head and pelvic wall of mother. This may lead to *hypoxia of the fetus*. If hypoxia persists for more than 5 min, it may damage fetal brain.

(b) ***Coiling of cord around fetal head:*** In about one-fifth of all deliveries, if the cord is long, it may *encircle the neck of the fetus and may cause strangulation*.

(c) ***Short cord and premature separation of placenta:*** A short cord may create difficulty in parturition by pulling the placenta, leading to its separation.

(d) ***Velamentous umbilical cord insertion with vasa previa:***

In velamentous cord insertion, the *umbilical vessels* are inserted into the chorioamniotic membrane, and hence travel between amnion and chorion toward placenta. The vessels are not protected by Wharton's jelly, hence *susceptible to compression and rupture*.

The velamentous cord insertion is very risky with vasa previa when exposed umbilical vessels cross cervix as they may rupture with membranes during labor (Fig. 10.21).

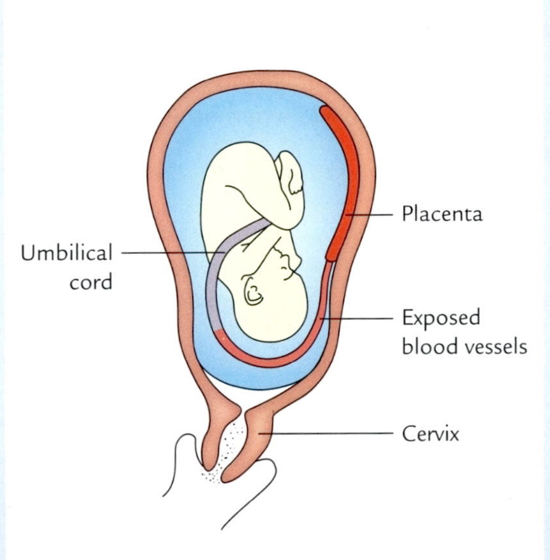

Fig. 10.21 Velamentous umbilical cord insertion with vasa previa.

MULTIPLE PREGNANCY

The pregnancy carrying more than one fetus is termed as multiple pregnancy (i.e., number of fetuses > 1).

Recently the incidence of multiple pregnancies has increased due to increased use of *in vitro* fertilization (IVF).

Classification: Multiple pregnancy is classified into following types depending on the number of fetus:

Number of Fetus	Type	Incidence
2	Twins	1:89
3	Triplets	$1:89^2$
4	Quadruplets	$1:89^3$
5	Quintuplets	$1:89^4$

Because the incidence of twins is quite common, the following description deals and discusses only twins.

Twins

Nurturing of two conceptuses/embryos/fetuses at the same time is termed as ***twinning*** (or twins).

Types of Twinning

There are two types of twins: (a) monozygotic and (b) dizygotic.

The arrangement of fetal membranes in twins varies considerably, depending on the type of twins.

Dizygotic (fraternal) twins (Fig. 10.22) AN 80.4

About two-thirds of twins are dizygotic (fraternal) twins. Their incidence increases with maternal age (7–10 per 1000 births).

They result from the fertilization of two different oocytes by two different sperms. The resultant two zygotes form two blastocysts – each of which implants separately into the uterine endometrium. These twins are not genetically alike. They do not look alike and can be of different sex. In such twins, the placenta, chorionic, and amniotic sacs are separate and independent. These twins have totally different genetic constitutions, they have no more resemblances than any other two brothers and sisters (siblings).

N.B. Sometimes two placentae are so close together that they fuse. In this condition, sometimes each dizygotic twin possesses two different types of red blood cells (**erythrocyte mosaicism**) because of exchange of red blood cells between two placentae.

- In humans, the **dizygotic twins** are more frequent than the **monozygotic twins** (3:1 ratio).
- In twin births, **twin boys are the most common**, next common are a boy and a girl, and least common are twin girls.

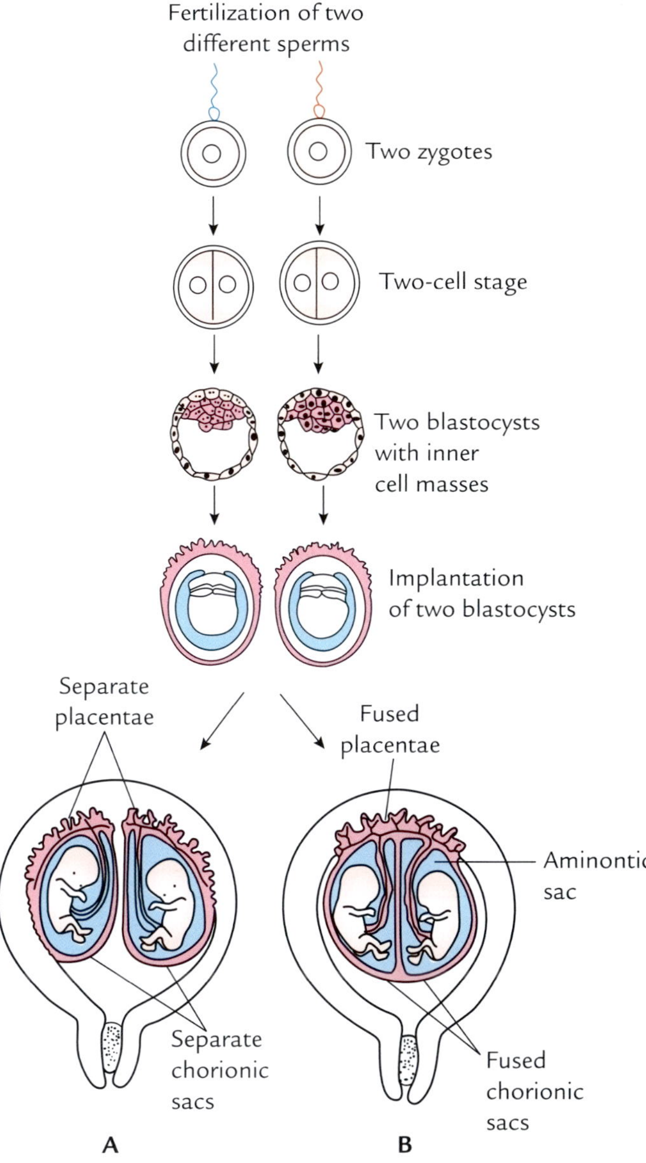

Fig. 10.22 Dizygotic twins. (A) Separate amniotic sacs, chorionic sacs, and placentae. (B) Fused chorionic sacs and placentae.

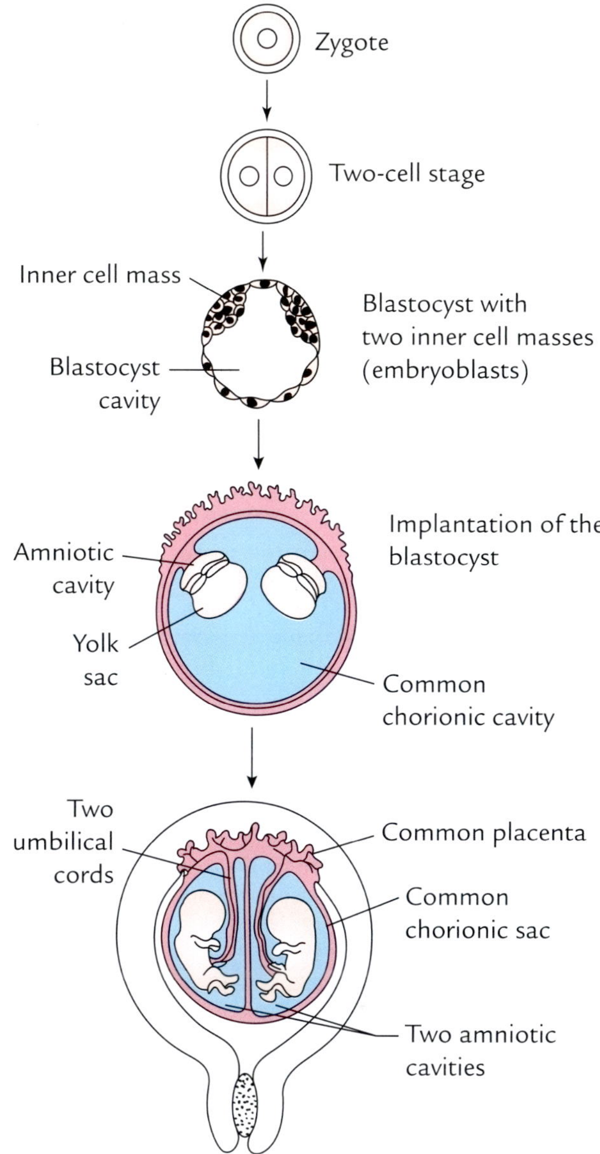

Fig. 10.23 Monozygotic twins.

Monozygotic (identical) twins (Fig. 10.23) AN 80.4

The monozygotic twins result from fertilization of one oocyte by one sperm. The resultant zygote forms a blastocyst in which inner cell mass (**embryoblast**) splits into two parts. Each part develop a separate embryo. Therefore, the monozygotic twins are genetically identical. These twins are of the same sex and look alike. They have *common chorionic and amniotic sacs*. The placenta is however one but with two umbilical cords.

Sometimes two independent placentae are formed, which may fuse with each other but do not have anastomosis of blood vessels.

N.B. The cells formed by first few mitotic divisions (cleavage) are totipotent, i.e., each cell is capable to form one embryo. If two cells of two-cell stage of cleavage separate, they develop independently. In this condition, the twins have separate amniotic and chorionic sacs as in dizygotic twins.

The zygote normally develops till morula stage. But when it is converted into blastocyst, two inner cell masses (two embryoblasts) form within it. Each of which develops into a separate fetus. In this condition, the two fetuses have a common placenta, but each lies in an independent amniotic sac.

The differences between the monozygotic and dizygotic twins are given in Table 10.2.

N.B. Twins have a high incidence of morbidity and mortality due to preeclampsia, congenital anomalies, premature delivery, etc.

Table 10.2 Differences between monozygotic and dizygotic twins

Monozygotic Twins	Dizygotic Twins
• Form from single zygote	Form from two zygotes
• Incidence is more common	Incidence is less common
• Genetically identical	Genetically not identical
• Twins are of the same sex	Twins are of the same sex or of different sex
• Resemblance is similar	Resemblance is just like any other two siblings
• Mostly have two amniotic sacs, one chorionic sac, with single placenta	Mostly have two amniotic sacs, two chorionic sacs, and two placentas
• Are often called conjoined twins	Not seen as conjoined twins

CLINICAL CORRELATION

Congenital Anomalies of Twins

1. ***Conjoint (Siamese) twins:*** This condition is seen in monozygotic twins. In this case, the inner cell mass (embryoblast) does not completely split, and hence two fetuses are joined to each other by a tissue bridge.

   Classification of conjoint twins: The conjoint twins are classified into following four types based on the site and extent of fusion (Fig. 10.24).

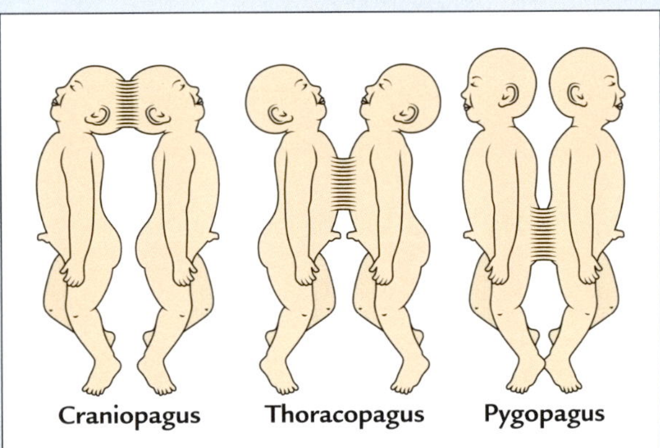

Fig. 10.24 Types of conjoined twins.

   (a) *Craniopagus:* Fusion of heads
   (b) *Thoracopagus:* Fusion of thorax
   (c) *Cephalothoracopagus:* Fusion of head and thorax
   (d) *Pygopagus:* Fusion of sacral regions

   The conjoint twins can be separated only if they have no vital parts in common.

N.B. Pagus = Fastened

2. ***Parasitic twin:*** When one member of identical conjoint twins remains rudimentary due to poor blood supply and grows like a parasite from the body of the well-developed co-twin, it is termed **parasitic twin** (Fig. 10.25).

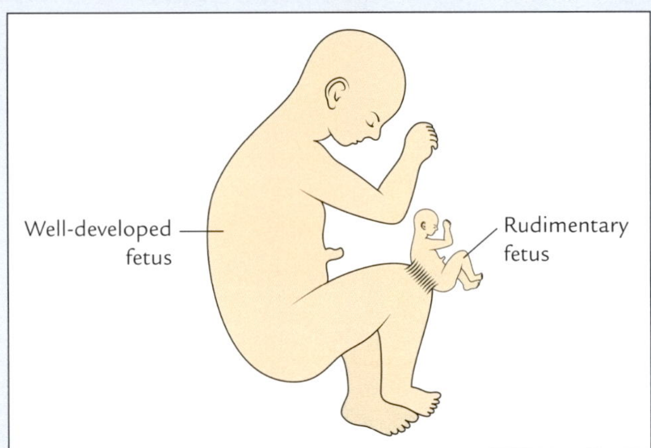

Fig. 10.25 Parasitic twins.

   Occasionally, the parasitic twin may be completely enclosed within the body of the co-twin. In this condition, the fetus is termed **fetus in fetu.**

3. ***Fetus papyraceous:*** It is a rare condition in which one member of twin dies and get compressed and mummified between the healthy growing fetus and uterine wall (Fig. 10.26).

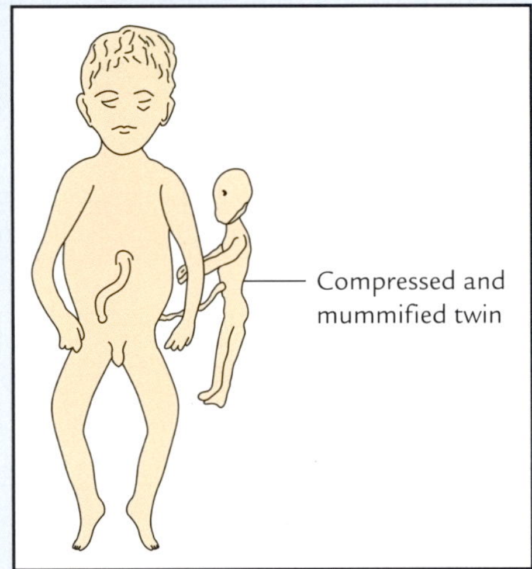

Fig. 10.26 Fetus papyraceous.

Clinical significance of multiple pregnancies

The risk of chromosomal anomalies and fetal mortality is higher in multiple pregnancies. The number of fetuses is directly proportional to the increase in risk.

GESTATIONAL AGE OF KEY DEVELOPMENTAL EVENTS

Developmental Event	Time of Occurrence
➢ Amnion	Day 8
➢ Yolk sac, chorion	Day 9
➢ Allantois	Day 16
➢ Placenta, connecting stalk, umbilical cord	Day 12
➢ Extraembryonic mesoderm	Day 12
➢ Extraembryonic coelom	Day 13
➢ Formation of primary villi	Day 12
➢ Secondary yolk sac	Day 14

GOLDEN FACTS TO REMEMBER

➢ **Bag of waters**	Double-walled chorioamniotic sac filled with amniotic fluid, which protects the fetus and breaks during birth releasing its fluid.
➢ **Decidua**	Uterine endometrium in a pregnant woman
➢ **Most unique feature of placenta**	Only organ that develops from two different individuals (mother and fetus)
➢ **Three main functions of placenta**	(a) Transport of gases and nutrients (b) Metabolism (e.g., synthesis of glycogen) (c) Endocrine secretion (e.g., human chorionic gonadotropin, etc.)
➢ **Number of cotyledons in fully developed placenta**	15–20
➢ **Weight of placenta at full term**	500 g
➢ **Total surface area of placental membrane**	14 m^2 (i.e., equal to absorptive area of the gastrointestinal tract)
➢ **Langer's layer**	Cytotrophoblast
➢ **Syncytiotrophoblast**	Multinucleated mass of cells derived from trophoblast
➢ **Following the birth of a baby the placenta is shed off**	After about half an hour
➢ **Definitive placenta is formed at the end of**	Second month of intrauterine life (IUL)
➢ **Hyrtl's anastomosis**	Only anastomosis between two umbilical arteries

CLINICAL PROBLEM SOLVING

PROBLEMS

1. An ultrasound of a pregnant woman with 7 months of gestation revealed **excessive accumulation of fluid in the amniotic cavity. Name the clinical condition and give its embryological basis.**
2. **Thyrotoxic mothers give birth to babies with normal thyroid function.** Why? Give the embryological basis.
3. **Pregnant women are advised not to take drugs during pregnancy without prescription by a specialist.** They are also advised to avoid cigarette, smoking, and ingestion of alcohol during pregnancy. Why?
4. In what condition, the **leakage of fetal blood** or **syncytial tissue** in the mother may lead to immune responses such as **erythroblastosis fetalis**? Explain in detail.
5. Out of following two techniques: **amniocentesis and chorionic villus biopsy**, which technique can detect genetic disorder in fetus earlier?
6. **The fetus possesses paternal antigens, which should act as foreign antigens to the tissue of the uterine wall of the mother, but mother tolerates these antigens of fetus until pregnancy reaches the full term. Why?**

SOLUTIONS

1. The **excessive accumulation of amniotic fluid** in the amniotic sac is called **polyhydramnios** (or hydramnios). This clinical condition occurs due to esophageal atresia and CNS defects (anencephaly) because of which fetus is unable to swallow the amniotic fluid. The high incidence of polyhydramnios (25%) is noted in diabetic mothers. In 35% cases, the cause is not known.
2. This is because the **placental membrane** acts as a **barrier** for the passage of maternal hormones such as ACTH and TSH into the fetal blood.
3. This is because alcohol and certain drugs such as thalidomide, phenytoin, diazepam, etc., can cross the placental barrier and cause congenital anomalies in the fetus.

   Alcohol consumption and cigarette smoking may be hazardous for embryo. Smoking may be responsible for the low birth weight, and alcohol may be responsible for certain congenital anomalies such as mental retardation, microcephaly, etc.
4. Erythroblastosis fetalis/hemolytic disease of newborn. For details see p. 106.
5. Both these techniques are used to detect the genetic disorders such as **Down syndrome** by examining the chromosomes in the fetal cells. The **amniocentesis** is usually performed at the **14th or 15th week of pregnancy** to obtain the amniotic fluid. The **chorionic villus biopsy** is a technique used to detect the genetic disorder much earlier than amniocentesis permits. The chorionic villus biopsy can provide genetic information at **10 to 12 weeks of gestation.**
6. The mother does not reject the fetus because maternal tissue fails to recognize HLA antigens of trophoblastic cells as the entire trophoblastic shell is covered or coated by the layer of **fibrinoid material (Nitabuch layer). The fibrinoid material is negatively charged and hence repels the negatively charged material lymphocytes.**

11 Integumentary System and Mammary Glands

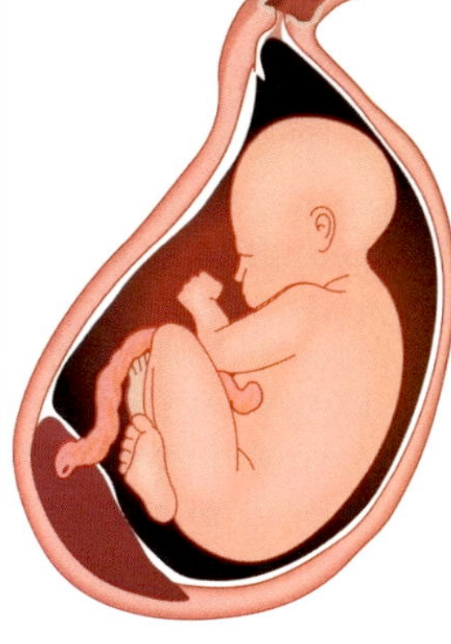

LEARNING OBJECTIVES

After studying this chapter, the student should be able to:

- Describe the development of various layers of skin.
- Describe **vernix caseosa** and its functional significance.
- Discuss the formation of **epidermal ridges** and **dermal papillae** and their functional significance.
- Define **dermatoglyphics** and enumerate the four basic types of dermatoglyphic patterns of the digits.
- Define the skin and its appendages. AN 72.1
- Describe the development of breast (mammary gland) and discuss its various congenital anomalies. AN 9.3

DEVELOPMENT OF SKIN AND ITS APPENDAGES

OVERVIEW

The **skin and its appendages** (sebaceous glands, sweat glands, hair, and nails) constitute the **integumentary system.** The skin is the largest organ of the body and covers more than 76,000 cm^2 (300 $inches^2$) of the body surface of an average adult. It consists of two layers: a superficial layer (the **epidermis**) and a deep layer (the **dermis** or **corium**).

The skin develops from two sources: (a) the **epidermis** develops from surface ectoderm and (b) the **dermis** develops from the underlying mesoderm. In addition to the above two sources, the melanoblasts (dendritic cells) of epidermis develop from the **neural crest cells.**

The **appendages of skin** (e.g., sebaceous and sweat glands, hair, and nails) are derived from the epidermis.

Development of Skin

The skin develops from two main sources, viz. surface ectoderm and underlying mesoderm.

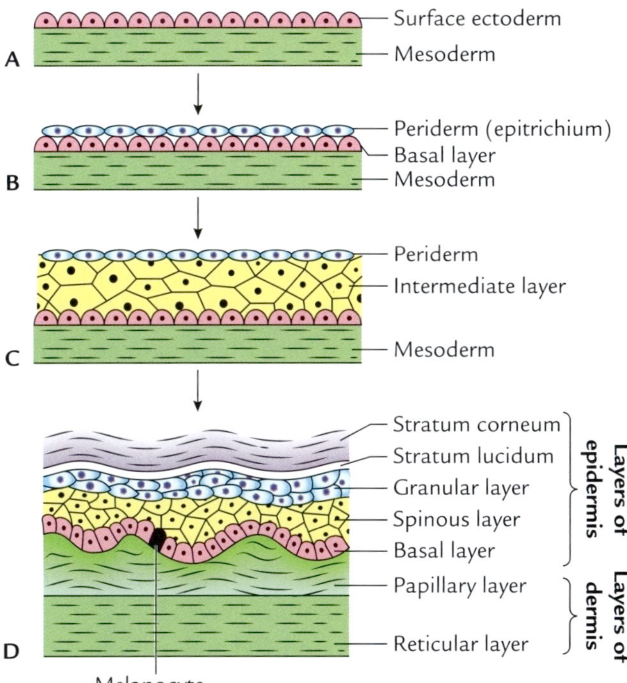

Fig. 11.1 Stages of development of skin.

Epidermis (Fig. 11.1)

The epidermis develops from surface ectoderm. Initially, the surface ectoderm consists of a single layer of cells (Fig. 11.1A). In the 2nd month, these cells proliferate and form a second layer of flattened cells called **periderm/epitrichium.**

The epidermis now consists of two layers: superficial layer of flattened cells (**periderm**) and deep layer of cuboidal cells (**basal layer**) (Fig. 11.1B).

The cells of periderm are cast off during 2nd month of intrauterine life (IUL).

With further proliferation of cells in the basal layer, a third **intermediate layer** is formed (Fig. 11.1C).

The **basal layer** functions as a germinative layer and is called **stratum germinativum**. The cells of the basal layer proliferate and differentiate to form the various layers (strata) of the epidermis.

Formation of Four Layers of Epithelium

At the end of 4th month, the **epidermis** consists of four layers. From deep to superficial, these four layers are

1. **Basal layer (stratum germinativum)**
2. **Spinous layer (stratum spinosum)**
3. **Granular layer (stratum granulosum)**
4. **Horny layer (stratum corneum).**

N.B. The cells of **periderm** undergo *keratinization* to form stratum corneum and *desquamation* to form **vernix caseosa**.

1. The **basal layer** consists of columnar cells. These cells constantly divide mitotically and move superficially to renew the epidermis approximately in every 27 days.
2. The **spinous layer** consists of numerous irregular prickle cells (cells with spine-like processes).
3. The **granular layer** consists of three or four rows of flattened cells. The cytoplasm of the cells of the granular layer contains *keratohyalin granules* as a result of keratinization.

   The cells superficial to granular layer are cells with scanty nuclei and form a homogeneous layer called **stratum lucidum.** Histologically, this layer appears clear. It exists only in lips and thick skin of the soles and palms.
4. The **horny layer** consists of several layers of flattened scale-like cells that are continuously shed off.

The **melanoblasts** (**dendritic cells**) derived from neural crest invade the basal layer during the 3rd month of IUL and soon become melanocytes. They synthesize melanin pigments and provide color to skin and hair.

N.B. The periderm disappears when the stratum corneum is formed.

Formation of epidermal ridges and dermal papillae

The stratum germinativum of epidermis proliferates and projects into the dermis to form **epidermal ridges.** The parts of dermis projecting between the epidermal ridges are called **dermal papillae** (Fig. 11.2).

The epidermal ridges and dermal papillae interlock with each other at junction of epidermis and dermis (dermoepidermal junction). As a result of this interlocking, the surfaces of pulp of fingertips produce epidermal ridges. These ridges produce **fingerprints.**

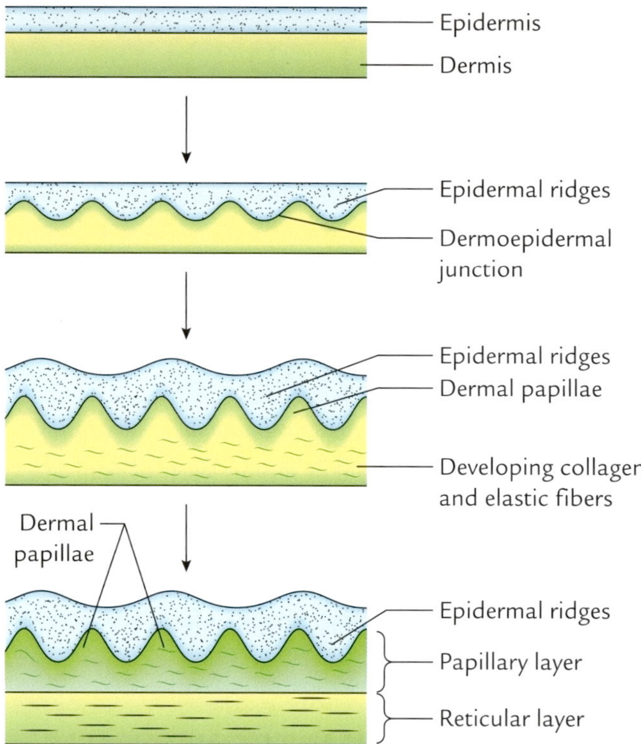

Fig. 11.2 Formation of epidermal ridges and dermal papillae.

CLINICAL CORRELATION

Fingerprints: These are impressions of ectodermal ridges on the tips of fingers and toes which form the typical patterns, the development of which is genetically controlled and these patterns are unique for each individual including identical twins. This forms the basis of personal identification from the fingerprints for the **medicolegal purpose.** In children with chromosomal abnormalities, the ectodermal patterns on the hands and fingers are used as a diagnostic tool. For example, these patterns are abnormal in mongolism or **trisomy 21.**

The study of **epidermal ridge pattern** is called **dermatoglyphics** and it can be used as one of the diagnostic tools in various genetic disorders.

The four basic types of dermatoglyphic patterns in the digits are (Fig. 11.3): (a) **arch**, (b) **whorl**, (c) **loop**, and (d) **composite** (i.e., combination of earlier three patterns).

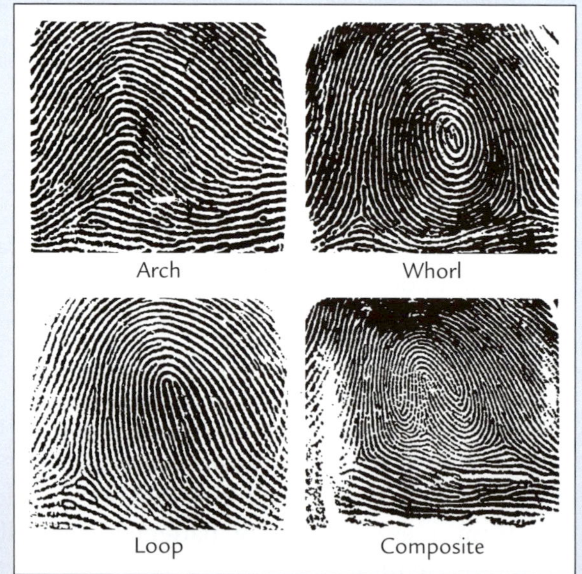

Fig. 11.3 Four basic types of dermatoglyphic patterns on the tips of fingers.

Dermis

The **dermis** develops from mesenchyme lying underneath the surface ectoderm. This mesenchyme is derived from three sources: (a) paraxial mesoderm, (b) somatopleuric layer of lateral plate mesoderm, and (c) neural crest cells.

The mesenchymal cells differentiate into connective tissue cells that form **connective tissue fibers** (collagen and elastic fibers) and amorphous **ground substance** of the connective tissue.

During the 3rd and 4th months, dermis forms many irregular ridges called dermal papillae, which project into the epidermis and interdigitate with the **epidermal ridges**. The dermis differentiates into two layers:

1. Superficial papillary layer
2. Deeper reticular layer

Most of the dermal papillae of **papillary layer** of dermis contain a small loop of capillary plexus and a sensory receptor (sensory nerve end organ). The loops of capillary plexus provide nourishment to the epidermis and to the sensory nerve end organ.

The deeper reticular layer of dermis contains large amount of fatty tissue.

The blood vessels in the dermis develop initially as endothelium-lined structures that differentiate from the mesenchyme. These primordial vessels give rise to the capillaries (**angiogenesis**). The angiogenesis of the dermis is completed by the end of the first trimester of pregnancy.

CLINICAL CORRELATION

1. ***Ichthyosis*** (Gr. ***Ichthys*** = fish): It is a clinical condition characterized by dryness of skin with fish-like scaling in part of or entire body. It occurs due to excessive keratinization of the skin.
   In severe cases, ichthyosis may result in a **grotesque appearance**, e.g., **harlequin fetus**.
2. ***Albinism:*** It is a clinical condition characterized by reduced or absence of pigmentation in the skin, hair, and eyes (retina lacks pigment; however, iris usually shows some pigmentation). In most cases, it occurs due to abnormal synthesis of melanin by the melanocytes.

N.B. The generalized albinism is an autosomal recessive disorder, whereas localized albinism is autosomal dominant disorder.

3. ***Vitiligo:*** It is a clinical condition characterized by patchy loss of pigmentation in the skin and overlying hair. It results from loss of melanocytes due to an autoimmune disorder.

Development of Hair (Fig. 11.4)

The hairs or pili (L. ***Pilus*** = hair) begin to develop early in the fetal life (7–12 weeks).

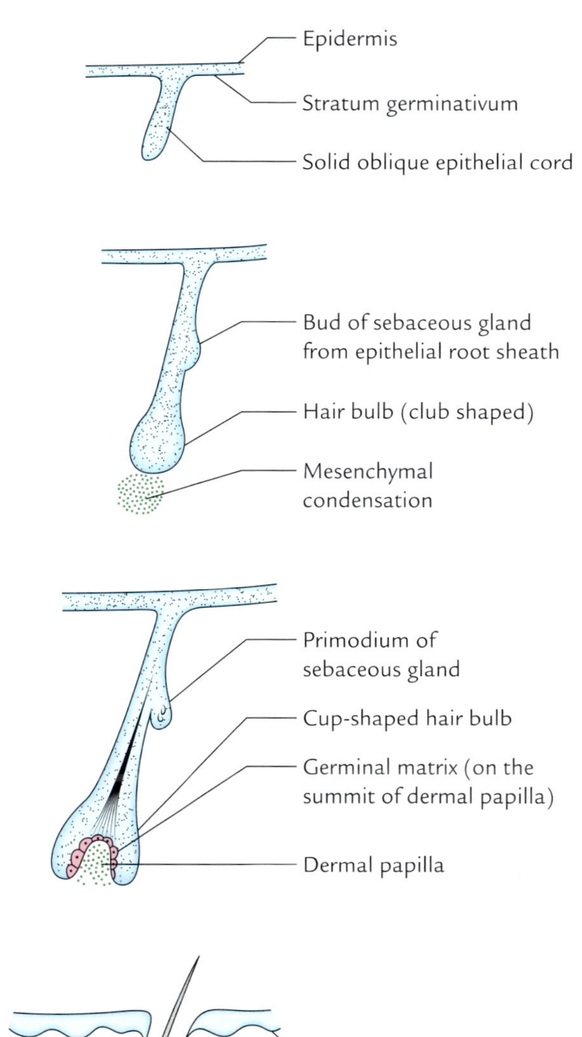

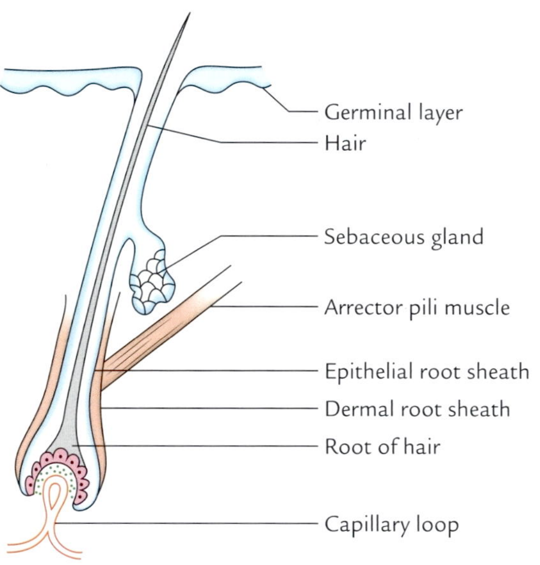

Fig. 11.4 Development of hair.

Each hair develops from downgrowth of the epidermis into underlying dermis. The cells of the stratum germinativum proliferate to form a solid epithelial cord that extends obliquely downward in the dermis to form **hair bud**. The terminal part of the hair bud becomes club shaped and forms the **hair bulb**. It is invaginated by the mesenchymal condensation of the dermis and the hair bulb now becomes **inverted cup-shaped structure**. The dermis within the cup-shaped hair bulb is called **dermal papilla**. The cells of the hair bulb at the summit of dermal papilla form the **germinal matrix** that later produces hair.

The peripheral cells of developing hair follicle form **epithelial root sheath**. The dermis condenses around this sheath to form **dermal root sheath**.

The cells of the germinal matrix proliferate to form **root of the hair**. As the root grows, it is pushed outside the hair follicle on the surface of skin as a **shaft of the hair**. The root and shaft of hair become keratinized.

The melanoblasts migrate into the hair bulbs and differentiate into **melanocytes**. Melanin formed by these melanocytes is transferred to proliferating cells of the germinal matrix. This melanin is responsible for the color of hair.

First hairs that appear are fine, soft, lightly pigmented, and silky. They help to hold the vernix caseosa on the skin surface. These hairs are called **lanugo**.

The lanugos (downy hairs) are replaced by **coarser hairs** during the perinatal period, which persists over most of the body except in axillary and pubic regions where they are replaced at puberty by even coarser **terminal hair**. In men, similar coarse hairs appear on the face (e.g., moustache and beard) and often on the chest.

The **definitive hair** grows to a certain length and then cease to grow, e.g., hairs of eyelashes, eyebrows, pubic, and axillary regions.

At certain sites, e.g., scalp of males and females and the face of males, the hair grows continuously throughout life. These are called **angora**.

Arrector Muscle of Hair (Arrector Pili Muscle)

The small bundle of smooth muscle fibers differentiate from the mesenchyme surrounding the hair follicle usually on one side. They attach the dermal root sheath of hair follicle and papillary layer of the dermis to form **arrector pili muscle**. The contraction of arrector pili muscles causes **goose bumps**.

CLINICAL CORRELATION

1. ***Hypertrichosis*** (excessive hairiness) results due to unusual abundance of hair follicles or due to excessive hair growth either in small isolated area, especially over lower lumbar region covering a spina bifida occulta defect, or all over the body.
2. ***Congenital alopecia/atrichia*** (absence or loss of hair) may occur alone but usually associated with other abnormalities of epithelial derivatives, viz. **teeth** and **nails**.

Glands of the Skin

There are two types of glands in the skin: sebaceous glands and sweat glands. Both these types of glands are derived from the epidermis and grow into the dermis.

Sebaceous Glands (Fig. 11.4)

The sebaceous gland develops as a **bud from the epithelial root sheath of hair follicle**. The bud grows into the surrounding dermis and divides into a number of branches to form primordia of several alveoli and their associated ducts. The cells in the center of alveoli (acini) degenerate to produce an oily secretion called **sebum**. It is released into the hair follicle and from here it passes to the surface of the skin.

It mixes with desquamated peridermal cells to form greasy material – the **vernix caseosa** covering the body of fetus.

Sweat Glands (Fig. 11.5)

The sweat glands are of two types: **eccrine** and **apocrine**.

Eccrine sweat glands are found in the skin of most parts of the body. The *eccrine sweat gland* develops before birth as downgrowth of the epidermis into the underlying dermis. The cells of stratum germinativum proliferate to form a solid mass of epithelial cells that extend downward in the underlying dermis to form the bud of sweat gland. This downgrowth elongates and its terminal part becomes coiled. Later this solid downgrowth is canalized to form lumen. The terminal coiled part of downgrowth forms *secretory part of the sweat gland*, whereas the proximal straight part forms *duct of the sweat gland*. The site of beginning of downgrowth from the surface epithelium forms *pore of the duct of the sweat gland*. The eccrine sweat glands start functioning shortly after birth.

Apocrine sweat glands are found in the axilla, pubic, and perineal regions, and areolae of nipples. *They begin to develop during puberty*. They develop from same epidermal buds that form the hair follicles. Consequently, these glands open into the hair follicles instead of opening on the skin surface.

N.B. The sweat produced by apocrine sweat glands contains **lipids**, **proteins**, and **pheromones**. The odor produced from these sweat glands is due to breakdown of these products. It is thought to act as a **sexual attractant**.

The difference between eccrine and apocrine sweat glands is given in Table 11.1.

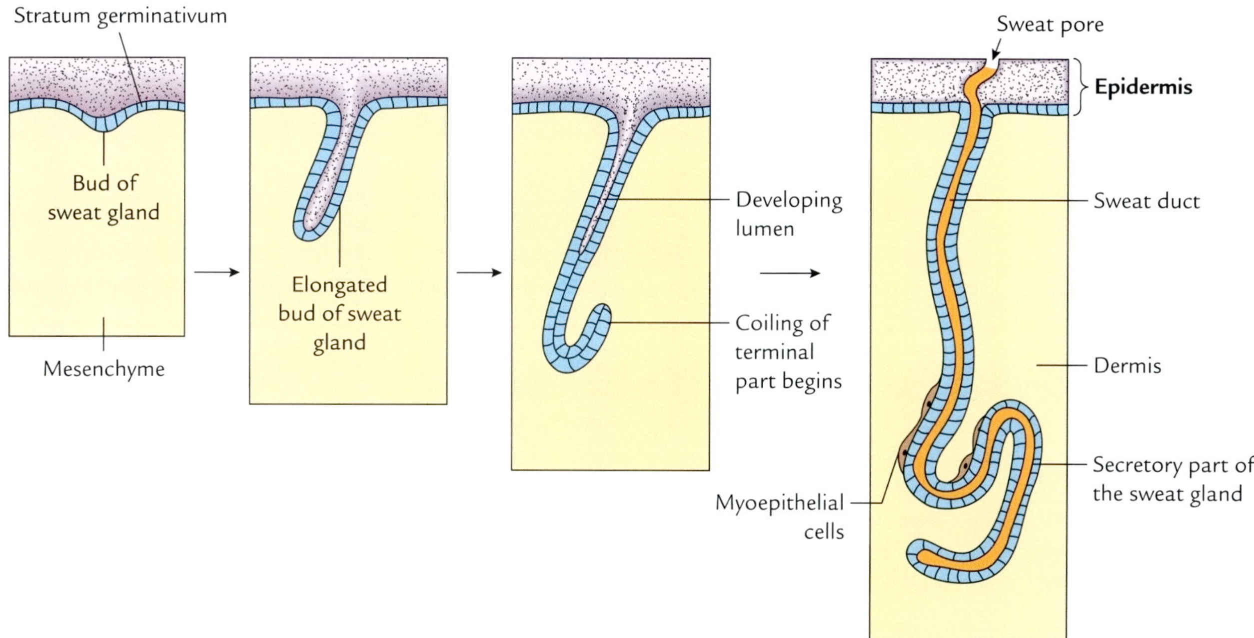

Fig. 11.5 Development of sweat glands.

Table 11.1 Difference between eccrine and apocrine sweat glands

Eccrine Sweat Gland	Apocrine Sweat Gland
• Found over most parts of the body	• Confined to axilla, pubic, and perineal regions, and areolae of the nipples
• Develops before birth	• Develops after birth at puberty
• Develops directly from surface epithelium	• Develops from epidermal bud that produces hair follicle
• Pours its secretion directly on the skin surface	• Pours its secretion in the hair follicles just above the opening of sebaceous gland
• Secretes by merocrine mechanism (exocytosis)	• Secretes by apocrine mechanism (a portion of secretory cells is shed/pinched off and incorporated into the secretion)
• Secretion is watery and involved in temperature control	• Secretion is thick and produces an odor that acts as a sexual attractant

Vernix Caseosa

It is a white greasy substance which covers the body of fetus. The vernix caseosa is formed by the exfoliation of peridermal cells and oily secretions of sebaceous glands.

Functions

1. Protection of fetal skin from toxic substances of urine within amniotic fluid.
2. Facilitates the process of parturition.

Development of Nails (Fig. 11.6)

The nail develops on the tips of fingers approximately at 10 weeks of IUL, whereas on toenails at 14 weeks of IUL.

Initially, the ectoderm at the tip of each digit thickens to form primordium of nail – the **primary nail field.** Subsequently, these nail fields migrate onto the dorsal aspect of terminal parts of the digits carrying their innervation from the nerves of ventral aspect. The nail fields are now surrounded proximally and laterally by U-shaped fold of ectoderm – the **nail folds**. The formation of nail fold defines certain structures in the terminal part of the digit-like **nail groove** and **nail bed.**

The cells of germinal layer at the base of proximal nail groove proliferate to form a thick layer of cells called **germinal matrix.**

The cells of germinal matrix proliferate, get keratinized, and form **nail plate**, which corresponds to the stratum lucidum of the epidermis. With continued proliferation of germinal matrix, the nail plate grows and slides over the nail bed. With the formation of the nail plate, the part of epidermis overlapping proximal part of the developing nail is called **eponychium**. This eponychium degenerates and exposes the nail, except at its base where it persists as cuticle. The epidermis below free margin of the nail is called **hyponychium**. The part of the nail in the groove is called **root of the nail.**

Points to Note

- The development of fingernails precedes that of toenails by approximately 4 weeks.

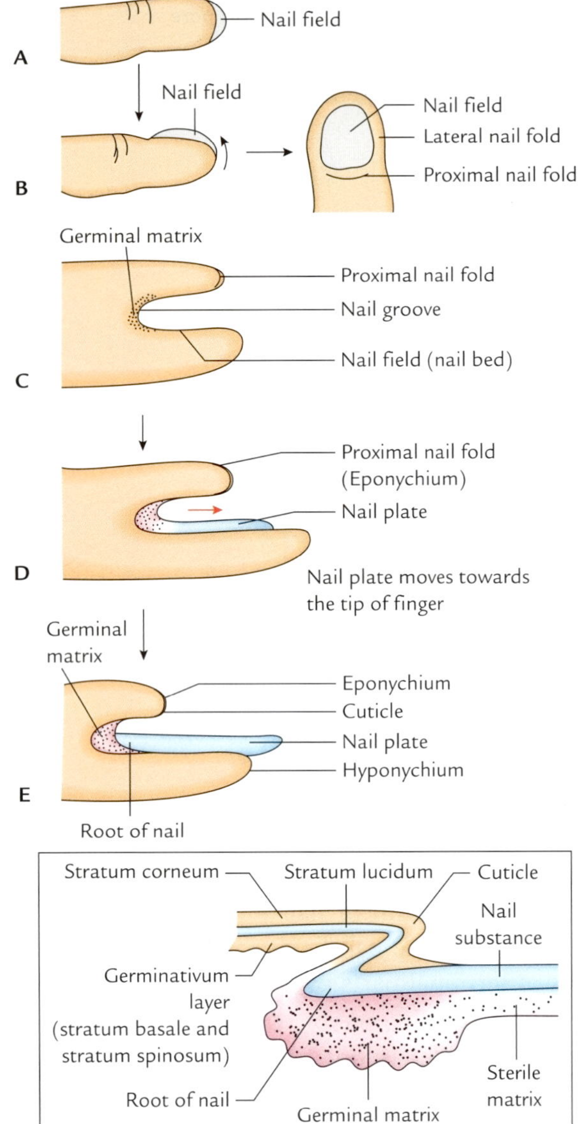

Fig. 11.6 Stages of development of a fingernail. Figure in the inset shows the detailed structure. Note that fingernail reaches the end of the finger by 32 weeks (8 months).

- The fingernails grow at the rate of about 1 mm per week; the growth rate of toenails is somewhat slower.
- The fingernails reach the fingertips at about 32 weeks. The toe nails reach the toe tips at about 36 weeks.
- The growth area of the nail is **nail matrix**, which is exhibited on the surface as **lunula** (half-moon-shaped area) at the base of the nail.

N.B. Morphologically, the nail substance corresponds to the **stratum lucidum**.

CLINICAL CORRELATION

Anonychia (absence of nails at birth): It is extremely rare and occurs due to failure of **nail fields** to form or failure of the proximal nail fold to form **nail plates**. Anonychia may be restricted to one or more nails.

DEVELOPMENT OF MAMMARY GLANDS (FIG. 11.7)

OVERVIEW

The fully developed mammary glands are located on the front of female chest. They are responsible for production of milk to feed the baby. Both males and females possess rudimentary mammary glands at birth, but in females they develop into two hemispherical bulges at/after puberty under the influence of estrogen. However, it remains rudimentary in males.

The breasts are secondary sexual organs in females.

The mammary glands are modified and **specialized apocrine sweat glands** and therefore develop from the surface ectoderm as follows:

- In the 4th week, the surface ectoderm thickens on either side of the ventral aspect of the embryo along the line extending from the axilla to the upper part of the thigh. Just below the inguinal region to form **mammary ridge line** or **milk ridge/line.**
- About 15–20 **mammary buds** develop as solid downgrowth of the epidermis into the underlying mesenchyme along the mammary ridge on each side.
- Normally, the mammary ridge and associated mammary buds disappear, except in the pectoral region.
- In the pectoral region, the mammary bud presents a surface depression called **mammary pit.**
- About 15–20 epithelial cords grow inwards from the bottom of the pit into the underlying dermis. The epithelial cords are **primordia of lactiferous ducts.**
- The deeper ends of the epithelial cords subdivide further and terminate as ampullated ends – the **primordia of ductules and alveoli.**
- At the end of fetal life, the epithelial cords and their branches are canalized and form lactiferous ducts.
- Initially, the lactiferous ducts open into the bottom of the mammary pit.
- Shortly before birth, the pit is evaginated by the growth of underlying mesoderm and forms the nipple.
- The full development of breasts occurs at about 19 years of age.

The growth in size of breast at puberty occurs due to the growth of its ducts and secretory acini. The proliferation of adipose tissue adds to its size and smooth rounded contour.

N.B. In some animals, e.g., **bitches**, a series of mammary glands develop on either side of midline on the ventral aspect of the trunk (**polymastia**).

The polymastia is common in lower mammals. Its persistence in human is an example of **atavism**.

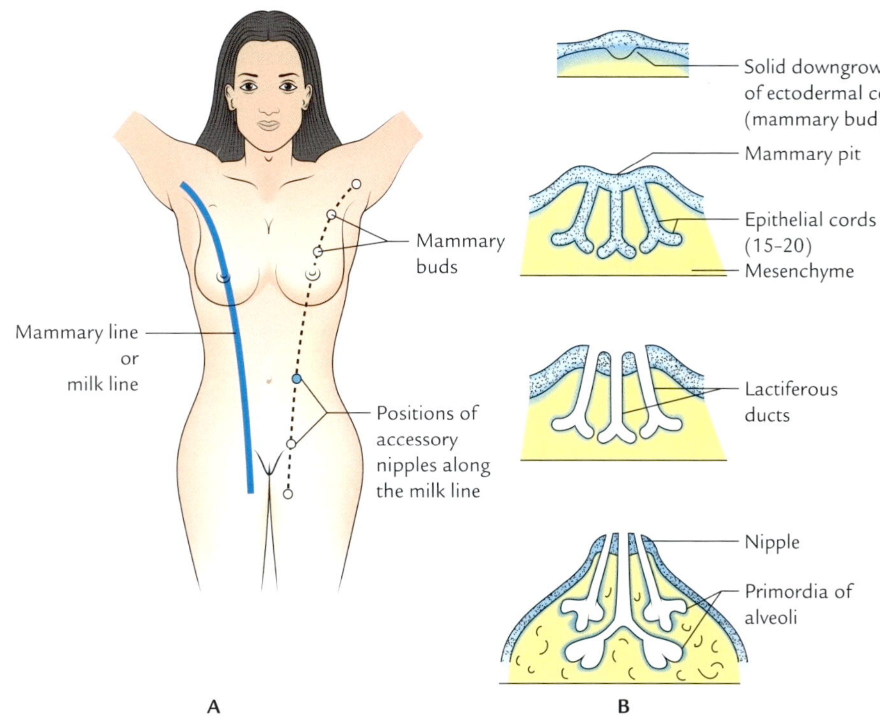

Fig. 11.7 Development of mammary gland. (A) Mammary ridge (left side) and positions of accessory nipples (right side). (B) Stages of development of mammary glands.

CLINICAL CORRELATION

Developmental (congenital) anomalies of the mammary glands

1. ***Amastia (absence of breast) and athelia*** (absence of nipple): This condition occurs due to failure of formation of mammary ridge or failure of formation of mammary bud. Clinically, it presents as the absence of breast on one or both sides. Bilateral complete absence of mammary glands is a rare anomaly.
2. ***Polythelia (presence of supernumerary nipples):*** They may be found along the milk line/ridge, but are most commonly seen in the region of axilla.
3. ***Polymastia (accessory breasts):*** In 1% to 5% cases, accessory breast develops from buds along the milk line/ridge. The occurrence of accessory breasts is less common than polythelia.
4. ***Inverted (or crater) nipple:*** It occurs due to failure of evagination of the mammary pit. In such a case, lactiferous ducts open into a pit causing **difficulty in suckling**.

GESTATIONAL AGE OF KEY DEVELOPMENTAL EVENTS

Developmental Event	Gestational Age
➢ Epiderm/epitrichium	2nd month
➢ Four-layered epidermis	3rd month
➢ Dermal papilla	3rd and 4th months
➢ Ectodermal mammary ridge/ milk line	4 weeks
➢ Full development of breast	19 years

GOLDEN FACTS TO REMEMBER

➢ **Dermatoglyphics**	Study of the patterns of the epidermal ridges on the tips of digits and toes
➢ **Most important factor responsible for different skin color**	Amount of melanin in skin in different individuals
➢ **Milk ridge**	Ectodermal ridge extending from axillary region to the inguinal region
➢ **First evidence of development of breast**	Development of ectodermal milk ridge
➢ **Most common site of accessory/ supernumerary nipples**	Region of axilla
➢ **Witch milk/ neonatal milk**	Milk expelled from mammary gland of newborn (both sexes)
➢ **Full development of breast in female occurs at the age of**	19 years

CLINICAL PROBLEM SOLVING

PROBLEMS

1. **Although the developing fetal skin is constantly exposed to amniotic fluid, which has high urine content, it is still not affected.** Why?
2. **What is nevus?** Give its embryological basis.
3. **What is witch milk?** Give its embryological basis.
4. **What is gynecomastia?** Give its embryological/anatomical basis.
5. **An adult female has an accessory breast in her axilla.** Give its embryological basis.

SOLUTIONS

1. Because the fetal body (skin) is covered by vernix caseosa (L. *Vernix* = Varnish), a white creamy biofilm.
2. The nevus is a birthmark that appears at birth or shortly thereafter. The nevus occurs due to persistence of some primitive blood capillaries. There are three main types of nevi: (a) capillary nevus, (b) strawberry nevus, and (c) port-wine nevus.
   - **Capillary nevus** is a flat pink or pinkish-brown area.
   - **Strawberry nevus** is a bright red raised area up to 10 cm (4 inches) across.
   - **Port-wine nevus** is a purplish-red area, often extensive, which occurs singly on the face or neck (Fig. 11.8).
3. The rudimentary mammary glands of newborns are often enlarged and secrete some milk called **witch milk**. This occurs due to action of maternal hormones that cross the placental barrier and affect the developing fetal breasts.
4. The **gynecomastia** is a clinical condition where rudimentary mammary glands in males may increase in size as in females and may even secrete milk (Gr. *Gyne* = woman + *Mastos* = breast) (Fig. 11.9). It occurs due to the development of rudimentary lactiferous ducts into male mammary tissue. During mid-puberty, about two-thirds of boys present varying degrees of gynecomastia. It is caused by decreased ratio of testosterone to estradiol.
5. The mammary gland (breast) develops from a bud arising from **mammary ridge** in the pectoral region. Occasionally, a mammary bud might develop at an accessory site along the mammary ridge, usually in the axillary region. It is called **accessory breast**.

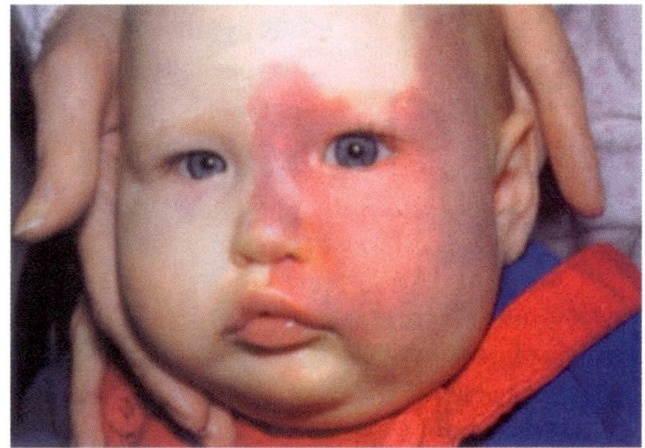

Fig. 11.8 Port-wine nevus in an infant. (*Source:* This figure was published in Publication *Short Cases in Clinical Medicine*, 4th edition by A.B.M. Abdullah, ISBN: 9788131226698, page 24, Chapter 1, Copyright Elsevier, 2009.)

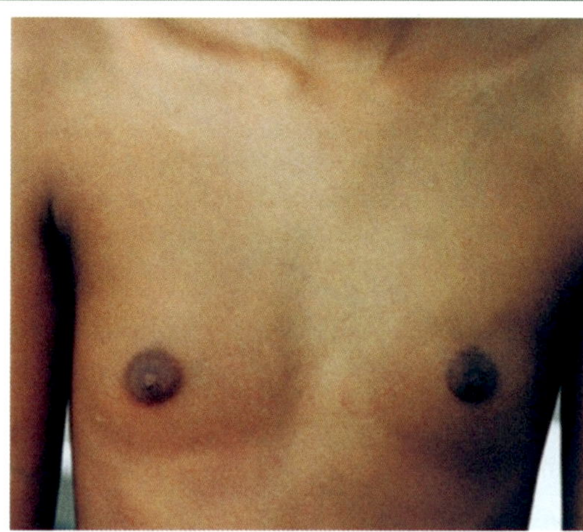

Fig. 11.9 Bilateral gynecomastia. (*Source:* This figure was published in Publication *The Developing Human: Clinically Oriented Embryology*, 8th edition by Keith L. Moore and T.V.N. Persaud, ISBN: 9781416037064, page 444, Fig. 19.6, Copyright Elsevier, 2008.)

12 Skeletal System, Development of Bones, Axial Skeleton, Limbs, and Joints

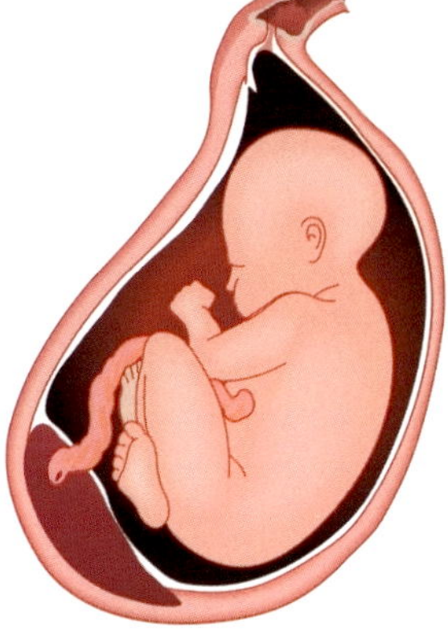

LEARNING OBJECTIVES

After studying this chapter, the student should be able to:

- Define ossification and discuss the differences between membranous and cartilaginous ossification.
- Classify the bones of a body according to their ossification.
- Write short notes on *spina bifida, achondroplasia, fontanelles, anencephaly*, and *clubfoot*.
- Give brief description of somites and their role in development of vertebral column.
- Explain the embryological basis of nucleus pulposus.
- Discuss the basic concepts of development of upper and lower limbs. AN 13.8, AN 20.10
- Describe briefly the stages of development of a typical long bone and discuss the medicolegal significance of ossification center at the lower end of the femur.

OVERVIEW

The skeletal system consists of bones and cartilages. Both bones and cartilages develop from mesenchyme (loose tissue of mesoderm).

The **mesenchyme**-forming bones and cartilages are derived from following three sources:

1. **Paraxial mesoderm** (main source)
2. **Parietal layer of lateral plate mesoderm**
3. **Neural crest cells**

Whatever may be the source of origin of mesenchyme, the general process of formation of **cartilages** and **bones** is the same.

FORMATION OF CARTILAGE

The cartilage is formed by **chondrocytes.** The mesenchymal cells become closely packed (**mesenchymal condensation**) in an area where the cartilage is to be formed. During 5th week these cells then proliferate and differentiate into cartilage-forming cells called **chondroblasts.** The chondroblasts form the collagen fibers and ground substance of the matrix (intercellular substance). Some chondroblasts get imprisoned within the intercellular substance of the developing cartilage and are called **chondrocytes.** Depending upon the presence and predominance of collagen or elastic fibers, the cartilages are classified into three types: *fibrocartilage*, *hyaline cartilage*, and *elastic cartilage*.

The **hyaline cartilage** has a homogeneous, glassy, bluish, and transparent appearance. The collagen fibers present in the matrix are fine and not seen easily. Because fibrils present in the matrix have same refractive index as that of ground substance.

The **elastic cartilage** is pliable and imparts yellowish tinge. The intercellular substance of elastic cartilage, as the name indicates, is permeated by **elastic fibers.**

The mesenchymal cells surrounding the surface of developing cartilage form the **perichondrium.**

The **fibrocartilage** is a dense, fasciculated, and opaque white tissue. The collagen fibers present in fibrocartilage are numerous and arranged in parallel bundles.

N.B. Fibrocartilages are devoid of perichondrium.

FORMATION OF BONES

All the bones are mesodermal in origin. They are formed either directly from the mesenchyme or from preformed cartilaginous model. **The process of bone formation is called ossification.** The processes of bone formation from mesenchyme and cartilage are termed **membranous and cartilaginous ossifications**, respectively.

Membranous Ossification (Fig. 12.1)

At the site where the **membrane bone** is to be formed, the mesenchyme condenses to form a membrane-like structure (**mesenchymal model**). Some cells of mesenchymal model differentiate into **osteoblasts.** The osteoblasts lay down the matrix of bone called **osteoid.** The osteoid tissue consists of collagen fibers and ground substance. The osteoid tissue under the influence of

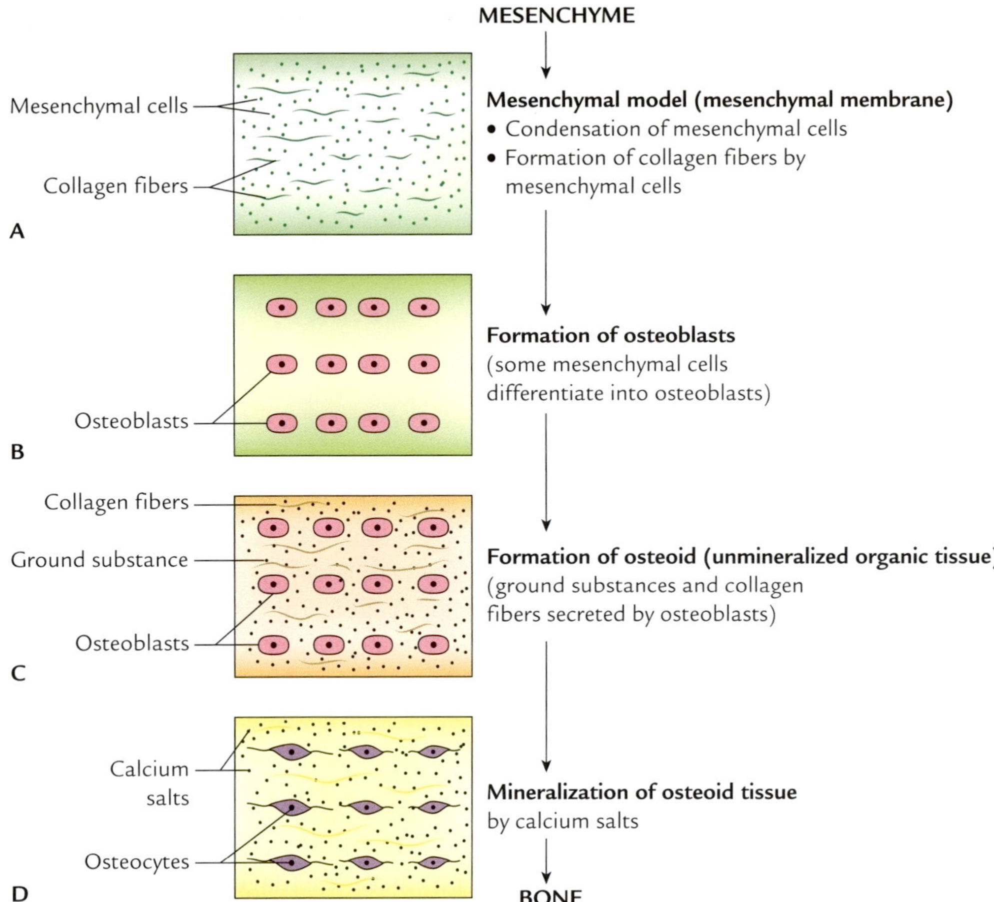

Fig. 12.1 Membranous ossification.

osteoblasts becomes mineralized with calcium salts and becomes the bone. The osteoblasts are trapped in the bone that is formed around it and are converted into **osteocytes.** The bone formed by membranous ossification is in the **form of spicules or trabeculae** that are arranged irregularly with spaces between them. This type of bone is called **spongy bone.** In the spaces of spongy bone, the mesenchyme differentiates into **hemopoietic tissue.** On the surface of the spongy bone, osteocytes lay down a layer of compact bone.

The bones of the cranial vault and face are formed by membranous ossification.

Bone Mineralization

It is a process by which organic bone matrix (**osteoid**) becomes mineralized by inorganic salts, especially by calcium phosphate crystals.

For mineralization to occur the osteoblasts secrete/release:

1. ***Osteocalcin and alkaline phosphatase***, which release calcium salts from their substrates.
2. ***Matrix vesicles*** (membrane-bound vesicles), which concentrate the calcium and phosphate in osteoid. The matrix vesicles are most important factors for mineralization of bone.

Cartilaginous (Endochondral) Ossification (Fig. 12.2)

In this type of bone formation, the *preformed cartilaginous models of bones are converted into bones.* Usually, **long bones** (viz. ***humerus, radius, ulna, femur, tibia***, etc.) are formed in this way. The process starts in the diaphysis of shaft of long bones; this is called **primary center of ossification**. The cartilage cells enlarge and matrix surrounding them gets calcified under the influence of an enzyme (**alkaline phosphatase**) secreted by cartilage cells. The cartilage cells die and disappear, leaving behind the empty spaces (**primary areolae**). The cells on the surface of cartilage, i.e., cells of perichondrium (primordium of periosteum) differentiate into **osteoblasts**. These osteoblasts along with blood vessels (**periosteal bud**) migrate inward. Most of the calcified cartilage is absorbed, leaving behind only thin layers of calcified matrix (thin bars of calcified matrix)

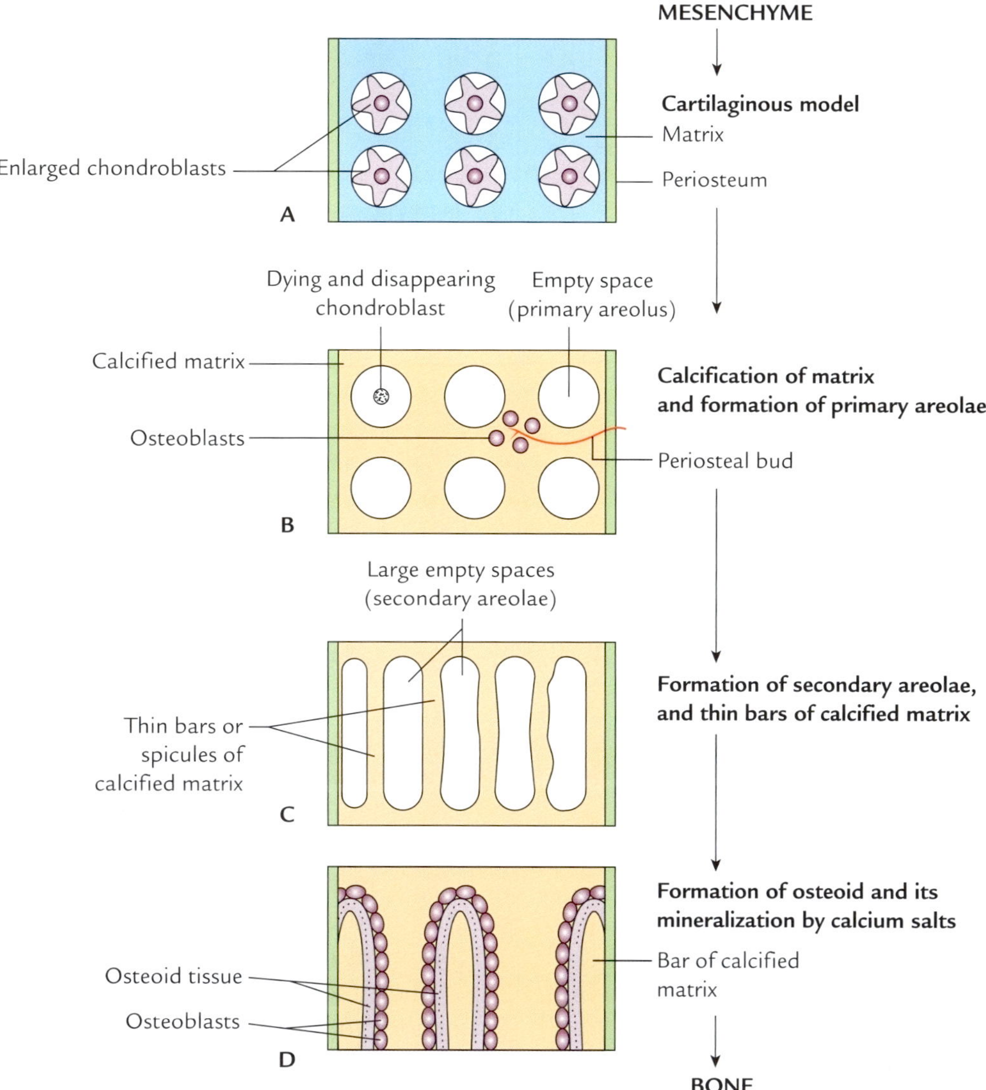

Fig. 12.2 Important stages of cartilaginous ossification.

around the enlarged spaces (**secondary areolae**). The new bone (osteoid) is laid down on the surface of these **bars or spicules of calcified cartilage** by the osteoblasts. The mineralization of osteoid tissue leads to bone formation. The process of ossification spreads to other parts of cartilage and is replaced by bone. Note that when the cartilage cells die, the calcified matrix of cartilage acts only as a support for the developing trabeculae of bone. With bone formation, the perichondrium is called periosteum.

N.B. The process of bone formation by osteoid tissue in case of cartilaginous ossification is same as that in the membranous ossification.

For details of ossification, refer to ***General Anatomy with Systemic Anatomy, Radiological Anatomy, Medical Genetics, Third Edition*** by Dr Vishram Singh.

The bones of base of skull and long bones of limbs are formed by cartilaginous (endochondral) ossification.

N.B. Some bones of the body are formed by both membranous and cartilaginous ossification (i.e., membranocartilaginous ossification) such as mandible and clavicle.

CLINICAL CORRELATION

1. **Cleidocranial dysostosis** (Fig. 12.3): It is a congenital abnormality in which there is complete or partial absence of the clavicles. In the event of bilateral absence of clavicles, both the shoulders of the individual nearly touch each other. It is accompanied by defective ossification of cranium with large fontanelles and delayed closing of sutures. This condition occurs due to defective intramembranous ossification.
2. **Achondroplasia/dwarf** (Fig. 12.4): It is an inherited autosomal dominant trait. The mutation in FGFR3 gene leads to abnormal endochondral ossification. As a result, the individual is abnormally short (dwarf) with short curved arms and legs, dorsal kyphosis, and lumbar lordosis; however, the head and trunk remain normal (also see pp. 136 and 358).

Continued

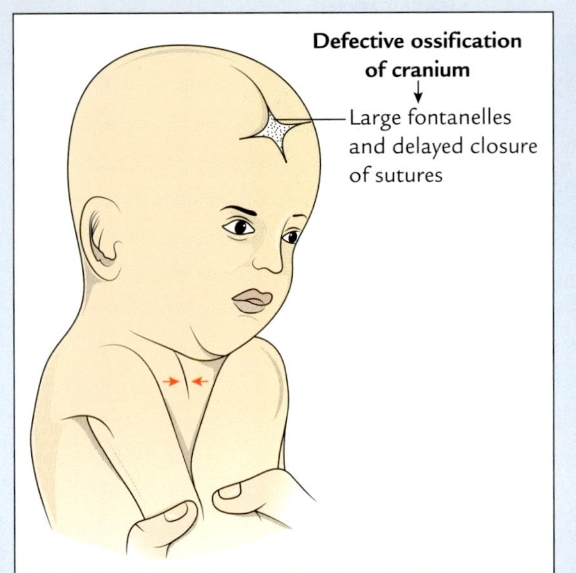

Fig. 12.3 Cleidocranial dysostosis (congenital absence of the clavicles). Note approximation of the shoulders.

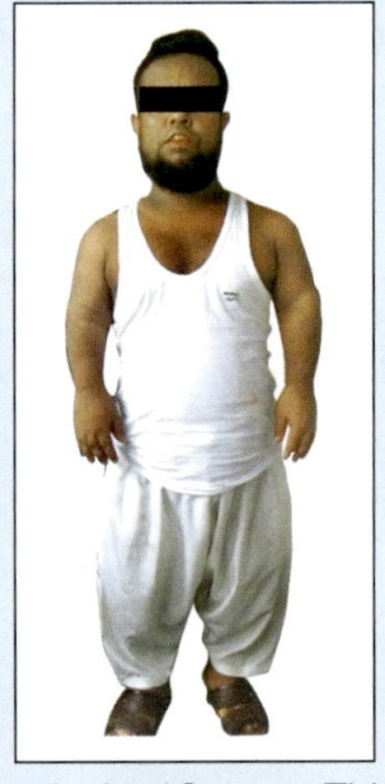

Fig. 12.4 Achondroplasia. (*Source:* This figure was published in Publication Short Cases in Clinical Medicine, 4th edition by A.B.M. Abdullah, ISBN: 9788131226698, Chapter 5, Copyright Elsevier, 2009.)

DEVELOPMENT OF AXIAL SKELETON

The axial skeleton consists of skull (cranium), vertebral column, sternum, and ribs. (Development of skull being a little difficult for students is discussed at the end of this section.)

Development of Vertebral Column

The vertebral column develops from somites derived from paraxial mesoderm. Each somite differentiates into two parts, the ventromedial part called **sclerotome** and a dorsolateral part called **dermomyotome** (for details see p. 142). The sclerotomes take part in the development of the vertebral column.

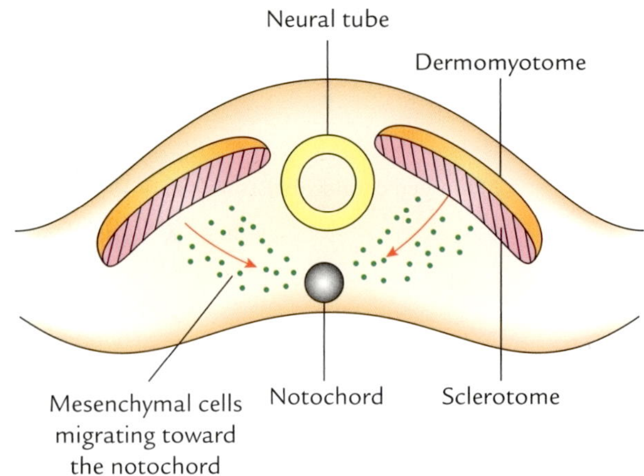

Fig. 12.5 Differentiation of somites into sclerotome (ventromedial part) and dermomyotome (dorsolateral part). Note the migration of mesenchymal cells toward the notochord (red arrows).

Development of Vertebrae

During 4th week of intrauterine life (IUL), the cells of sclerotome become large, polymorphic, and get loosely arranged to form **mesenchyme.** The mesenchymal cells have the potential to differentiate into fibroblasts, chondroblasts, and osteoblasts (bone-forming cells).

The mesenchymal cells from the sclerotomes migrate medially toward notochord to form the vertebral column as follows (Fig. 12.5):

The mesenchymal cells condense (a) around the notochord to form the **centrum**, (b) around the neural tube to form right and left **neural (vertebral) arches**, and (c) in the body wall adjacent to the proximal part of neural arches to form **costal processes.**

The adult derivatives of these structures are as follows:

- The **centrum** forms the **vertebral body.**
- The **vertebral arches** form **pedicles, laminae, spine, articular processes**, and **transverse processes.**
- The **costal processes** form the **costal elements of the transverse processes.**

The costal elements of transverse processes in the thoracic region form ribs (Fig. 12.6).

The relative contribution of centrum, neural arch, and costal element (process) to the vertebrae in different regions is shown in Fig. 12.7.

Intersegmental Position of Vertebrae and Segmental Position of Intervertebral Discs (Figs 12.8 and 12.9)

The mesenchymal cells derived from sclerotomes migrate medially and surround the notochord and neural tube, but the mesenchyme derived from each somite maintains its segmental character (i.e., *it can be seen as*

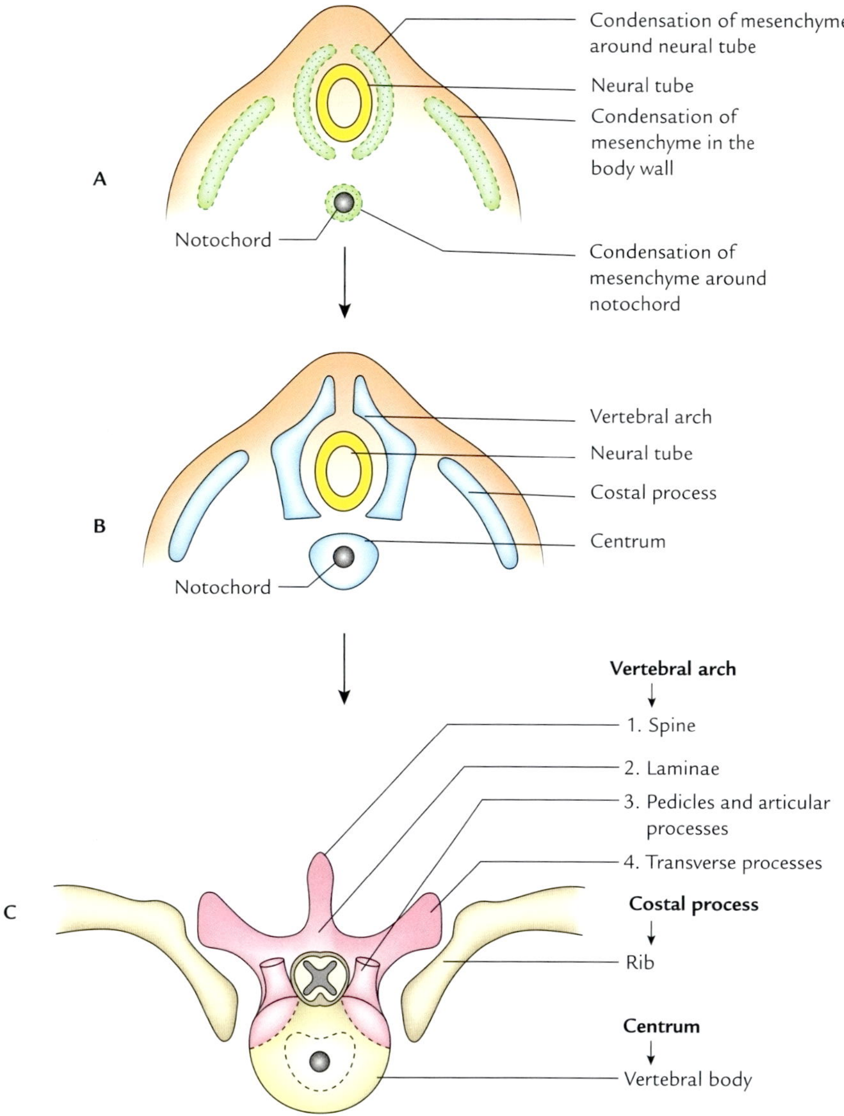

Fig. 12.6 Development of typical thoracic vertebra.

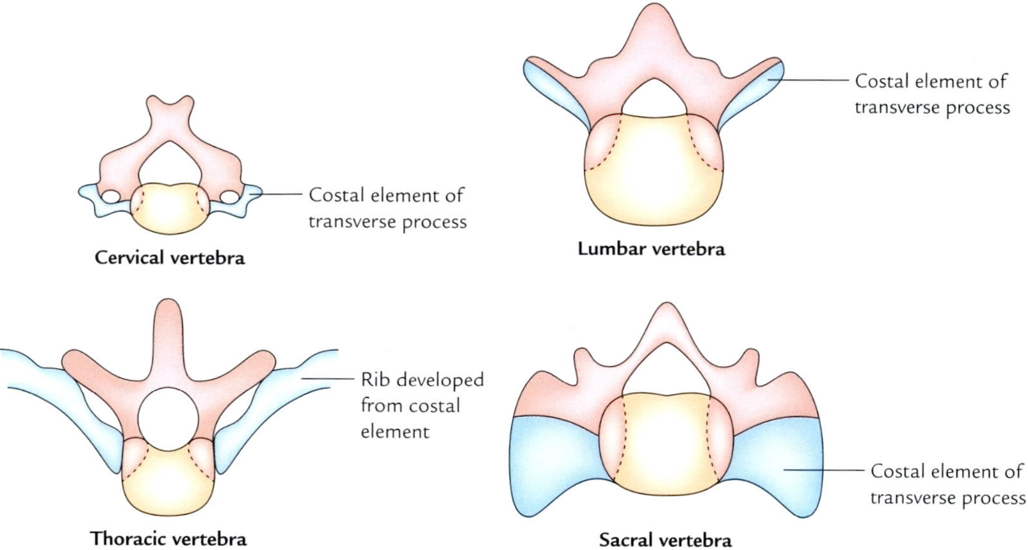

Fig. 12.7 Position of costal elements (rudimentary costal processes) in the transverse processes of cervical, lumbar, and sacral vertebrae. Note the development of rib from the costal process in the thoracic region.

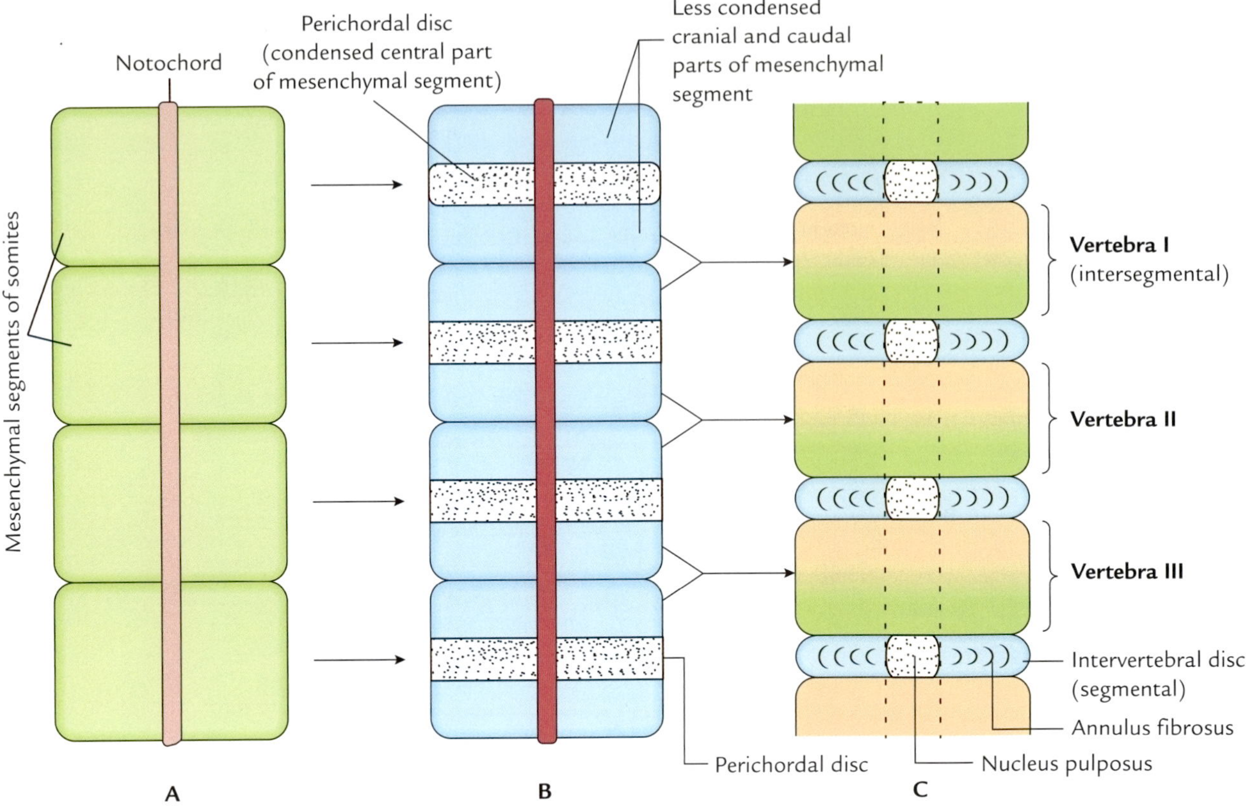

Fig. 12.8 Development of vertebral bodies and intervertebral discs. (A) Mesenchymal segments around the notochord. (B) Differentiation of mesenchymal segment into three parts: condensed central part and less dense cranial and caudal parts. (C) Resegmentation due to the formation of vertebra from adjoining two less condensed parts of two adjacent mesenchymal segments (somites).

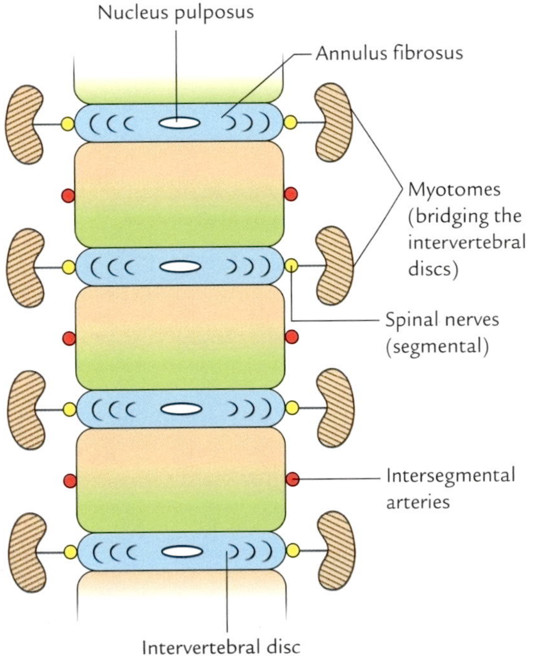

Fig. 12.9 Vertebrae are formed by the upper and lower halves of two successive sclerotomes. The myotomes bridge the intervertebral discs so that they can move the vertebral column.

a distinct mesenchymal segment in developing vertebral column [Fig. 12.8A]) even after migration.

Initially, the mesenchymal cells in each segment are uniformly distributed.

Later, the mesenchymal cells in the central part of each segment become condensed to form **perichordal disc.** The parts above and below the perichordial disc remain less dense (Fig. 12.8B). The body of each vertebra is formed by fusion of adjoining less condensed parts of the two sclerotomes (somites). The **vertebra is thus an intersegmental structure** being derived from two mesenchymal segments representing sclerotomes (somites). The part of notochord trapped in the body of the vertebra degenerates and disappears.

The **perichordal disc** forms the peripheral part of the intervertebral disc (**annulus fibrosus**). The **notochord** trapped within the perichordial disc persists and forms the central part of the intervertebral disc – the **nucleus pulposus.** The **intervertebral disc and nucleus pulposus are therefore segmental structures.**

The resegmentation of mesenchymal segments (sclerotomes) into definitive vertebrae causes myotomes to bridge the intervertebral disc, and this provides them the capacity to move the spine.

Embryological basis of nucleus pulposus AN 79.5

The nucleus pulposus is the inner core of intervertebral disc. It is made up jelly-like material, which allows the vertebral column (intervertebral discs) to withstand the forces of compression.

Embryologically, it is derived from notochord trapped within the perichordal discs – a condensed central part of mesenchymal segments of embryonic vertebral column.

Salient Features of Development of Vertebral Column

1. **Vertebrae are intersegmental structures** because each vertebra is derived from portions of two adjacent somites (e.g., caudal half of one somite and cranial half of the other somite below it).
2. **Transverse processes and ribs are intersegmental**, and hence separate the muscles derived from two adjoining myotomes.
3. **Spinal nerves are segmental** and hence emerge between the two adjacent vertebrae.

N.B. Each vertebra is formed by caudal half of one somite and cranial half of other somite below it. The **patterning of shapes of different vertebrae** is regulated by ***Hox*** **genes**.

Ossification of a Typical Vertebra (Fig. 12.10)

The newly formed vertebra is cartilaginous. This cartilaginous model of vertebra is soon converted into bone by ossification. The vertebrae ossify by the three primary centers of **ossification**: one for each vertebral (neural) arch and one for the centrum. At birth, each vertebra consists of three bony parts: two vertebral arches and a centrum connected by a cartilage. The vertebral arches fuse posteriorly by 3–5 years of age to form **spinous process.** The vertebral arches articulate with the centrum at cartilaginous **neurocentral joints**, which disappear by 3–6 years of age. Posterolateral part of body on each side receives a contribution from the neural arch. The line of junction between part derived from the centrum and part derived from the neural arch represents the site of **neurocentral joint**.

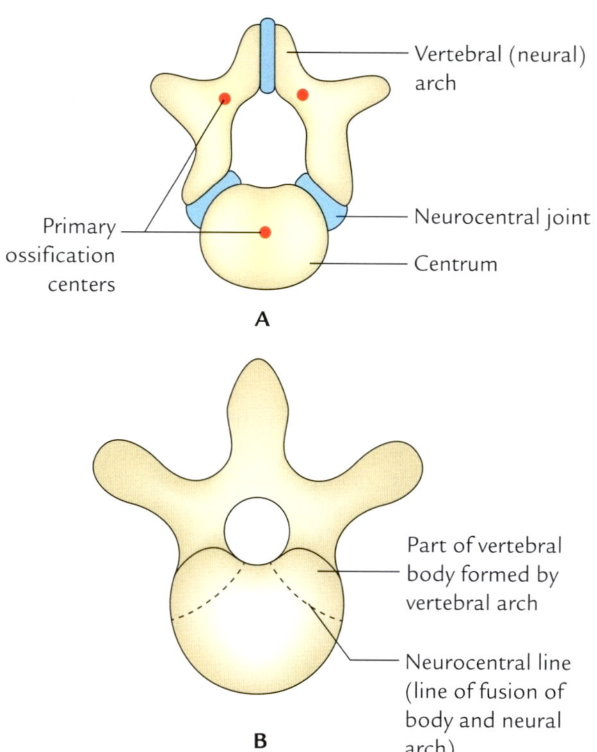

Fig. 12.10 Ossification of typical vertebra. (A) Three parts of vertebra joined by cartilage at birth. (B) Fusion of three parts.

CLINICAL CORRELATION

A. **Spina bifida** AN 79.5

It is a large gap in vertebra dorsally that occurs when two embryonic neural arches fail to fuse with each other. It is one of the most serious vertebral defects. This defect occurs in 1 per 1000 births and may be prevented in many cases by giving folic acid to mothers prior to conception. It occurs more frequently in girls than boys. Depending upon the severity of lesion, the spina bifida is divided into following types (Fig. 12.11).

1. ***Spina bifida occulta*** (closed spina bifida): The bone defect is covered by skin and no neurological deficit occurs. The skin at the site is pigmented, with hairy patches, fatty lump, or a dermal sinus.

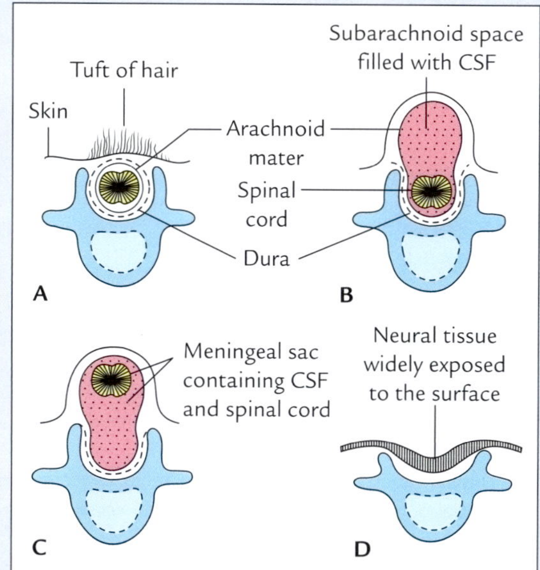

Fig. 12.11 Types of spina bifida. (A) Spina bifida occulta. (B) Spina bifida with meningocele. (C) Spina bifida with meningomyelocele. (D) Spina bifida with rachischisis.

Continued

2. ***Spina bifida with meningocele:*** The bone defect is covered by skin but the meninges herniate through the gap to form meningeal sac filled with cerebrospinal fluid (CSF).
3. ***Spina bifida with meningomyelocele:*** The bone defect is covered by skin but the meninges and spinal cord herniate through the gap.
4. ***Spina bifida aperta*** (spina bifida with rachischisis): This is the most severe form of spina bifida. There is no skin covering. The neural tube is open and lies on the surface of the back of the body.

N.B. The **prenatal diagnosis of spina bifida** can be made by ultrasonography and by detecting elevated levels of α-fetoprotein in the amniotic fluid.

B. Some other congenital anomalies of the vertebrae (Fig. 12.12)

1. ***Hemivertebra*** (Fig. 12.12A): At times the vertebral body ossifies from two separate primary centers. In such an event if one center fails to appear, only half of the vertebra will form. This may lead to a clinical condition called **congenital scoliosis** (i.e., lateral bending of the spine).

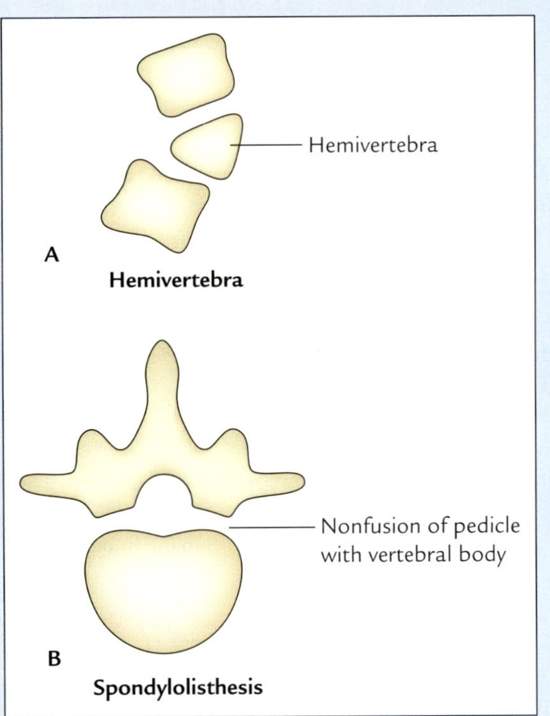

Fig. 12.12 Some congenital anomalies of the vertebra.

2. ***Congenital fusion of vertebral bodies***
   (a) Occipitalization of atlas vertebra: It occurs due to fusion of atlas vertebra with occipital bone.
   (b) Sacralization of the fifth lumbar vertebra: It occurs due to partial or complete fusion of the fifth lumbar vertebra with the sacrum.
   (c) Lumbarization of the first sacral vertebra: It occurs due to partial or complete fusion of first sacral vertebra with the fifth lumbar vertebra.
3. ***Spondylolisthesis*** (Fig. 12.12B): It occurs when the pedicles of vertebral arch fail to fuse with the vertebral body. This allows the vertebral body to slip anteriorly over the body of the vertebra below. This condition commonly affects the L5 vertebra. As a result, the body of the fifth lumbar vertebra slips forward over the sacrum.

Development of Ribs

The ribs develop from **costal processes in the thoracic region**. The costal processes at first elongate to form cartilaginous costal arches, which are then ossified to form the ribs.

In **cervical, lumbar, and sacral regions**, the costal processes remain rudimentary and are represented by a small part of the transverse process of each vertebra called **costal element**.

CLINICAL CORRELATION

Accessory ribs

1. ***Accessory lumbar rib:*** It is the commonest rib anomaly. However, it does not attract much attention of clinicians as it is symptomless.
2. ***Accessory cervical rib:*** It occurs only in 0.5%–1% of the cases. It can be unilateral or bilateral. It develops from the costal element of seventh cervical vertebra. The accessory cervical ribs may exert pressure on lower trunk of brachial plexus and subclavian artery leading to a clinical condition called **superior thoracic outlet syndrome**. For details, see ***Clinical and Surgical Anatomy*** by Dr Vishram Singh.

Development of Sternum (Fig. 12.13)

At first, two mesenchymal vertical plates, one on either side of midline, develop in anterior body wall due to condensation of somatic mesoderm. These plates are called **mesenchymal sternal bars** (Fig. 12.13A). Later, two sternal bars are converted into cartilage to form **cartilaginous sternal bars**. The two cartilaginous sternal bars start fusing with each other in a craniocaudal sequence (Fig. 12.13B). After their fusion, the **cartilaginous model of the sternum** is formed. It consists of **manubrium**, **body** (made up of four segments called **sternebrae**), and **xiphoid process**. The cartilaginous model of sternum gets ossified to form the sternum.

Manubrium and body ossify by five double centers from above downward during 5th, 6th, 7th, 8th, and 9th months. The upper pair of centers forms manubrium and the lower four pairs of centers form four sternebrae that fuse with each other from below upward. The fusion is complete by 25 years of age. The xiphoid process ossifies late in life. The center for xiphoid process appears during the 3rd year or later and fuses with the body of sternum at about 40 years.

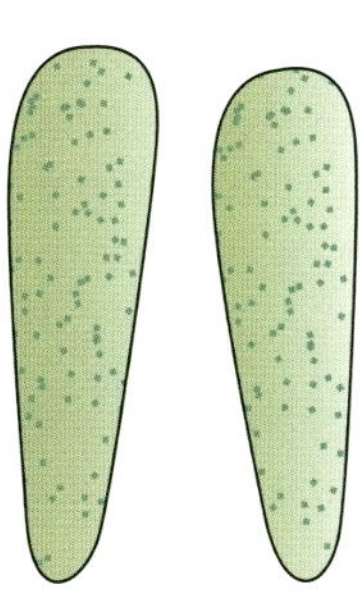

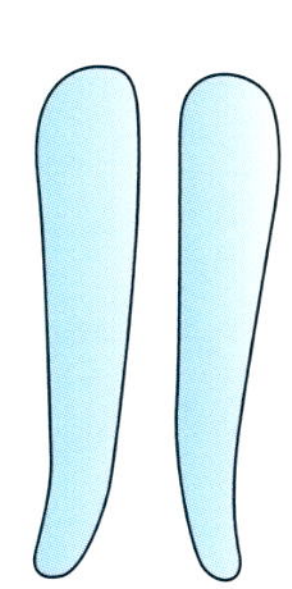

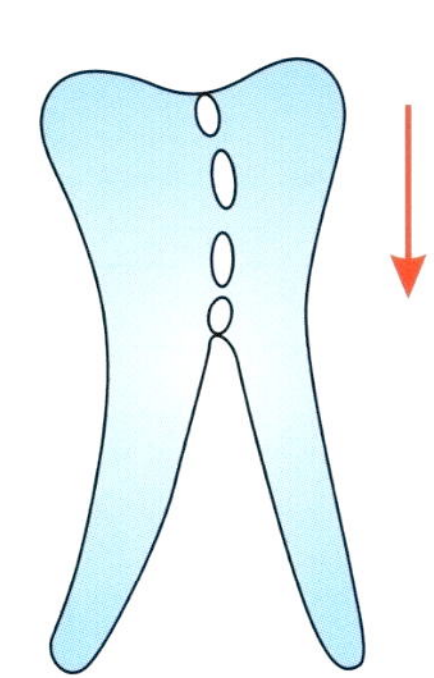

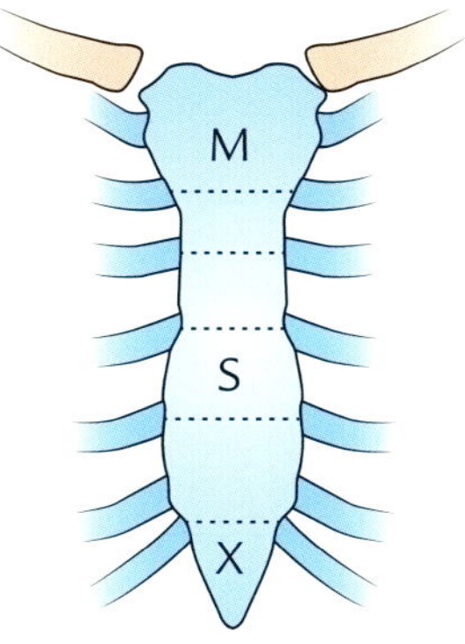

Fig. 12.13 Stages of development of sternum. M, manubrium; S, sternebrae; X, xiphoid process.

CLINICAL CORRELATION

1. ***Sternal foramen and sternal cleft*** (Fig. 12.14): It occurs when the two sternal bars fail to fuse completely. The defect ranges from *sternal foramen* to *sternal cleft*. The latter may be associated with *ectopia cordis*. It is fairly common but of no clinical significance, if small. Fusion of the two sternal bars is often incomplete in the caudal part producing the *bifid xiphoid process* or a *hole in xiphoid process*.

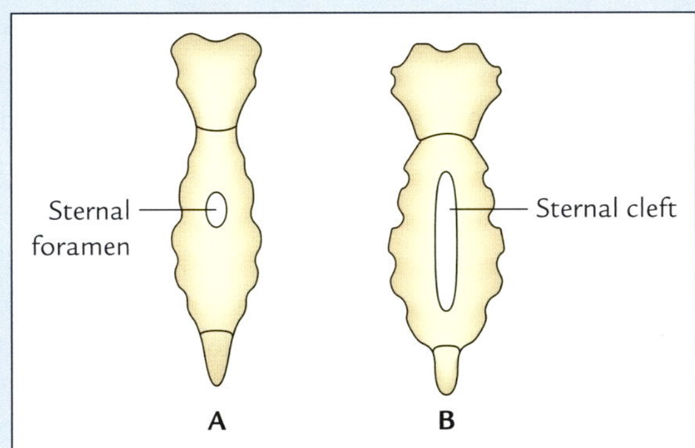

Fig. 12.14 (A) Sternal foramen. (B) Sternal cleft.

2. ***Funnel chest (pectus excavatum)*** (Fig. 12.15): It is the most common congenital anomaly of the chest. In this condition, the chest is compressed anteroposteriorly and sternum is pushed backward compressing the heart. Clinically, it presents as a depression in the anterior median region of the chest wall that may extend from manubrium to the xiphoid process. An early surgical intervention is recommended not only to improve cosmetic appearance but also to alleviate cardiopulmonary restriction.

   The funnel chest occurs because lower half of the sternum and attached costal cartilages are pulled inward due to abnormally short tendon of diaphragm.

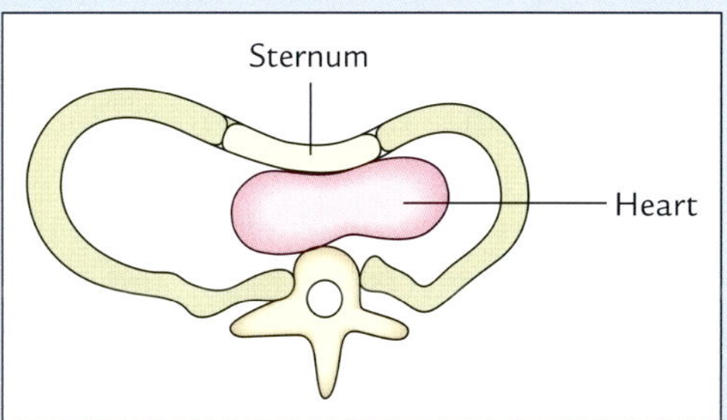

Fig. 12.15 Funnel chest.

3. ***Pigeon chest (pectus carinatum)*** (Fig. 12.16): In this condition, the upper part of the sternum and related costal cartilages project forward in the midline as in birds (e.g., pigeon), and hence the name pigeon chest.

   In this case, the chest is compressed from side to side causing forward projection of the sternum and related cartilages.

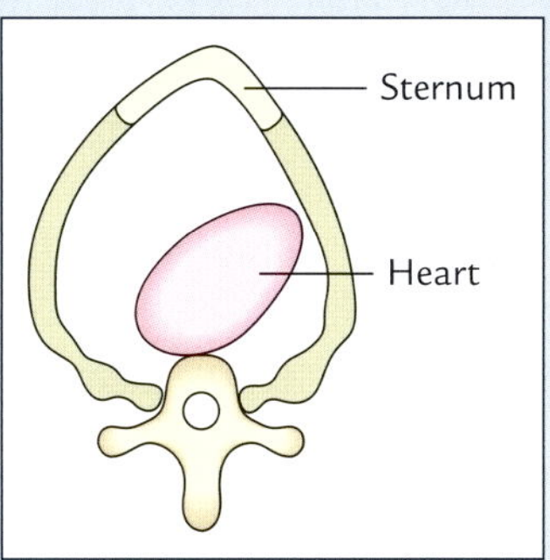

Fig. 12.16 Pigeon chest.

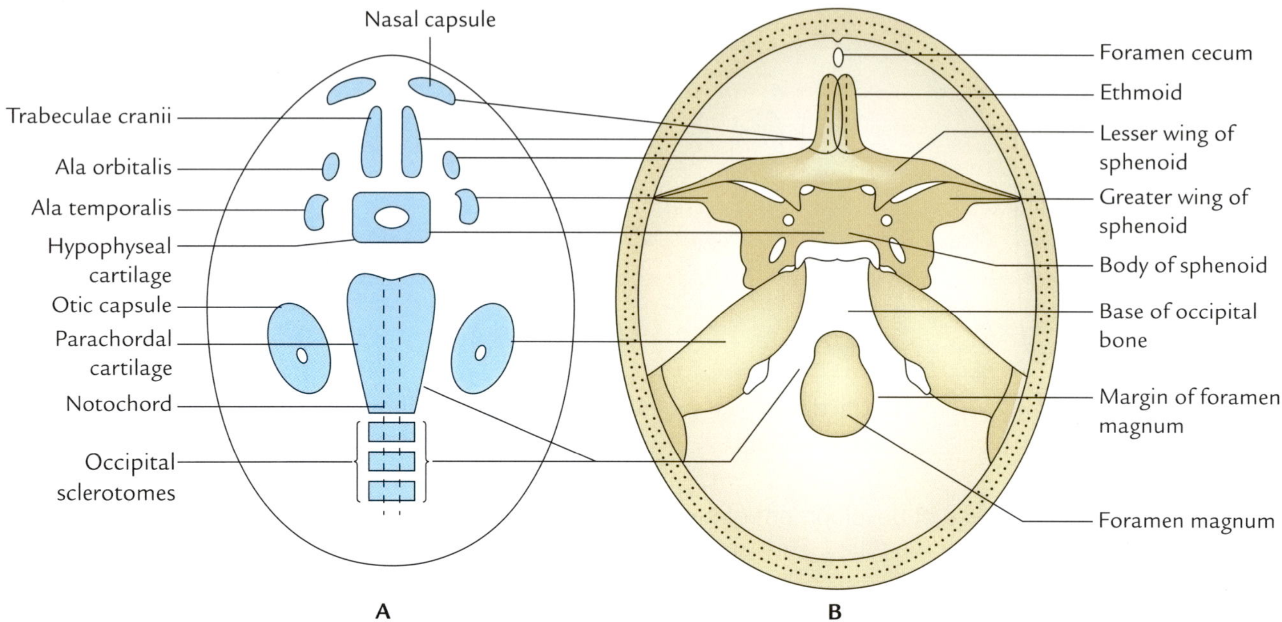

Fig. 12.17 Development of the base of the skull (dorsal view). (A) Cartilages that form cartilaginous neurocranium. (B) Bones of the base of the skull formed by various cartilages of neurocranium by endochondral ossification.

Development of Skull

The skull (cranium) develops from mesenchyme around the developing brain. The skull (cranium) is divided in two parts: (a) **neurocranium** that encloses cranial cavity and protects the brain and (b) **viscerocranium** that forms the skeleton of the face.

Neurocranium

The neurocranium consists of a cartilaginous portion that forms the **base of the skull** and a membranous portion that forms **cranial vault**.

Base of skull (Fig. 12.17)

The base of skull, at first, is cartilaginous (cartilaginous neurocranium). It is formed by the fusion of several cartilages. These cartilages are formed by chondrification of mesenchyme below the brain.

The various cartilages that form the cartilaginous neurocranium are as follows:

1. *Parachordal cartilage (basal plate):* It forms around cranial end of notochord.
2. *Hypophyseal cartilage:* It forms around developing pituitary gland.
3. *Trabeculae cranii (two in number):* They form in front of hypophyseal cartilages.
4. *Ala orbitalis:* It develops on either side lateral to the trabeculae cranii.
5. *Ala temporalis:* It develops on either side lateral to the hypophyseal cartilage.
6. *Otic capsules:* They develop around otic vesicles – the primordia of internal ears.
7. *Nasal capsules:* They develop around nasal sacs.

The bones of the base of skull derived from these cartilages are given in Table 12.1.

The cartilaginous base is subsequently ossified to form the base of the skull.

Table 12.1 Adult derivatives of various cartilages forming the cartilaginous base of developing skull

Embryonic Structure	Adult Derivatives
Trabeculae cranii and nasal capsules	Ethmoid bone
Hypophyseal cartilage	Body of sphenoid
Ala orbitalis	Lesser wing of sphenoid
Ala temporalis	Greater wing of sphenoid
Parachordal plate and cartilages derived from four occipital somites (sclerotomes)	Base of the occipital bone including boundaries of foramen magnum
Otic capsule	Petrous and mastoid parts of the temporal bone

Cranial vault (vault of skull) (Fig. 12.18)

The vault of skull develops from mesenchyme on superior and lateral aspects of developing brain (**membranous neurocranium**). This mesenchyme is derived from the neural crest cells and paraxial mesoderm.

The vault of the skull is first membranous in nature that later undergoes membranous ossification to form a number of flat membranous bones, which together form the vault (top) of the skull.

The primary centers appear where the bones start ossifying and grow toward the periphery by forming needle-like bony spicules.

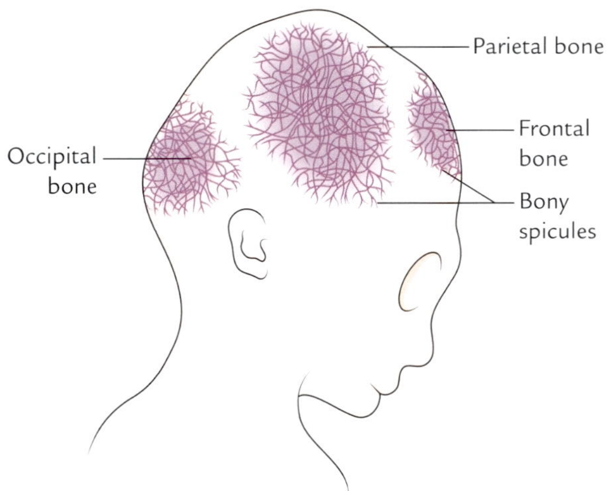

Fig. 12.18 Spread of bony spicules from primary ossification centers in the flat bones of skull in a 3-month-old fetus.

Viscerocranium (Fig. 12.19)

The major part of viscerocranium develops from the mesenchyme derived from first (having maxillary and mandibular processes) and second pharyngeal arches. This mesenchyme undergoes membranous ossification to form the bones of the facial skeleton.

The mandibular process of the first pharyngeal arch contains Meckel's cartilage. The mesenchyme around the Meckel's cartilage condenses and ossifies by membranous ossification to form the mandible.

The Meckel's cartilage disappears; however, its perichondrial sheath remains in the form of sphenomandibular ligament. The maxillary process of first pharyngeal arch gives rise to maxilla, zygomatic bone, and part of the temporal bone.

The dorsal tip of the mandibular process along with the second pharyngeal arch gives rise to three ear ossicles, namely, **malleus**, **incus**, and **stapes** (see Fig. 14.8, p. 153). The lacrimal and nasal bones are derived from neural crest cells.

N.B. Initially, the neurocranium is larger than viscerocranium (face) due to the absence of paranasal air sinuses and smaller size of the bones of the face, especially jawbones.

The bones of the skull are formed by membranous ossification, or cartilaginous ossification, or both (vide supra). Accordingly, the bones of the skull are of three types: membranous bones, cartilaginous bones, and membranocartilaginous bones (Table 12.2).

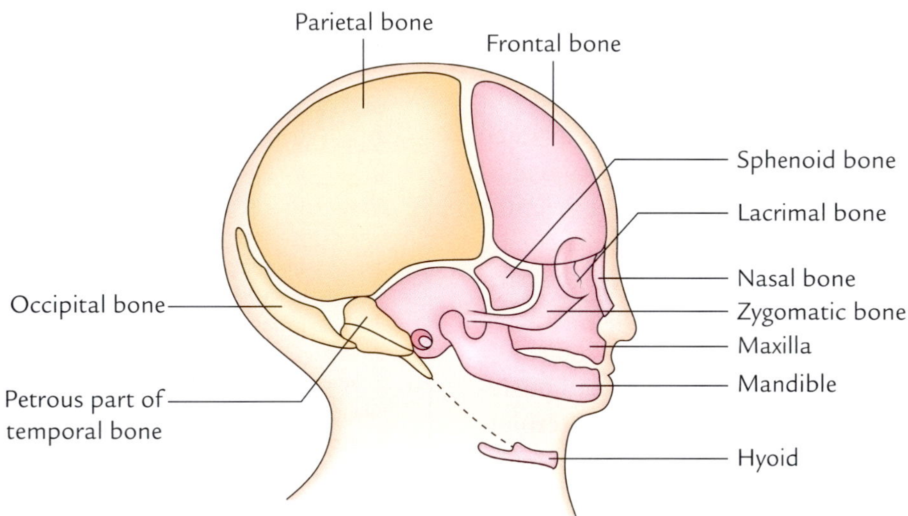

Fig. 12.19 Skeletal structures of the head and face. The mesenchyme of these bones is derived from neural crest (pink) and paraxial mesoderm (somites and somitomeres) (orange).

Table 12.2 Types of bones of skull according to their development (ossification)

Membranous Bones (Ossify in Membrane)	Cartilaginous Bones (Ossify in Cartilage)	Membranocartilaginous Bones (Ossify Both in Membrane and Cartilage)
• Frontal • Parietal • Maxilla (excluding premaxilla) • Zygomatic • Nasal • Lacrimal • Vomer	• Ethmoid • Inferior nasal concha	• Occipital (part above the superior nuchal line is membranous and the remaining part is cartilaginous) • Sphenoid (lateral parts of greater wings and pterygoid processes are membranous and rest is cartilaginous) • Temporal (squamous) and tympanic parts are membranous, whereas petromastoid part and styloid process are cartilaginous • Mandible (condylar and coronoid processes are cartilaginous and the rest of the mandible is membranous)

Newborn Skull

The newborn skull presents two striking features:

1. Small viscerocranium (facial skeleton) as compared to neurocranium.
2. Presence of fontanelles.

Factors responsible for disproportion between viscerocranium and neurocranium

Relatively, the huge size of **neurocranium** is due to fast and enormous development of brain. The brain reaches 25% of its adult size at birth and 75% by the age of 4 years.

The face (**viscerocranium**) is small because of small size of facial bones, particularly the jaws (maxillae and mandibles) and virtual absence of paranasal air sinuses.

N.B. With the eruption of teeth and development of paranasal air sinuses, the face loses its babyish look.

Fontanelles (Fig. 12.20)

The fontanelles are soft membranous areas in the vault of newborn skull. They are also sometimes termed **soft spots.** At birth, the flat bones of the skull are separated from each other by narrow seams of fibrous tissue called **sutures.** At sites where more than two bones meet the sutures are wide and are called **fontanelles.** There are **six fontanelles at birth** – one at each angle of the parietal bone. Thus, two are located in the median plane on top of the skull and two on either side of the skull.

The two median fontanelles are **anterior** and **posterior**, and two paired lateral fontanelles are **anterolateral (or sphenoid)** and **posterolateral (or mastoid).** The most prominent of these is **anterior fontanelle.** It is diamond shaped and located where two halves of the frontal bone and two parietal bones meet. All the fontanelles except anterior fontanelle are closed within 3 or 4 months after birth. The anterior fontanelle is usually closed between 2nd and 3rd years of age.

Functions of fontanelles

1. Allow bones of the skull to overlap (**molding**) during parturition to facilitate the baby birth.
2. Permit postnatal growth of skull bones, especially bones of the vault to increase the cranial capacity.
3. Allow postnatal development of the brain.

Clinical significance of fontanelles. In first few years after birth, palpation of anterior fontanelle provides following valuable information to the clinician:

1. As to whether ossification of the skull is proceeding normally or not.
2. As to whether intracranial pressure is normal or not, i.e., the depressed (sunken) fontanelle indicates **dehydration** and bulging fontanelle indicates **increased intracranial pressure.**

CLINICAL CORRELATION AN 79.5

1. ***Anencephaly*** (Fig. 12.21): In this condition, major portion of the cranial vault fails to form (**cranioschisis**). It occurs if anterior neuropore of neural tube fails to close. The brain tissue is exposed to amniotic fluid and gradually degenerates. Children with such severe skull and brain defects cannot survive (i.e., *anencephaly is incompatible with extrauterine life*). If not, stillborn infants with anencephaly survive only few hours or weeks.

   Anencephaly is the most serious birth defect seen in stillborn infants. It is easily diagnosed by ultrasonography and raised serum α-fetoprotein level. The therapeutic abortion should be performed with mother's consent.
2. ***Encephalocele:*** It occurs due to small defects in the skull through which meninges and/or brain tissue herniate. Depending upon severity, the encephalocele is divided into three types: meningocele, meningoencephalocele, and meningohydroencephalocele (Fig. 12.22).

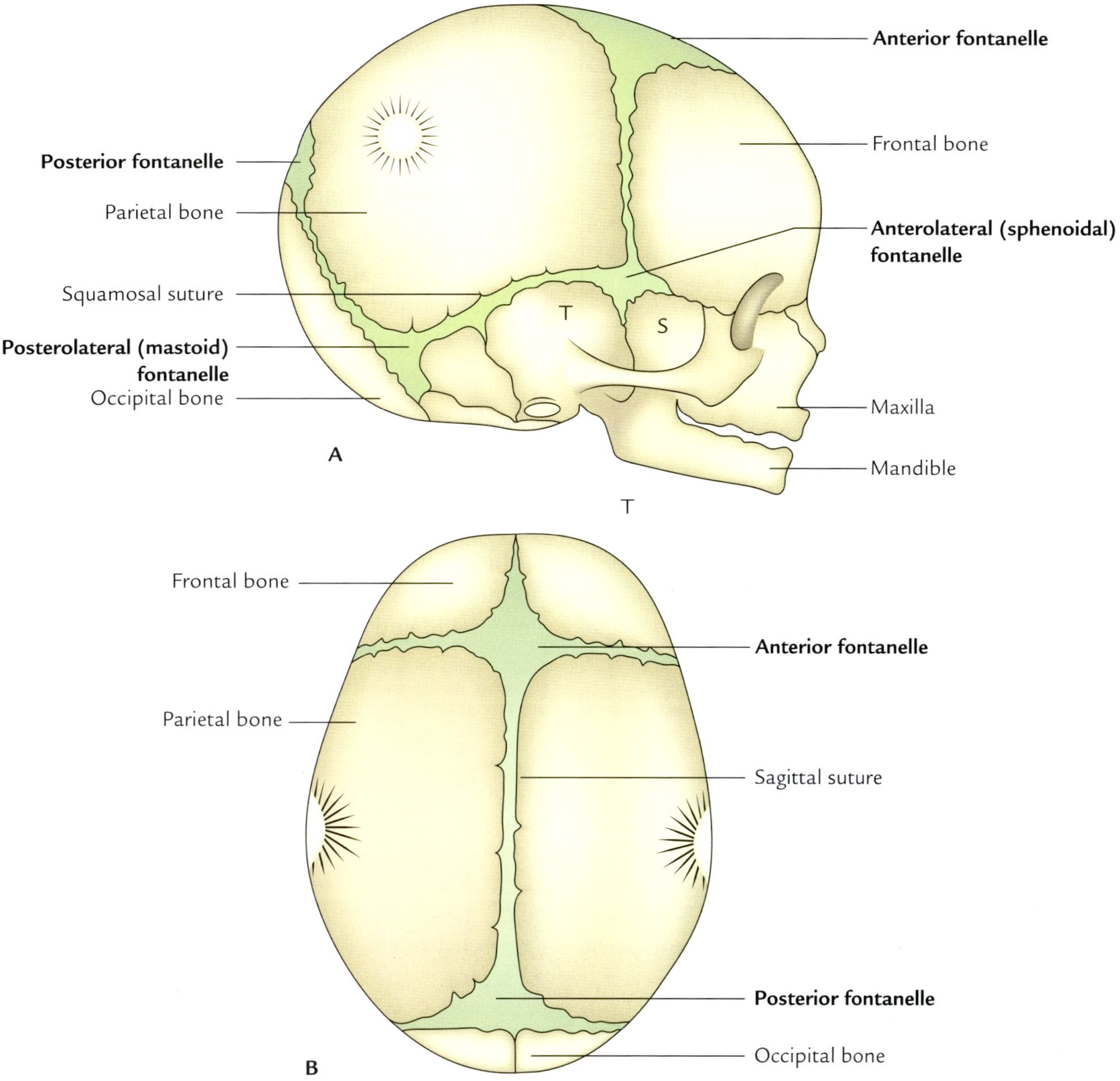

Fig. 12.20 Fetal skull showing six fontanelles. (A) Right lateral view. (B) Superior view. T, temporal bone; S, greater wing of sphenoid.

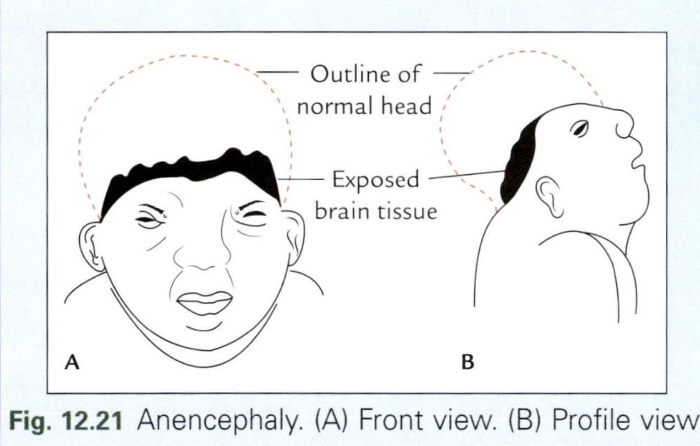

Fig. 12.21 Anencephaly. (A) Front view. (B) Profile view.

3. ***Abnormalities of the shape of the skull***
   (a) *Scaphocephaly:* Boat-shaped skull due to frontal and occipital expansions. It occurs due to early closure of the sagittal suture (57% of cases).
   (b) *Brachiocephaly:* Short skull due to premature bilateral synostosis (closure) of the coronal suture.
   (c) *Plagiocephaly:* It occurs due to premature closure of coronal and lambdoid sutures on one side only. It results in grossly unequal curvatures of skull on two sides.
   (d) *Acrocephaly:* Pointed skull due to premature closure of the coronal suture.
   (e) *Microcephaly:* Small skull due to failure of proper development of the brain.

Continued

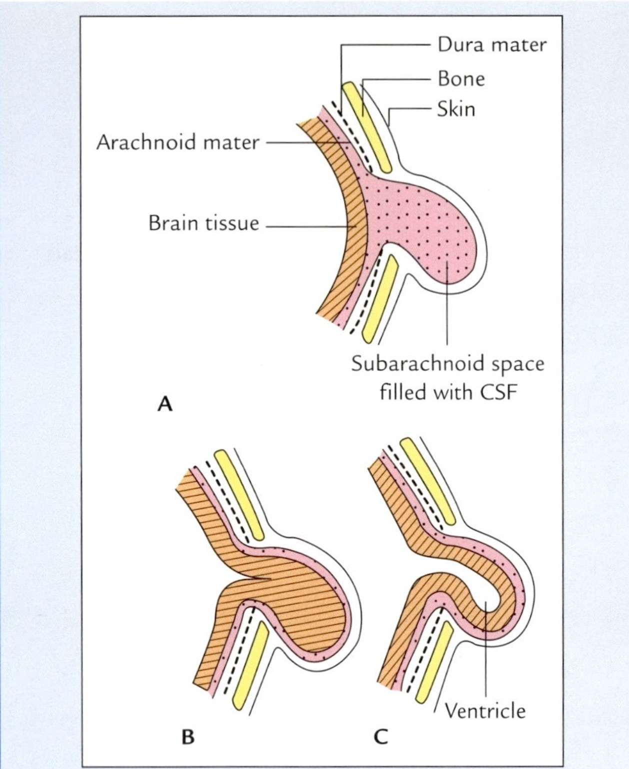

Fig. 12.22 Schematic diagrams showing (A) meningocele, (B) meningomyelocele, and (C) meningohydroencephalocele.

DEVELOPMENT OF APPENDICULAR SKELETON

The appendicular skeleton consists of pectoral and pelvic girdles and limb bones.

The lateral plate mesoderm migrates into limb buds and condenses along the central axis to form skeletal components of the limbs.

The bones in the limbs develop in a proximodistal sequence and are regulated by ***Hox* genes.**

It is necessary for students to first understand the development of limbs before they understand the development of the appendicular skeleton.

Development of Upper and Lower Limbs AN 13.8, AN 20.10

The limb buds appear as outpouchings from the ventrolateral aspects of the body wall at the end of the 4th week of embryonic development (Fig. 12.23). The **forelimbs** appear first followed by **hind limbs** 1 or 2 days later.

The various stages in the development of upper limb are as follows (Fig. 12.24):

The ectoderm at the tip of the limb bud thickens to form **apical ectodermal ridge** (AER).

In the 6th week of embryonic development, the terminal part of the limb bud becomes flattened to form **hand and foot plates**, and are separated from the

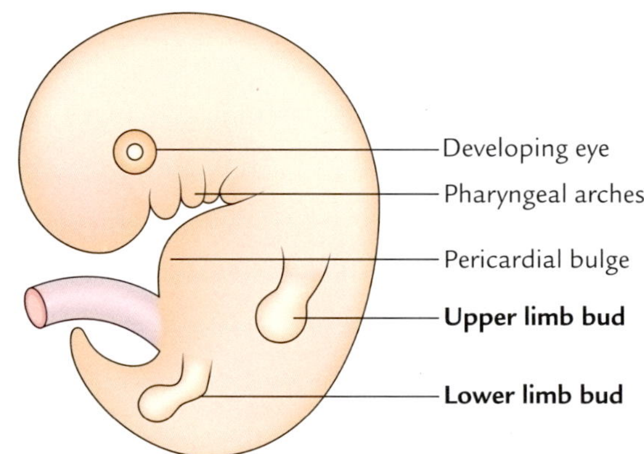

Fig. 12.23 A 12.5–15.75 mm embryo showing limb buds.

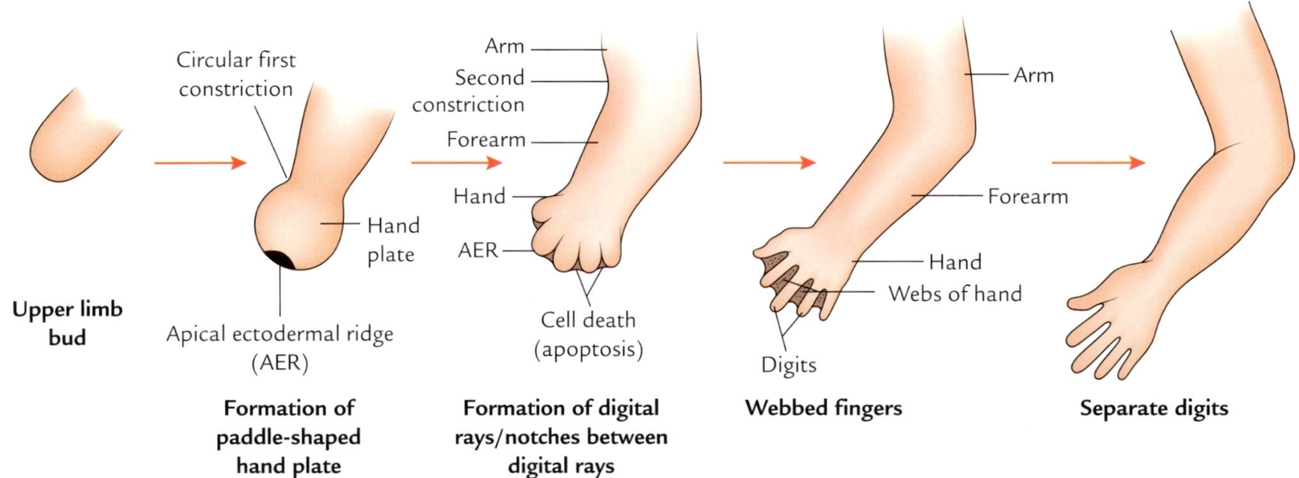

Fig. 12.24 Stages in the development of upper limb.

rest of the limb bud by a circular constriction. The expanded plate exhibits five longitudinal mesodermal condensations or **digital rays.** Later, second constriction divides the rest of the limb bud into two segments. Now main parts of the limb become recognizable (e.g., **arm**, **forearm**, and **hand** in upper limb; and **thigh**, **leg**, and **foot** in lower limb). Now the digits are formed in the hand and foot plates following cell death in the ectodermal ridges.

Rotation of Limb Buds

Initially, the limb buds are paddle shaped and each bud has **preaxial** and **postaxial border**, with the former being directed toward the cranium (head).

The digit formed along the preaxial border is **thumb** in the upper limb and **great toe** in the lower limb.

The limbs now rotate. The **upper limb rotates 90° laterally**, and as a result, its preaxial border and thumb come to lie on the lateral side. On the other hand, the **lower limb rotates 90° medially**, and as a result, its preaxial border and great toe come to lie on the medial side.

N.B. The development of upper and lower limbs is similar except the following facts:
1. The development of lower limb starts 1 or 2 days later to that of the upper limb.
2. During the 7th week of gestation, the upper limb rotates 90° laterally, whereas the lower limb rotates 90° medially (Fig. 12.25).

Arrangement of Dermatomes in the Upper and Lower Limbs

Area of skin supplied by a single spinal nerve and therefore by a single spinal segment is termed **dermatome.**

1. The upper limb develops from the body wall opposite C4, C5, C6, C7, C8, T1, and T2 spinal segments, and hence innervated by corresponding spinal nerves.

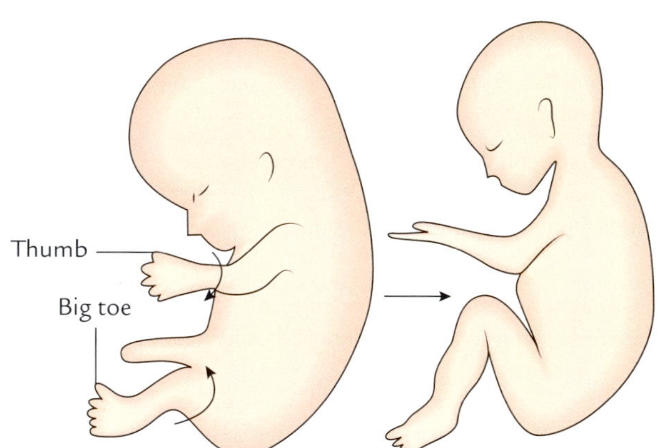

Fig. 12.25 Relation of limb buds during embryonic development.

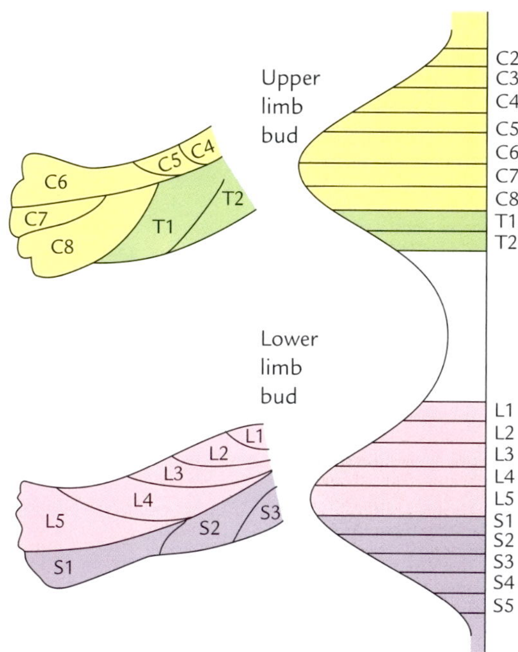

Fig. 12.26 Arrangement of dermatomes in the upper and lower limbs of the embryo.

2. The lower limb develops from the body wall opposite L2, L3, L4, L5, S1, and S2 spinal segments, and hence innervated by the corresponding spinal nerves.

The arrangement of dermatome in the upper and lower limbs of the embryo is shown in Fig. 12.26.

N.B. The positioning of limbs along the craniocaudal axis in the body wall is regulated by ***Hox*** **genes.**

Development of Upper Limb Bones AN 13.8

All the bones of upper limb, namely, **scapula, clavicle, humerus, radius, ulna, carpals, metacarpals**, and **phalanges**, develop from somatic layer of lateral plate mesoderm.

The sequence of events of formation of upper limb bones is as follows (Fig. 12.27)

1. During the 5th week, the mesenchyme derived from lateral plate mesoderm migrates along the central axis of limb bud and condenses to form **mesenchymal models of bones.**
2. During the 6th week, the **mesenchymal models of bones** undergo chondrification to form **hyaline cartilage models of bones.**
3. The hyaline cartilage models undergo **ossification** to form **bones.**

Ossification

All the bones of the upper limb are formed by **endochondral ossification**; however, clavicle is formed by both **membranous (mainly) and endochondral ossification.**

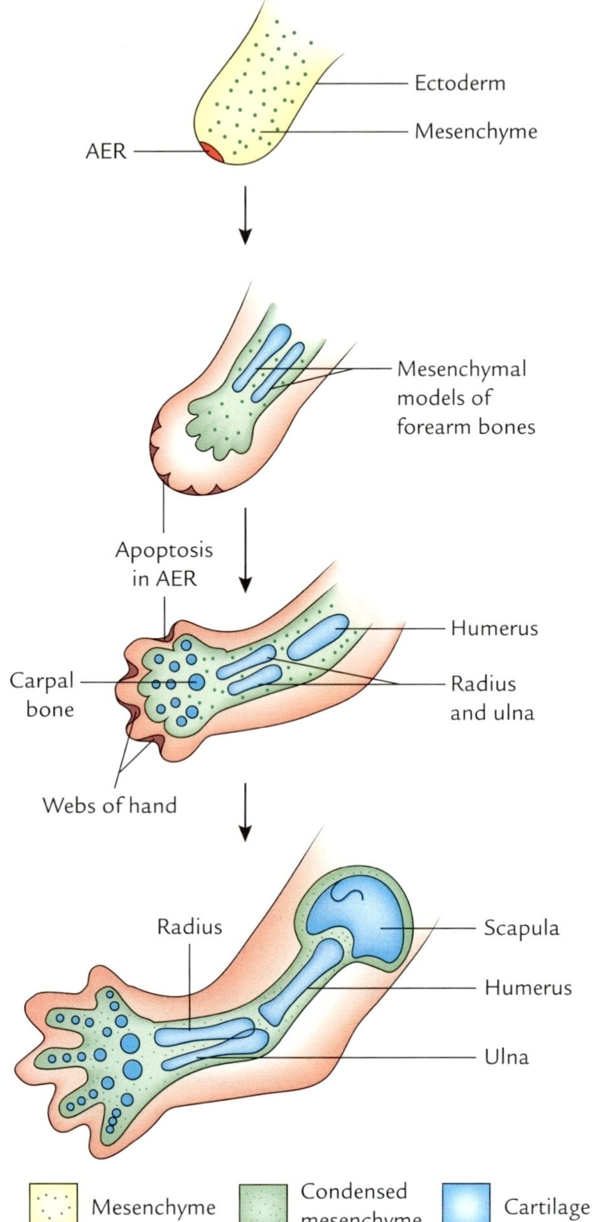

Fig. 12.27 Stages in the development of upper limb bones.

The clavicle is the first bone to ossify in the entire body. For ossification of individual bones, refer ***Textbooks of Osteology***. However, as a classical example of ossification, only ossification of long bone is given here. The ossification of a typical long bone occurs as follows (Fig. 12.28):

1. During the 8th week, primary center of ossification appears in the middle of the long bone.
2. During childhood, secondary centers appear at the ends of long bone.
3. The primary center forms the diaphysis of long bone, whereas the secondary centers form the epiphyses of long bone.
4. The bone formed by the primary center in the diaphysis does not fuse with the bone formed by the secondary center in the epiphysis. They remain separated from each other by a plate of cartilage called **epiphyseal cartilage**. The growth of bone in length occurs at the epiphyseal cartilage. Hence, it is also called **growth plate**. When the epiphyseal cartilage ossifies, the growth of bone ceases.

Development of Lower Limb Bones

AN 20.10

Like upper limb, all the bones of lower limb, namely, hip bone, femur, tibia, fibula, tarsals, metatarsals, and phalanges, develop from somatopleuric layer of lateral plate mesoderm.

The sequence of events involved in development of bones of lower limb is same as in upper limb.

Ossification

The bones of the lower limb ossify in the same fashion as those of the upper limb.

N.B. The primary centers of ossification of limb bones appear at different times in different bones, but most of them appear between 7th and 12th weeks, i.e., virtually all primary centers of ossification are present at birth and most of the secondary centers appear after birth.

CLINICAL CORRELATION

1. ***Medicolegal importance of ossification center at the lower end of femur:*** The secondary center of ossification at the lower end of femur usually appears during the last month of intrauterine life. Therefore, visibility of this center in radiograph (Fig. 12.29) is used as a medicolegal evidence to confirm the fact that newborn infant found dead was near full-term and viable.
2. ***Achondroplasia:*** It is the most common type of dwarfism (shortness of stature). It occurs due to defective **endochondral ossification** at the epiphyseal plates of cartilage, particularly of long bones. It occurs in about 1 in 26,000 live births. The limbs become bowed and short; trunk remains normal and head is enlarged with bulging forehead (also see p. 358).
3. ***Amelia:*** In this condition, there is a complete absence of a limb. The absence of all four limbs is rare and called as **tetra-amelia**.
4. ***Phocomelia:*** In this condition, rudimentary hands and feet are directly attached to the trunk.
5. ***Meromelia:*** In this condition, limbs are malformed. There is congenital absence of part of limbs (Fig. 12.30).

N.B. **Amelia**, **phocomelia**, and **meromelia** are characteristically seen in children whose mothers have used an antiemetic drug – **thalidomide** – between the 6th and 8th week of gestation. Hence, children with these abnormalities are called **thalidomide babies**.

6. ***Syndactyly (webbed fingers or toes):*** It is the common limb anomaly and results from failure of hand and foot webs to degenerate between the digits.
7. ***Polydactyly:*** In this condition, there is a **supernumerary digit** in hand or foot, most commonly the thumb that may have an extra phalanx. It is the most common congenital anomaly of the hand and may occur due to mutation of autosomal dominant genes (Fig. 12.31).

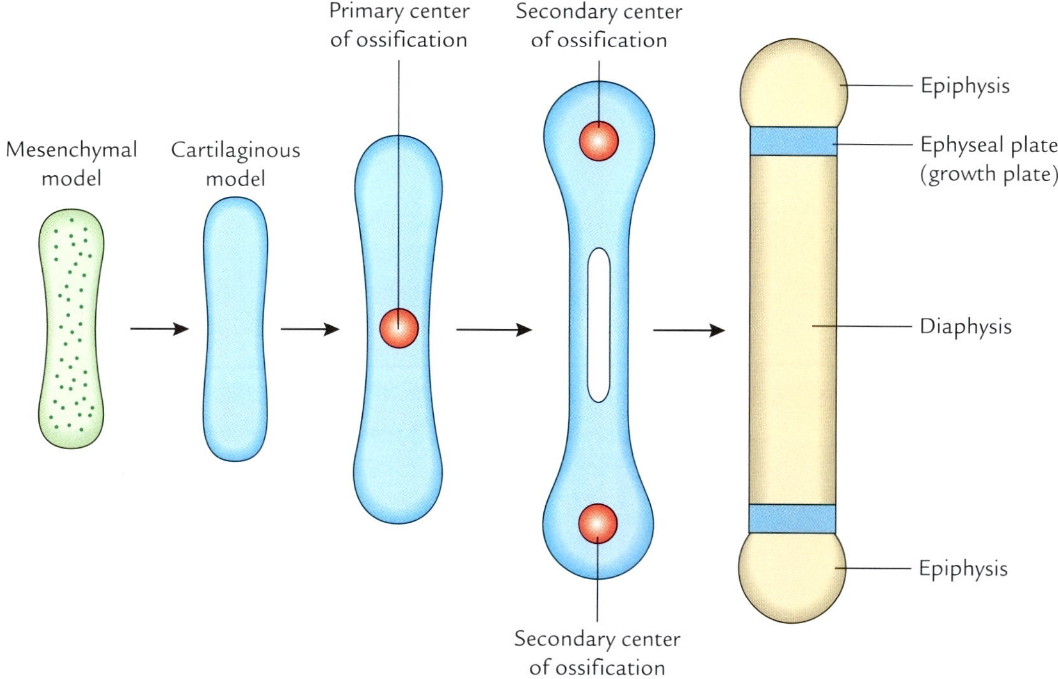

Fig. 12.28 Stages of ossification of a typical long bone.

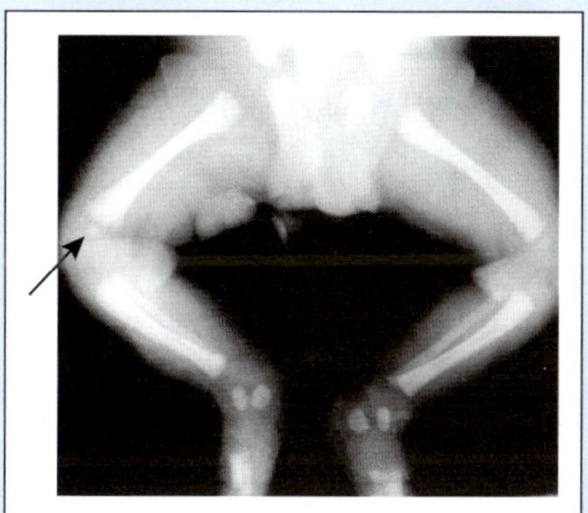

Fig. 12.29 Radiograph of a full-term child showing the presence of secondary center of ossification at the lower end of the femur (arrow). (*Source:* This figure was published in Publication *Textbook of Forensic Medicine and Toxicology*, 5th edition by Krishan Vij, ISBN: 9788131226841, Fig. 7.1, Copyright Elsevier, 2011.)

8. ***Lobster claw hand or foot:*** In this condition, third digit is missing and the second and fourth digits are separated by a wide cleft. Medial two digits are fused; lateral two digits may also be fused.
9. ***Talipes or clubfoot:*** Any deformity of foot involving talus is called **talipes** or **clubfoot**. There are various types but **talipes equinovarus** is the most common type of club foot occurring about 1 in 1000 births. In this condition, the foot is turned medially and is inverted. This prevents normal weight bearing. It results from abnormal positioning or restricted movements of fetus's lower limbs in utero.
10. ***Congenital dislocation of hip:*** In this condition, the joint capsule is lax at birth and there is underdevelopment of acetabulum. The dislocation almost always occurs after birth. It occurs in about 1 in 1500 newborn infants and is more common in female babies.

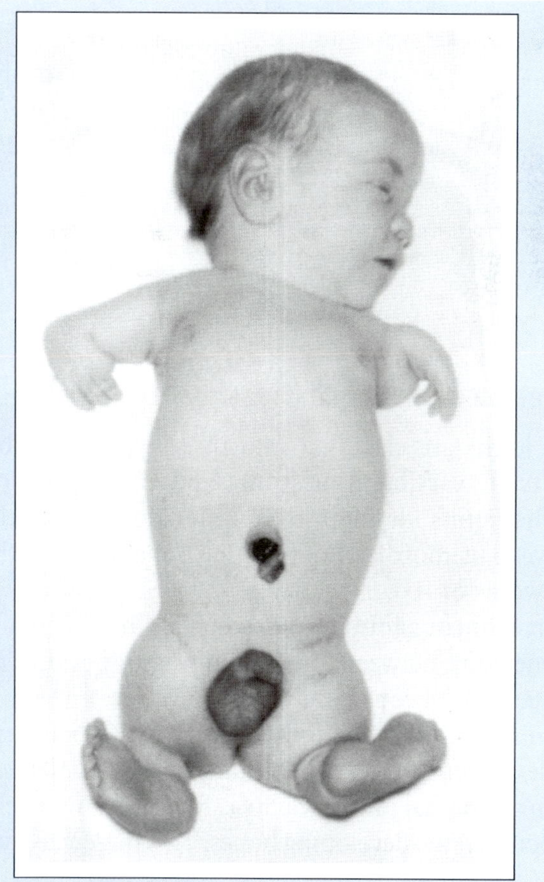

Fig. 12.30 Meromelia. (*Source: From Moore KL:* The vulnerable embryo: causes of malformation in man. *Manitoba Med Rev.* 43:306, 1963.)

Continued

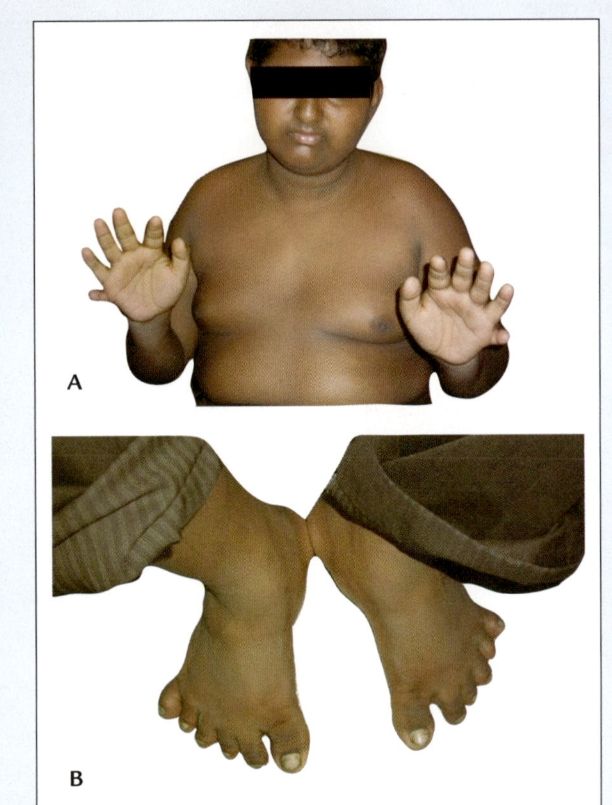

Fig. 12.31 Polydactyly. (A) Supernumerary digit in hand (six fingers). (B) Supernumerary digit in foot (six toes). (*Source:* This figure was published in Publication Short Cases in Clinical Medicine, 4th edition by A.B.M. Abdullah, ISBN: 9788131226698, Chapter 1, Copyright Elsevier, 2009.)

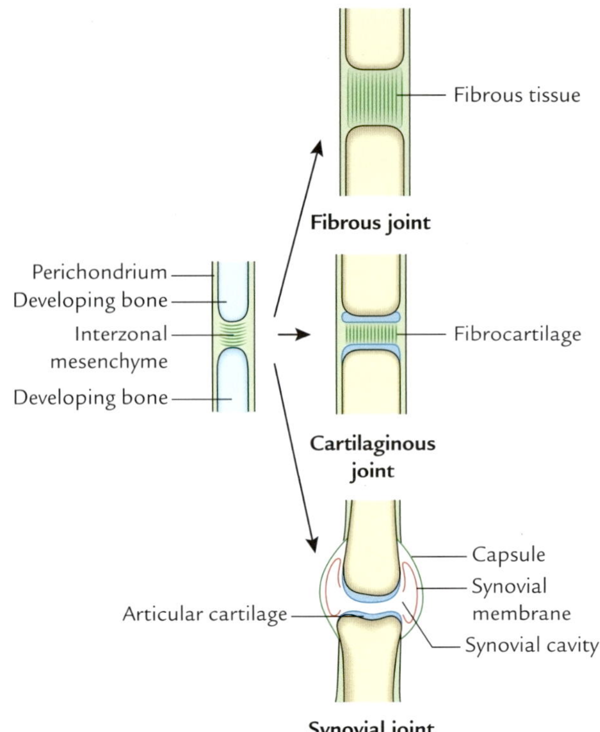

Fig. 12.32 Development of joints.

Development of Joints (Fig. 12.32)

The joints are classified into three types: (a) **fibrous joints**, (b) **cartilaginous joints**, and (c) **synovial joints**.

The joints develop from interzonal mesenchyme between primordia of developing bones during 6th and 7th weeks of IUL.

1. In a **fibrous joint (syndesmosis)**, intervening mesenchyme between the developing bones differentiates into fibrous tissue.
2. In a **cartilaginous joint**, mesenchyme between the developing bones differentiates into a cartilage.
3. In a **synovial joint**, a cavity is formed in mesenchyme between the developing bones. This mesenchyme also gives rise to synovial membrane, joint capsule, and other ligaments of the joint.
   - Central part of mesenchyme breaks to form **joint cavity**.
   - Peripheral part of mesenchyme **capsule and ligaments**.
   - Part which lines capsule forms **synovial membrane**.

GESTATIONAL AGE OF KEY DEVELOPMENTAL EVENTS OF LIMBS

Developmental Event	Gestational Age
➤ Upper limb buds	4th week
➤ Lower limb buds	4th week + 1 or 2 days
➤ Joints	6th–7th weeks
➤ Rotation of limbs	7th week
➤ Digits of hands and feet	8th week
➤ Primary centers of ossification in long bone	7th–12th weeks
➤ Secondary centers of ossification of lower end of femur	At birth

GOLDEN FACTS TO REMEMBER

- **Most important factor responsible for mineralization** — Membrane vesicles released by osteoblasts
- **Most severe birth defect in stillborn babies** — Anencephaly
- **Most serious vertebral defect** — Spina bifida
- **Most severe form of spina bifida** — Spina bifida aperta (spina bifida with rachischisis)
- **Commonest accessory rib** — Lumbar rib[a]
- **Most common congenital anomaly of the chest** — Funnel chest
- **Most prominent (largest) fontanelle** — Anterior fontanelle
- **First bone to start ossifying in the body** — Clavicle
- **Most common congenital defect due to defective endochondral ossification** — Achondroplasia (dwarfism)
- **Most common type of club foot** — Talipes equinovarus
- **Most common limb anomaly of fingers and toes** — Polydactyly (supernumerary finger or toe)
- **Mutant genes involved in achondroplasia, brachydactyly, or osteogenes is imperfecta** — HOX, BMP, SHH, WNT7, FGFR3, etc.

[a]Clinically, cervical rib is the commonest accessory rib.

CLINICAL PROBLEM SOLVING

PROBLEMS

1. All cervical spinal nerves emerge out of the vertebral canal through intervertebral foramina except **C1, spinal nerve which emerges out between the base of skull and first cervical vertebra**. Give the embryological basis.
2. Give the **embryological basis of various deformities of shape of heads in newborns.**
3. A mother noticed a difference in lengths of the legs of her 12-month-old daughter while she was standing up. Give the embryological basis.
4. A newborn baby has **clubfoot**. What is clubfoot and what is **its most common variety**? Give its embryological basis.
5. A pregnant mother took **thalidomide** – an antiemetic drug – during her pregnancy. What congenital anomalies are likely to occur in the newborn baby?
6. What are the factors that cause **congenital limb defects**? Give an example of defect associated with each factor.
7. In a breech (buttock first) presentation, delivery is more difficult than in vertex (head first) presentation. Give the embryological basis.

SOLUTIONS

1. This is because in the cervical region, fourth occipital sclerotome fuses with cranial portion of first cervical sclerotome to form base of the occipital bone. As a result, the C1 spinal nerve emerges out of the vertebral canal through a gap between occipital bone and atlas (C1) vertebra.
2. The developing bones of the skull are separated by narrow seams of fibrous tissue called **sutures**.

   Premature closure of one or more sutures (**craniosynostosis**) causes deformities in shape of head of the newborn (for details see p. 133).
3. The difference in the lengths of legs of her daughter is due to **congenital dislocation of the hip joint**, which is about eight times more common in female infants than male. It occurs due to congenital laxity of capsule of the hip joint and underdevelopment of acetabulum. The congenital dislocation of hip always occurs after birth and becomes obvious only when baby attempts to stand at about 12 months after birth.
4. The **clubfoot** is a congenital anomaly of the foot in which the foot is turned inward, adducted, and plantar flexed. The foot is fixed in the tiptoe position, resembling the foot of a horse (L. *Equinus* = horse). The most common type of clubfoot is **talipes equinovarus**. It is thought to occur due to abnormal positioning of fetus's lower limb in utero and follows a multifactorial pattern of inheritance.
5. The newborn baby of the mother who took thalidomide during her pregnancy is likely to suffer from following congenital anomalies of its limbs: (a) amelia, (b) phocomelia, and (c) meromelia (also see p. 136).
6. The congenital anomalies of limbs are caused by the following factors:
   (a) Genetic factors such as chromosomal abnormalities due to mutant genes, e.g., brachydactyly (short digits).
   (b) Environmental factors such as thalidomide, e.g., amelia, meromelia, and phocomelia (for details see p. 136).
   (c) Combination of genetic and environmental factors (multifactorial inheritance), e.g., congenital dislocation of the hip.
   (d) Ischemia, e.g., reduction in size of limbs.
7. During normal parturition, molding of the fetal skull is such that occipital bone is usually pressed under two parietal bones. In addition, one parietal bone overlaps the other. The depressed parietal bone comes to lie against the sacral promontory of the mother.

   In case of breech delivery, the molding does not occur and as a result the delivery is more difficult.

13 Muscular System

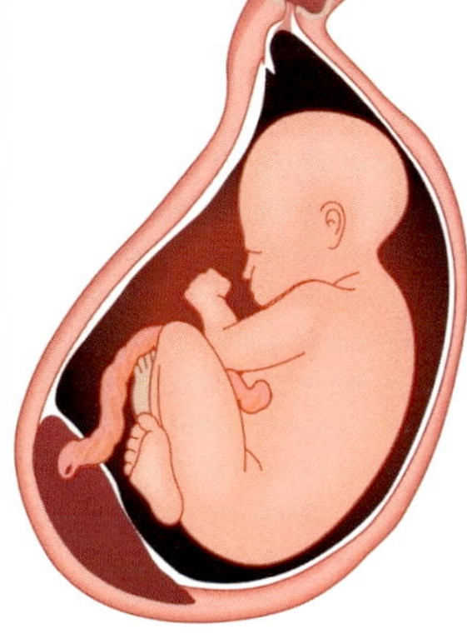

LEARNING OBJECTIVES

After studying this chapter, the student should be able to:

- Give the source of development of skeletal, smooth, and cardiac muscles.
- Discuss the myogenesis of the skeletal muscle.
- Give the embryological basis of multinucleated nature of skeletal muscle fibers.
- Give the embryological basis that extrinsic muscles of eye are supplied by III, IV, and VI cranial nerves.
- Give the embryological basis that all muscles of tongue are supplied by twelfth cranial nerve.

OVERVIEW

All muscles of the body develop from mesoderm except the **muscles of iris, arrector pili** of skin, and **myoepithelial cells** of glands, which develop from ectoderm.

Muscles are classified into three types: skeletal (striated or **voluntary**), smooth (unstriped or **involuntary**), and **cardiac** (structurally striated but functionally smooth muscle).

- The **skeletal muscles** of limbs and trunk develop from somites (paraxial mesoderm/somatic mesoderm).
- The **smooth and cardiac muscles** develop from splanchnic mesoderm.

DEVELOPMENT OF SKELETAL MUSCLES

The skeletal muscles of axial skeleton, body wall, limbs, and head develop from somites and somatomeres that extend from occipital to sacral region (Fig. 13.1). Each somite differentiates into two distinct zones: **sclerotome** and **dermomyotome**. The sclerotome forms bones of axial skeleton. The dermomyotome consists of two components: a deeper part called **myotome** and a superficial part called **dermatome.** The myotome forms muscular tissues, whereas the dermatome forms dermis of skin (Fig. 13.2).

Muscles of eyeball (extraocular muscles) develop from **preotic myotomes**, muscles of tongue develop from **occipital myotomes**, muscles of limbs develop from myotomes present in the upper and lower limb bud regions, and muscles of the body wall develop from myotomes in the trunk region (Fig. 13.2).

Myogenesis (muscle formation) of skeletal muscle (Fig. 13.3): The mesenchymal cells differentiate into primordial muscle cells called **myoblasts.** This differentiation includes elongation of cell and its nucleus. The myoblasts fuse with each other end-to-end to form an elongated multinucleated cylindrical syncytial cell called **myotube.** The myotubes synthesize **actin**, **myosin**, and **other muscle proteins.** These proteins aggregate to form **myofilaments** and **myofibrils.** At this stage, the myotubes are called **muscle fibers.** A number of these muscle fibers are bound together by connective tissue to form **individual muscles**, which secondarily get attached to skeletal elements.

N.B.

- During myogenesis, myofilaments and myofibrils develop in the cytoplasm of muscle fibers.
- All the skeletal muscles develop by birth.
- Mitotic activity of myoblasts ceases after birth. Therefore, all the muscle fibers that an individual is destined to have are formed by birth.

Development of Skeletal Muscles in Different Regions of the Body

In the human body, the skeletal muscles are divided into following groups:

- Muscles of the body wall (trunk)
- Muscles of head and neck
- Extraocular muscles
- Muscles of tongue
- Muscles of limbs

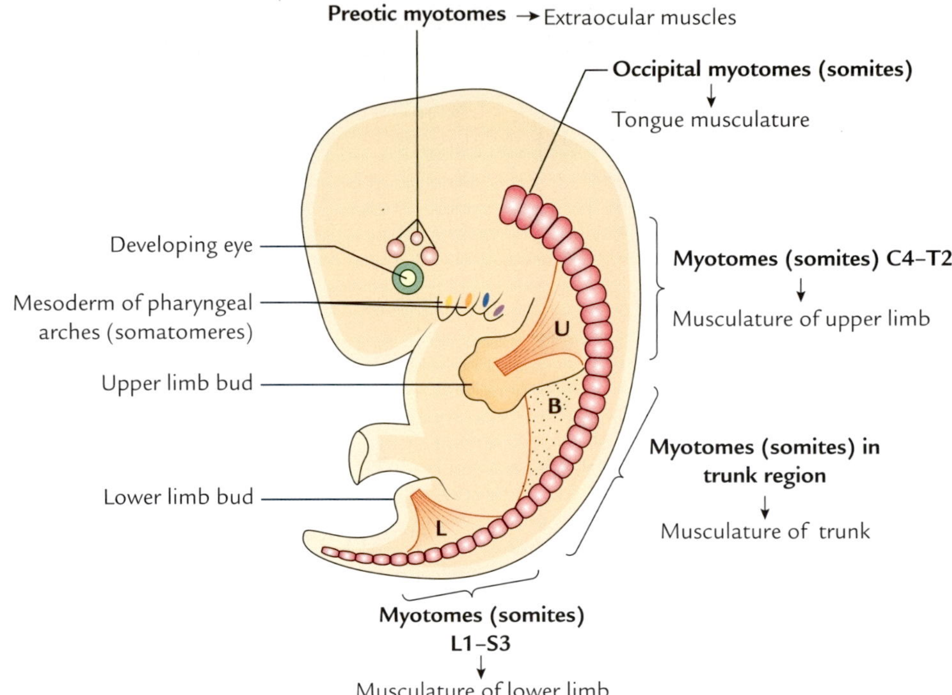

Fig. 13.1 Myotomes derived from somites and somatomeres in different regions of the body which form skeletal muscles. U, musculature of upper limb; B, musculature of trunk; L, musculature of lower limb.

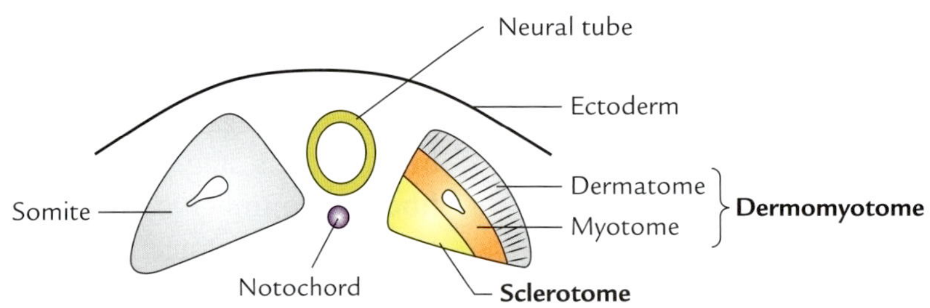

Fig. 13.2 Somite (on the left side) and its subdivisions (on the right side).

Muscles of the Body Wall (Figs 13.4 and 13.5) AN 52.4

Muscles of the body wall are derived from **myotomes** (somites) of the trunk region. Each myotome is supplied by a single spinal nerve. Each myotome divides into two parts: a smaller dorsal part called **epaxial part** (**epimere**) and a larger ventral part called **hypaxial part** (**hypomere**). The muscles derived from **epimere** are supplied by dorsal ramus of spinal nerve and muscles derived from **hypomere** are supplied by ventral ramus of spinal nerve.

The **epimeres of myotomes** form extensor muscles of the vertebral column (e.g., erector spinae).

The hypomeres of myotomes extend ventrolaterally along the somatopleuric layer of coelomic cavity and form the following muscles of the body wall:

1. Three layers of muscles in the thorax, namely, external intercostal, internal intercostal, and intercostal intimus (transversus thoracis).
2. Three layers of muscles in the abdomen, namely, external oblique, internal oblique, and transversus abdominis.
3. Longus colli, longus capitis, and scalene muscles in the neck. *The scalene muscles in the neck represent intercostal muscles.* On each side of midline on the ventral aspect of body, three primitive muscles of

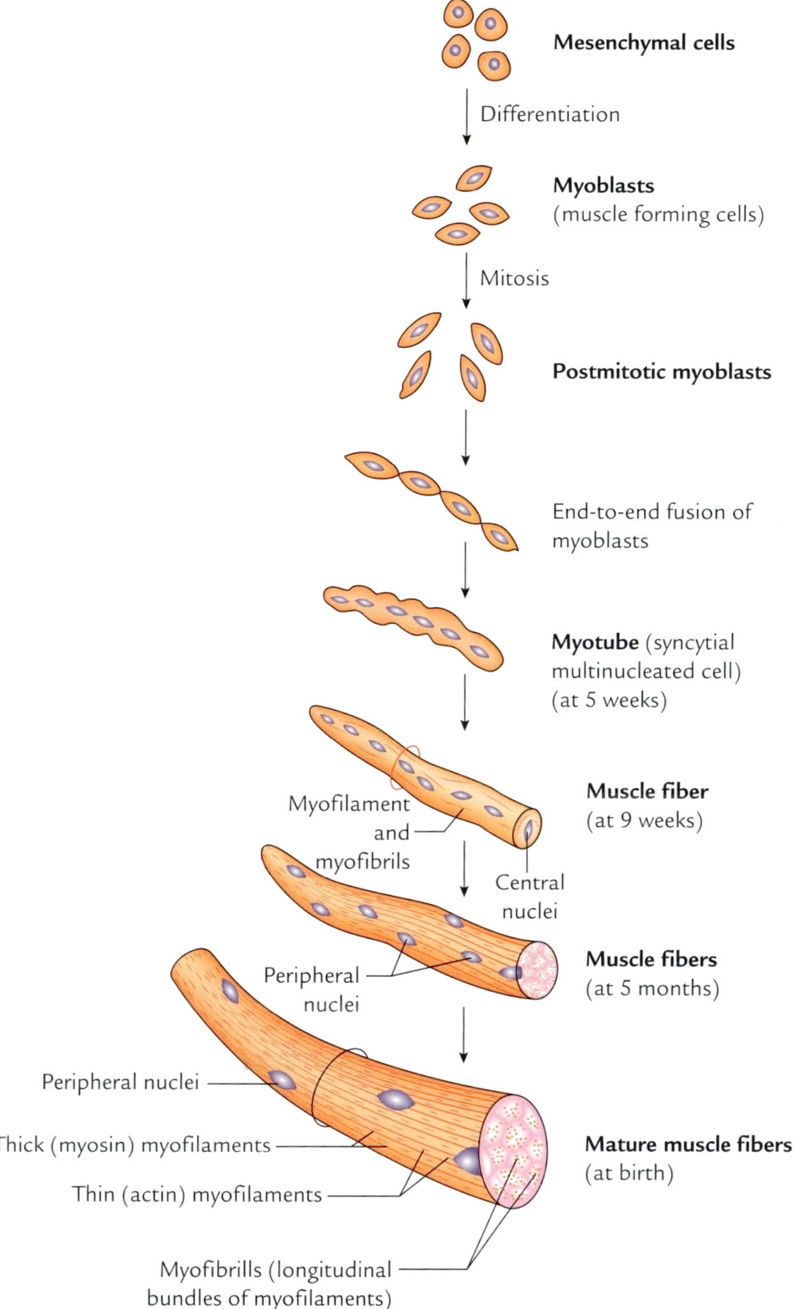

Fig. 13.3 Myogenesis of a skeletal muscle.

the body wall fuse to form the longitudinal column of muscle. This longitudinal column of muscle in humans is represented by

(a) rectus abdominis in abdomen,
(b) rectus sternalis in thorax (present sometimes only), and
(c) infrahyoid muscles in the neck.

N.B. The innermost muscle of primitive body wall in the thoracic region (e.g., transversus thoracis) is gradually peeled off by developing lung buds and subsequently blends with septum transversum to form **diaphragm**.

Muscles of Head and Neck

1. **Extraocular muscles (extrinsic muscles) of eyeball** (Fig. 13.6): These muscles develop from **three preotic myotomes** that are arranged around developing eye. The muscles derived from these myotomes are innervated by **third**, **fourth**, and **sixth cranial nerves;** hence, the extraocular muscles are supplied by third, fourth, and sixth cranial nerves.
2. **Muscles of tongue** (Fig. 13.6): These develop from precervical somites called **occipital somites.** The

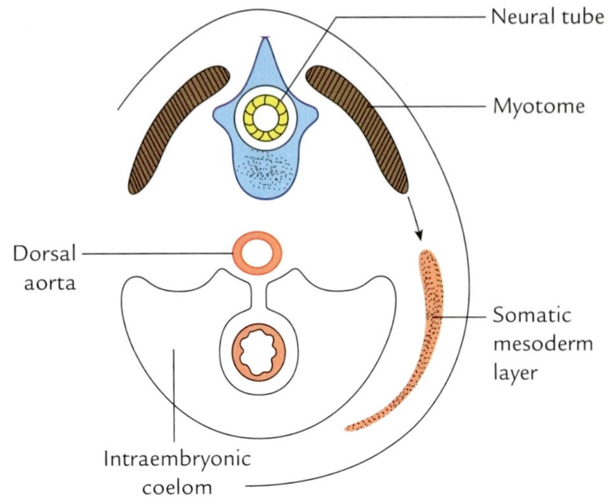

Fig. 13.4 Migration of cells of myotome in ventral direction.

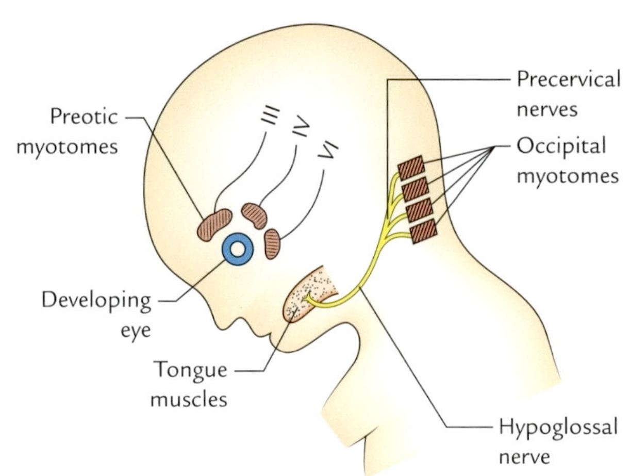

Fig. 13.6 Development of the muscles of tongue and extrinsic muscles of the eye.

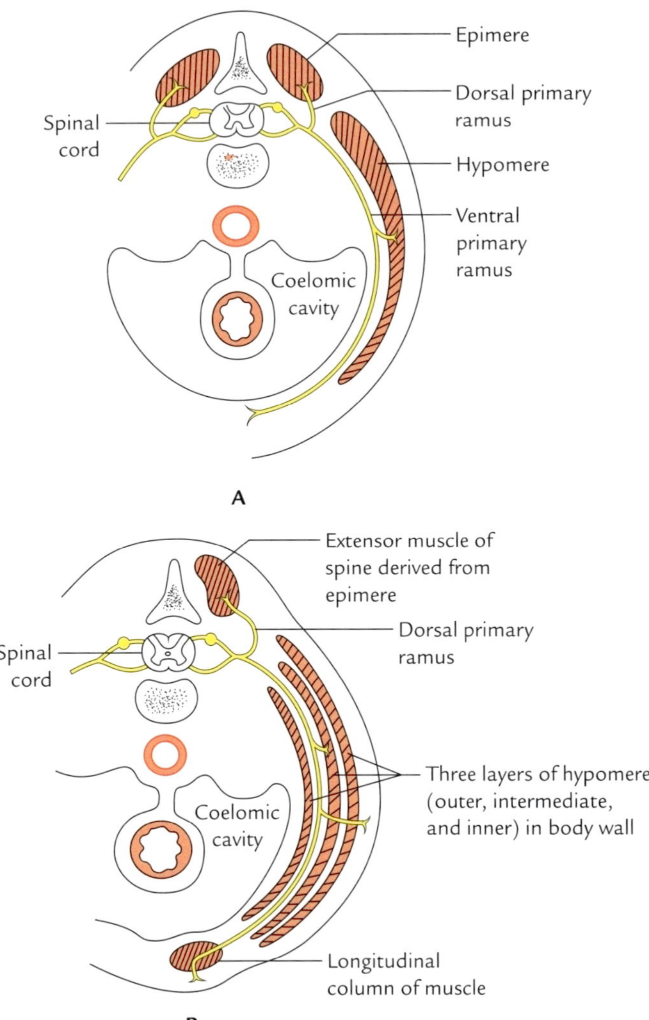

Fig. 13.5 (A) Subdivision of myotome into epimere and hypomere, and their innervation by dorsal primary ramus and ventral primary ramus, respectively. (B) Formation of three separate muscle layers from hypomere and ventral longitudinal muscles.

occipital myotomes are innervated by **precervical nerves** that subsequently fuse to form composite **hypoglossal nerve.** When the tongue develops in the floor of pharynx, the occipital myotomes migrate forward along **epipericardial ridge**, invade substance of the developing tongue, and form all intrinsic and extrinsic muscles of the tongue except palatoglossus. Therefore, the hypoglossal nerves supply all the intrinsic and extrinsic muscles of the tongue except palatoglossus, which truly speaking is not a muscle of the tongue but that of a palate.

3. **Muscles of pharyngeal arches:** These develop from mesoderm of pharyngeal arches derived from somatomeres. The muscles derived from mesoderm of pharyngeal arches are muscles of mastication, facial expression, pharynx, and larynx. These muscles are innervated by nerves of the respective pharyngeal arches. The muscles of pharyngeal arches are described in detail in Chapter 14.

Muscles of Limbs (Fig. 13.7)

Muscles of limbs develop from myotomes present in the upper and lower limb bud regions. The mesoderm derived from these myotomes migrates into the limb bud during the 5th week and forms **anterior** and **posterior condensations.**

The **anterior condensation** of mesoderm gives rise to flexor and pronator muscles of the upper limb and extensor and adductor muscles of the lower limb.

The **posterior condensation** of mesoderm gives rise to **extensor and supinator muscles of the upper limb** and flexor and abductor muscles of the lower limb.

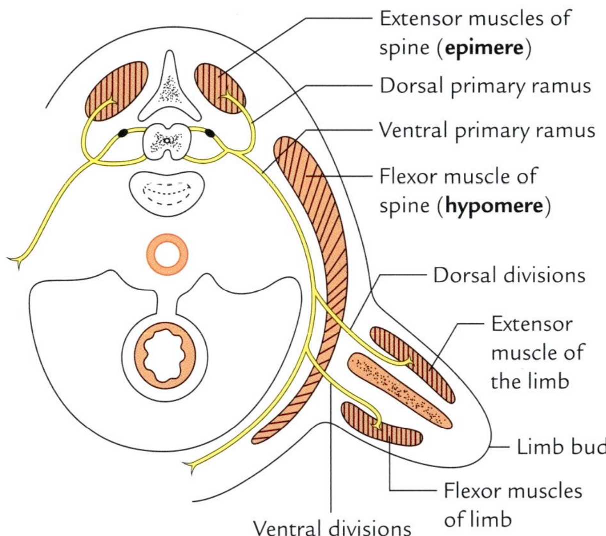

Fig. 13.7 Development of musculature into the limb bud. Note the extensor (dorsal) and flexor (ventral) components of limb musculature.

N.B. The upper limb bud lies opposite the lower five cervical and upper two thoracic (C4 through C8 and T1-2) segments, whereas the lower limb lies opposite the lower four lumbar and upper two sacral (L2 through L5 and S1-2) segments. Hence, the muscles of upper limb are innervated by lower five cervical and upper two thoracic segments, whereas the muscles of lower limb are supplied by lower four lumbar and upper two sacral spinal segments.

As the limb buds are formed, various spinal nerves enter into the mesenchyme. At first these nerves enter as isolated dorsal and ventral divisions of ventral primary rami (Fig. 13.7), but soon these divisions unite to form large dorsal and ventral nerves. Thus, radial nerve, which supplies to the extensor muscle, is formed by the union of dorsal divisions, whereas the ulnar and median nerves, which supply the flexor muscles, are formed by the union of ventral divisions.

CLINICAL CORRELATION

1. ***Duchenne muscular dystrophy (DMD):*** It is a hereditary disease of skeletal muscles that usually affects males (for details see p. 359).
2. ***Congenital anomalies of the skeletal muscles***
   (a) *Partial or complete absence of one or more muscles:* It is a rather common phenomenon. One of the best examples is partial or complete absence of pectoralis major muscle. The other examples are palmaris longus, serratus anterior, and quadratus femoris.
   (b) *Congenital torticollis:* It is congenital shortening of the sternocleidomastoid muscle, which occurs due to excessive stretching of this muscle during delivery. The excessive stretching causes hemorrhage in the muscle and subsequent shortening due to fibrosis.

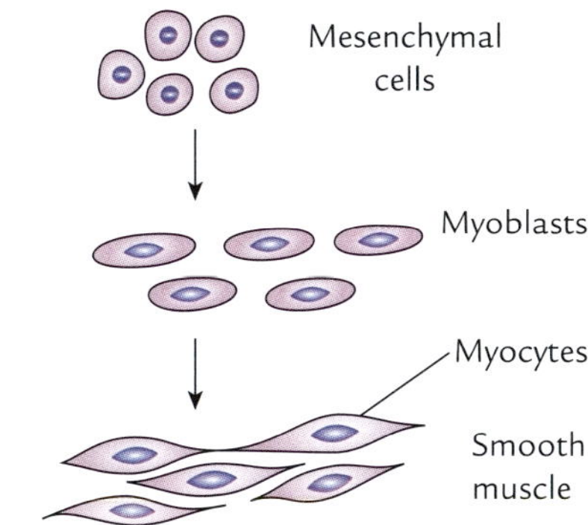

Fig. 13.8 Myogenesis of smooth muscle.

DEVELOPMENT OF SMOOTH (INVOLUNTARY) MUSCLES

1. The smooth muscle in the wall of digestive and respiratory tracts develops mainly from **splanchnic mesoderm** surrounding primordia of digestive and respiratory tracts.
2. The smooth muscle in the wall of most of the blood and lymph vessels develops in situ from surrounding splanchnic mesoderm.
3. Muscles of iris (**sphincter** and **dilator pupillae**), arrector pili muscles of skin, and myoepithelial cells of sweat and mammary glands develop from mesenchymal cells derived from ectoderm. The muscles of iris develop from ectoderm of the optic cup.

N.B. **Axiom:** Mesenchyme present anywhere in the body is a potential source of smooth muscle tissue.

Myogenesis of the Smooth Muscle (Fig. 13.8)

The mesenchymal cells differentiate into myoblasts. The myoblasts become spindle shaped and their nuclei become oval. The myoblasts do not fuse with each other as in skeletal muscle; consequently, muscle fibers of smooth muscle remain mononucleated.

The contractile elements develop in the cytoplasm of the muscle fiber but are nonsarcomeric.

DEVELOPMENT OF CARDIAC MUSCLE

The cardiac muscle develops from **myoepicardial mantle**, which is formed by thickening of **splanchnic mesoderm** surrounding the developing heart tube.

Myogenesis of the Cardiac Muscle (Fig. 13.9)

The cardiac muscle fibers develop from differentiation and growth of single myoblasts, unlike skeletal muscle fibers that develop from fusion of a number of myoblasts. The growth of cardiac muscle fibers occurs due

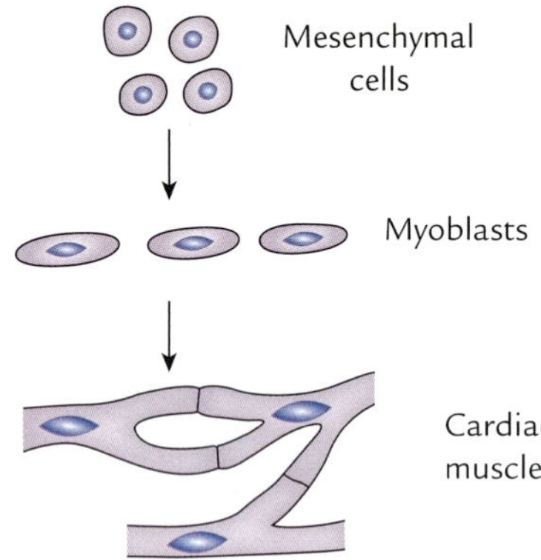

Fig. 13.9 Myogenesis of cardiac muscle.

to the formation of new myofilaments and myofibrils. **The cardiac muscle fibers elongate and give rise to numerous side branches.** The side branches as well as ends of one cardiac muscle fiber adhere to side branches and ends of other cardiac muscle fibers, but the intervening cell membranes persist (i.e., they do not disintegrate). These sites of adhesion of the cell membranes between cardiac muscle fibers persist as **intercalated discs.** Therefore, the cardiac muscle does not form true syncytium.

The myofibrils around the central nucleus of the cardiac muscle fibers present cross-striated appearance.

N.B. Late in the embryonic period, some myoblasts develop cardiac muscle fibers that have relatively few myofibrils and relatively larger diameters than the typical cardiac muscle fibers. These **atypical cardiac muscle fibers** form bundles called **Purkinje fibers**, which form conducting system of the heart.

GESTATIONAL AGE OF KEY DEVELOPMENTAL EVENTS

Developmental Event	Gestational Age
➢ Muscles begin to develop during	6th week
➢ All skeletal muscles develop by	Birth
➢ Heart/cardiac muscle becomes recognizable in	4th week

GOLDEN FACTS TO REMEMBER

➢ **First hallmark in muscle development**	Elongation of nuclei and cell bodies of mesenchymal cells
➢ **Myoblasts**	Embryonic muscle cells
➢ **All the skeletal muscle fibers in humans are formed**	By birth (since mitotic activity of myoblasts ceases after birth)
➢ **Contractile cells in the body other than those in skeletal, cardiac, and smooth muscles**	(a) **Myoepithelial cells** (associated with secretory acini) (b) **Myofibroblasts** (involved in wound healing) (c) **Myoid cells** (found around seminiferous tubules)
➢ **Rectus abdominis muscle of abdomen in the thorax is represented by**	Rectus sternalis
➢ **Occipital group of segmental nerves are represented by**	Hypoglossal nerve
➢ **Occipital myotome which disappears soon after its formation**	First occipital myotome
➢ **Best example of partial or complete absence of skeletal muscle**	Pectoralis major
➢ **Most common type of muscular dystrophy**	Duchenne muscular dystrophy (DMD)
➢ **Most skeletal muscles develop from**	Myotomes
➢ **Most smooth muscles develop from**	Splanchnic mesoderm
➢ **Cardiac muscle develops from**	Splanchnic mesoderm

CLINICAL PROBLEM SOLVING

PROBLEMS

1. What is **Duchenne muscular dystrophy**? Give its embryological basis and discuss its clinical presentation.
2. A newborn female infant presents with an absence of right anterior axillary fold and displacement of her right nipple below and toward the axilla. What is the most probable clinical diagnosis? Discuss its functional and cosmetic implications.
3. Discuss the **molecular regulation of development of muscle**.
4. **The human baby takes several months after birth to crawl, while babies of most mammals can walk or even run within few hours after birth. Why?**

SOLUTIONS

1. The **Duchenne muscular dystrophy (DMD)** is a clinical condition characterized by **progressive muscle weakness and wasting**. It generally leads to death of an individual in his teens or 20s due to cardiac or respiratory failure.

   The DMD is an X-linked condition caused by a **recessive allele**. Men who have only defective allele of the DMD gene from the mother suffer from this disease (for details see p. 359).

2. The most likely clinical diagnosis is **Poland syndrome**. This syndrome is characterized by partial (often sternal part) or complete absence of pectoralis major muscle. The absence of pectoralis major is occasionally associated with the absence of mammary gland and/or hypoplasia of the nipple. In this case, the cause of abnormal surface feature is the absence of pectoralis major. The affected individuals may present shortness of middle digits (**brachydactyly**) and fusion of digits (**syndactyly**).

   Loss of the pectoralis major muscles produces little or no functional loss as other muscles associated with shoulder joint compensate for the loss of the pectoralis major, but disfigurement of the chest is a cause of concern, particularly in females.

3. The molecular signals for muscle cell induction arise from tissues adjacent to prospective muscles cells. The myogenic cells express two types of genes: ***Myo*D** (a helix–loop–helix transcription factor) and ***MYFs*** (myogenic regulator factors).

   Following induction, myogenic cells enter the cell cycle (i.e., undergo mitosis). The ***Myo*D** genes remove myogenic cells from the cell cycle (i.e., mitosis stops) and switch on muscle-specific genes (***MYF***) to form **postmitotic myoblasts**.

N.B. **The damaged muscles fail to regenerate because they develop from postmitotic myoblasts.**

4. The development of skeletal muscle tissue begins to develop from specialized mesodermal cells (myoblasts) during the 4th week of intrauterine life. At 9th week, primitive myofilaments develop in the cytoplasm of developed muscle fibers. The muscles of entire muscular system get differentiated and correctly positioned by the 8th week. The orientation of developing muscle is preceded and influenced by cartilaginous models of bones. The muscles of the trunk and limbs are supplied by spinal nerves.

   It is not certain when skeletal muscles are sufficiently developed to sustain contractions but by week 17, the fetal movements (known as **quickening**) are strong enough to be recognized by mother.

   Muscle coordination is an ongoing process of achieving a fine neural control of muscle fibers, i.e., 1 year after birth in humans, whereas in lower mammals such as quadrupeds it is achieved before birth. This is the reason why human baby takes several months to crawl, whereas babies of lower animals can walk or even run immediately after birth.

14 Development of Head, Neck, and Pharyngeal Apparatus

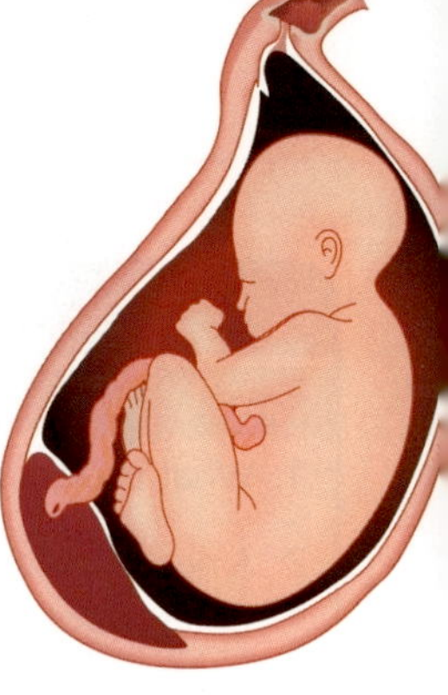

LEARNING OBJECTIVES

After studying this chapter, the student should be able to:

- Define pharyngeal arches, and enumerate their number and source of development.
- Discuss the nerves and arteries of pharyngeal arches.
- Define the components of pharyngeal arch, and enumerate the derivatives of these components in each pharyngeal arch.
- Discuss the developmental components of a pharyngeal apparatus and its congenital anomalies. AN 43.4
- Describe pharyngeal clefts, pouches, and membranes, and enumerate their derivatives.
- Describe the embryological basis of branchial cyst and branchial fistula.

OVERVIEW

The **development of head and neck region** occurs during 4th to 8th week of embryonic period. The **neck** is formed as a result of elongation of region between stomodeum and pericardial bulge due to descent of developing heart. It begins with the development of pharyngeal arches during 4th week of intrauterine life (IUL).

The pharynx is funnel-shaped upper part of foregut. It is flattened dorsoventrally and has a floor (ventral wall), roof (dorsal wall), and two lateral walls.

The lateral wall from superficial to deep consists of ectoderm, mesoderm, and endoderm.

Early in the **4th week of intrauterine** development, a series of surface elevations appear in the lateral wall of primitive pharynx caudal to stomodeum. These elevations are termed **pharyngeal arches** (Figs 14.1 and 14.2). The *pouches* between these arches on the inner aspect of the pharyngeal wall are termed **pharyngeal pouches**, and the grooves between these arches on the outer aspect of the pharyngeal wall are called **pharyngeal clefts**. The thin segments of lateral wall between pharyngeal cleft and pouch are called **pharyngeal membranes**.

Initially, the pharyngeal arches are confined in the lateral wall of the primitive pharynx. But gradually they extend ventrally and fuse with their counterparts of the opposite side in floor of the primitive pharynx to form horseshoe-shaped cylindrical bars (Fig. 14.7B).

Initially, there are six arches. The **fifth arch** is small and rudimentary and soon disappears. Some authorities even say that it just appears to disappear. Thus, only **five pharyngeal arches** remain. The pharyngeal arches are numbered craniocaudally as 1, 2, 3, 4, and 6 (Figs 14.1, 14.2, 14.3, and 14.7).

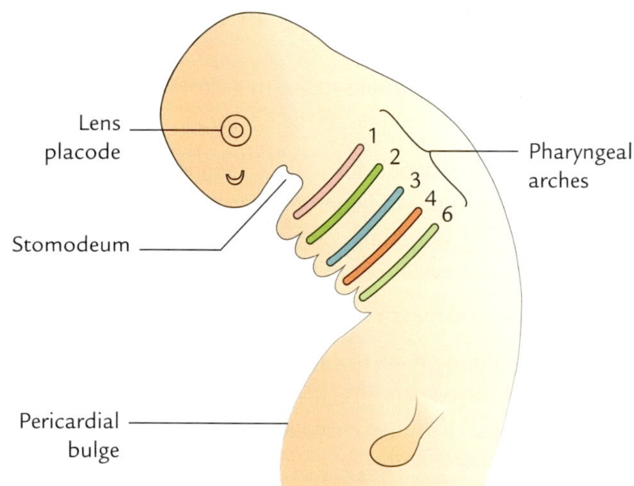

Fig. 14.1 Pharyngeal arches.

Pharyngeal Apparatus

The **pharyngeal apparatus** consists of *pharyngeal arches, pharyngeal pouches, pharyngeal clefts (grooves),* and *pharyngeal membranes.* All these structures largely contribute to the *formation of head and neck region* (e.g., face, neck, definitive mouth, pharynx, and larynx).

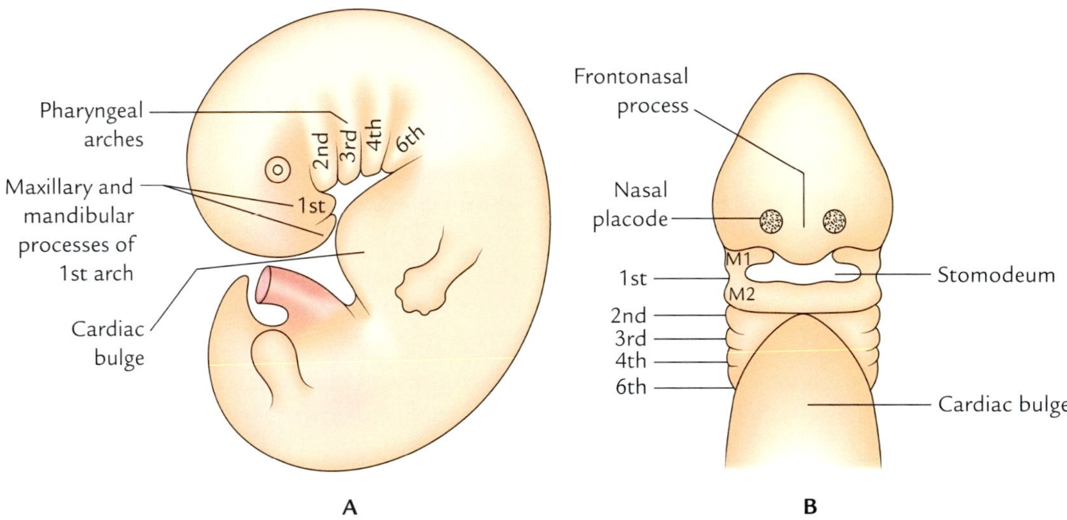

Fig. 14.2 Formation of pharyngeal arches. (A) Lateral view. (B) Frontal view. Note that the first pharyngeal arch consists of maxillary and mandibular processes. M1 = maxillary process, M2 = mandibular process.

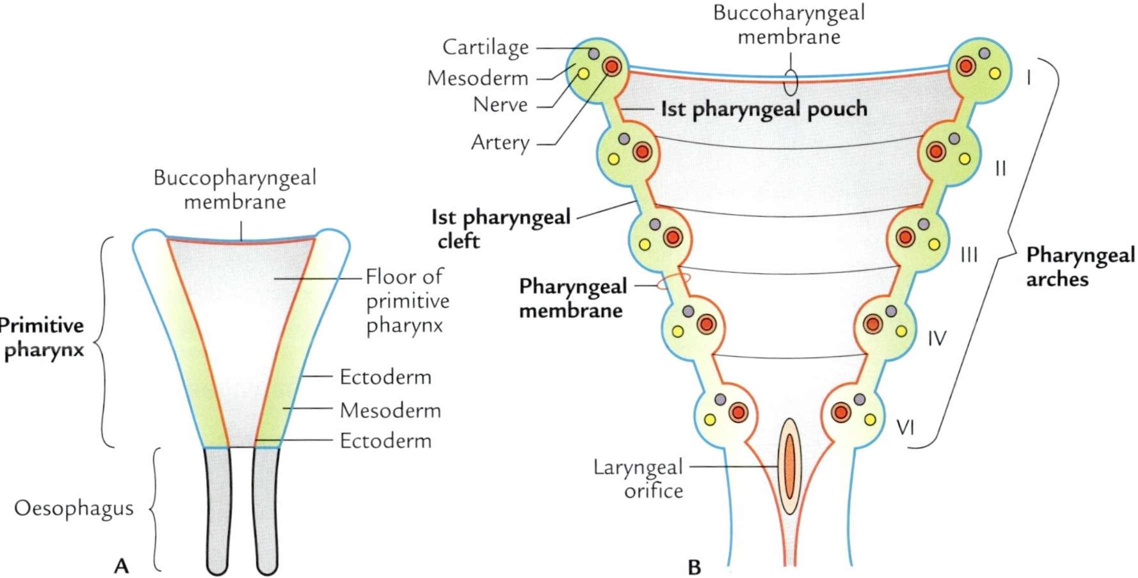

Fig. 14.3 Primitive pharynx (as seen in coronal section). (A) Before the formation of pharyngeal arches. (B) After the formation of pharyngeal arches.

COMPONENTS OF PHARYNGEAL APPARATUS (FIG. 14.3)

1. **Pharyngeal arches:** *Five in number* and present in the lateral wall and floor of the primitive pharynx. They consist of a central core of mesoderm, lined externally by ectoderm and internally by endoderm.
2. **Pharyngeal clefts (grooves):** *Four in number* and present externally between the arches. They are lined by **ectoderm.**
3. **Pharyngeal pouches:** *Four in number* and located internally between the two pharyngeal arches. They are lined by **endoderm.**
4. **Pharyngeal membranes:** Four in number and located between the two adjacent arches where pharyngeal cleft and pouches are opposed to each other.

PHARYNGEAL ARCHES

Pharyngeal arches appear due to proliferation of mesoderm in the wall of primitive pharynx. They form horseshoe-shaped cylindrical bars in its lateral and ventral walls. These provide support to the wall of primitive pharynx ventrolaterally.

Each pharyngeal arch consists of a **core of mesoderm**, derived from paraxial mesoderm and neural crest cells. It is covered externally by ectoderm and internally by endoderm.

The cells of mesodermal core of pharyngeal arches are pluripotent and differentiate into an artery, skeletal element (e.g., cartilage), and muscle masses. In addition, each arch is traversed by a nerve.

Components of a Pharyngeal Arch

A typical pharyngeal arch consists of the following components (Fig. 14.4):

- A **cartilaginous bar/rod** (*skeletal element*) derived from neural crest mesenchyme.
- A **muscle mass** derived from mesodermal core of the pharyngeal arch.
- A **pharyngeal arch artery** that connects with the corresponding horn of aortic sac (truncus arteriosus) of primitive heart.
- A **nerve** derived from hind brain vesicle.

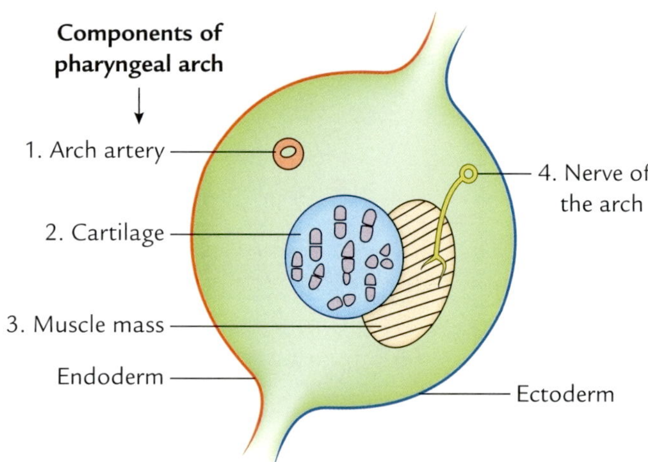

Fig. 14.4 Structures of pharyngeal arch.

FATE OF PHARYNGEAL ARCH COMPONENTS

The **arch mesoderm** derived from paraxial mesoderm gives rise to most of the muscles of head and neck region, whereas the arch mesoderm derived from neural crest cells gives rise to skeletal elements and connective tissue of the head and neck region.

A **cartilaginous rod of arch** forms the skeletal derivatives of the arch. Part of cartilage forms permanent skeletal elements (e.g., bone and cartilage) and part of it disappears. Sometimes the cartilage disappears, but its perichondrium persists to form ligament/raphe.

The **arch arteries** are connected ventrally to ventral aorta. They pass around the primitive pharynx to open in the dorsal aorta.

The **nerve of arch** provides motor innervation to muscles derived from arch and sensory innervation to skin and mucosa derived from the arch, respectively.

The arch arteries develop into major arteries close to the heart. (These are described in detail in Chapter 23.)

N.B. Morphologically, each pharyngeal arch is supplied by two nerves. The nerve that runs along cranial border of the arch is known as **post-trematic nerve** and nerve that runs along its caudal border is called **pretrematic nerve**. In human beings, the pretrematic nerves disappear from all arches except first arch where it persists as **chorda tympani nerve**. Some authorities consider that the *tympanic branch of glossopharyngeal nerve* and *auricular branch of vagus nerve* represent the pretrematic branches of these nerves (Fig. 14.5).

1. Muscles of the Pharyngeal Arches

The mesoderm of each arch gives rise to muscles. These muscles either are attached to the skeletal elements developed from the same arch or migrate elsewhere. However, all these muscles are supplied by nerve of the

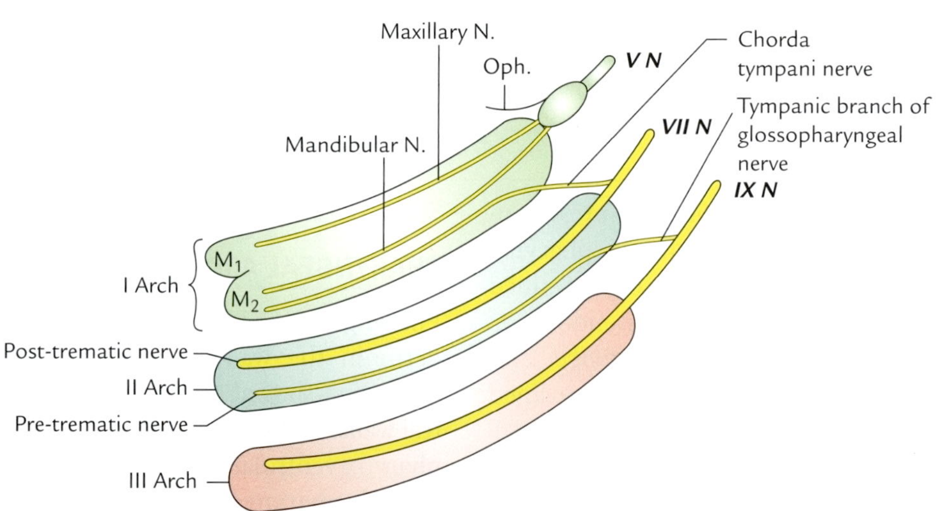

Fig. 14.5 Arrangement of post-trematic and pretrematic nerves.

arch from which they develop. Hence, nerve supply of the muscle indicates its origin from the particular arch.

Muscles of First Arch

The muscles derived from first arch are muscles of mastication (namely, temporalis, masseter, lateral pterygoid, and medial pterygoid), anterior belly of digastric, mylohyoid, tensor tympani, and tensor palati.

All these muscles of first arch are supplied by mandibular nerve.

Muscles of Second Arch

The muscles derived from second arches are muscles of the facial expression, posterior belly of digastric, stylohyoid, and stapedius.

All these muscles of second arch are supplied by facial nerve.

Muscles of Third Arch

The only muscle derived from the third arch is stylopharyngeus.

Muscles of third arch are supplied by glossopharyngeal nerve.

Muscles of Fourth and Sixth Arches

The muscles derived from fourth arch are cricothyroid, levator veli palati, and constrictors of the pharynx.

These are supplied by superior laryngeal nerve.

The muscles derived from sixth arch are intrinsic muscles of the larynx.

These are supplied by recurrent laryngeal nerve.

2. Nerves of the Pharyngeal Arches (Fig. 14.6)

Nerve of the First Arch

Trigeminal nerve (CN V) (maxillary and mandibular divisions) is the nerve of the first arch. The first arch is also supplied by the **chorda tympani nerve**, *a pretrematic branch of the facial nerve* – the nerve of second arch.

Motor branches from mandibular nerve supply muscles derived from the first arch (see Table 14.1, p. 154).

Sensory branches from maxillary and mandibular nerves supply the skin of face, mucous membrane of the nasal cavity, oral cavity, soft palate and tongue, and teeth of upper and lower jaw.

The chorda tympani nerve supplies taste fibers to the anterior two-thirds of tongue.

Nerve of the Second Arch

Facial nerve (CN VII) is the nerve of the second arch and supplies the motor branches to all the muscles derived from the second arch (see Table 14.1, p. 154).

Nerve of the Third Arch

Glossopharyngeal nerve (CN IX) is the nerve of the third arch. Its motor component supplies stylopharyngeus muscle, whereas its sensory component supplies mucous membrane of the pharynx.

Nerves of the Fourth and Sixth Arches

Superior laryngeal nerve, a branch of vagus nerve, is the nerve of the fourth arch, and **recurrent laryngeal nerve**, also a branch of the vagus, is the nerve of the sixth arch.

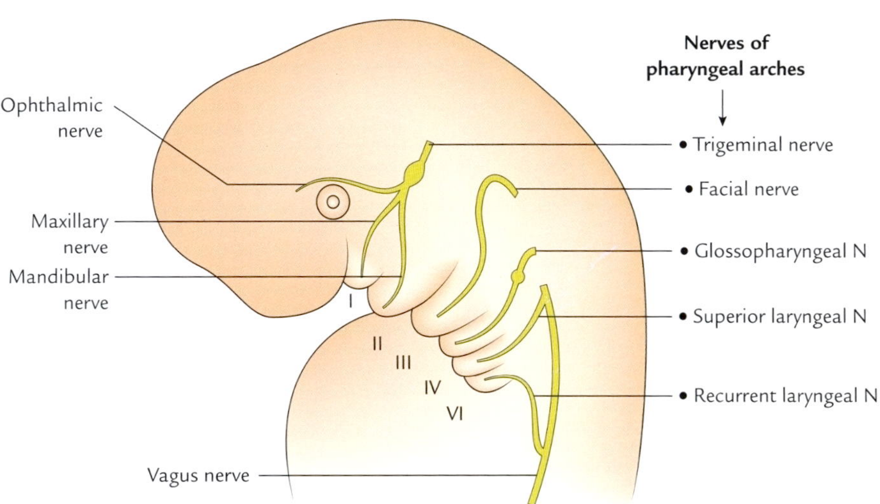

Fig. 14.6 Nerves of pharyngeal arches.

Superior laryngeal nerve supplies cricothyroid muscle of the larynx, whereas the recurrent laryngeal nerve supplies rest of the intrinsic muscles of the larynx.

Sensory branches from both these nerves supply mucus membrane of the larynx. Superior laryngeal nerve supplies the mucus membrane above vocal cords, whereas recurrent laryngeal nerve supplies the mucous membrane below vocal cords.

3. Cartilages of the Pharyngeal Arches and Their Derivatives (Figs 14.7 and 14.8)

Each cartilage is horseshoe shaped with its ends directed dorsally. The dorsal ends lie at a higher level than the ventral part of the arch (Fig. 14.7).

First Arch Cartilage

The first arch cartilage is called **Meckel's cartilage**. It forms in the ventral portion of the first arch called **mandibular process**. The dorsal end of this cartilage lies close to developing middle ear cavity.

The dorsal end of Meckel's cartilage persists and forms two small bones: **malleus and incus** – the ear ossicles that are then incorporated in the middle ear cavity.

The ventral part of Meckel's cartilage largely disappears. The local mesenchyme lying around ventral part of the Meckel's cartilage ossify by membranous ossification to form **mandible**.

The **intermediate part of the Meckel's cartilage** between ear ossicles and mandible disappears but its perichondrium persists to form two ligaments: (a) **anterior ligament of malleus** and (b) **sphenomandibular ligament.**

N.B.
- **Mandible** is not formed from the Meckel's cartilage but is molded around it by membranous ossification of surrounding mesoderm.
- The mesenchyme of dorsal portion – the maxillary process of the first pharyngeal arch – gives rise to **premaxilla, maxilla, zygomatic bone,** and **part of the temporal bone** by membranous ossification.

Second Arch Cartilage

The second arch cartilage is called **Reichert's cartilage.** The dorsal end of the second arch cartilage ossifies to form the third ear ossicle – the **stapes.** It is later incorporated into the middle ear cavity. Caudal to stapes, the second arch cartilage forms **styloid process of the temporal bone.** The ventral part of the Reichert's cartilage ossifies to form **lesser cornu** and **upper part of body of the hyoid bone.** The part of cartilage between hyoid bone and styloid process disappears but its perichondrium persists to form **stylohyoid ligament.**

Third Arch Cartilage

The third arch cartilage is located in the ventral part of the arch. The ventral part of the third arch cartilage ossifies to form **greater cornu** and the **lower part of the body of hyoid bone.** The rest of the cartilage disappears.

Fourth and Sixth Arch Cartilages

Fourth and sixth arch cartilages fuse with each other. Together these form all the cartilages of the larynx,

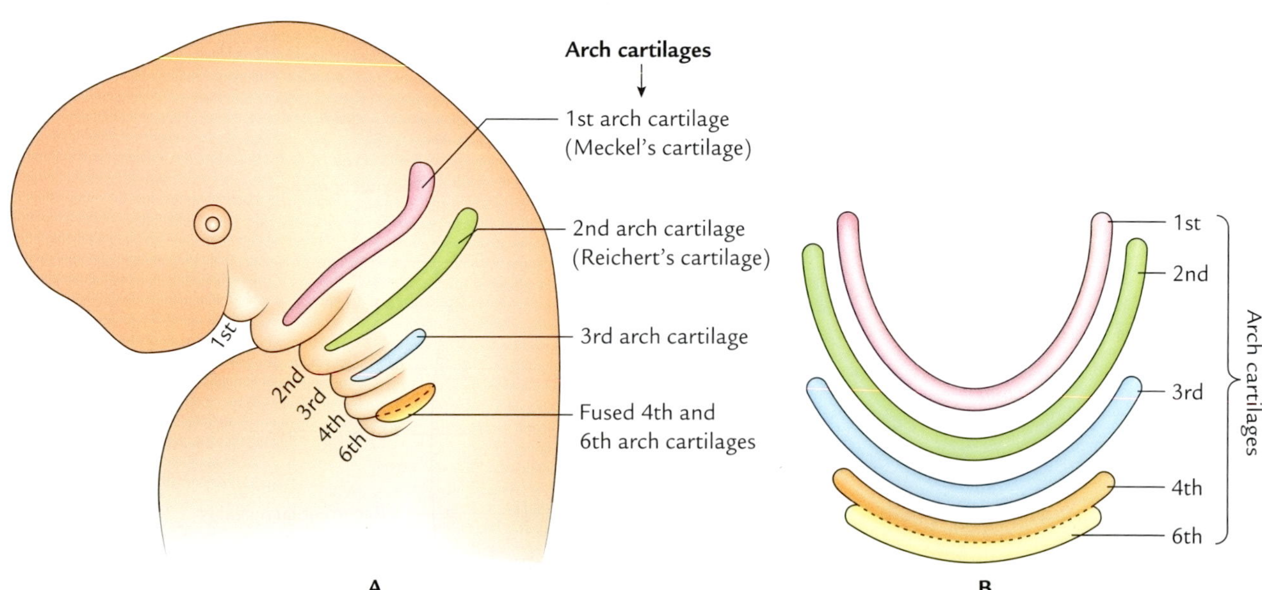

Fig. 14.7 Cartilages of pharyngeal arches. (A) Lateral view. (B) Frontal view. Note that cartilages of fourth and sixth pharyngeal arches are fused.

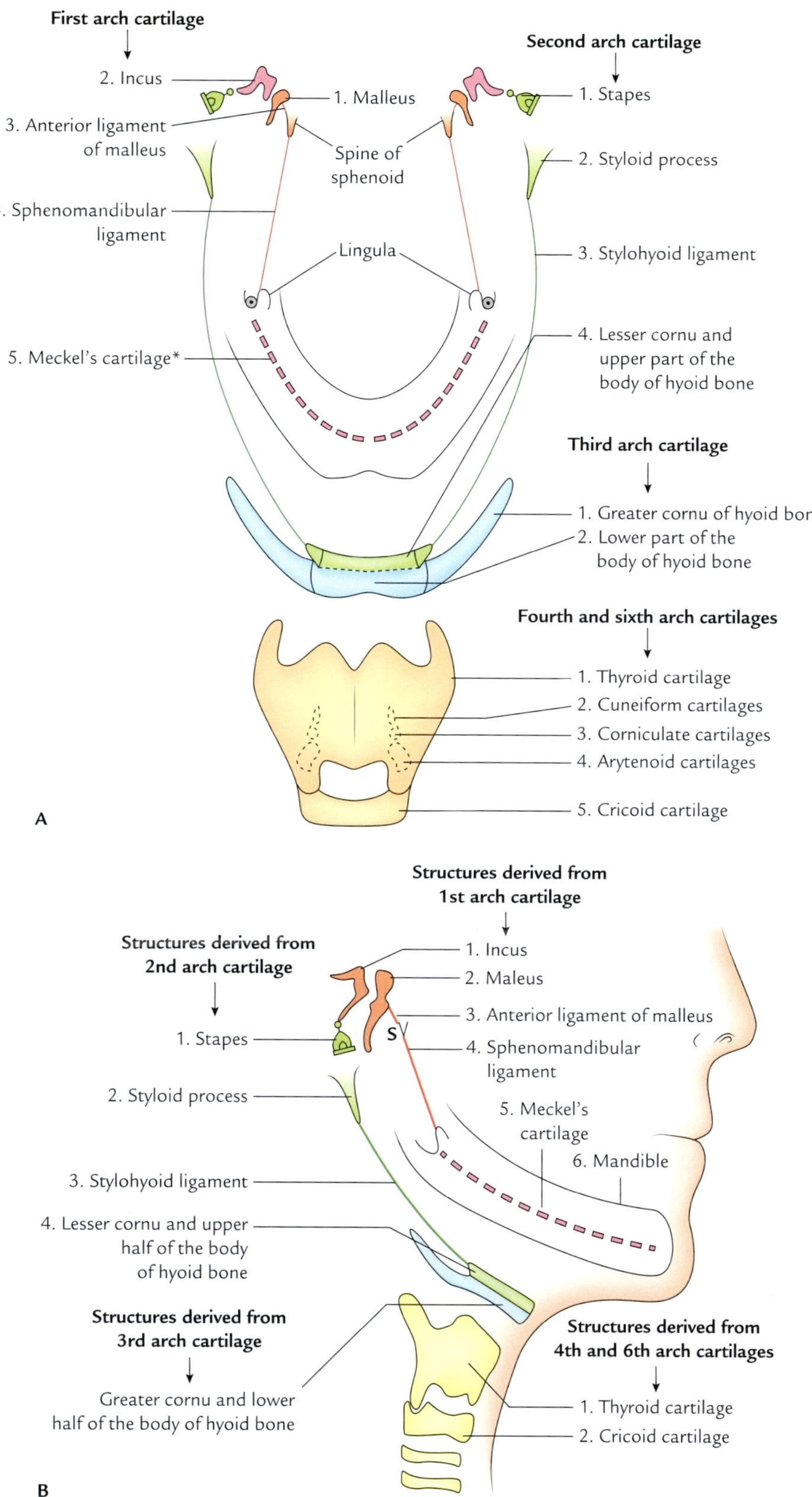

Fig. 14.8 Skeletal derivatives from various pharyngeal arch cartilages: (A) Frontal view. (B) Side view. Structures derived from first arch cartilage (red color), structures derived from second arch cartilage (green color), structures derived from third arch cartilage (blue color), and structures derived from fourth and sixth arch cartilages (yellow color). *Ventral part of Meckel's cartilage largely disappears and mandible develops from local mesenchyme by intramembranous ossification.

Table 14.1 Main derivatives of the pharyngeal arches

Pharyngeal Arch	Nerve/Nerves	Muscles	Skeletal Derivatives
First arch/ mandibular arch	Mandibular nerve	**Muscles of mastication** (temporalis, masseter, medial, and lateral pterygoids), mylohyoid, anterior belly of digastric, tensor veli palatini, and tensor tympani	Malleus, incus, anterior ligament of malleus, sphenomandibular ligament, and mandible from Meckel's cartilage
Second arch	Facial nerve	**Muscles of facial expression** (buccinator, auricularis, occipitofrontalis, platysma, orbicularis oris, and orbicularis oculi), posterior belly of digastric, stylohyoid, and stapedius	Stapes, styloid process, stylohyoid ligament, lesser cornu of the hyoid bone, and upper part of body of the hyoid bone from Reichert's cartilage
Third arch	Glossopharyngeal nerve	Stylopharyngeus	Greater cornu and lower part of body of the hyoid bone from third arch cartilage
Fourth and sixth arches	**Superior laryngeal nerve**, a branch of vagus nerve (nerve of fourth arch) **Recurrent laryngeal nerve**, a branch of vagus nerve (nerve of sixth arch)	Cricothyroid, levator palati, constrictors of pharynx, and intrinsic muscles of the larynx	Laryngeal cartilages (thyroid, cricoid, arytenoid, corniculate, and cuneiform) from fourth and sixth arch cartilages

namely, **thyroid, cricoid, arytenoid, corniculate**, and **cuneiform cartilages** except **epiglottis**, which develops from the caudal part of hypobranchial eminence (for details see p. 217).

The skeletal derivatives of pharyngeal arches are shown in Fig. 14.8. The main structures derived from pharyngeal arches are given in Table 14.1.

4. Arteries of Pharyngeal Arches

Each pharyngeal arch has its own artery that connects the **aortic sac** with the **dorsal aorta**. (Described in detail in Chapter 23.) The fate of pharyngeal arch arteries is given in Table 14.2.

Table 14.2 The fate of pharyngeal arch arteries

Arch Artery	Derivatives
First arch artery	Maxillary artery
Second arch artery	Hyoid and stapedial arteries in fetal life
Third arch artery	(a) Common carotid artery (b) Internal carotid artery
Fourth arch artery	(a) Aortic arch (on the left side) (b) Subclavian artery (on the right side)
Sixth arch artery	(a) Ductus arteriosus (on the left side) (b) Pulmonary artery (on the right side)

CLINICAL CORRELATIONS

First arch syndromes

These syndromes occur due to lack of migration of neural crest cells into the first pharyngeal arch. Clinically, they present with various facial anomalies called **first arch syndromes**. The important first arch syndromes are (a) **Treacher Collins syndrome**, (b) **Pierre Robin syndrome**, and (c) **DiGeorge syndrome**.

The first two are most important first arch syndromes.

1. ***Treacher Collins syndrome (mandibulofacial dysostosis):*** It is inherited as an *autosomal dominant trait*, i.e., caused by an autosomal dominant gene. It occurs in about 1/85,000 births. Clinically, it presents as (Fig. 14.9)
   - malar hypoplasia (due to underdevelopment of zygomatic bones),
   - mandibular hypoplasia (underdeveloped lower jaw),
   - down slanting palpebral fissures, and
   - deformed external ears.
2. ***Pierre Robin syndrome:*** It is an autosomal recessive disorder and occurs in approximately 1/85,000 births. The affected infant usually presents triad of anomalies: (a) micrognathia (small mandible), (b) cleft palate, and (c) glossoptosis (posteriorly placed tongue). The primary defect is small mandible.
3. ***DiGeorge syndrome:*** It is caused due to microdeletion on the long arm of chromosome 22. This leads to abnormal development of neural crest cells. It occurs in 1/25,000 births and represents the most severe example of disorders related to pharyngeal arches. Infants born with *DiGeorge syndrome* are without thymus and parathyroid glands, and have defects in their cardiac outflow tracts. Clinically, it presents as
   - fish mouth deformity (shortened philtrum),
   - low set notched ears, and
   - increased susceptibility to infection.

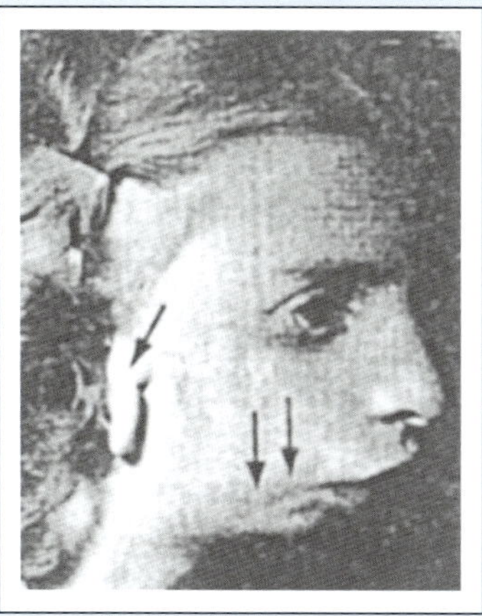

Fig. 14.9 Treacher Collins syndrome. (*Source:* This figure was published in Publication Recognizable Patterns of Human Malformation: Genetic, Embryologic and Clinical Aspects, 3rd edition by David W. Smith, ISBN: 9780721683812, Copyright Elsevier, 1982.)

PHARYNGEAL POUCHES (FIG. 14.10)

There are four pairs of pharyngeal pouches. These are evaginations of endodermal, lining of the interior of primitive pharynx between the two *arches*. The pharyngeal pouches are numbered in craniocaudal direction. Thus, the first pouch is between the first and second arch, the second pouch is between the second and third arch, and so on.

First Pharyngeal Pouch

The first pharyngeal pouch elongates to form a diverticulum called **tubotympanic recess.** The distal part of this recess expands, whereas the proximal part remains tubular. The distal expanded part of tubotympanic recess comes in contact with the first pharyngeal groove. The distal expanded part of tubotympanic recess forms the **middle ear cavity** (tympanum) and **mastoid antrum.**

The proximal tubular part of tubotympanic recess forms the **pharyngotympanic** (eustachian/auditory) **tube**, which forms a communication between nasopharynx and tympanic cavity (middle ear).

Second Pharyngeal Pouch

It forms the endodermal lining of the tonsil. The endoderm of the second pouch proliferates to form a number of tiny solid buds that extend into the underlying mesoderm. The mesoderm condenses around these buds. The central core of these buds breaks down to form **tonsillar crypts.**

The endoderm of the second pharyngeal pouch forms the stratified squamous, nonkeratinized epithelium lining, the medial surface of the tonsil and tonsillar crypts. The mesoderm forms lymphoid tissue, fibrous capsule, and connective tissue elements of the tonsil.

The second pouch is mostly obliterated by developing palatine tonsil. In adults, part of this pouch remains as **intratonsillar cleft** (crypta magna).

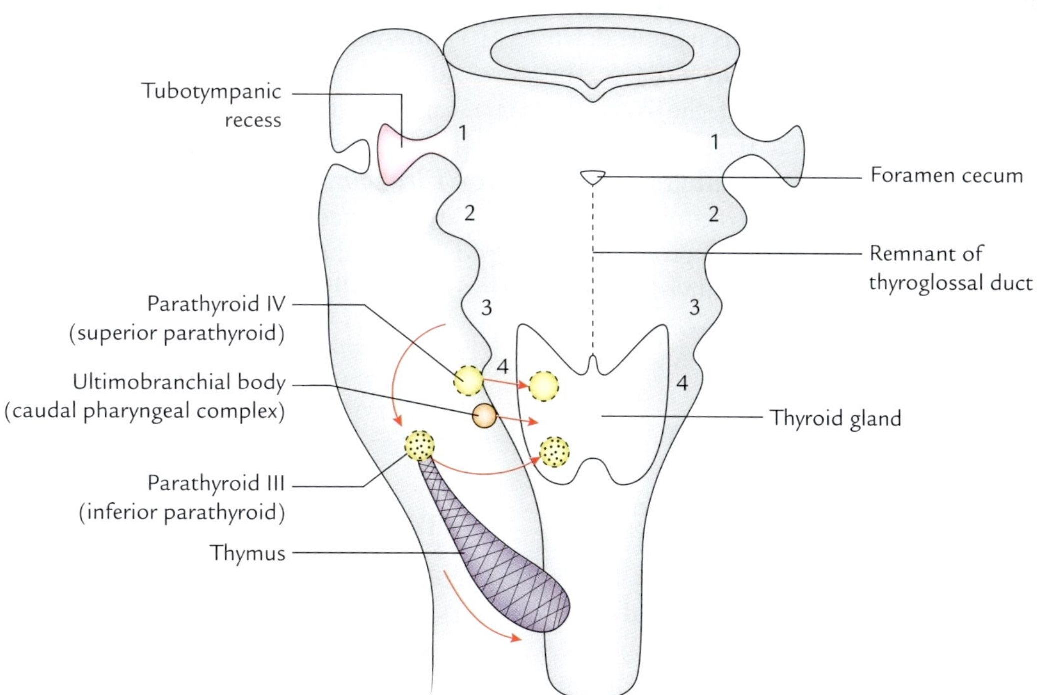

Fig. 14.10 Migration of parathyroid and thymus glands. Note that the thyroid glands originate at the level of foramen cecum and descend to the level of first tracheal ring. 1, 2, 3, 4 stand for first, second, third, and fourth pharyngeal pouches.

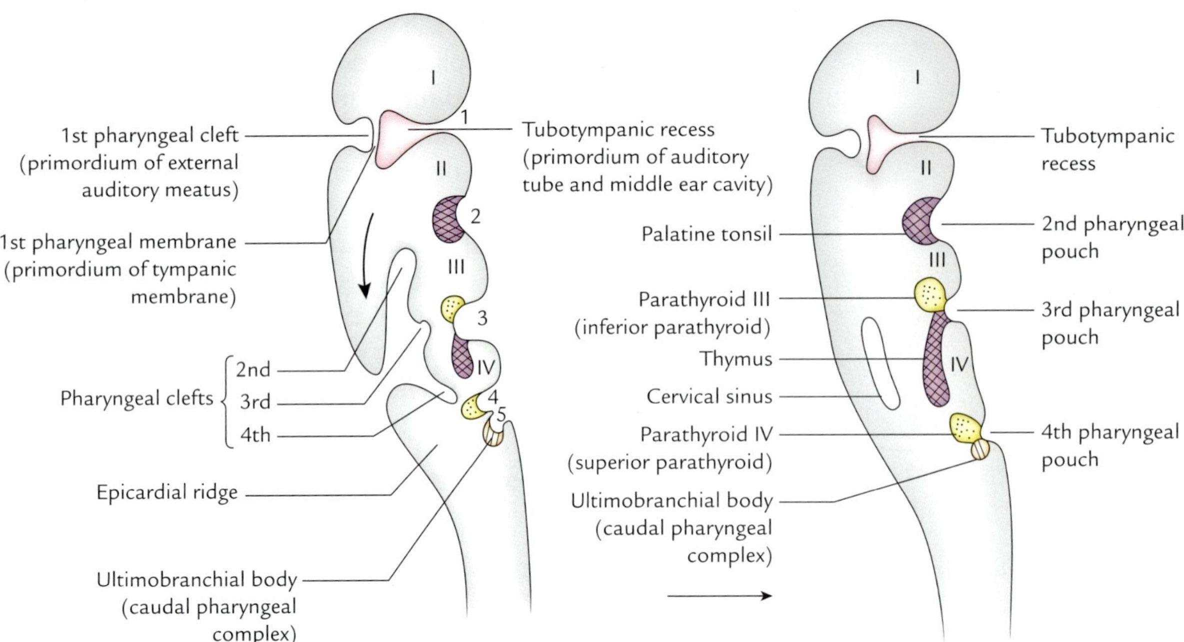

Fig. 14.11 Structures derived from pharyngeal pouches and pharyngeal clefts and formation of cervical sinus. Note that the second arch grows over the third and fourth arches, thus burying the second, third, and fourth pharyngeal clefts to form the cervical sinus.

N.B. According to some authorities, the dorsal part of second pharyngeal pouch along with dorsal part of first pharyngeal pouch forms the tubotympanic recess and ventral part of second pharyngeal pouch forms the tonsil.

Third Pharyngeal Pouch (Fig. 14.11)

The third pharyngeal pouch expands and differentiates into **dorsal bulbar part** and **ventral tubular part.** The communication of the third pouch with the pharynx narrows down and ultimately the pouch is cut off from the pharynx. The pouch is now lying in the mesoderm outside the pharynx.

The endoderm of **dorsal bulbar part** of the third pouch proliferates to form **inferior parathyroid gland** or **parathyroid III.** The endoderm of ventral tubular part of the third pouch proliferates and gives rise to **thymus.** The developing thymus and parathyroid glands later on lose their connection with pharynx.

Fourth Pharyngeal Pouch (Fig. 14.11)

The fourth pouch expands and differentiates into **dorsal bulbar part** and **ventral tubular part.** The communication of the fourth pouch with the pharynx becomes narrow and soon disappears.

The endoderm of the dorsal bulbar part of the fourth pouch proliferates to form **superior parathyroid gland (parathyroid IV).**

Parathyroid III, developing from third pouch, migrates caudally along with thymus. Hence, its position is lower than the parathyroid IV developing from the fourth pouch (Fig. 14.11).

Caudal Pharyngeal Complex (Fig. 14.11)

The fifth pouch appears for a very brief period and gets incorporated with the fourth pouch, to form the **caudal pharyngeal complex.**

It consists of three components:

(a) ***Thymic element***, which gets incorporated into developing thymus.
(b) ***Lateral thyroid element***, which fuses with the median thyroid element derived from thyroglossal duct and arrests the further migration of median thyroid element.
(c) ***Ultimobranchial body*** provides the path for migration of neural crest cells.

The neural crest cells that migrate into this complex form **parafollicular or "C" cells of the thyroid gland.**

N.B. In some species the fifth pouch develops as an ultimobranchial body, as a hollow vesicle in neck that forms **calcitonin-producing cells.**

The derivatives of pharyngeal pouches are given in Table 14.3 and shown in Figs 14.10 and 14.11.

PHARYNGEAL CLEFTS (GROOVES)

There are **four pharyngeal clefts** (grooves) (1, 2, 3, and 4). These are invaginations of surface ectoderm between the pharyngeal arches.

In the region of pharyngeal membrane, the pharyngeal wall is very thin but consists of three layers. From inside out these are endoderm, mesoderm, and ectoderm (cf., embryonic disc and tympanic membrane).

Table 14.3 Derivatives of pharyngeal pouches

Pouch	Derivatives
First pouch	• Pharyngotympanic tube • Tympanic (middle ear) cavity
Second pouch	• Palatine tonsil (lining) • Intratonsillar cleft
Third pouch	• Inferior parathyroid gland • Thymus
Fourth pouch	• Superior parathyroid gland • Caudal pharyngeal complex[a] (ultimopharyngeal body)

[a]The **neural crest cells** that migrate into caudal pharyngeal complex (ultimobranchial body) form parafollicular/C cells of the thyroid gland.

Only the first pharyngeal cleft has a definitive fate and gives rise to the **external auditory meatus** – whereas all other clefts (2, 3, and 4) are obliterated.

Cervical Sinus

It is a temporary depression on the side of neck of embryo containing 2nd, 3rd, and 4th pharyngeal clefts. During the 5th week of IUL, the mesenchyme of second pharyngeal arch grows rapidly and extends downward, to overlap the second, third, and fourth pharyngeal clefts (grooves). Later it fuses with the epicardial ridge. Thus, second, third, and fourth pharyngeal clefts get concealed under the surface and form a slit-like cavity – the **cervical cyst** that is lined by ectoderm. The cervical cyst soon disappears as the neck develops. Consequently, the side of the neck that was so far marked by the pharyngeal grooves now becomes smooth (Fig. 14.11).

CLINICAL CORRELATION

Cervical cyst/branchial cyst (Fig. 14.12): Normally, the cervical sinus disappears as the neck develops, but if it fails to obliterate, it leads to the formation of **branchial cyst/cervical cyst**.

The branchial cyst appears as spherical swelling along the anterior border of the sternocleidomastoid at the junction of its upper one-third and lower two-thirds, below and behind the angle of mandible.

- It contains fluid and cellular debris derived from desquamated epithelial lining of the cervical cyst.
- ***Branchial sinus***
  It could be external or internal.
  (a) *External branchial sinus:* It occurs if cervical cyst opens on the body surface. The external branchial sinus opens along the anterior border of the sternocleidomastoid (Fig. 14.12).
  (b) *Internal branchial sinus:* It occurs if cervical cyst opens into the floor of intratonsillar cleft.
- ***Branchial fistula***
  It occurs if *cervical cyst* opens both externally and internally. It is rarely formed. It passes deep between the external and internal carotid arteries (**carotid fork**) and opens into the **tonsillar fossa**. Externally it opens on the surface of neck along the anterior border of sternocleidomastoid. Such a branchial fistula occurs due to rupture of membrane between the second pharyngeal cleft and second pharyngeal pouch (Fig. 14.13).

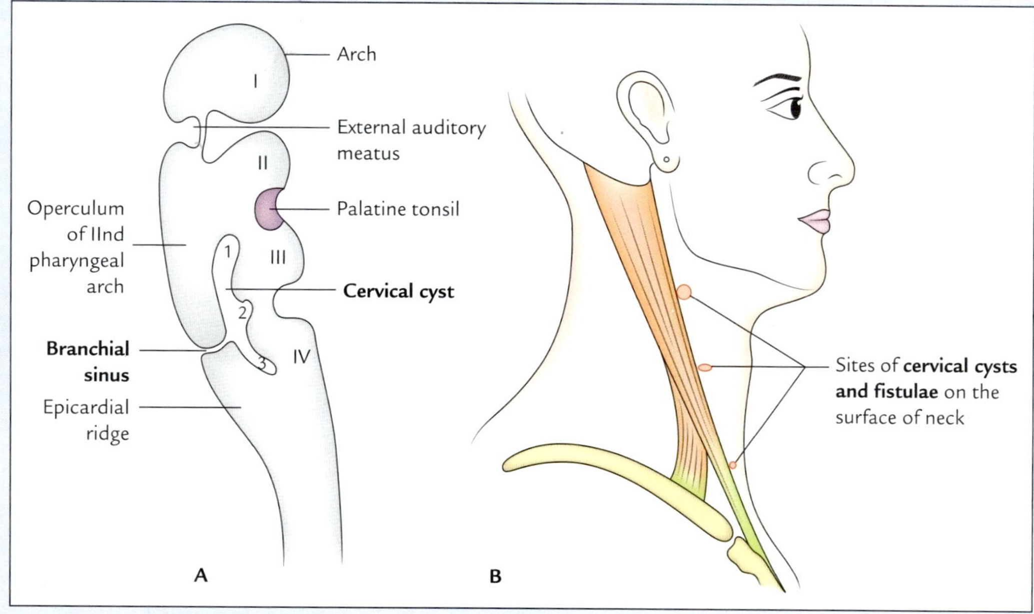

Fig. 14.12 (A) Cervical cyst opening at the side of neck by way of fistula. (B) Localization of branchial cysts and fistulae in front of sternocleidomastoid. The numerals 1, 2, and 3 stand for second, third, and fourth pharyngeal clefts.

Continued

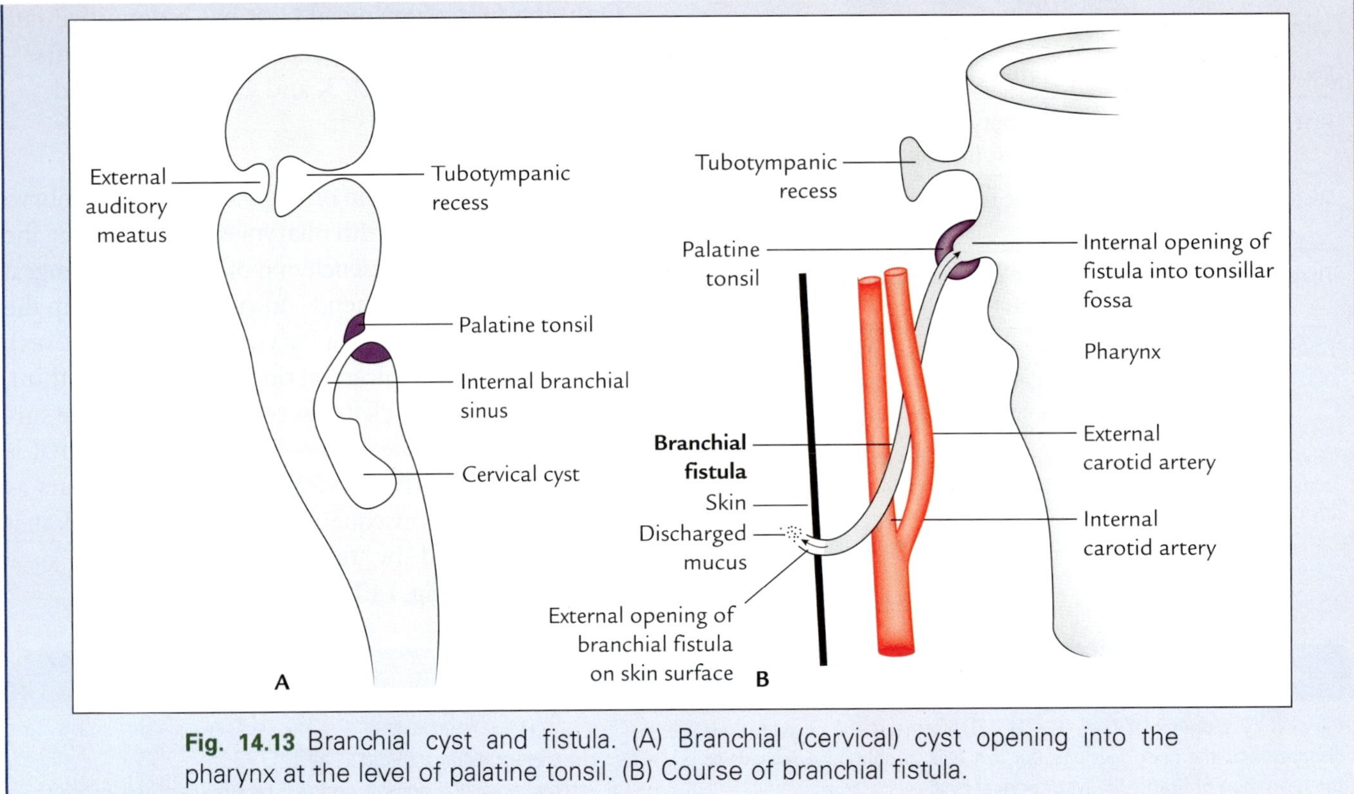

Fig. 14.13 Branchial cyst and fistula. (A) Branchial (cervical) cyst opening into the pharynx at the level of palatine tonsil. (B) Course of branchial fistula.

PHARYNGEAL MEMBRANES

There are four pharyngeal membranes (1, 2, 3, and 4). They are located between the pharyngeal arches and are initially formed of two layers: (a) an inner layer formed by the *endodermal lining of the pouch* and (b) an outer layer formed by the *ectodermal lining of the pharyngeal cleft*. Later these two layers become separated by thin layer of mesoderm. Now **it consists of three layers: outer layer of ectoderm, middle layer of mesoderm, and inner layer of endoderm** (cf., arrangement of layers in the trilaminar embryonic disc and tympanic membrane).

Only the first pair of the pharyngeal membrane forms the **definitive structure** – the *tympanic membrane*; the remaining pharyngeal membranes disappear.

The derivatives of pharyngeal clefts and membranes are given in Tables 14.4 and 14.5.

Table 14.4 Derivatives of pharyngeal clefts

Pharyngeal Clefts	Adult Derivatives
First	• External auditory meatus • Outer ectodermal layer of tympanic membrane
Second Third Fourth	Obliterate/disappear

Table 14.5 Derivatives of pharyngeal membranes

Pharyngeal Membranes	Adult Derivatives
First	Tympanic membrane
Second Third Fourth	Obliterate/disappear

GESTATIONAL AGE OF KEY DEVELOPMENTAL EVENTS

Developmental Event	Gestational Age
➢ Pharyngeal arches develop early in the	4th week
➢ Pharyngeal clefts becomes visible during	4th and 5th weeks
➢ Lymphatic nodules in the palatine tonsil develop at	20th week
➢ Parathyroid glands develop during	5th week
➢ Histogenesis of parathyroid glands:	
(a) Chief cells differentiate during	Embryonic period
(b) Oxyphil cells differentiate during	5–7 years after birth

GOLDEN FACTS TO REMEMBER

➢ **Each pharyngeal arch is supplied by one nerve *except***	First arch, which is supplied by two nerves (a) Trigeminal nerve (CN V) (maxillary and mandibular divisions) (b) Chorda tympani nerve – a branch of facial nerve (CN VII)
➢ **Only pharyngeal arch that has two processes**	First arch (it presents maxillary and mandibular processes)
➢ **All the cartilages of larynx develop from fourth and sixth arch cartilages *except***	Epiglottis, which develops from the caudal part of hypobranchial eminence
➢ **Meckel's cartilage**	First pharyngeal arch cartilage
➢ **Reichert's cartilage**	Second pharyngeal arch cartilage
➢ **Two most important first arch syndromes**	Treacher Collins syndrome and Pierre Robin syndrome
➢ **All the pharyngeal membranes disappear *except***	First pharyngeal membrane which gives rise to the tympanic membrane
➢ **All the pharyngeal clefts disappear *except***	First pharyngeal cleft which gives rise to the external auditory meatus
➢ **Most common location of branchial cyst/ fistula**	Just below the angle of jaw anterior to sternocleidomastoid muscle

CLINICAL PROBLEM SOLVING

PROBLEMS

1. A mother took her 11/2-year-old son to a pediatrician and complained that her child has an **intermittent discharge of pus from a small opening on the side of her son's neck.** On physical examination, the pediatrician found **a small dimple in the neck at the junction of middle one-third and lower one-third of the anterior edge of the sternocleidomastoid muscle.** The area around it was swollen and red. What is the most likely diagnosis? Give its embryological basis.
2. A male infant was born with a very **small mandible, reduced malar prominences, down-slanting palpebral fissures**, and **malformed external ears.** What is the most likely diagnosis? Give its embryological basis.
3. A male infant was born with a very **small mandible (micrognathia), cleft palate**, and **posteriorly placed tongue (glossoptosis).** What is the most likely diagnosis? Give its embryological basis.
4. A pediatrician was called to examine a child with a **very small philtrum of the upper lip** (**fish mouth deformity**) and **low-set notched ears.** The child had numerous episodes of pneumonia. The pediatrician diagnosed this as **DiGeorge syndrome.** Give its embryological basis.

SOLUTIONS

1. The most likely diagnosis is **branchial sinus or fistula.** It is a rare congenital anomaly, which occurs when the **cervical sinus** fails to disappear and ruptures on the surface of the neck. The branchial fistula may also occur if the second pharyngeal arch fails to grow caudally over the third and fourth arches, and thus leaving second, third, and fourth pharyngeal clefts open on the surface of the neck by a narrow canal. When branchial sinus is infected, it becomes swollen, painful, and starts discharging mucoid material (for details see p. 157).
2. The most likely diagnosis is **Treacher Collins syndrome.** It occurs due to an **inherited autosomal dominant disorder** due to mutation of **TCOF1 gene** located on chromosome 5 (for details see p. 154).
3. The most likely diagnosis is **Pierre Robin syndrome.** It is an autosomal recessive disorder which mostly occur due to mutation of **SOXG gene** located on chromosome 17. It occurs in 1/85,000 births (for details see p. 154).
4. The **DiGeorge syndrome** occurs when the third and fourth pharyngeal pouches fail to differentiate into thymus and parathyroid glands. The loss of thymic tissue compromises the immune system, especially **defective T-cell function**, which leads to numerous infections, e.g., **pneumonia.** It occurs in 1/2000–3000 births and is caused by the **deletion of long arm** of **chromosome 22.** Hence, it is also called **22q deletion syndrome.**

15 Development of Tongue and Thyroid Gland

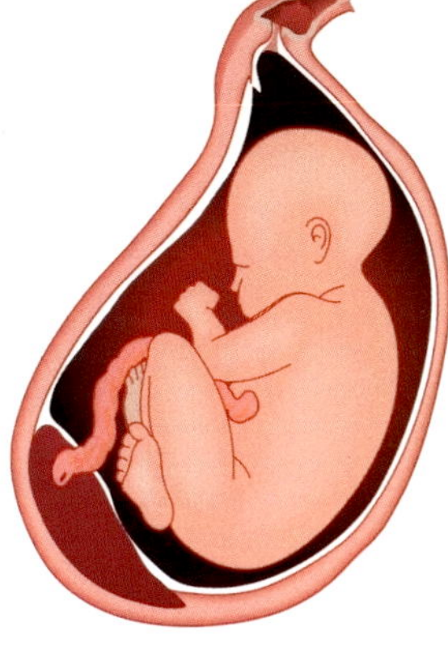

LEARNING OBJECTIVES

After studying this chapter, the student should be able to:

- Describe the development of tongue in brief and give the embryological basis of its nerve supply. AN 39.1, AN 43.4
- Give the development al basis of congenital anomalies of tongue. AN 43.4
- Describe the development of thyroid gland and give the embryological basis of its congenital anomalies. AN 43.4
- Give the embryological basis of (a) tongue tie, (b) lingual thyroid, (c) thyroglossal cyst and fistula, and (d) ectopic thyroid.

DEVELOPMENT OF TONGUE AN 43.3

OVERVIEW

The **tongue** is divided into two parts: **oral part** (anterior two-third) and **pharyngeal part** (posterior one-third).

- The **oral part** of tongue develops from three swellings associated with first pharyngeal arch. These swellings are of two types: **two lateral lingual swellings** and **one median swelling** – the **tuberculum impar** (Fig. 15.1).
- The **pharyngeal part** of tongue develops from another median swelling called **hypobranchial eminence** or **copula of His** associated with second, third, and fourth pharyngeal arches (Fig. 15.1).
- Muscles of tongue develop from **occipital myotomes**.

The tongue develops in the floor of developing mouth from first, second, third, and fourth pharyngeal arches. At the end of the 4th week of intrauterine life (IUL), a small median triangular swelling called **tuberculum impar** develops in the floor of primitive pharynx, just cranial to **foramen cecum.***

Soon after the appearance of tuberculum impar, the **two lateral oval swellings** called **lingual swellings** develop one on each side of tuberculum impar. The two lateral lingual swellings are placed slightly distal to the tuberculum impar, and hence they are also called **distal tongue buds** (Fig. 15.1A).

Caudal to tubercular impar, a second large median swelling called **hypobranchial eminence** (**copula of His**) develops in the floor of primitive pharynx in relation to second, third, and fourth pharyngeal arches. The hypobranchial eminence soon subdivides into large cranial part and small caudal part (Fig. 15.1B).

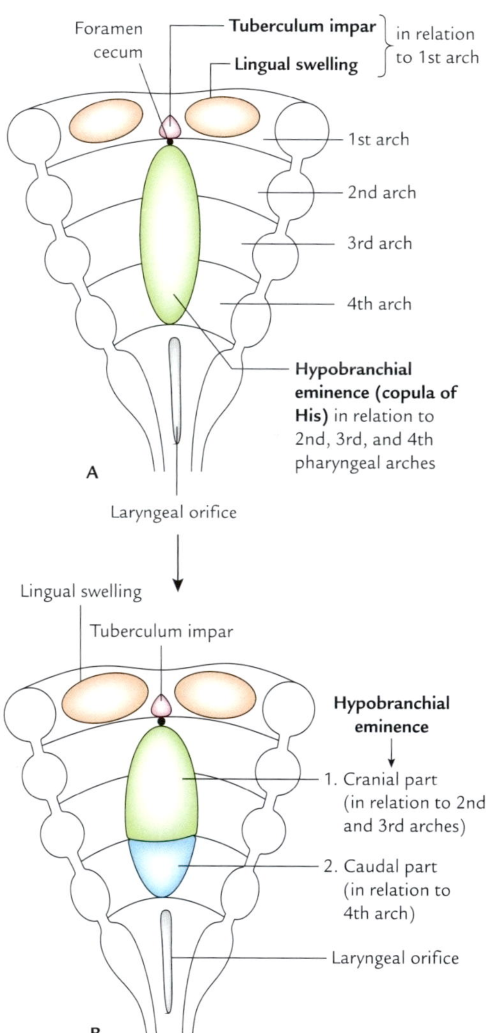

Fig. 15.1 Development of tongue. (A) Appearance of four swellings (tuberculum impar, two lingual swellings, and hypobranchial eminence), which give rise to the various parts of the tongue. (B) Subdivision of hypobranchial eminence into cranial and caudal parts.

*__Foramen cecum:__ A blind foramen in the floor of primitive pharynx, which marks the site of development of thyroid gland.

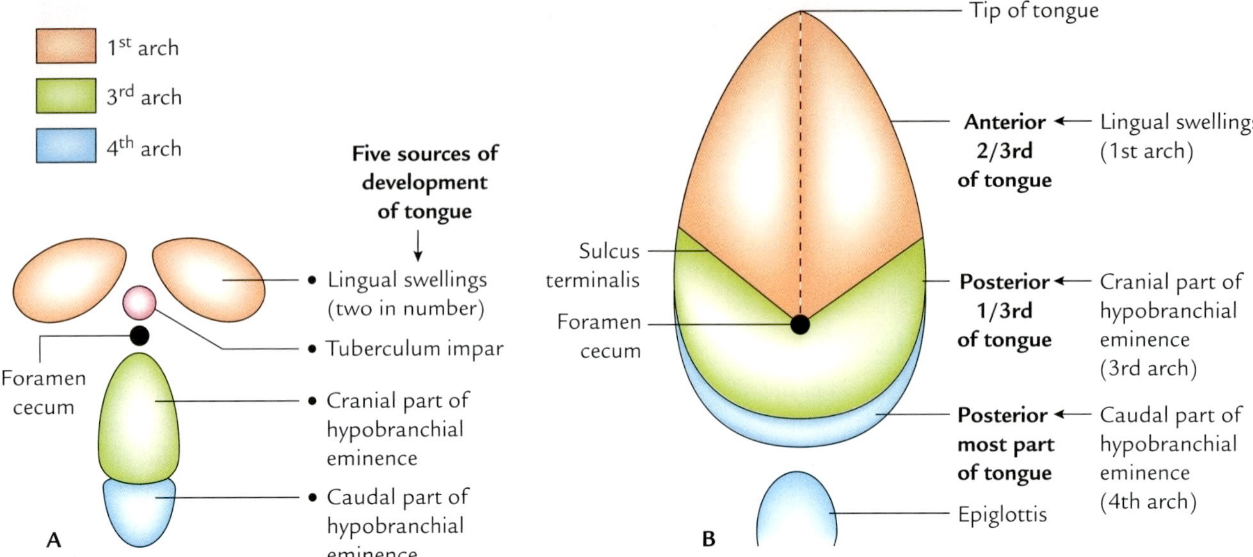

Fig. 15.2 Schematic diagrams to show the development of various parts of the tongue from different sources. (A) Five sources of development. (B) Definitive tongue.

Development of Various Parts of Tongue (Fig. 15.2)

The two **lateral lingual swellings** overgrow the tuberculum impar and merge with each other to form **anterior two-third of the tongue**. The line of fusion of two lingual swellings in the median plane forms **median sulcus** on the dorsal surface of the tongue.

The tuberculum impar does not form any recognizable part of the adult tongue.

Since mucous membrane covering the anterior two-third of the tongue develops from the first pharyngeal arch, it is innervated by **mandibular branch** of trigeminal nerve – the nerve of first arch.

The posterior one-third of the tongue including circumvallate papillae develops from cranial part of hypobranchial eminence.

The line of fusion of the anterior two-third and posterior one-third of the tongue is indicated by a V-shaped groove – the **sulcus terminalis**. Since the mucous membrane of the posterior one-third of tongue (including vallate papillae) develops from the third pharyngeal arch, it is supplied by **glossopharyngeal nerve** – the nerve of third arch.

The **posterior-most part of the tongue and epiglottis** develops from the caudal part of the hypobranchial eminence. Since the mucous membrane of the posterior-most part of tongue and epiglottis develop from fourth pharyngeal arch, it is supplied by the **superior laryngeal nerve** – the nerve of the fourth arch.

During this sequence of events, the third arch mesoderm grows over the mesoderm of the second arch and fuses with the mesoderm of the first arch. Thus, the second arch gets buried underneath the third arch and thereby gets excluded from the tongue development (Fig. 15.3).

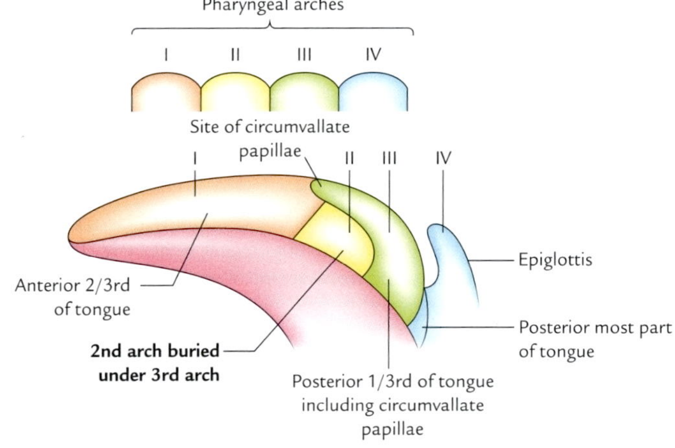

Fig. 15.3 Overgrowth of third arch over the second arch. Note second arch is buried under third arch.

The **muscles of tongue** develop from myoblasts that migrate into developing tongue from the **occipital myotomes**. The hypoglossal nerve – the nerve of occipital myotomes – accompanies the myoblasts during their migration to the pharyngeal arches and innervates the muscles of tongue as they develop (Fig. 15.4). The migration of the occipital myotomes to the developing tongue explains the course of the hypoglossal nerve. Some muscles of tongue probably develop **in situ**.

N.B. At birth, both the anterior and posterior parts of the tongue are located within the oral cavity; later, the posterior third of tongue descends into the oropharynx by 4 years of age and forms its anterior

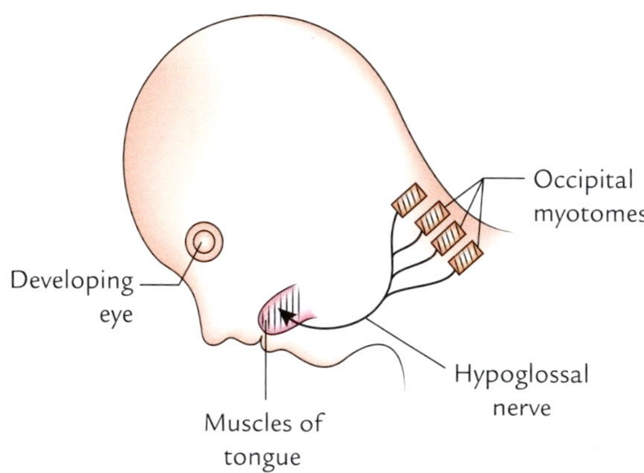

Fig. 15.4 Development of muscles of the tongue.

wall (pharyngeal part of the tongue). Consequently, in adults, the anterior part of tongue is located in the oral cavity and posterior part of tongue is located in the oropharynx.

Correlation of Nerve Supply of Tongue With Its Development

The correlation of nerve supply of the tongue with its development is given in Table 15.1.

N.B. Taste sensations from anterior two-third of the tongue are carried by chorda tympani nerve, from posterior one-third by glossopharyngeal nerve, and from posterior-most part by the internal laryngeal nerve.

The beer is tasted at the posterior-most part of the tongue, which is supplied by the internal laryngeal nerve. For this reason, the internal laryngeal nerve is also called **beer drinker's nerve.**

Points to Remember

1. **Mucous membrane** of the tongue is derived from the endoderm of the primitive foregut.
2. **Taste buds** are formed in relation to the terminal branches of nerves carrying taste sensations.
3. **Muscles of the tongue** develop from occipital myotomes.
4. **Fibroareolar tissue** that binds the tongue muscles develops from mesenchyme of the pharyngeal arches.

Relation of Anterior Part of Tongue With the Floor of the Mouth (Fig. 15.5)

The tongue develops from endodermal lining of the floor of mouth (primitive pharynx). First, the tongue forms a recognizable swelling in the middle. Later a sulcus called **linguogingival sulcus** develops on either side of this swelling and separates the developing tongue from the floor of the mouth.

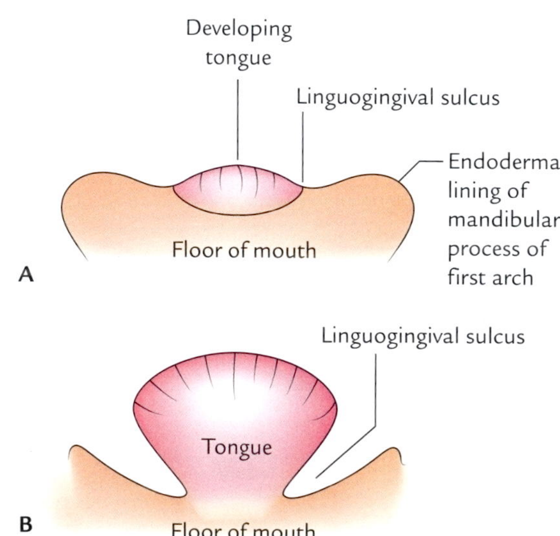

Fig. 15.5 Separation of tongue from the floor of the mouth (i.e., from the rest of the mandibular processes). (A) Development of tongue and linguogingival sulci in the region of mandibular process. (B) Separation of tongue from the floor of the mouth by deepening of linguogingival sulci.

Table 15.1 Embryological basis of nerve supply of the tongue

Structure	Source of Development	Nerve Supply
A. **Mucosa of Tongue**		
a. Mucous membrane and taste buds of anterior two-third of the tongue	• Endodermal lining of first arch and submerged second arch	• *Lingual nerve* (a branch of mandibular nerve – a nerve of first arch carrying general sensations) • *Chorda tympani nerve* (a branch of facial nerve – the nerve of second arch carrying special [taste] sensations)
b. Mucous membrane and taste buds of posterior one-third of the tongue	• Endodermal lining of the third arch	• *Glossopharyngeal nerve* – the nerve of third arch carrying general and special (taste) sensations
c. Mucous membrane and taste buds of the posterior-most part of the tongue	• Endodermal lining of the fourth arch	• *Superior laryngeal nerve* – the nerve of fourth arch carrying general and special (taste) sensations
B. **Musculature of Tongue** Muscles of tongue	Occipital myotomes	Hypoglossal nerve – the nerve of occipital myotomes supplies all muscles of tongue, except palatoglossus

CLINICAL CORRELATION

Congenital anomalies of the tongue AN 43.4

1. ***Aglossia*** (absence of tongue): It is very rare and occurs due to complete agenesis of tongue primordia.
2. ***Hemiglossia*** (half tongue): It occurs if one of the lingual swellings fails to develop.
3. ***Microglossia:*** Tongue is too small.
4. ***Macroglossia:*** Tongue is too large.
5. ***Tongue tie (ankyloglossia)*** (Fig. 15.6): It occurs when frenulum of tongue extends to the tip of the tongue, thus preventing its protrusion and causing difficulty in speech (For details see Clinical Problem No. 2 on page 167).

   N.B. Occasionally, the tongue may be adherent to the palate (ankyloglossia superior).

6. ***Bifid tongue:*** In this condition, the anterior portion of the tongue splits into two parts. It is caused by failure of fusion of two lingual swellings. (cf. The tongue of snake is always bifid.)
7. ***Lingual thyroid:*** It is a clinical condition in which thyroid tissue is present in the tongue, either under the mucosa or within the muscles.
8. ***Fissuring of tongue and hypertrophy of the lingual papillae:*** It is a characteristic of infants with **Down syndrome**.

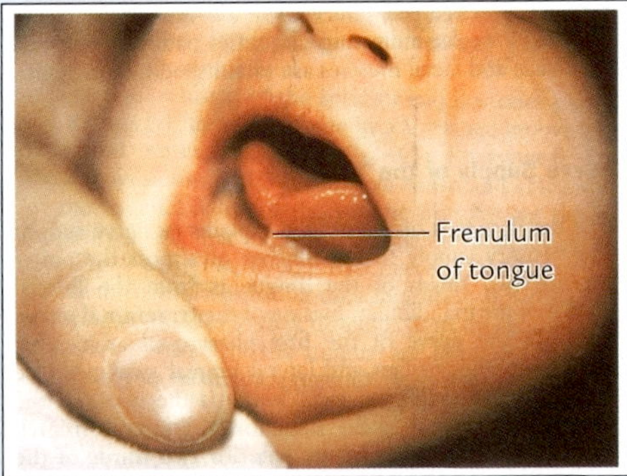

Fig. 15.6 Tongue tie (ankyloglossia). (*Source: The Developing Human: Clinically Oriented Embryology*, 8th edition by Keith L. Moore and T.V.N. Persaud, ISBN: 9781416037064, page 178, Fig. 9.25, Copyright Elsevier, 2008.)

DEVELOPMENT OF THYROID GLAND (FIG. 15.7)

AN 43.4

OVERVIEW

The thyroid gland develops from endodermal diverticulum – the **thyroglossal duct** that forms in the **floor of primitive pharynx**. The site of formation of this diverticulum is seen in adults as the **foramen cecum**.

The **parafollicular cells or C cells** of thyroid gland develop from **neural crest cells** that migrate into **ultimobranchial body of caudal pharyngeal complex** formed by fusion of fourth and fifth pharyngeal pouches. For details, see p. 156.

The thyroid gland begins to develop during the 3rd week of IUL as an endodermal thickening in the midline of the floor of primitive pharynx between the **tuberculum impar** and **copula.**

This thickening forms a small outpouching (i.e., becomes depressed) below the surface to form a diverticulum called **thyroglossal duct**. This duct first grows downward and slightly forward across the tongue and then descends on the front of the neck. In the neck, first it passes in front of the hyoid bone, then winds around its lower border to become **retrohyoid**, and finally descends below the hyoid bone with a slight inclination to one side, usually to the left.

By the end of the 7th week of IUL, it reaches to its definitive position where its tip becomes a solid mass of cells and soon bifurcates. The proliferation of cells of this bifid tip of thyroglossal duct gives rise to **two lobes of the thyroid gland** that are connected to each other by an **isthmus**. The isthmus of the thyroid gland lies anterior to developing second and third tracheal rings. The **parafollicular or C cells** in the lateral lobes of the thyroid gland are contributed by neural crest cells of caudal pharyngeal complex.

The connecting link between the thyroid gland and the floor of primitive pharynx – the **thyroglossal duct** – gets obliterated and disappears. The proximal opening of the thyroglossal duct persists as a small pit on the dorsum of tongue as **foramen cecum**.

In 50% people, a **pyramidal lobe** differentiates from the distal end of the thyroglossal duct, which is often attached to the hyoid bone by a band of fibrous tissue and/or smooth muscle – the **levator glandulae thyroideae**.

N.B. The thyroid gland is the first endocrine gland to develop. It starts functioning by the end of the 3rd month.

Histogenesis of Thyroid Gland

The thyroid primordium consists of solid mass of endoderm cells. It breaks up into a network of epithelial cords as it is invaded by the surrounding mesenchyme. Later, these cords divide in smaller cell groups/clusters. A lumen soon forms in each of these cell clusters and cells get arranged around a lumen, thus forming **thyroid follicles. By the end of the 3rd month (12th week), follicular cells start producing colloid – a source of thyroxine and triiodothyronine** in the lumen. At the same time, **parafollicular cells** (C cells) derived from neural crest cells in the **caudal pharyngeal complex** start producing **calcitonin**. The C cells of thyroid gland are so named because they produce **calcitonin hormones**.

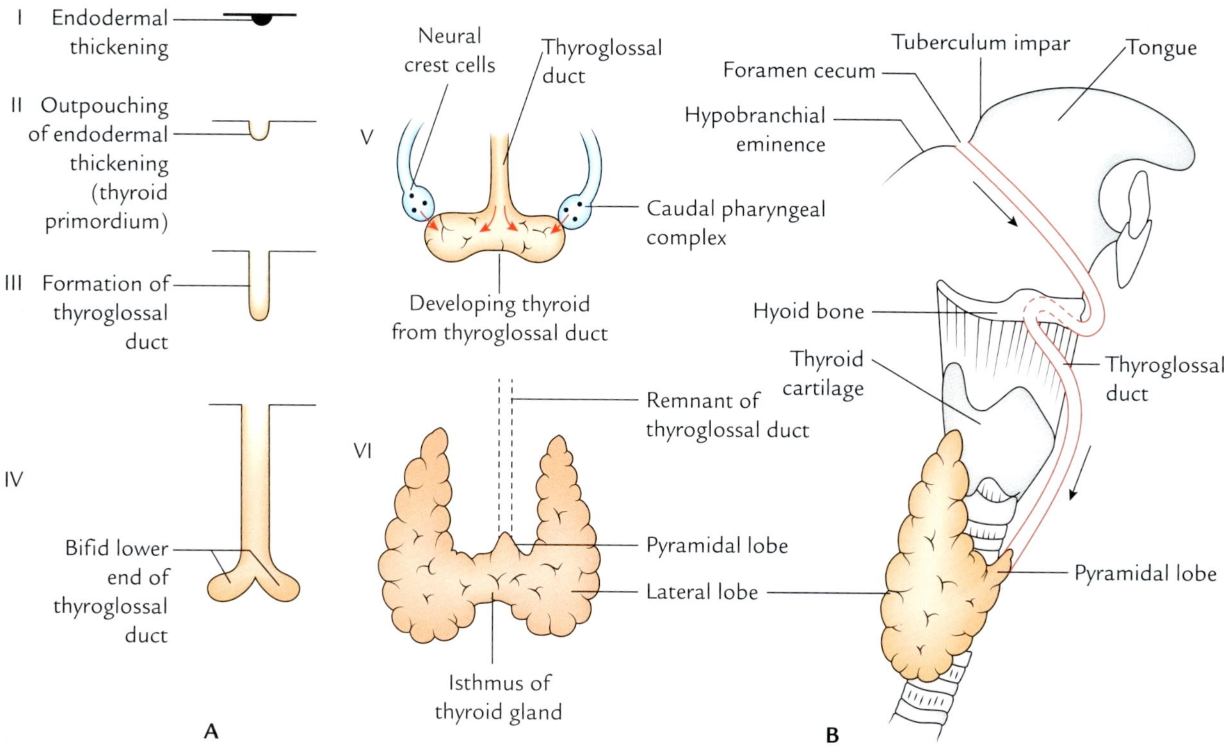

Fig. 15.7 Development of the thyroid gland. (A) Stages of development. (B) Pathway of the thyroglossal duct (arrows).

CLINICAL CORRELATION

Congenital anomalies of the thyroid AN 43.4

1. ***Anomalies of position of thyroid:*** The important anomalous positions of the thyroid are as follows:
   (a) *Lingual thyroid:* The thyroid tissue infrequently forms anywhere along the course of the thyroglossal duct (Fig. 15.8). But the *commonest abnormal site of thyroid tissue formation* is the tongue, where it is termed *lingual thyroid*. It may be just below the mucosa of dorsum of tongue at the foramen cecum or within the muscles of the tongue. The lingual thyroid is seen in as many as 10% of the autopsies. The lingual swelling due to lingual thyroid may cause difficulty in swallowing (Fig. 15.8).
   (b) *Sublingual thyroid* (Fig. 15.9): It is a thyroid tissue present high in the neck above, at, or just below the hyoid bone.

N.B. The sublingual thyroid always and invariably forms the only functioning thyroid tissue. If it is removed by mistake, then after its removal the patient is left at the mercy of thyroid drug regime for the rest of his/her life.

   (c) *Intrathoracic thyroid:* Sometimes, the whole gland or part of it may lie in the thorax (intrathoracic thyroid).
2. ***Ectopic thyroid tissue:*** The small masses of thyroid tissue may be present at the abnormal sites, e.g., in **larynx, trachea, esophagus, pericardium, pleura,** and **ovaries.**

N.B. **Lateral aberrant thyroids:** Truly speaking, the lateral aberrant thyroid does not exist. Earlier, the ectopic thyroid tissue in relation to cervical lymph node was described as an aberrant thyroid. Now it has been established that this thyroid tissue formed in relation to the cervical lymph node is actually metastasis in these nodes from *occult carcinoma of the thyroid.* When the carcinoma of the thyroid is less than 1.5 cm in diameter, it is termed *occult carcinoma of thyroid.*

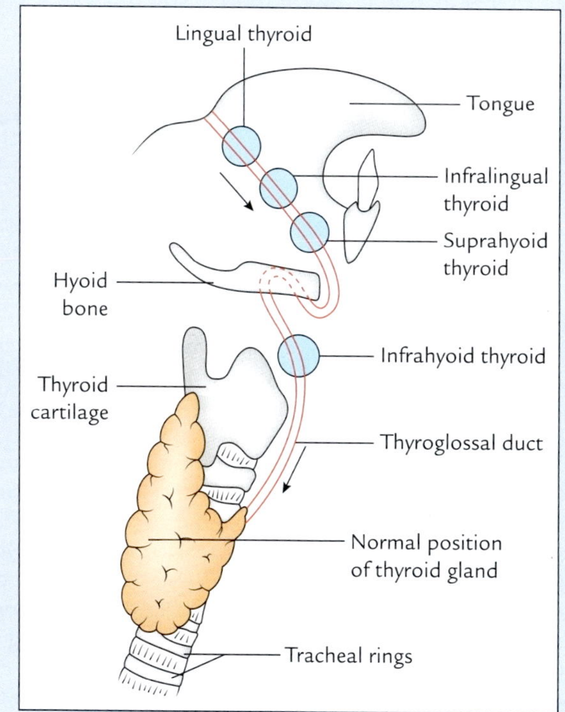

Fig. 15.8 Path of thyroglossal duct. Note the possible locations of thyroid tissue and thyroglossal cysts in this path.

Continued

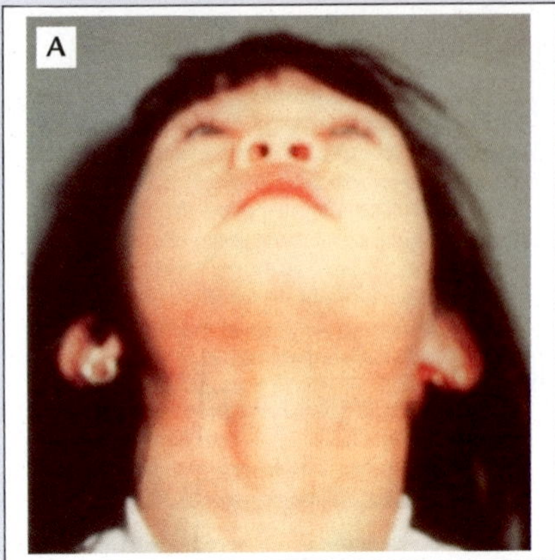

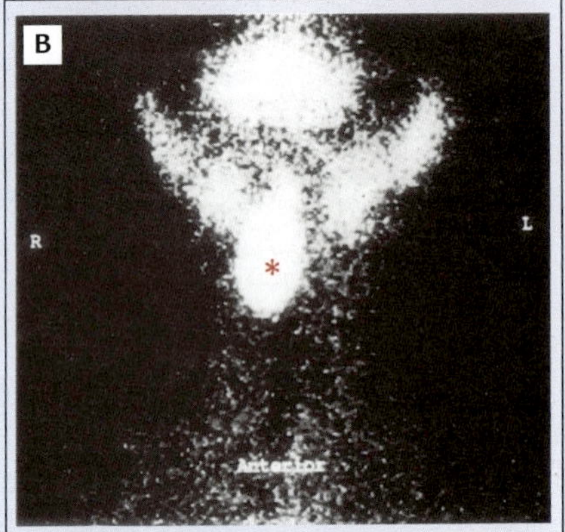

Fig. 15.9 Sublingual thyroid. (A) Surface view. (B) Technetium-99m scan showing sublingual thyroid gland (*). (*Source: The Developing Human: Clinically Oriented Embryology*, 8th edition by Keith L. Moore and T.V.N. Persaud, ISBN: 9781416037064, page 177, Fig. 9.23, Copyright Elsevier, 2008.)

3. ***Anomalous lobes and shapes***
   (a) One of the lateral lobes of thyroid gland may be missing. Thyroid hemiagenesis is commonly seen on the left side.
   (b) *Pyramidal lobe:* It often arises from upper aspect of the isthmus, usually on the left side. It may arise from one of the lobes or may be detached from thyroid. It may be too small or too large to reach the hyoid bone.
   (c) Isthmus may be absent.
4. ***Thyroglossal cyst or fistula*** (Fig. 15.8): The thyroglossal cyst may form anywhere along the course of the thyroglossal duct. Normally, the thyroglossal duct atrophies and disappears but a part of it may persist and form a cyst called thyroglossal cyst. The thyroglossal cysts are always formed in the midline of the front of the neck and observed by the age of 5 years. If thyroglossal cyst ruptures, it communicates to the exterior by a secondary opening on the surface of the neck and it is called thyroglossal fistula.
5. ***Accessory thyroid:*** Sometimes, small nodules of thyroid tissue are found in close proximity to the thyroid gland. They are often of insufficient size to maintain the normal function if the thyroid gland is removed.

N.B.

- When the thyroid tissue is present in an anomalous position, the thyroid gland may or may not be present at its normal site.
- In surgical removal of thyroglossal cyst or fistulae, it is essential to remove all remnants of the thyroglossal duct. Also, remember that the thyroglossal duct is intimately related to the hyoid bone.

GESTATIONAL AGE OF KEY DEVELOPMENTAL EVENTS

Development Event	Gestational Age
➢ Development of tongue begins during	4th week
➢ Development of tongue completes at	6th month
➢ Development of thyroid begins during	3rd week (24th day)
➢ Thyroglossal duct reaches to its definitive position by the end of	7th week
➢ Thyroid gland starts functioning at the end of	3rd month
➢ Reflex pathways between taste buds and muscles of facial expressions are established by	7th month of IUL

GOLDEN FACTS TO REMEMBER

➢ **Age at which baby can distinguish between sweet and bitter tastes**	First 3 months after birth
➢ **First indication of development of tongue**	Appearance of tuberculum impar
➢ **First lingual papillae to develop**	Vallate and foliate papillae
➢ **Beer drinker's nerve**	Internal laryngeal nerve
➢ **First endocrine gland to develop**	Thyroid gland (it develops approximately 24 days after fertilization)
➢ **First endocrine gland to start functioning**	Thyroid gland starts functioning at the end of 3rd month of IUL
➢ **At birth, whole of tongue is located**	In the oral cavity
➢ **Commonest site of abnormal position of thyroid tissue**	Tongue (e.g., lingual thyroid)

CLINICAL PROBLEM SOLVING

PROBLEMS

1. **Although the tongue develops from first, second, third, and fourth pharyngeal arches, the facial nerve (nerve of second arch) does not provide the general sensory innervation to the tongue.** Why?
2. **What is tongue tie? Give its embryological basis.**
3. **Facial responses of fetus can be induced by tasting bitter substances by mother at 26–28 weeks of IUL. Embryologically, what does it indicate?**
4. A 17-year-old girl consulted her physician about a small swelling in the anterior part of her neck just inferior to the hyoid bone. A probable diagnosis of thyroglossal cyst was made by the physician. What is the embryological basis of thyroglossal cyst and also tell with what other entity/condition such a swelling may be confused with? What precautions should be taken by a surgeon before removing the **thyroglossal cyst**?

SOLUTIONS

1. It is because the third arch mesoderm (**copula**) grows over the mesoderm of the second arch to fuse with the mesoderm of the first arch and thus burying the second arch mesoderm. Therefore, facial nerve, the nerve of second arch, does not provide the general sensory innervation to the tongue. However, its **chorda tympani nerve**, a branch of facial nerve, does provide the special sensory innervation (taste sensation) to anterior two-third of the tongue. This is because the taste buds develop in relation to terminal branches of the nerves carrying taste sensations.
2. **Tongue tie:** It is a clinical condition that occurs due to overdevelopment of frenulum linguae. As a result, apical part of the tongue is anchored to the floor of the mouth by **frenulum linguae.** Clinically, it presents as disturbed speech due to restriction of movements of the tongue.

N.B. Along the front and sides of primitive tongue, an endodermal **alveololingual sulcus** develops, which gradually separates the tongue from the floor of the primitive mouth. If this separation is incomplete, the apical part of the tongue remains attached to the floor of the mouth by the frenulum linguae (**tongue tie**).

3. The taste buds of tongue develop during 11–12 weeks of IUL by inductive interaction between the epithelial cells of the tongue and invading gustatory nerves cells from **nerves of taste**, namely, **chorda tympani**, **glossopharyngeal**, and **superior laryngeal**. The fetal facial responses induced by bitter-tasting substances at 26–28 weeks of IUL indicate that reflex pathways between the taste buds and muscles of facial expression are established by this age.
4. The **thyroglossal duct** extends from foreman cecum to jugular notch in the median plane of front of the neck. Normally, it atrophies and disappears. A remnant of duct may form a cyst anywhere along the course of the thyroglossal duct called **thyroglossal cyst**.

A **thyroglossal cyst** may be confused with abnormal position of thyroid tissue.

It is important for a surgeon to differentiate a thyroglossal cyst from an abnormal thyroid tissue, which may also be present anywhere along the course of thyroglossal duct to prevent inadvertent removal of the thyroid tissue. Because this may be the only thyroid tissue present, failure to do so may leave the person to suffer permanently from **hypothyroidism**.

16 Development of Face, Nose, and Palate

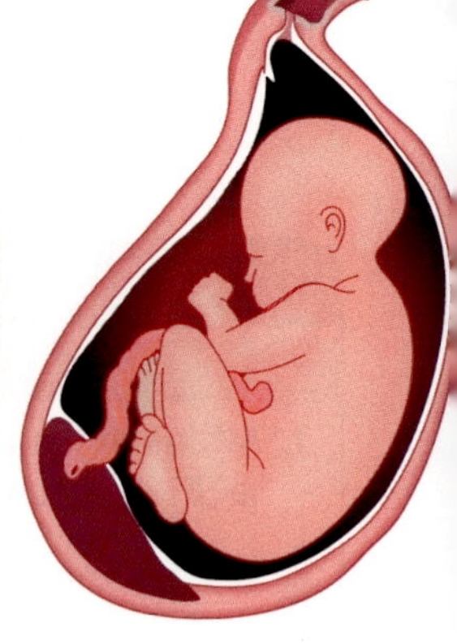

LEARNING OBJECTIVES

After studying this chapter, the student should be able to:

- Describe the development of face in brief and discuss the associated common congenital anomalies. AN 43.4
- Describe the development of palate in brief and give the embryological basis of cleft palate and cleft lip. AN 43.4
- Write short notes on (a) development of upper lip, (b) intermaxillary segment, and (c) nasolacrimal duct.

DEVELOPMENT OF FACE

OVERVIEW

The development of face includes formation of mouth, forehead, nose, upper lip, lower lip, and cheeks.

The face develops from five swellings/processes that form around the primitive mouth (stomodeum). These processes are as follows (Fig. 16.1A):

- **Single frontonasal process**
- **Paired maxillary processes**
- **Paired mandibular processes**

Frontonasal process forms forehead, nose, and philtrum of the upper lip.

Maxillary processes form lateral parts of the upper lip and upper parts of the cheeks.

Mandibular processes form lower lip, chin, and lower parts of the cheeks.

The development of face occurs between 4 to 8 weeks of embryonic period. At the end of 4th week, the **stomodeum (primitive mouth)** forms as a small pit between the bulging forebrain vesicle and the pericardial bulge. Simultaneously five swellings (**facial primordia**) appear around the primitive mouth (stomodeum).

The **five facial primordia** consist mainly of mesenchyme (derived from neural crest cells) covered by an ectoderm.

1. The **frontonasal process** is formed by the proliferation of mesenchyme lying ventral to forebrain vesicle and forms forehead, external nose, nasal cavity, nasal septum, and middle part of the upper lip border of the stomodeum.
2. The paired **maxillary processes** of first arch form the lateral parts of the upper border of the stomodeum.
3. The paired **mandibular processes** of the first arch form the whole lower border of the stomodeum.

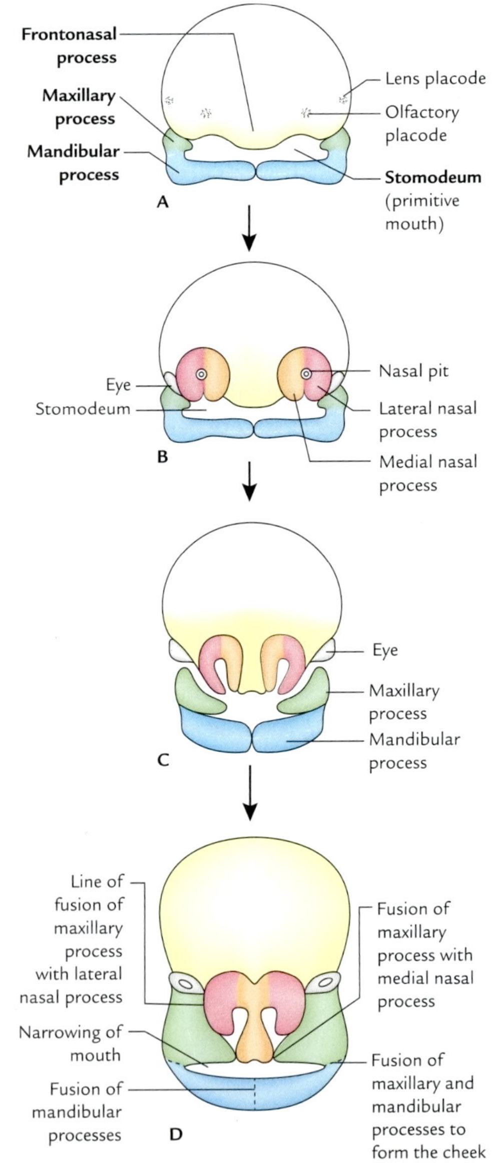

Fig. 16.1 Development of face.

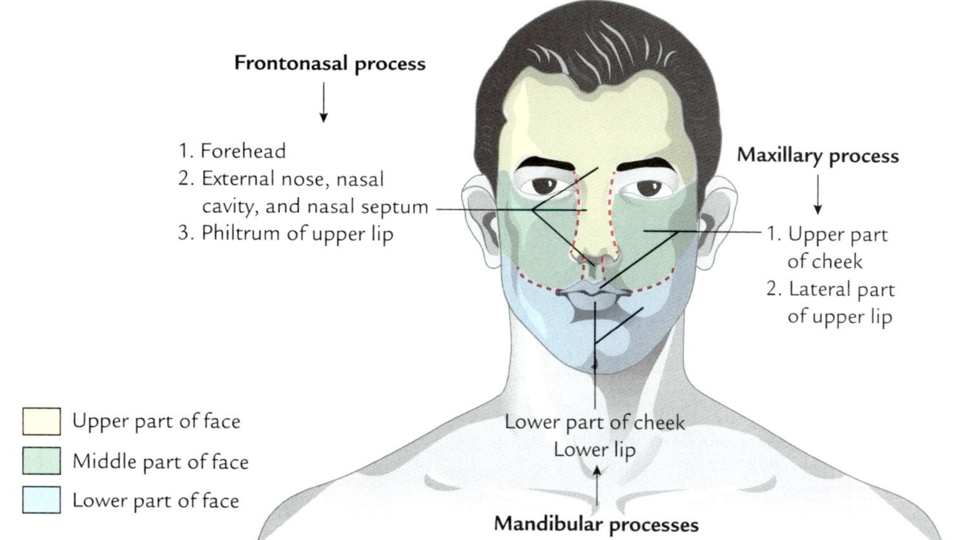

Fig. 16.2 Development of the various parts of face from frontonasal, maxillary, and mandibular processes.

Further Development of Various Parts of the Face (Fig. 16.2)

1. The **frontonasal process** (proper) forms forehead and bridge of nose.
   - On each side of the median plane in the ventrolateral part of frontonasal process, the surface ectoderm thickens to form an ectodermal elevation – the **olfactory placode.** The olfactory placodes invaginate into the underlying mesoderm to form **olfactory pits** or **nasal pits.** The pits are continuous with the stomodeum below. The mesenchyme around margins of nasal pits proliferates to form **horseshoe-shaped elevations.** Medial half of horseshoe-shaped elevation is called **medial nasal process** and lateral half is called **lateral nasal process.**

   The **medial nasal processes** extend more toward the stomodeum and form two globular processes that are separated by a small triangular notch.

   These processes fuse with each other to form **intermaxillary segment.** This segment is divided into 3 parts. From superficial to deep these are:
   - **Labial**
   - **Upper jaw component**
   - **Palatal component**

   The labial component forms the **philtrum of upper lip**. The intermaxillary segment is discussed in detail on page 173.

   (a) **Nasal pits** grow deeper to form **nasal cavities.**

   (b) **Median nasal processes** form dorsum of nose, **primitive nasal septum, crest and tip of nose,** and **philtrum of the upper lip.**

   (c) Lateral **nasal processes** form sides and alae of nose.
2. The **two maxillary processes** grow medially below developing eyes and fuse with the lateral nasal process to form the **lateral part of the upper lip** and **upper part of the cheek.**
3. The **two mandibular processes** form the **lower lip** and **lower part of the cheek.**
4. The surface opening of stomodeum forms the **oral fissure.** Lateral angles of the oral fissure are formed by fusion of maxillary and mandibular processes.

N.B. **Developmental enigma of upper lip:** The upper lip develops from three sources – the median part, the **philtrum** from globular process derived from frontonasal processes, and lateral parts from two maxillary processes.

- The mesodermal basis of **lateral parts of the upper lip** is derived from the mesenchyme of the maxillary processes, and skin over these parts is derived from ectoderm covering these processes.
- The mesodermal basis of the median part of the upper lip (**philtrum**) is derived from the mesenchyme of the frontonasal process. The ectoderm overlying the maxillary processes overgrows the mesoderm of the philtrum to form skin over it (Fig. 16.3).
- According to the recent clinical and embryological evidence, the upper lip is entirely formed from the maxillary processes. The lower parts of medial nasal processes become deeply positioned and get covered by medial extensions of maxillary processes to form the philtrum. Hence, sensory innervation of upper lip is derived from maxillary nerves.

Embryological Basis of Innervation of Structures in the Region of Head and Face (Fig. 16.4)

- *Sensory innervation*

  a. The upper part of face is derived from *frontonasal process*, hence supplied by the *ophthalmic nerve* (V_1).

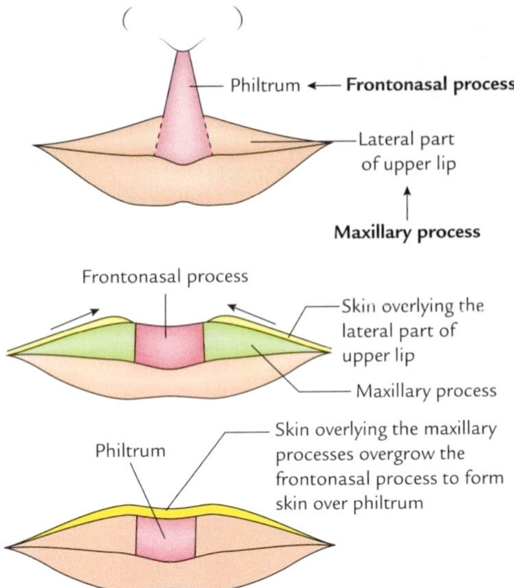

Fig. 16.3 Diagram showing how skin covering maxillary processes (forming lateral parts of lips) overgrows over the frontonasal process to form the skin covering the philtrum.

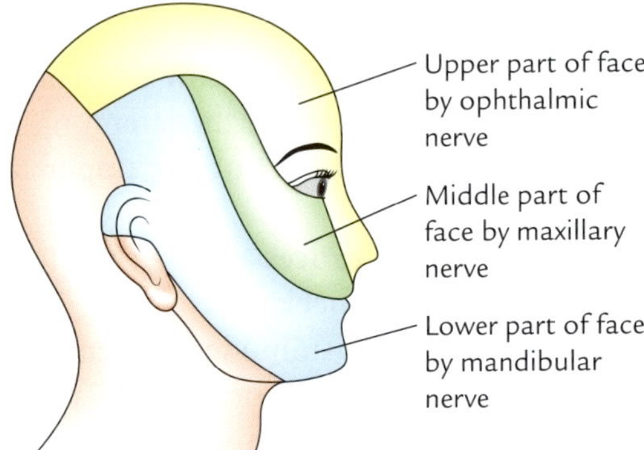

Fig. 16.4 Embryological basis of the sensory innervations of the face by three divisions of trigeminal nerve.

b. The middle part of face is derived from *maxillary processes*, hence supplied by the *maxillary nerve* (V_2).
c. The lower part of face is derived from *mandibular processes*, hence supplied by the *mandibular nerve* (V_3).
   The details are given in Table 16.1.

- ***Motor innervation***
  The muscles of face are derived from mesoderm of *second pharyngeal arch*, hence supplied by the *facial nerve*.

Development of Nasolacrimal Duct and Sac (Fig. 16.5)

On either side, the maxillary process grows medially and fuses with the lateral nasal process.

- The line of fusion of maxillary and lateral nasal processes presents a groove called **nasolacrimal groove**. This groove is lined by surface ectoderm.

Table 16.1 Correlation of sensory nerve supply of various components of face and their source of development

Component of Face	Develops From	Nerves
Forehead	Frontonasal process	Ophthalmic division of Vth CN (V_1)
Nose	Frontonasal process	Ophthalmic division of Vth CN (V_1)
Cheek		
(a) Upper part	Maxillary process	Maxillary division of Vth CN (V_2)
(b) Lower part	Mandibular process	Mandibular division of Vth CN (V_3)
Upper lip	Fusion of maxillary processes of two sides with the frontonasal process[a]	Maxillary division of Vth CN (V_2)
Lower lip	Fusion of mandibular processes of two sides	Mandibular division of Vth CN (V_3)

[a]The skin of the philtrum of the upper lip is derived from skin overlying the maxillary processes; hence, it is supplied by the maxillary nerve.

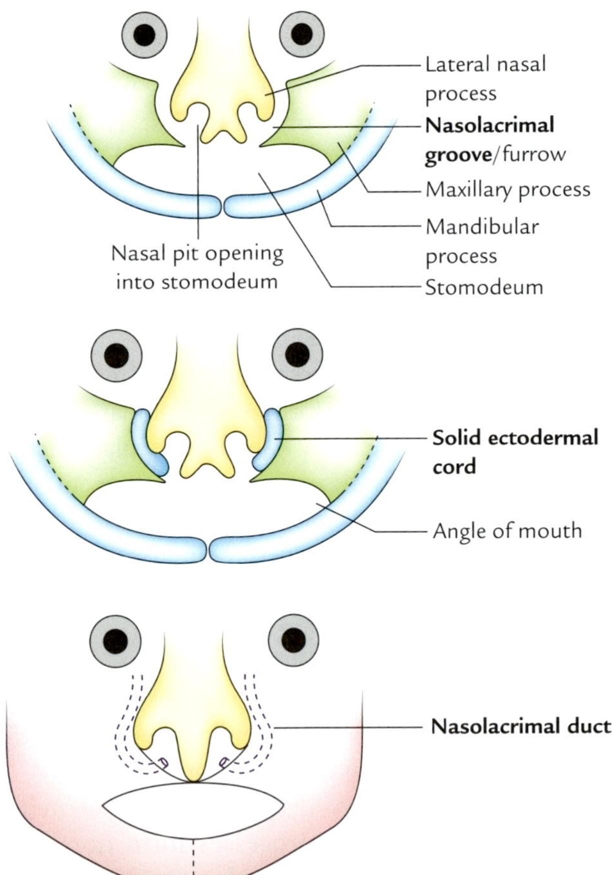

Fig. 16.5 Development of nasolacrimal duct.

- The ectoderm in floor of this groove proliferates to form a solid epithelial cord (**ectodermal cord**). Later on, this epithelial cord is detached from the surface ectoderm and gets canalized to form **nasolacrimal duct.**
- The upper end of nasolacrimal duct widens to form the **lacrimal sac**.
- The nasolacrimal duct becomes completely patent only after birth. The nasolacrimal duct communicates secondarily with the nasal cavity at its caudal end and with the conjunctival sac at its cephalic end.
- In adults, the nasolacrimal duct runs from medial angle of the eye to inferior meatus of the nasal cavity.

DEVELOPMENT OF NOSE

The nose consists of **external nose** and **nasal cavities.**

a. **Development of external nose** (Fig. 16.6)
   The external nose develops from five facial processes, namely frontonasal process, two medial nasal processes, and two lateral nasal processes, as follows:
   - ***The frontonasal process*** forms the ***bridge of the nose.***
   - ***Two fused medial nasal processes*** form ***dorsum and tip of the nose.***
   - ***Two lateral nasal processes*** form ***sides and alae of the nose.***

b. **Development of nasal cavities** (Figs 16.7 and 16.8)
   The **nasal cavities** develop from ectodermal **nasal pits.** The *nasal pits* deepen dorsally during the 6th week of intrauterine life to form **nasal sacs.** Each nasal sac grows dorsoventrally to developing forebrain to form **primitive nasal cavity**. Dorsal end of primitive nasal cavity is separated from oral cavity by **oronasal membrane.** At the end of 6th week, this membrane ruptures to form **primitive choanae** and as a result the nasal cavity communicates with the primitive oral cavity. The primitive choanae lie at the junction of primitive nasal and oral cavities, immediately behind **primary palate.** Later with further growth of primitive nasal cavity (**definitive nasal cavity**) and formation of secondary palate, the **definitive choanae** lie at junction of the nasal cavity and the nasopharynx.

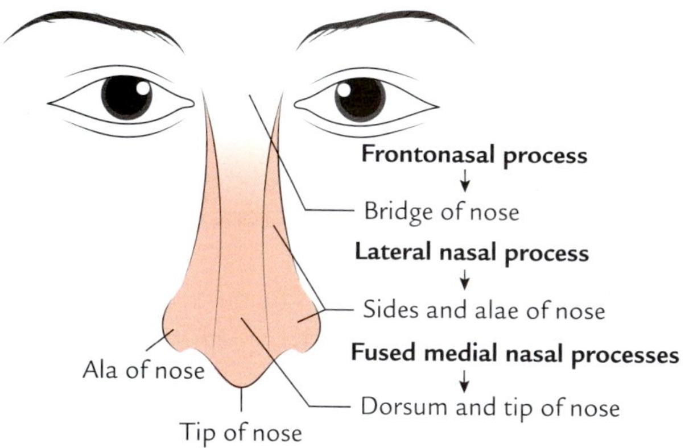

Fig. 16.6 Development of external nose.

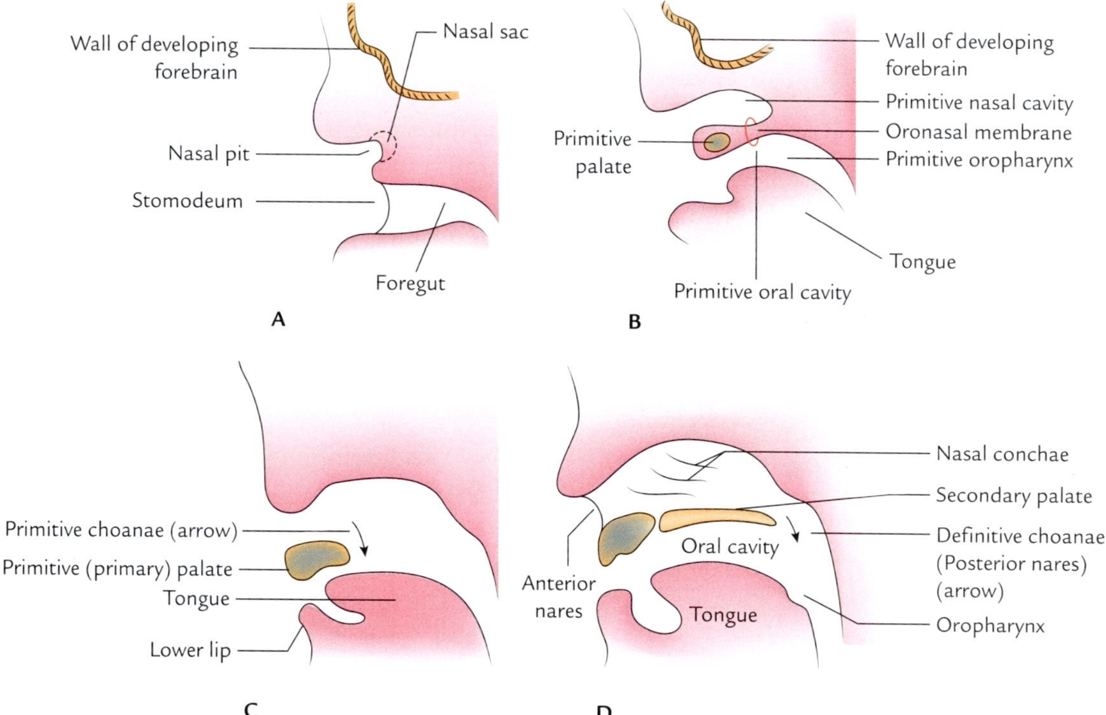

Fig. 16.7 Development of the nasal cavity.

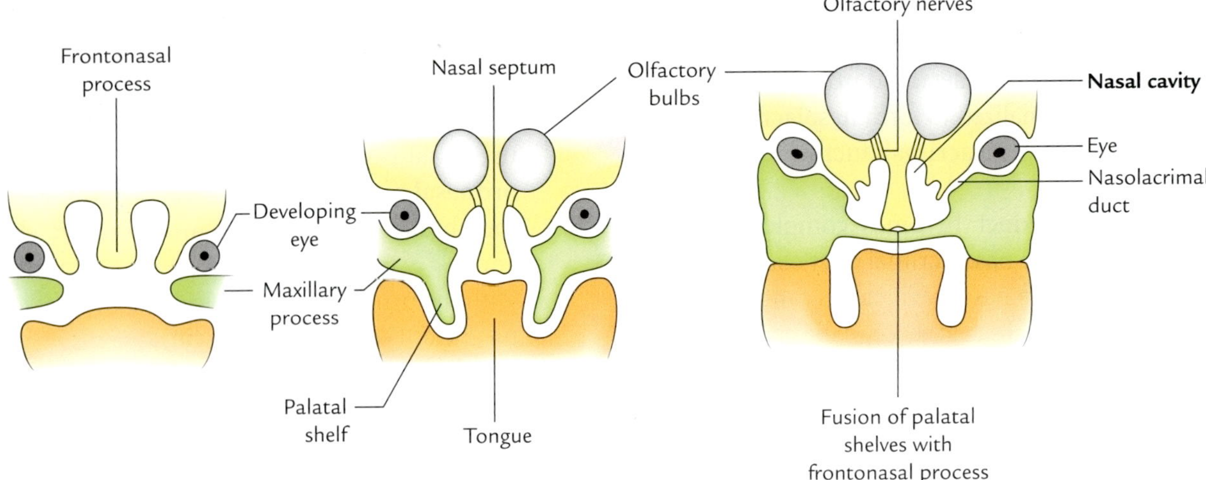

Fig. 16.8 Formation of the nasal septum and palatine shelves.

External openings of the nasal pits persist as **external nares**. While these changes are occurring, the following events take place:

- The **superior, middle,** and **inferior nasal conchae** develop as curved elevations from the lateral wall of the nasal cavity.
- Ectoderm lining the roof of the nasal cavity becomes specialized to form **olfactory epithelium**, which provides origin of olfactory nerves (Fig. 16.8).

The nasal septum develops from medial nasal processes. The formation of nasal septum and palatine shelves are shown in Fig. 16.8.

The development of various components of the nose is summarized in Table 16.2.

Development of Paranasal Air Sinuses

The paranasal air sinuses develop as **diverticula from the walls of the nasal cavities**. They grow into surrounding bones, namely *maxilla, ethmoid, frontal,* and *sphenoid*, and become air filled. They are named after the name of the bone that they invade, namely *maxillary air sinus* in maxillary bone, *frontal air sinus* in frontal bone, *ethmoidal air sinuses* in ethmoid bone, and *sphenoidal air sinuses* in sphenoid bone. The primitive openings of diverticula persist as orifices of the adult sinuses. The lining of paranasal air sinuses is ectodermal as that of the nasal cavity.

All the sinuses begin to develop before birth except frontal air sinuses, which begin to develop after birth.

Maxillary air sinuses are first to develop, and they appear as shallow groove on the medial surface of each maxilla during the 3rd month of intrauterine life.

The frontal air sinuses develop by 5th or 6th postnatal year.

The paranasal air sinuses reach their maximum size at puberty and subserve following functions:

1. Contribute to definitive shape of face
2. Reduce weight of skull
3. Add resonance to the voice

Table 16.2 Development of the various components of the nose and their source of development

Components	Develop From
• Dorsum and tip of nose	Frontonasal process
• Nasal cavities	Nasal sacs formed by elongation of nasal pits
• Nasal septum	Frontonasal process
• Nostrils (anterior nares)	Nasal pits
• Choanae (posterior nares)	Rupture of oronasal membrane (in the 2nd month)

OTHER DEVELOPMENTAL EVENTS OF FACE

Lens Placode

The sites of development of lens placodes indicate the sites of development of the eyes in the region of the face. Here, only a brief account of their development is given. The development of the eye is described in detail in Chapter 28.

The surface ectoderm at the sites of development of eyes thickens to form *lens placodes – primordia of eye lenses.* The formation of lens placode is induced by underlying developing optic vesicles from the forebrain. The developing eyeballs produce bulges at these sites. These bulges at first lie in angles between the maxillary and lateral nasal processes, but later due to narrowing of maxillary processes they come forward.

Intermaxillary Segment of Face

The **intermaxillary segment** is a wedge-shaped mass of mesenchyme formed by the fusion of two medial nasal processes deep to philtrum of upper lip. From superficial to deep, it is divided into three parts: (a) ***labial component***, (b) ***upper jaw component***, and (c) ***palatal component***.

Derivatives of intermaxillary segment

1. **Philtrum of upper lip** from **labial component**.
2. **Alveolar process of upper jaw** lodging four incisor teeth from **upper jaw component.**
3. **Triangular primary palate premaxilla** from **palatal component**.

DEVELOPMENT OF PALATE

Embryologically, the palate consists of two parts: **primary palate** and **secondary palate.** The primary palate develops from the **frontonasal process** and secondary palate develops from the **maxillary processes.**

Development of palate begins in the 6th week and completes by the end of the 12th week. The palate develops in two stages:

1. Development of primary palate
2. Development of secondary palate

Development of Primary Palate (Fig. 16.9)

The primary palate is formed by fusion of two medial nasal processes of the frontonasal process at a deeper level. The fusion of these processes (at a deeper level) forms a wedge-shaped mass of mesenchyme opposite upper jaw in the mid-region carrying four incisor teeth called **primary palate.** It ossifies to form **premaxilla.**

Development of Secondary Palate (Fig. 16.10)

It is the main part of definitive palate. It is formed by the fusion of two shelf-like outgrowths called **palatine shelves**

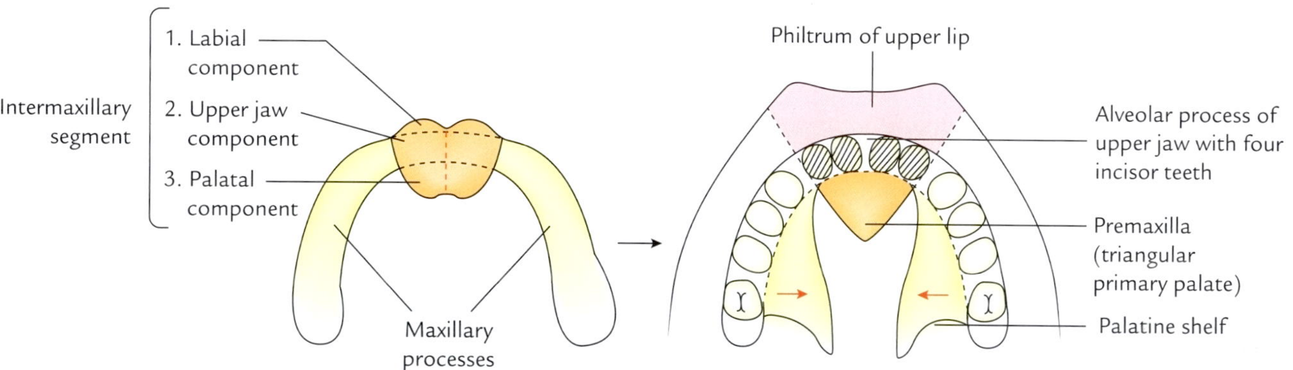

Fig. 16.9 Intermaxillary segment and maxillary processes. Note that intermaxillary segment gives rise to (A) philtrum of the upper lip, (B) median part of maxillary bone with its four incisor teeth, and (C) triangular primary palate.

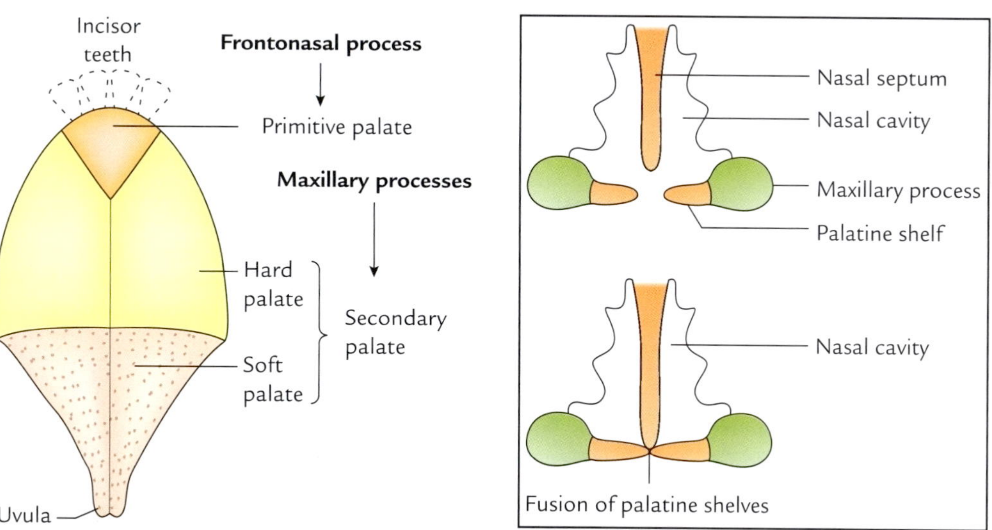

Fig. 16.10 Development of definitive palate. Note derivation of its various parts from different sources. Figure in the inset (on the right side) shows separation of nasal cavities from each other and from the oral cavity.

from inner aspects of the maxillary processes. The palatine shelves appear in the 6th week of development. Initially, they grow downward and medially on each side of and below the tongue. Later, during the 7th and 8th week, they assume horizontal position above the tongue and fuse with each other to form the **secondary palate**.

The secondary palate is the primordium of most of hard part and whole of soft part of the adult palate.

Once the palatine shelves are fused, the ossification extends from the maxillae and palatine bones into these shelves to form the hard palate. The posterior parts of these processes that extend posteriorly beyond the nasal septum fail to ossify and form the **soft palate**, including its soft conical projection – **uvula**.

Development of Permanent Palate

Anteriorly, the secondary palate fuses with the primary palate by a **Y-shaped suture** and each limb of Y passes between the lateral incisor and canine teeth. Junction between the primitive and secondary palates is represented in adults by **incisive fossa** into which two incisive foramina open.

The nasal septum grows down and joins superior aspect of anterior three-fourth of the hard palate in the midline. The nasal septum develops as a downgrowth from the frontonasal process. The fusion between nasal septum and secondary palate begins anteriorly during the 9th week and is completed posteriorly by the 12th week.

The *anterior three-fourth of permanent palate* ossifies in the membrane and forms the ***hard palate***.

The *posterior one-fourth of the permanent palate* that fails to join with the nasal septum and fails to ossify as well forms the **soft palate**. The soft palate hangs as a curtain to form the posterior margin of the hard palate.

The components of adult palate and their sources of development are summarized in Table 16.3.

Table 16.3 Development of various components of the adult palate

Component	Source of Development (i.e., Develops From)
1. **Hard palate**	
(a) In front of incisive fossa (premaxilla) carrying four incisor teeth	Fused medial nasal processes of frontonasal process
(b) Behind the incisive fossa	Fusion of palatine shelves (palatal processes) of maxillary processes of two sides
2. **Soft palate**	Unossified part of fused palatine shelves (palatal processes) of two maxillary processes, which extend posteriorly beyond the nasal septum

CLINICAL CORRELATION

1. ***Cleft lip:*** It commonly occurs in the upper lip. The incidence of cleft lip is 1 in 1000 births and 60%–80% of children involved are males. The cleft upper lip presents three varieties (Fig. 16.11):
   (a) *Unilateral cleft lip:* It occurs due to failure of fusion of maxillary process with the medial nasal process of the same side.
   (b) *Bilateral cleft lip:* It occurs due to failure of fusion of maxillary processes with the frontonasal process.

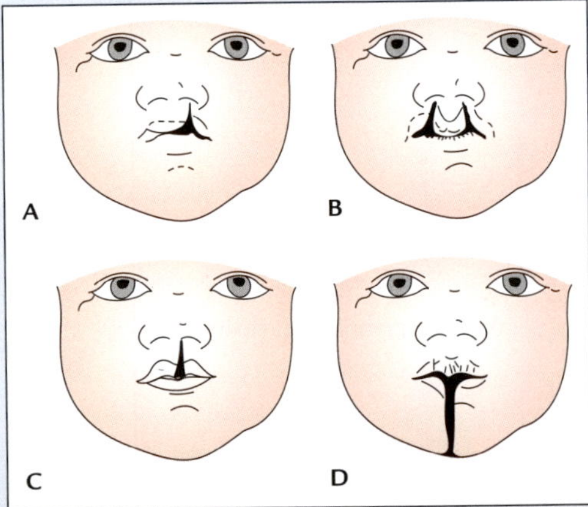

Fig. 16.11 Types of cleft lip. (A) Unilateral cleft of upper lip. (B) Bilateral cleft of the upper lip. (C) Median cleft of the upper lip (hair lip). (D) Cleft of lower lip.

   (c) *Central cleft lip/hair lip:* It occurs due to failure of development of philtrum of the upper lip from the frontonasal process.
   Very rarely, the two mandibular processes may fail to fuse in the midline to cause *cleft lower lip*.
2. ***Cleft palate:*** The defective fusion of various segments of palate gives rise to clefts in the palate. These vary considerably in degree, leading to varieties of cleft palate as follows:
   (a) **Complete cleft palate** (Fig. 16.12)

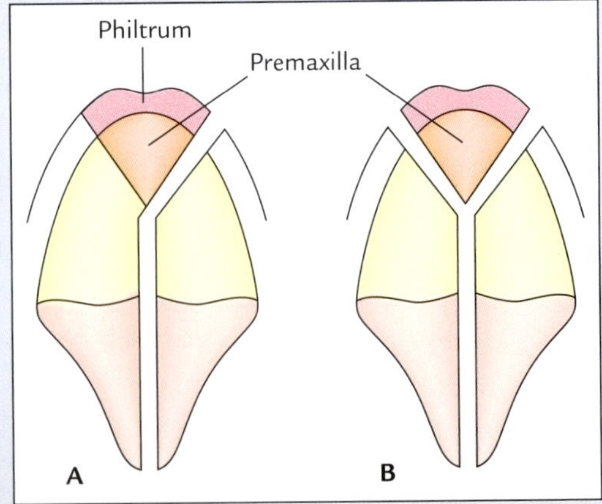

Fig. 16.12 Complete cleft palate. (A) Unilateral. (B) Bilateral.

- *Unilateral complete cleft palate* occurs if maxillary process on one side does not fuse with the premaxilla. It is always associated with the cleft lip on the same side.
- *Bilateral complete cleft palate* occurs if both the maxillary processes fail to fuse with the premaxilla. In this type, secondary palate is divided into two equal halves by a median cleft with an anterior V-shaped cleft separating the premaxilla completely.

(b) **Incomplete or partial cleft palate** (Fig. 16.13): The following types may occur:
- *Bifid uvula:* Cleft involving only uvula; it is of no clinical importance.
- *Cleft of the soft palate:* Involving uvula and adjoining part of the soft palate.
- *Cleft of the soft palate:* Involving uvula, whole of the soft palate, and extends into the hard palate.

Clinical photographs of cleft lip and **cleft palate** are shown in Fig. 16.14.

3. ***Microstomia*** (small mouth) and ***macrostomia*** (large mouth): Lateral angles of oral fissure are formed at the junction of the maxillary and mandibular processes. Initially, the lateral angle of mouth extends much laterally close to auricle. Subsequently, in normal conditions the angles of mouth gradually shift medially by fusion between the maxillary and mandibular processes till normal adult position is reached. The excessive fusion of these processes leads to *microstomia* and arrest of this fusion leads to *macrostomia.*
4. ***Oblique facial cleft*** (also called ***orbitofacial fissure*** Fig. 16.15): It is a rare congenital anomaly of the face, which occurs when maxillary process fails to fuse with the lateral nasal process. The fissure extends from medial angle of the eye to the upper lip. Consequently, the nasolacrimal duct is exposed to the exterior. This anomaly is usually bilateral.
5. ***Congenital anomalies of nose***
   a. **Bifid nose:** Sometimes, it occurs due to bifurcation of frontonasal process. It may be associated with median cleft lip. Occasionally, one half of the nose may be missing.
   b. **Proboscis** (Fig. 16.16): Rarely, the nose is present as an abnormal facial appendage below the forehead called **proboscis.** It is often associated with one median eye below it formed due to fusion of two eyes called **cyclops** (also see p. 332).

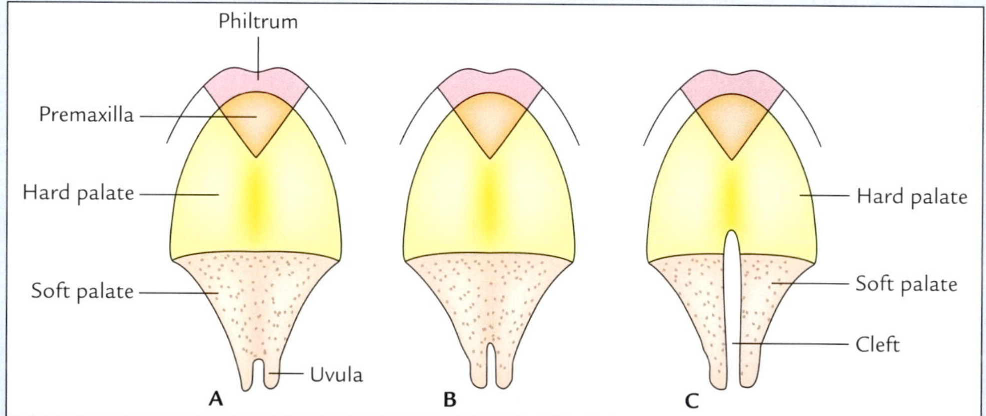

Fig. 16.13 Incomplete/partial cleft palate. (A) Bifida uvula. (B) Cleft of the soft palate involving uvula and adjoining part of the soft palate. (C) Cleft of the soft palate extending into the hard palate.

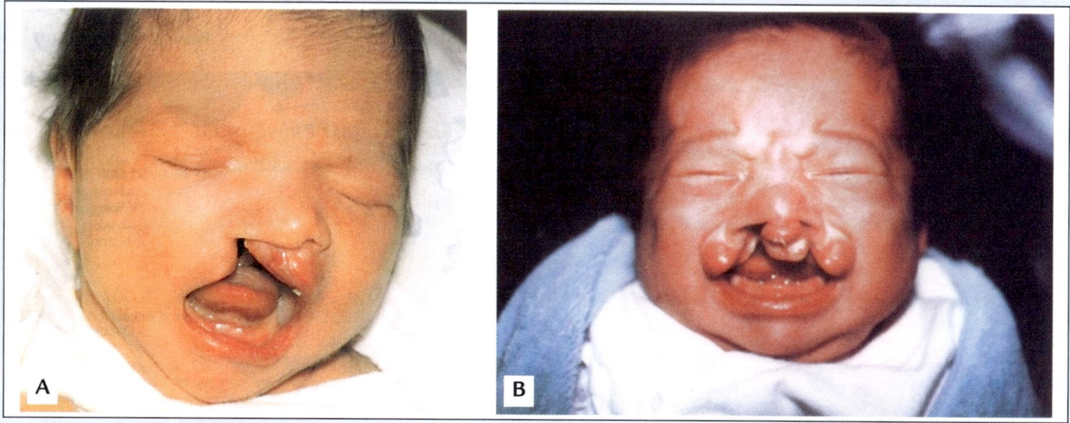

Fig. 16.14 Congenital anomalies of cleft lip and cleft palate. (A) Infant with unilateral cleft lip and cleft palate. (B) Infant with bilateral cleft lip and cleft palate. (*Source:* (A) *The Developing Human: Clinically Oriented Embryology*, 8th edition by Keith L. Moore and T.V.N. Persaud, ISBN: 9781416037064, page 190, Fig. 9.39, Copyright Elsevier, 2008; (B) The *Developing Human: Clinically Oriented Embryology*, 8th edition by Keith L. Moore and T.V.N. Persaud, ISBN: 9781416037064, page 192, Fig. 9.41, Copyright Elsevier, 2008.)

Continued

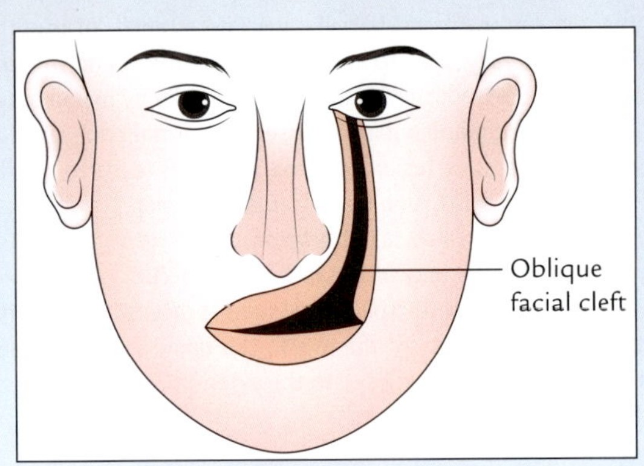

Fig. 16.15 Oblique facial cleft.

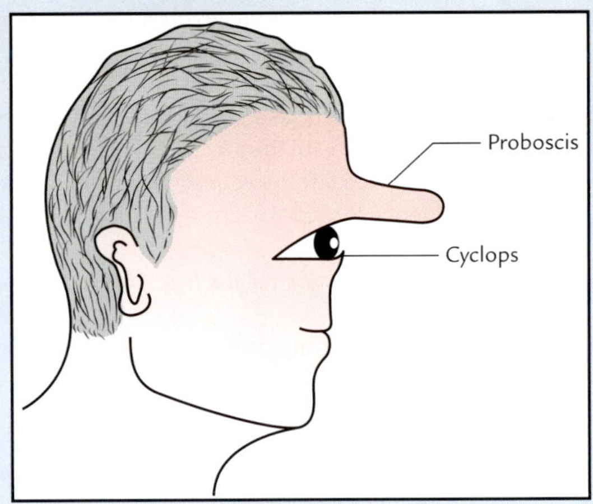

Fig. 16.16 Proboscis and cyclops. The proboscis is akin to mini trunk of an elephant.

GESTATIONAL AGE OF KEY DEVELOPMENTAL EVENTS

Developmental Event	Gestational Age
➢ Primordia of face around stomodeum appears at the end of	4th week
➢ Formation of nasal pit occurs in	6th week
➢ Development of palatine shelves	6th week
➢ Palatine shelves ascend and attain a horizontal position above tongue	7th and 8th weeks
➢ Development of palate	6th–12th weeks

GOLDEN FACTS TO REMEMBER

➢ **First part of the face to form**	Lower jaw and lower lip
➢ **Nasolacrimal duct and sac develop from**	Epithelial cord derived from ectodermal lining of the floor of nasolacrimal groove
➢ **Most common craniofacial congenital anomalies**	Cleft lip and cleft palate
➢ **Critical period of palate development**	End of 6th week to beginning of 9th week
➢ **Most common cleft lip**	Unilateral cleft upper lip
➢ **Most rare cleft lip**	Median cleft lower lip
➢ **Commonest cause of cleft lip with or without cleft palate**	Multifactorial inheritance (i.e., combination of genetic and environmental factors)
➢ **Commonest congenital anomaly of face**	Unilateral cleft upper lip

CLINICAL PROBLEM SOLVING

PROBLEMS

1. A baby was born with **unilateral cleft lip and cleft palate.** What is the **embryological basis** of unilateral cleft lip and cleft palate? Discuss symptoms from which the child suffers. Can it be seen in the first-trimester ultrasound screening?
2. **The cleft lip is often associated with the cleft palate. Give the embryological basis.**
3. Although the upper lip develops from two different sources (frontonasal process and maxillary processes), but general sensory innervation is provided only by nerves of maxillary processes (i.e., maxillary nerves). Why? Give the embryological basis.
4. **The clefts of the lip and palate are the most common congenital anomalies. Can they be recognized/identified before birth by ultrasonography?**
5. An epileptic mother who was treated with an anticonvulsant drug **phenytoin** during her pregnancy gave birth to a male child with **cleft lip associated with cleft palate**. Explain whether there is any evidence to suggest that this drug increases the incidence of these anomalies.

SOLUTIONS

1. The unilateral cleft lip is a gap between the philtrum and lateral part of the upper lip. It occurs when the maxillary process of first pharyngeal arch fails to fuse with the medial nasal process of the same side. It is often associated with cleft palate because the palate develops from same sources as that of the upper lip. The symptoms of the cleft lip and cleft palate are as follows:
   (a) Disfigurement
   (b) Inability to suckle
   (c) Interference with the speech, particularly with the formation of consonants, namely D, T, and G
   (d) Distortion of teeth

   Yes, it can be seen by ultrasonography during the **first-trimester ultrasound screening**.
2. The philtrum, alveolar arch bearing incisor teeth, and primary palate develop from (intermaxillary segments), whereas, the lateral part of the upper lip, associated alveolar arch, and secondary palate develop from the maxillary processes (palatine shelves) of the first pharyngeal arches.

   The cleft lip occurs due to nonfusion of frontonasal and maxillary processes; therefore, it often involves alveolar arch and palate due to a common source of development.
3. The skin overlying the mesenchymal masses of maxillary processes overgrows the mesenchymal mass of frontonasal process. Thus, the skin of whole upper lip is derived from the skin overlying the two maxillary processes, and hence it is supplied by two maxillary nerves (also see p. 170).

   N.B. **According to Frazer**, the human upper lip develops only from maxillary processes, whereas the frontonasal process (globular processes) grows deeply to form premaxilla/primary palate. This is substantiated by the fact that sensory innervation of the upper lip is provided by the maxillary nerves (vide supra).
4. The facial features of fetus become visible by beginning of the second trimester of pregnancy. Therefore, they can be recognized before birth by ultrasonography.
5. There is substantial clinical and experimental evidence that anticonvulsant drugs such as **phenytoin** if given during pregnancy increase the incidence of cleft lip and cleft palate, two- to threefold more as compared to the normal population.

17 Development of Oral Cavity (Mouth), Salivary Glands, and Teeth

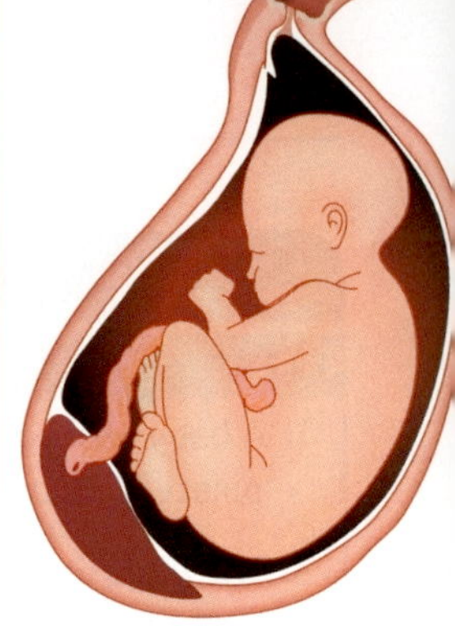

LEARNING OBJECTIVES

After studying this chapter, the student should be able to:

- Describe the development of oral cavity in brief.
- Describe the development of major salivary glands in brief.
- Describe the development of teeth in brief, and discuss various stages of their development.
- Give the embryological basis of (a) natal teeth and (b) dentigerous cyst.

DEVELOPMENT OF ORAL CAVITY

OVERVIEW

The oral cavity develops from two sources: (a) **stomodeum** – a surface depression lined by ectoderm and (b) a cephalic part of **foregut** lined by endoderm.

The oral cavity consists of two parts: (a) primitive oral cavity and (b) definitive oral cavity.

The ***primitive oral cavity*** develops from **ectodermal stomodeum,** whereas the ***definitive oral cavity*** develops from cephalic part of **endodermal foregut**. Initially, the two parts are separated from each other by **buccopharyngeal membrane.**

The two parts communicate with each other when buccopharyngeal membrane ruptures during the 3rd week of intrauterine life (IUL) (Fig. 17.1).

After rupture of **buccopharyngeal membrane,** the line of junction of ectodermal and endodermal parts cannot be defined.

N.B. **Imaginary location of buccopharyngeal membrane in adult:** If the buccopharyngeal membrane were to persist into the adults, it would occupy an imaginary plane extending downward obliquely from the body of sphenoid, through the soft palate to the inner surface of the body of mandible inferior to the incisor teeth.

Whole of **adult oral cavity** is derived from ectodermal stomodeum except floor of the mouth, which is derived from cephalic part of endodermal foregut.

Thus, epithelial lining of the cheeks, lips, gums, and hard palate is ectodermal in origin, whereas epithelial lining of tongue (developing in floor of the oral cavity), floor of mouth, most of the soft palate, and palatoglossal and palatopharyngeal folds is endodermal in origin.

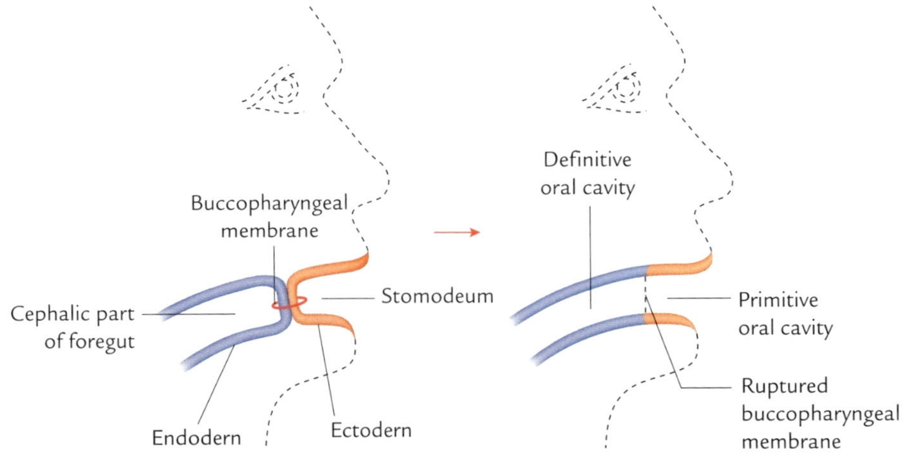

Fig. 17.1 Development of the oral cavity from stomodeum and cephalic part of the foregut.

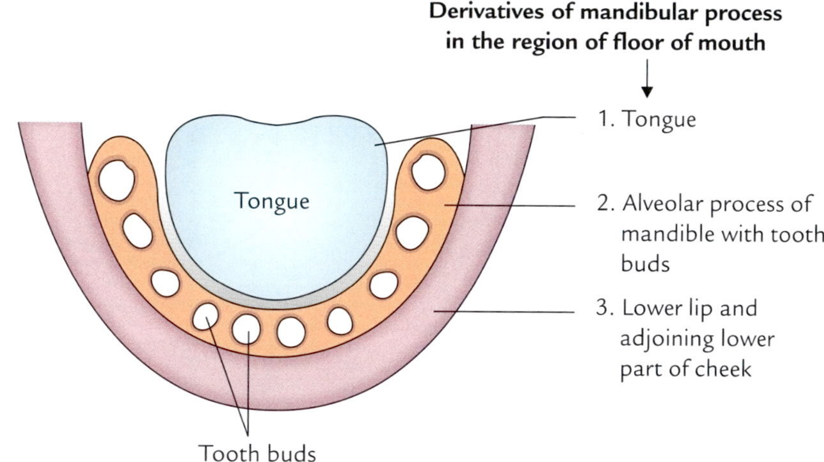

Fig. 17.2 Structures derived from mandibular processes in the region of the floor of the mouth.

Development of Floor

In the region of floor of mouth, mandibular processes form following three structures (Fig. 17.2):

1. Lower lip and adjoining parts of cheeks
2. Alveolar process of the lower jaw
3. Tongue

Initially, these structures are not demarcated from each other in the floor of the oral cavity. But soon the tongue begins to develop and forms a recognizable swelling, its anterior and lateral margins become separated from the floor of definitive mouth by development of an endodermal **linguogingival sulcus**.

Soon thereafter, ectodermal **labiogingival sulcus** appears far lateral to the *linguogingival sulcus*, which separates lips and cheeks from the gum and teeth of the lower jaw. As the linguogingival and labiogingival sulci deepen, area between the sulci is raised to form **alveolar process** (Fig. 17.3).

The ectodermal lining of the alveolar process thickens to form dental lamina. Soon series of thickened patches appear in the dental lamina, which extends into underlying mesoderm. The ectodermal projections are called *enamel organs*, which give rise to milk teeth.

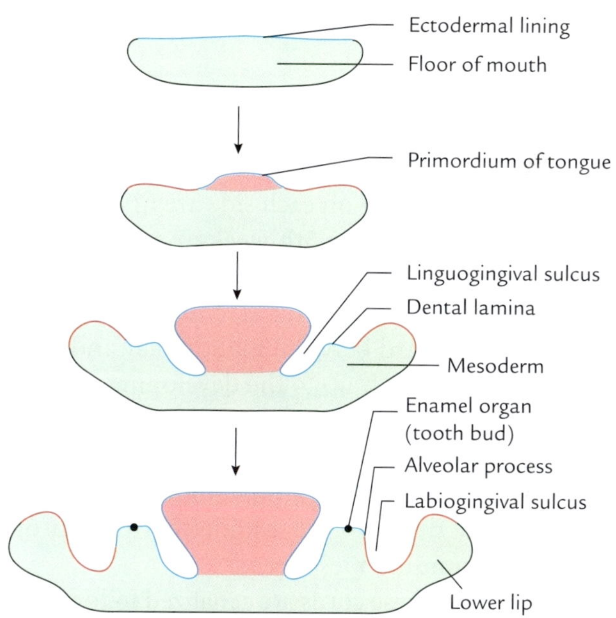

Fig. 17.3 Differentiation of the floor of the mouth into tongue, alveolar processes, and lips.

Development of Roof

The roof of the oral cavity is formed by palate (Fig. 17.4). For details see "development of palate" in Chapter 16, p. 173). The alveolar process of the upper jaw is separated from the upper lip and the cheek by the *labiogingival sulcus* similar to that of the lower jaw. Medial margin of the alveolar process of the upper jaw becomes defined only when the palate becomes well arched.

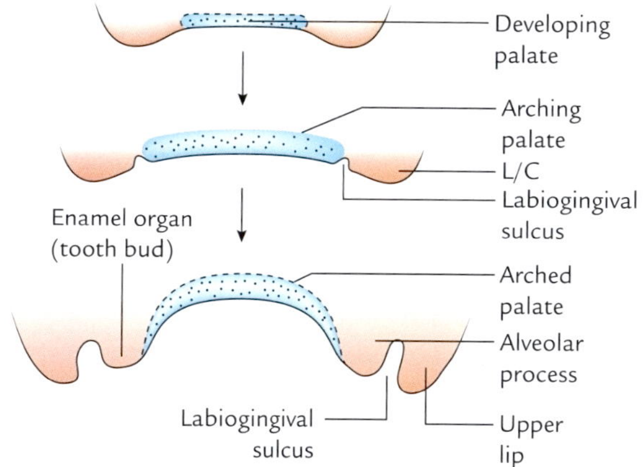

Fig. 17.4 Development of the roof of the oral cavity (L/C, lip or cheek).

DEVELOPMENT OF SALIVARY GLANDS

OVERVIEW

The salivary glands are tubuloacinar glands consisting of distal part of secretory acini and initial part of duct system. They develop as **solid outgrowth/buds from epithelial lining of the oral cavity (Fig. 17.5).** These outgrowths branch repeatedly and invade the surrounding mesenchyme. At first, the outgrowths and their branches are solid cords of epithelial cells. Later, they become canalized to form **duct system of gland.** The **secretory acini** of gland develop from rounded terminal ends of epithelial cords.

The capsules, septa, and connective tissues of the glands are formed from the surrounding mesoderm.

Major Salivary Glands

There are three pairs of major salivary glands: parotid, submandibular, and sublingual. They develop as outpouching of epithelial lining of oral cavity into surrounding mesoderm (Fig. 17.5).

Parotid Glands

The parotid gland, one on each side are first to appear. **They develop during the 5th week or early 6th week as an ectodermal outgrowth** from the cheek near the angle of the stomodeum. This ectodermal cord grows outward and upward between mandibular and maxillary processes to reach up to the developing ear. Later, the furrow is converted into a narrow tube, which forms the **parotid duct**. The medial end of the duct opens into the angle of primitive mouth, while from its lateral end the cords of ectodermal cells project into the surrounding mesoderm.

Subsequently, these cords are canalized to form **acini and ductules** of the parotid gland. Elongation of jaws causes elongation of the parotid duct; however, the gland remains at its site of origin. Later, the angle of mouth is shifted more medially due to fusion of mandibular and maxillary processes (Fig. 17.6).

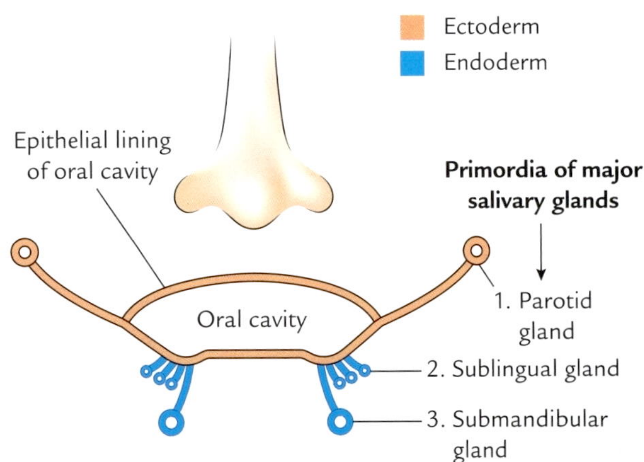

Fig. 17.5 Schematic diagram showing the sites of origin of parotid, submandibular, and sublingual glands.

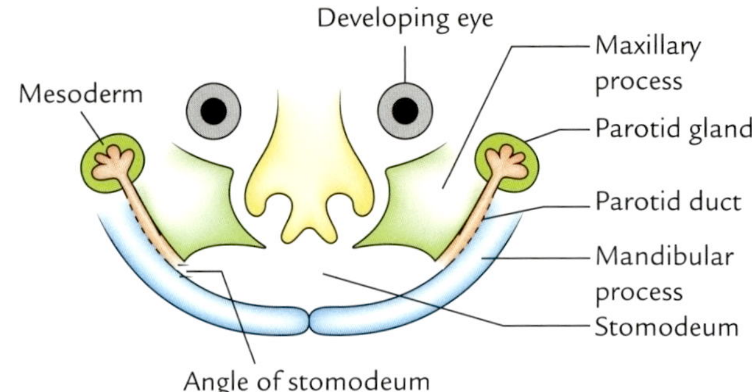

Fig. 17.6 Development of parotid glands.

In adults, the parotid gland opens into the vestibule of mouth opposite upper second molar tooth, which indicates position of angle of the primitive oral orifice.

Submandibular Glands

The submandibular glands, one on each side, **develop during later part of the 6th week** as a solid outgrowth of endoderm from the floor of stomodeum, actually floor of alveololingual groove/sulcus. The endodermal outgrowths grow posteriorly lateral to developing tongue. A linear groove forms lateral to the tongue that soon closes from behind to forward to form the **submandibular duct** that opens on the summit of **sublingual papilla** on each side of the frenulum linguae.

Sublingual Glands

The sublingual glands **develop in the 8th week**, about 2 weeks later than the other salivary glands; they develop as **multiple solid endodermal outgrowths** from the linguogingival sulcus and submandibular duct. Each outgrowth canalizes separately and opens independently on the summit of **sublingual fold.** Some of these ducts may join submandibular duct.

Minor Salivary Glands

Minor salivary glands are small submucosal glands that are distributed throughout the wall of the oral cavity, except gingivae. They develop in a similar fashion as the major salivary glands, except that they do not undergo branching at all or undergo very little branching. They open independently on the surface of oral mucosa.

The development of major salivary glands is summarized in Table 17.1.

Table 17.1 Development of major salivary glands

Gland	Source of Development	Time of Development
Parotid	Ectodermal outgrowth from cheek at an angle of stomodeum	5th week/early 6th week
Submandibular	Endodermal outgrowth from the floor of stomodeum/ linguogingival sulcus	6th week
Sublingual	Multiple endodermal outgrowths from the floor of linguogingival sulcus	8th week

DEVELOPMENT OF TEETH

OVERVIEW

In humans, two sets of teeth develop at different times of life (i.e., **humans are diphyodont**).

The first set called **deciduous teeth (primary dentition)** is temporary, and the second set called **permanent teeth (secondary dentition)** is permanent.

Teeth develop from **ectodermal oral epithelium** and the underlying **neural crest mesenchyme.** The tooth consists of *enamel, dentin, pulp, cementum,* and *periodontal ligament.* The *enamel of the tooth is derived from ectoderm, whereas all other tissues of tooth (namely dentin, pulp, cementum, and periodontal ligaments) are derived from neural crest mesenchyme.*

The teeth develop in relation to alveolar process involving reciprocal induction between neural crest mesenchyme and overlying ectodermal oral epithelium.

Stages of Development of Tooth (Figs 17.7 and 17.8)

For descriptive purposes, the development of tooth is divided into five stages: (1) dental lamina stage, (2) bud stage, (3) cap stage, (4) bell stage, and (5) apposition stage. The following text deals with the development of the lower incisor teeth.

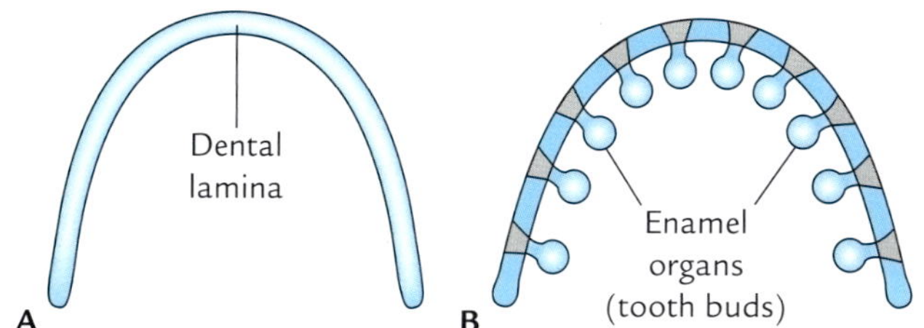

Fig. 17.7 Formation of dental lamina and tooth buds (enamel organs). Note the dental lamina acquires the shape of the alveolar arch.

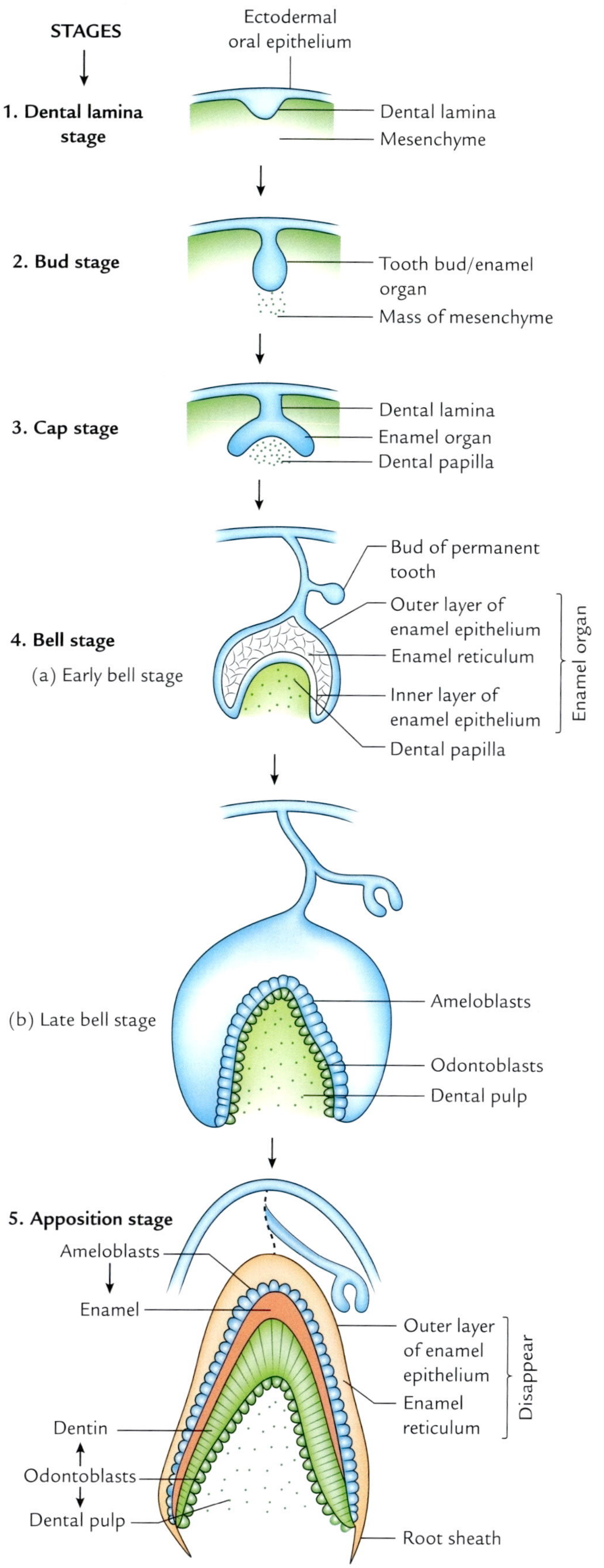

STAGES
Ectodermal oral epithelium
1. Dental lamina stage
Dental lamina
Mesenchyme
2. Bud stage
Tooth bud/enamel organ
Mass of mesenchyme
3. Cap stage
Dental lamina
Enamel organ
Dental papilla
4. Bell stage
(a) Early bell stage
Bud of permanent tooth
Outer layer of enamel epithelium
Enamel reticulum
Inner layer of enamel epithelium
Enamel organ
Dental papilla
(b) Late bell stage
Ameloblasts
Odontoblasts
Dental pulp
5. Apposition stage
Ameloblasts
Enamel
Dentin
Odontoblasts
Dental pulp
Outer layer of enamel epithelium
Enamel reticulum
Disappear
Root sheath

Fig. 17.8 The stages of development of tooth (1, 2, 3, 4).

1. Dental Lamina Stage

During the 6th week of development, the ectodermal epithelium lining of the convex "U"-shaped border of the alveolar processes of upper and lower jaws become thickened and projects into underlying mesoderm to form the **dental lamina.** Since the alveolar process is U shaped, the dental lamina is also U shaped (Figs 17.7A and 17.8A).

2. Bud Stage

The dental lamina now proliferates at 10 sites to produce local swellings called **dental buds/tooth buds** (**enamel organs**) that grow into the underlying mesenchyme. Thus, there are 10 such enamel organs (5 on each side) in each alveolar process. **These 10 enamel organs first form 20 deciduous teeth and later form permanent teeth when the deciduous teeth are shed off** (Figs 17.7B and 17.8B).

3. Cap Stage

The mass of underlying neural crest mesenchyme invaginates the tooth bud/enamel organ. As a result, the **enamel organ becomes cap shaped.** This mass of mesenchyme that invaginates the tooth bud is called **dental papilla** (Fig. 17.8C).

4. Bell Stage

The enamel organs differentiate into three layers:

1. Outer cell layer called **outer enamel epithelium**
2. Inner cell layer called **inner enamel epithelium**
3. Central core of loosely arranged cells called **enamel reticulum.**

As the enamel organ differentiates, the developing tooth assumes the shape of a bell, and hence it is called **bell stage** (Fig. 17.8D).

The cells of the inner layer enamel epithelium applied to dental papilla, become columnar and are now called ***ameloblasts.***

The mesodermal cells of dental papilla adjacent to ameloblasts arrange themselves as a continuous epithelial layer to form **odontoblasts.**

The ameloblasts derived from inner enamel epithelium of the **enamel organ** form the **enamel,** and the odontoblasts derived from **dental papilla** form the **dentin** and **dental pulp.**

Fig. 17.9 shows the photomicrographs of bell stage of developing lower incisor teeth.

5. Apposition Stage

The formation of the enamel and dentin occurs in this stage.

The ameloblasts lay down enamel (in the form of long prisms) on the outer surface of basement membrane separating ameloblasts and odontoblasts.

As the amount of enamel increases, the ameloblasts move toward the outer enamel epithelium. As a result, enamel reticulum and outer enamel epithelium disappear.

After the enamel is fully formed, ameloblasts also regress, leaving only a thin membrane – the **dental cuticle.** After the eruption of tooth, this membrane is gradually sloughed off.

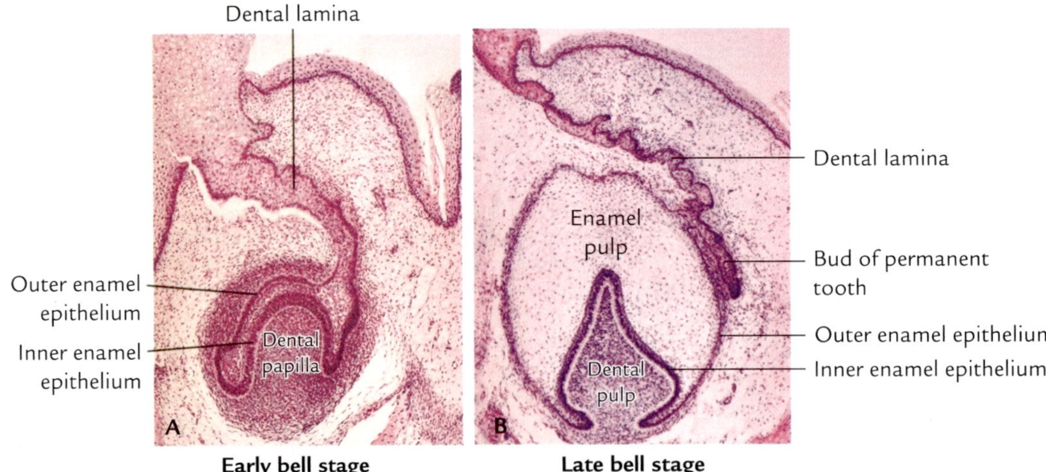

Fig. 17.9 Photomicrographs showing bell stage of development. (*Source: The Developing Human: Clinically Oriented Embryology*, 8th edition by Keith L. Moore and T.V.N. Persaud, ISBN: 9781416037064, page 451, Fig. 19.15, Copyright Elsevier, 2008.)

The odontoblasts produce **predentin** deep to the enamel. Later, predentin calcifies and forms second hardest tissue of body – **the dentin.** As the dentin thickens, cell bodies of odontoblasts regress, but their cytoplasmic processes called **odontoblastic processes** (**Tomes' processes**) remain trapped in the dentin.

Development of Root and Eruption of Tooth (Fig. 17.10)

The **root of the tooth** begins to develop after the formation of enamel and dentin is well advanced.

The outer and inner enamel epithelia come together at the neck of the tooth where they form a fold – the **Hertwig's epithelial root sheath.** This sheath grows in the mesenchyme and initiates the formation of the root.

The odontoblasts adjacent to root sheath produce dentin, which is continuous with that of the crown.

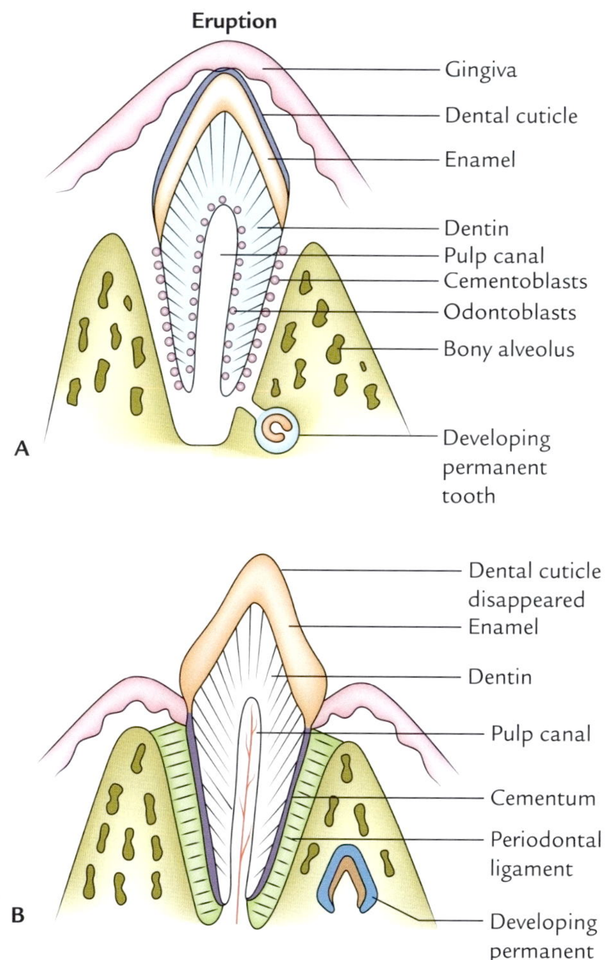

Fig. 17.10 Eruption of tooth. (A) Formation and elongation of root of tooth. (B) Eruption of crown of tooth through gingiva into oral cavity.

As more and more dentin is produced, the **pulp cavity** narrows and forms the **pulp canal.** The nerve and vessels pass to tooth through pulp canal.

The mesenchymal cells covering the root of tooth modifies to form **cementoblasts** that produce the cementum (a specialized bone) just before birth.

The mesenchyme cells of the outside cement layer (cementum) form the **periodontal ligament** that holds the root of the tooth firmly with the bony alveolar socket and also functions as a shock absorber. With further elongation of the root, the crown of the tooth is pushed through the overlying tissue of alveolus gingiva into the oral cavity, i.e., **eruption occurs.**

The characteristic features of the various stages of development of the teeth are summarized in Table 17.2.

Development of Permanent Teeth (Fig. 17.11)

The permanent teeth are 32 in number (16 in each jaw). They develop in a manner similar to that of deciduous teeth.

During the 3rd month of IUL, the dental lamina gives off a series of tooth buds on the lingual (medial) side of developing deciduous teeth. They give rise to permanent incisors, canines, and premolars.

Table 17.2 Stages of development of the tooth and their characteristic features

Stage	Characteristic Features
1. Dental lamina stage	Thickening of ectoderm overlying the alveolar process and its invagination into the underlying mesenchyme to form **dental lamina**
2. Bud stage	Proliferation of dental lamina at 10 centers/spots to form **tooth buds (enamel organs)**
3. Cap stage	• Tooth bud (enamel organ) is invaginated by the mesenchyme • Invaginated mesenchyme forms dental papilla • Tooth bud becomes cap shaped
4. Bell stage	• Histodifferentiation of ***ameloblasts*** from enamel organ and ***odontoblasts*** from the mesenchymal cells of pulp • Developing tooth assumes the shape of a bell
5. Apposition stage	Formation of enamel and dentin matrix

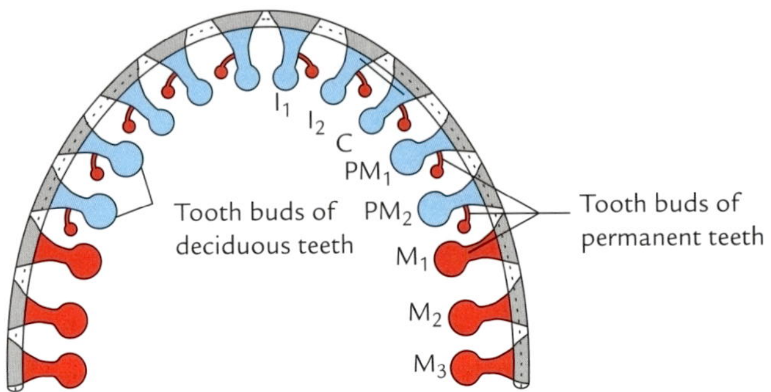

Fig. 17.11 Tooth bud (germs) of permanent teeth. Note buds of incisors, canines, and premolars are formed in relation to deciduous teeth, while buds of permanent molars arise from dental lamina posterior to the deciduous teeth. I, incisor; C, canine; PM, premolar; M, molar.

These buds remain dormant until about 6 years of postnatal life. As the tooth buds of permanent teeth grow, they push the deciduous teeth up from below. As a result, the deciduous teeth are shed off. As the permanent teeth grow, the roots of overlying deciduous teeth are reabsorbed by osteoclasts.

The permanent molars do not develop from tooth buds arising from dental lamina forming deciduous teeth, rather they are formed from tooth buds that arise directly from the dental lamina posterior to the region of lost milk teeth.

N.B. The tooth bud arising from dental lamina of first deciduous molar gives rise to first premolar, and tooth bud arising from second deciduous molar gives rise to second premolar (Fig. 17.11).

Thus, 20 deciduous or milk teeth are replaced by 32 permanent teeth.

- Deciduous teeth are two incisors, one canine, and two molars.
  The deciduous teeth begin to erupt at about 6 months of postnatal life, and all get erupted by the end of 2nd year or soon after. The teeth of the lower jaw erupt somewhat earlier than the corresponding teeth of the upper jaw.
- Permanent teeth are two incisors, one canine, two premolars, and three molars.
  The permanent teeth begin to erupt at about 6 years and all get erupted by the age of 18–25 years.

The approximate time of eruption of teeth (deciduous as well as permanent) and time of shedding of deciduous teeth are given in Table 17.3.

N.B. In general, mandibular teeth erupt before maxillary teeth, and girls' teeth generally erupt earlier than that of boys.

Table 17.3 Time of eruption and shedding of the teeth (after birth)

Tooth	Eruption Time	Shedding Time
Deciduous Teeth		
Central incisors	6–7 months	6–7 years
Lateral incisors	8–9 months	7–8 years
Canine	16–19 months	10–12 years
First molar	12–16 months	9–11 years
Second molar	20–24 months	10–12 years
Permanent Teeth		
Central incisor	7–8 years	Permanent teeth do not shed off
Lateral incisor	8–9 years	
Canine	10–12 years	
First premolar	10–11 years	
Second premolar	11–12 years	
First molar	6–7 years	
Second molar	12 years	
Third molar	18–25 years	

CLINICAL CORRELATION

Congenital anomalies of the teeth

1. ***Anodontia:*** The complete absence of tooth or teeth is called *anodontia*. In this condition, one or two teeth may be absent.
2. ***Supernumerary teeth (extra teeth):*** The extra tooth may be located posterior to normal teeth or wedged between the normal teeth disrupting positions of the teeth. The alignment of upper and lower teeth may be improper (**malocclusion**).
   Sometimes, the total number of teeth may be even less.
3. ***Natal teeth (eruption of teeth before birth):*** Sometimes, teeth are present at the time of birth. These are called *natal teeth*. Such teeth may cause injuries to nipple during breastfeeding. Usually, these are lower incisors.
4. ***Fused teeth:*** This condition occurs when a tooth bud divides or two tooth buds partially fuse with each other.
5. ***Impaction of tooth:*** In this condition, there is a delay in the eruption of tooth. It commonly involves last (third) molar tooth.
6. ***Anomalies of enamel formation***
   (a) The defective enamel formation may cause pits or fissures on the surface of the enamel of the tooth.
   (b) The enamel may be soft and friable, if there is hypocalcification. The enamel appears yellow or brown in color (**amelogenesis imperfecta**). This condition is often caused by vitamin D deficiency (rickets).
7. ***Dentinogenesis imperfecta (Fig. 17.12):*** It is an autosomal dominant genetic anomaly with a genetic defect located in most cases on chromosome 4q. In this condition, the teeth are brown or gray in color. Enamel wears down easily, and as a result, the dentin is exposed on the surface.
8. ***Discoloration of teeth:*** If infants and children are given tetracyclines, it is incorporated into the developing enamel causing yellow discoloration of teeth (both deciduous and permanent).
9. ***Dentigerous cyst:*** It is a cyst within mandible or maxilla and contains unerupted permanent tooth.

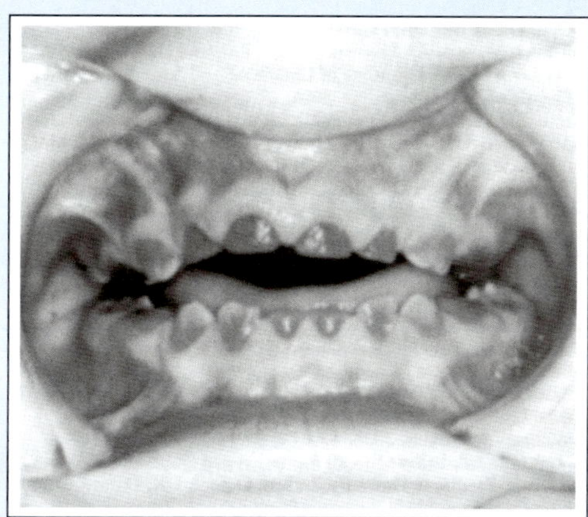

Fig. 17.12 Dentinogenesis imperfecta. (*Source: The Developing Human: Clinically Oriented Embryology*, 8th edition by Keith L. Moore and T.V.N. Persaud, ISBN: 9781416037064, page 455, Fig. 19.21, Copyright Elsevier, 2008.)

GESTATIONAL AGE OF KEY DEVELOPMENTAL EVENTS

Developmental Event	Gestational Age
➢ Buccopharyngeal membrane ruptures during	3rd week of IUL
➢ Parotid glands develop during	5th week of IUL
➢ Submandibular glands develop during	6th week of IUL
➢ Sublingual glands develop during	8th week of IUL
➢ Development of dental lamina occurs during	6th week of IUL
➢ Eruption of deciduous or milk teeth occurs	6–24 months after birth
➢ Buds of permanent teeth are formed during	3rd month after birth

GOLDEN FACTS TO REMEMBER

➢ **Two sources from which oral cavity forms**	(a) Stomodeum (b) Cephalic part of foregut
➢ **Primordia of ectodermal components of teeth**	Dental buds/enamel organs
➢ **Natal teeth**	Teeth present at birth
➢ **Amelogenesis imperfecta**	Defective formation of enamel (an autosomal dominant disorder)
➢ **Dentigerous imperfecta**	Defective formation of dentin (an autosomal dominant trait)
➢ **Whole oral cavity is derived from stomodeum *except***	Floor that is derived from foregut
➢ **Critical period of tooth development**	6–12 weeks
➢ **All the dental tissues (tissues of tooth) are derived from neural crest mesenchyme *except***	Enamel that is produced by ameloblasts derived from oral ectoderm
➢ **Hardest tissue in the body**	Enamel
➢ **Second hardest tissue in the body**	Dentin

CLINICAL PROBLEM SOLVING

PROBLEMS

1. **A baby was born with two mandibular incisor teeth. What are these teeth called and what problem they may cause?**
2. **Why are tetracyclines (a group of antibiotics) not prescribed to pregnant women** and children younger than 8 years?
3. Although the parotid gland **develops at the angle of primitive oral fissure, in adults the parotid gland is located far away from the oral fissure near the auricle. Give its embryological basis.**

SOLUTIONS

1. These teeth are called **natal teeth** (L. *Natus* = to be born). These are prematurely erupted primary (milk) teeth. The natal teeth may cause maternal discomfort during breastfeeding and may also injure the baby's tongue.

N.B. The **natal teeth** are teeth, which are already present at the time birth itself. They are different from **neonatal teeth**, which develop during first 30 days after birth.

2. This is because tetracyclines are extensively incorporated into the enamel and dentin of developing teeth, causing yellow discoloration and hypoplasia of the enamel.
3. This is because the parotid glands develop as an outgrowth of epithelium from the angle of oral fissure. **Initially, the angles of mouth extend much laterally, nearly up to the ear.** Subsequent fusion between maxillary and mandibular processes shifts the angles of the mouth more medially until they reach the adult position, but the parotid gland remains/located near auricle.

18 Digestive Tract, Foregut, Midgut, and Hindgut

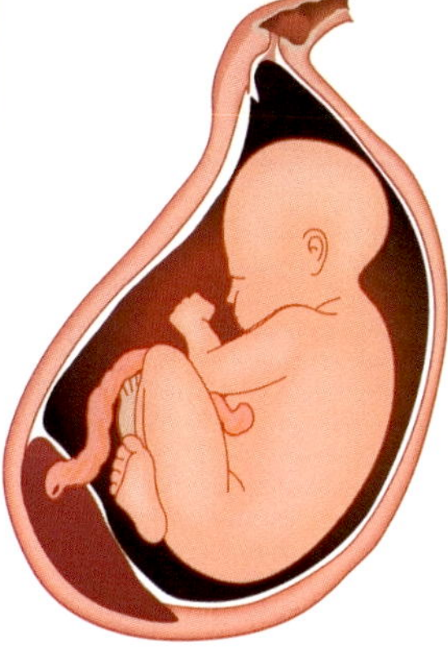

LEARNING OBJECTIVES

After studying this chapter, the student should be able to:

- Describe the development and congenital anomalies of foregut, midgut, and hindgut. AN 52.6
- Describe the development of primitive foregut in brief. Give its three subdivisions and their derivatives.
- Give the embryological basis of (a) tracheoesophageal fistula, (b) achalasia cardia, (c) rotation of stomach, (d) congenital pyloric stenosis, (e) exomphalos/omphalocele, and (f) congenital umbilical hernia.
- Write short notes on (a) Meckel's diverticulum, (b) subhepatic appendix, and (c) congenital megacolon (Hirschsprung disease).
- Describe the development of anal canal in brief and discuss the embryological basis of *imperforate anus.*

DIGESTIVE TRACT

OVERVIEW

The digestive tract (gastrointestinal tract) develops from ***primitive gut*** that is derived from the dorsal part of ***endodermal yolk sac.***

The primitive gut forms during the 4th week of intrauterine life (IUL) by the incorporation of a larger portion of the yolk sac (umbilical vesicle) into the embryonic disk during craniocaudal and lateral folding of embryo (Fig. 18.1). The tubular primitive gut extends in the median plane from *buccopharyngeal membrane* at its cranial end to *cloacal membrane* at its caudal end. It freely communicates with the remaining yolk sac by the **vitellointestinal duct.** The part of gut cranial to this communication is called **foregut**, part caudal to this communication is called **hindgut**, and part intervening between foregut and hindgut is called **midgut** (Fig. 18.1).

The cranial end of foregut is separated from the **stomodeum** by **buccopharyngeal membrane,** while the caudal end of hindgut is separated from the **proctodeum** by **cloacal membrane**.

At later stage of development, buccopharyngeal and cloacal membranes rupture and gut communicates to exterior at its both ends.

The endoderm of primitive gut forms the endothelial lining of all parts of the gastrointestinal tract except part of mouth and distal part of anal canal that are derived from ectoderm of *stomodeum* and *proctodeum,* respectively.

The muscular, connective tissue, and serous layers of wall of the digestive tract are derived from

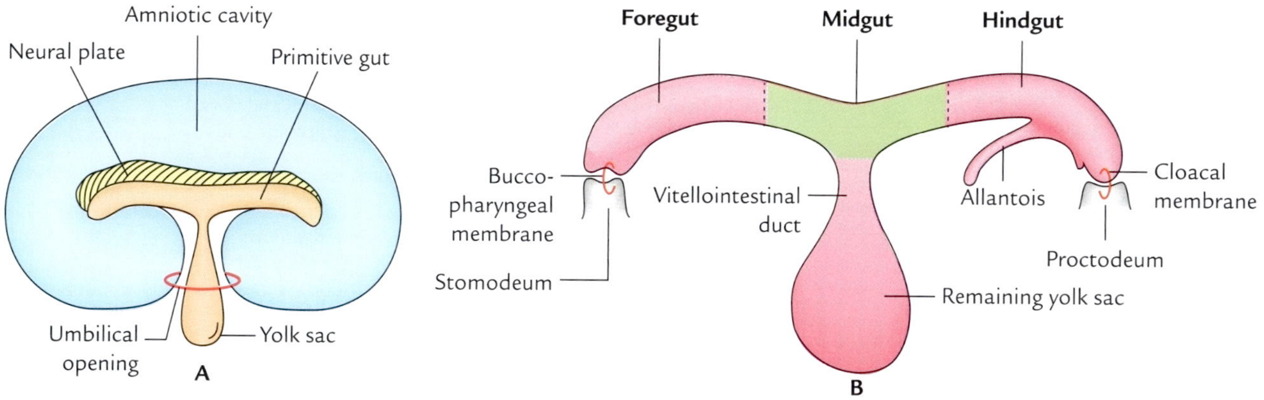

Fig. 18.1 Development of primitive gut. (A) The larger portion of yolk sac is taken inside the embryonic disk during its folding. Note that amniotic cavity covers the embryonic disk on all side except at the umbilical opening. (B) Subdivisions of primitive gut into foregut, midgut, and hindgut. Note that midgut communicates with the remaining yolk sac via vitellointestinal duct.

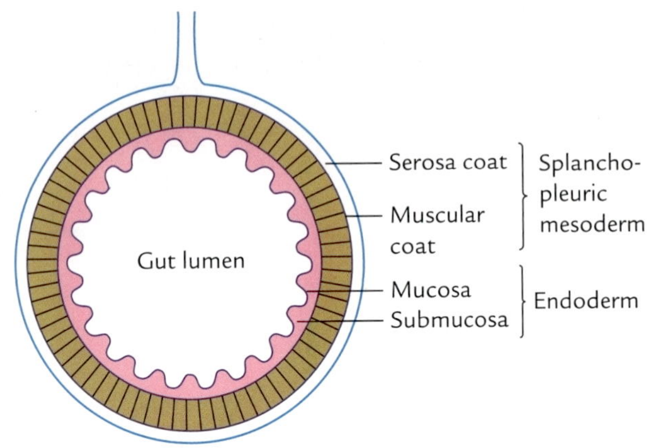

Fig. 18.2 Derivation of coats of the gut.

splanchnopleuric mesoderm surrounding the primitive gut derived from endoderm (Fig. 18.2).

While the primitive gut is being formed, the midline artery, **dorsal aorta**, gives off a series of ventral branches to the gut. Those in the region of midgut run right up to the yolk sac and are, therefore, termed **vitelline arteries.** Later most of these ventral branches of dorsal aorta disappear and only three of them remain: one of foregut (the **celiac artery**), one of midgut (the **superior mesenteric artery**), and one of hindgut (the **inferior mesenteric artery**) (Fig. 18.3).

The development of digestive (gastrointestinal) tract showing foregut, midgut, and hindgut along with primordia of structures derived from these is shown in Fig. 18.4.

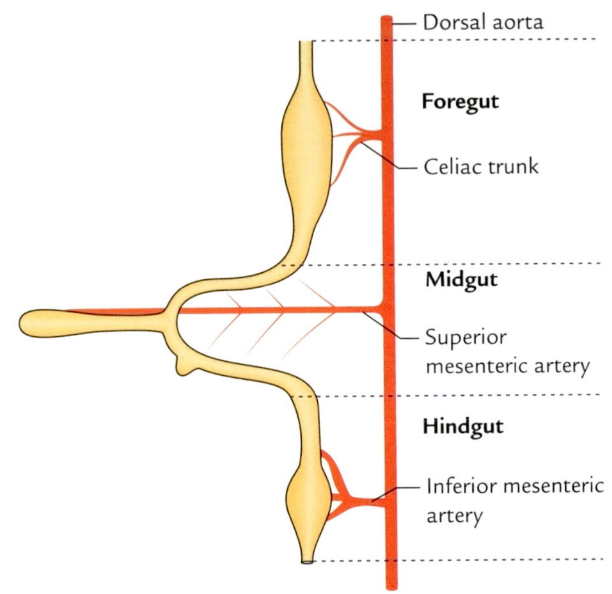

Fig. 18.3 Arteries supplying the three parts of the primitive gut (foregut, midgut, and hindgut).

N.B. **Molecular regulation** of regional differentiation of primitive gut to form its different parts is done by ***Hox* and *ParaHox*** genes and sonic hedgehog (SHH) signals.

The derivatives of the foregut, midgut, and hindgut are given in Table 18.1 and shown in Figs 18.4 and 18.5.

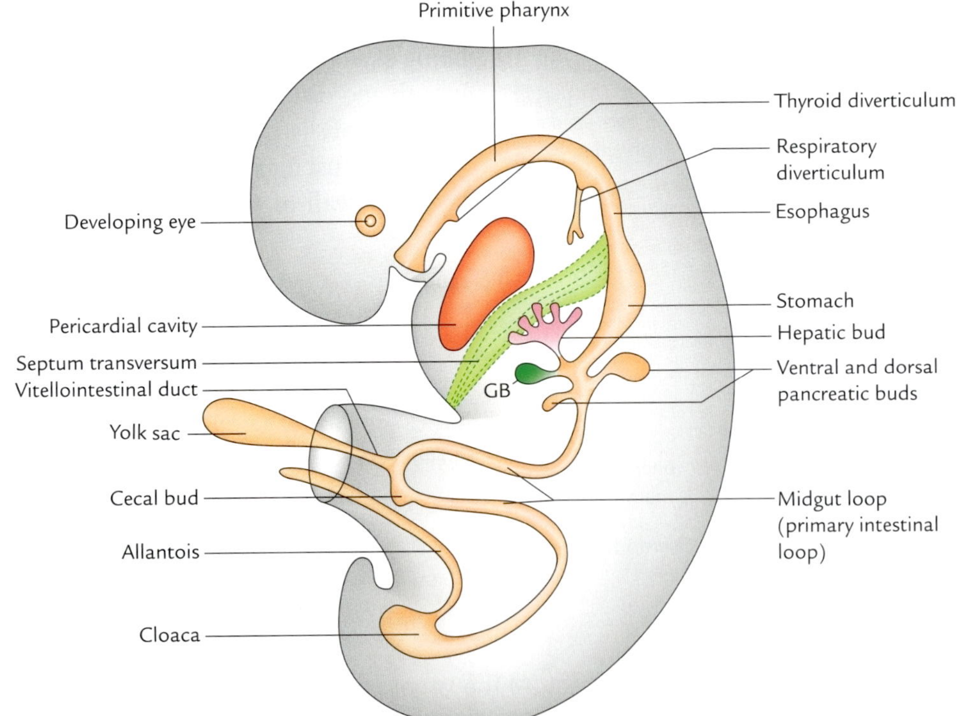

Fig. 18.4 Schematic diagram of 5-mm embryo showing the formation of the digestive tract. Note the subdivisions of digestive tract into foregut, midgut, and hindgut, and various derivatives originating from their endoderm. GB, gallbladder.

Table 18.1 Derivatives of three parts of the primitive gut

Part of Gut	Derivatives
Foregut	• Derivatives of primitive pharynx • Esophagus • Trachea and lung buds • Stomach • Proximal (upper) half of the duodenum (i.e., duodenum proximal to ampulla of Vater) • Liver • Pancreas • Extrahepatic biliary system } Endodermal outgrowths from duodenum
Midgut	• Distal (lower) half of the duodenum • Jejunum • Ileum • Cecum and appendix • Ascending colon • Right two-third of transverse colon
Hindgut	• Left one-third of transverse colon • Descending colon • Sigmoid (pelvic) colon • Rectum • Upper part of the anal canal

N.B. The junction between the foregut and midgut is known as **anterior intestinal portal**, whose position in adult gut corresponds with the termination of the bile duct in second part of the duodenum.

The junction between the midgut and hindgut is known as **posterior intestinal portal**, whose position in adult gut corresponds with the junction of proximal two-third and distal one-third of transverse colon. Fig. 18.5 shows various derivatives of abdominal part of the gut with location of anterior and posterior intestinal portals.

DEVELOPMENT OF FOREGUT DERIVATIVES AN 52.6

Esophagus

The esophagus develops from the part of foregut between the pharynx and the stomach. Ventrally at the pharyngo-esophageal junction, the foregut presents a median **laryngotracheal groove.** The groove bulges forward and caudally to form tracheobronchial (respiratory) diverticulum. The **tracheoesophageal septum** divides the foregut caudal to the pharynx into the esophagus and trachea (Fig. 18.6) (for details, see p. 216). Initially, the esophagus is short but later it elongates because of

1. Formation of neck
2. Descent of diaphragm
3. Descent of heart and lungs

Initially, the lumen of the esophagus is almost obliterated by the proliferation of endodermal cells. Later on, these cells breakdown and esophagus is recanalized.

The lining epithelium of the esophagus is derived from the endoderm of the foregut, while musculature as well as connective tissue of the esophagus is derived from splanchnic mesenchyme surrounding the foregut. *The **upper one-third part** of the esophagus has striated musculature, **middle one-third** has mixed (striated and smooth) musculature, and **lower one-third** has smooth musculature as in the rest of the gut.*

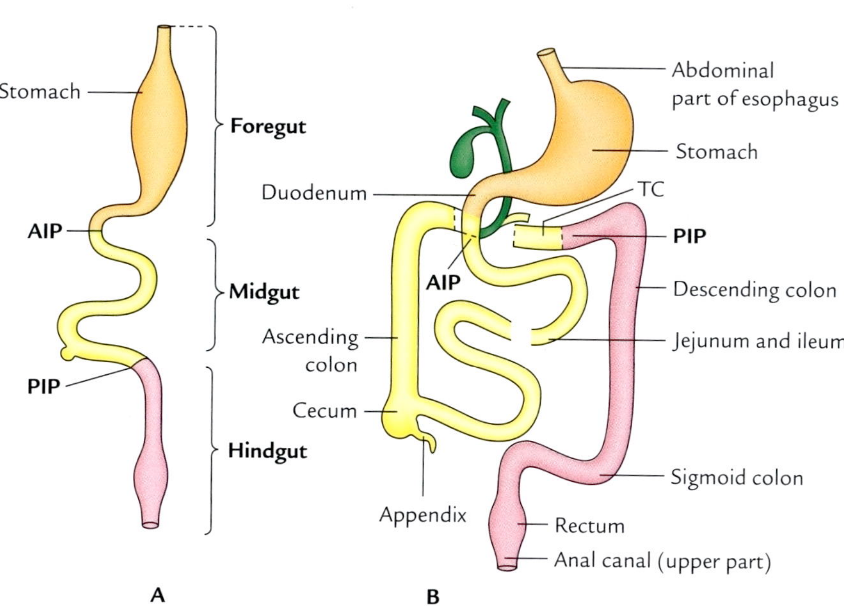

Fig. 18.5 Derivatives of various abdominal parts of the gut. (A) Primitive gut. (B) Adult gut. TC, transverse colon; AIP, anterior intestinal portal; PIP, posterior intestinal portal.

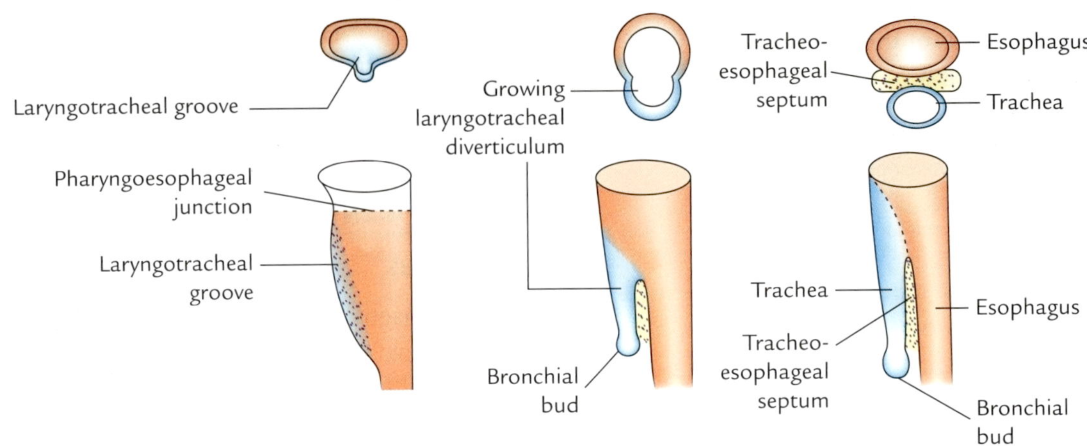

Fig. 18.6 Development of esophagus.

CLINICAL CORRELATION

Congenital anomalies of foregut

1. ***Esophageal atresia:*** It occurs due to failure of recanalization of the developing esophagus.
   - The esophageal atresia is often associated with **tracheoesophageal fistula**. It is produced by extreme posterior deviation of **tracheo-esophageal septum**.
   - In esophageal atresia, the fetus is unable to swallow amniotic fluid; hence, there is an abnormal increase in the amount of amniotic fluid, leading to a clinical condition called **polyhydramnios**.
   - A newborn with esophageal atresia accepts the first feed (i.e., milk or fluid diet) normally, but when given subsequent feed, it regurgitates through the mouth and nose; and this may cause respiratory distress and cyanosis.
   - The surgical correction (treatment) gives 85% survival rate.
2. ***Esophageal stenosis:*** In this anomaly, the lumen of the esophagus is narrow usually in lower third part. It is caused by incomplete esophageal recanalization and vascular abnormalities. Depending on grade and extent of stenosis, symptoms may be mild or severe. In severe cases, the symptoms are similar to that of esophageal atresia.

N.B. An **atresia** leads to **complete blockage**, while a **stenosis** leads to a **partial blockage**.

3. ***Tracheoesophageal fistula:*** It occurs due to failure of separation of tracheobronchial diverticulum from esophagus due to nonformation of tracheoesophageal septum (for details, see p. 217).
   In most of the cases (85%), the lower segment of esophagus communicates with the trachea. Clinically, it presents as follows:
   An infant vomits every feed that he/she is given. The presence of air in the stomach is the diagnostic sign of tracheoesophageal fistula (Fig. 18.7).
4. ***Achalasia cardia:*** It occurs due to failure of relaxation of the musculature in the lower part of the esophagus following loss of ganglionic cells in Auerbach plexus. Clinically, patient complains of difficulty in swallowing. On barium swallow, the lower part of esophagus presents pencil-shaped narrowing (**bird beak deformity**) (Fig. 18.8).
5. ***Dysphagia lusoria:*** See p. 258.
6. ***Short esophagus:*** It occurs when esophagus fails to elongate during development. When the esophagus fails to elongate, the stomach is pulled up into the esophageal hiatus of diaphragm causing **congenital hiatal hernia**.

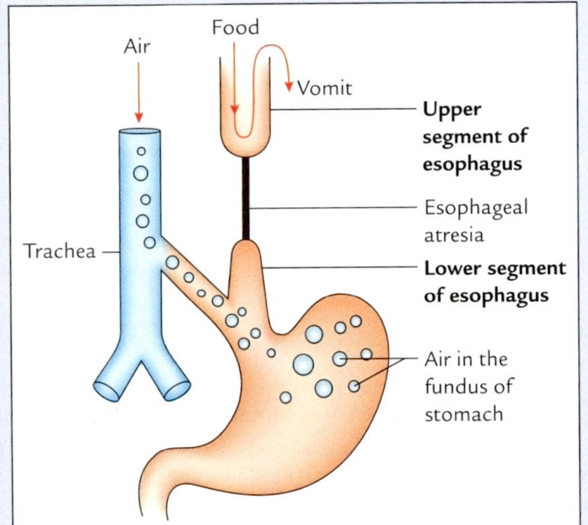

Fig. 18.7 Tracheoesophageal fistula.

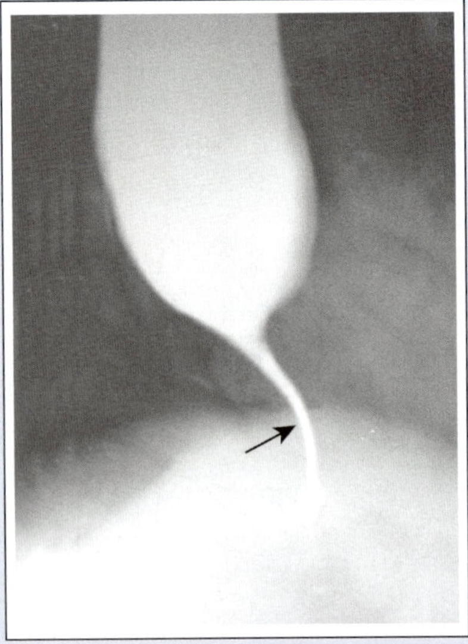

Fig. 18.8 Barium meal swallow showing characteristic bird's beak/rat tail appearance of esophagus. (*Source:* Plate 3.1B, Page 155, *Radiology in Medical Practice, Fifth edition*, ABM Abdullah. Copyright Elsevier Inc. 2016, All rights reserved.)

Stomach

The stomach appears as a fusiform dilatation of foregut distal to the esophagus in the 4th week of IUL.

This dilatation presents a **ventral border** and **dorsal border**, a **left surface** and a **right surface**, and an **upper end** and a **lower end**. The dorsal border provides attachment to dorsal mesentery (**dorsal mesogastrium**) that extends from the stomach to posterior abdominal wall. The ventral border provides attachment to ventral mesentery (**ventral mesogastrium**) that extends from the stomach to septum transversum and anterior abdominal wall.

Change in Shape and Position of Stomach (Fig. 18.9)

The **change in shape** of stomach occurs due to differential growth in its different regions.

Dorsal border grows much more than ventral border and forms **greater curvature** of the stomach, while the ventral border forms **lesser curvature** of the stomach.

The **changes in position** of the stomach can be easily explained by assuming that it rotates twice: (a) around a longitudinal axis and (b) around an anteroposterior axis.

Rotation of stomach

The stomach rotates twice: first around its **longitudinal axis** and then around its **anteroposterior axis** (vide supra). Line connecting cardiac and pyloric ends of stomach marks its **longitudinal axis.**

- First the stomach rotates 90° clockwise around its longitudinal axis (viewed from cranial end). As a result, its left surface now faces anteriorly and forms anterior surface. Similarly, its right surface faces

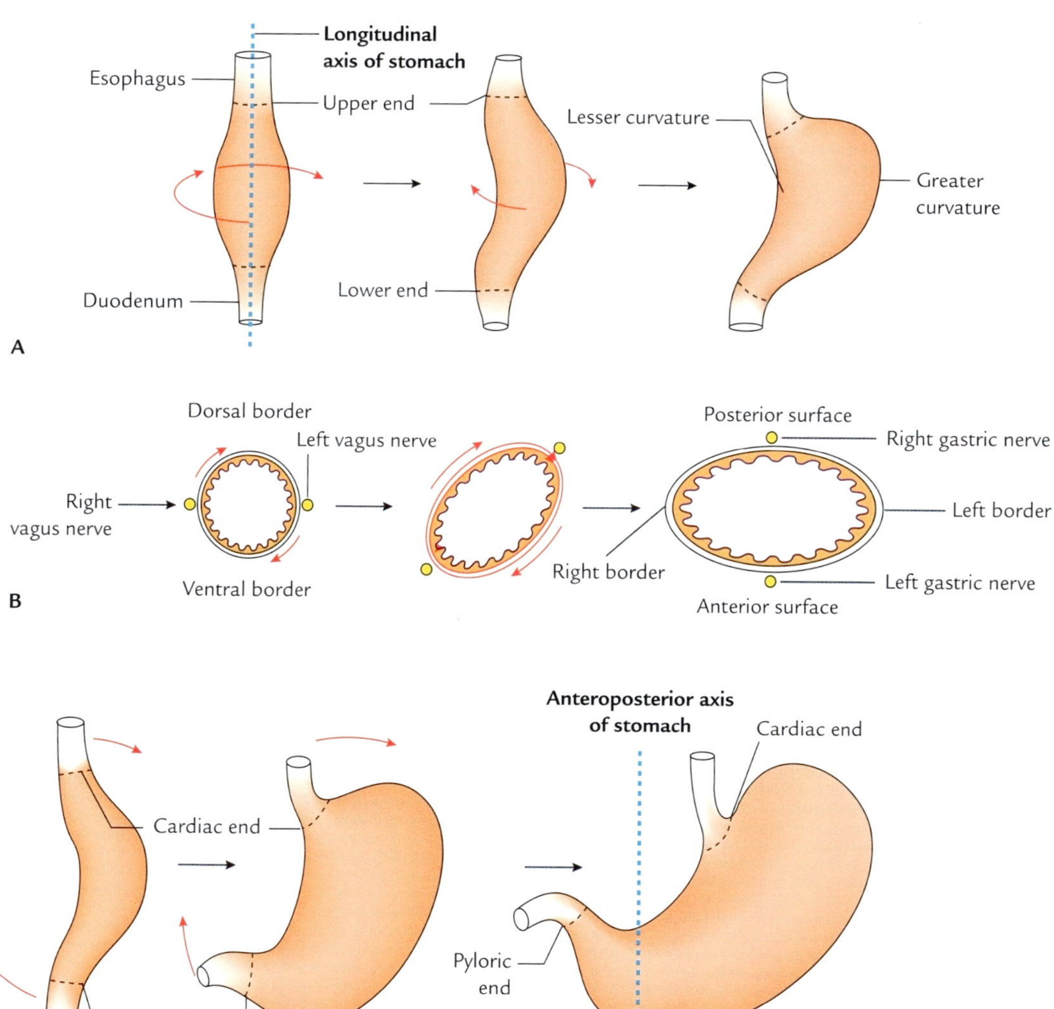

Fig. 18.9 Change in shape and position of stomach. (A) Rotation of stomach along its longitudinal axis as seen from the front. (B) Rotation of stomach along its longitudinal axis as seen in transverse section. (C) Rotation of stomach around the anteroposterior axis.

posteriorly to form posterior surface. For this reason, left vagus nerve initially supplying the left surface of stomach now supplies its anterior surface and right vagus nerve initially supplying the right surface now supplies its posterior surface.

- The cephalic and caudal ends of stomach originally lie in the midline.

Now the stomach rotates around its **anteroposterior axis.** As a result, the cardiac end of stomach originally lying in the midline moves to the left and slightly downward, and pyloric end originally lying in the midline moves to the right and slightly upward.

Change in the Mesenteries of the Stomach Due to Its Rotation (Figs 18.10 and 18.11)

Initially, the **ventral mesogastrium** of stomach extends from its lesser curvature to septum transversum and anterior abdominal wall. When liver develops in the septum transversum, the ventral mesogastrium is divided in two parts. The part extending from the stomach to the liver is called **lesser omentum**, and the part extending between the liver and anterior abdominal wall is called **falciform ligament** of the liver.

Initially, the dorsal mesogastrium of stomach extends from its greater curvature to the posterior abdominal wall. When the spleen develops from mesoderm lying between the two layers of dorsal mesogastrium, the dorsal mesogastrium is divided in two parts. The part extending from greater curvature (fundus) of the stomach to spleen forms the **gastrosplenic ligament**, while the part extending from spleen to posterior abdominal wall forms the **lienorenal ligament**. The dorsal mesogastrium attached to rest of greater curvature elongates and forms a large apron-like fold of peritoneum called **greater omentum.**

The rotation of stomach along its longitudinal axis pulls the dorsal mesogastrium to the left, creating a space behind the stomach called **lesser sac of peritoneum (omental bursa)** (Fig. 18.12). The development of lesser sac is described in detail in Chapter 21.

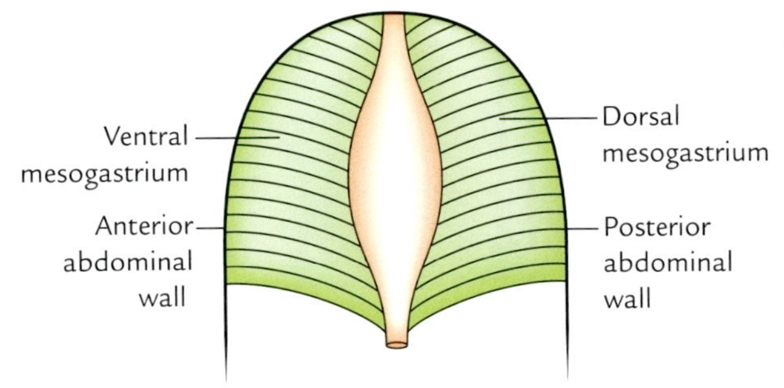

Fig. 18.10 Side view of stomach showing dorsal and ventral mesogastria.

Histogenesis of the Stomach

The **epithelial lining and gastric glands** of the stomach are derived from the endoderm of the primitive foregut, while the rest of the layers of the stomach (i.e., muscular and serous coats) are derived from surrounding splanchnic intraembryonic mesoderm.

- **Gastric glands** appear in the 3**rd** month of the IUL.
- **Oxyntic and zymogenic cells** appear in the **4th** month of IUL.

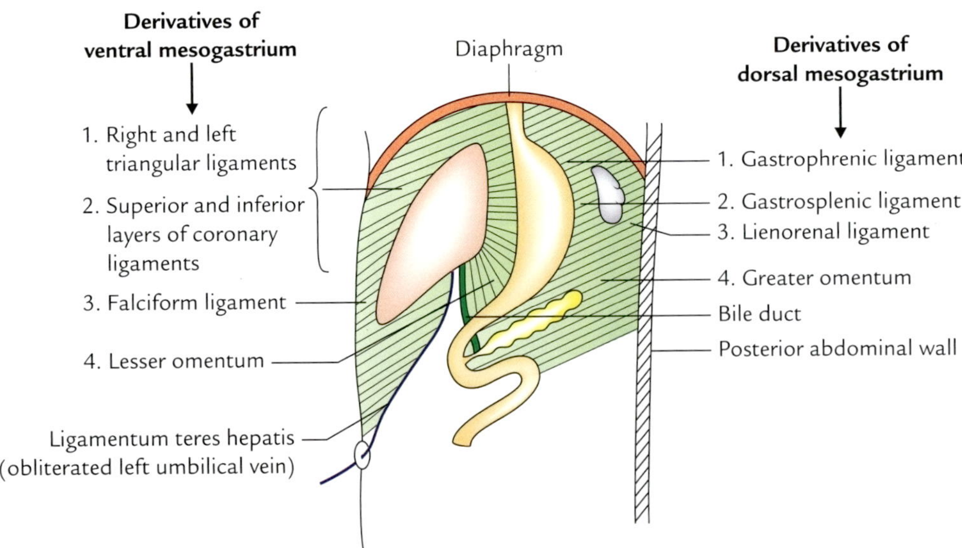

Fig. 18.11 Derivatives of ventral and dorsal mesogastria. Layers of coronary, and right and left triangular ligaments are not shown.

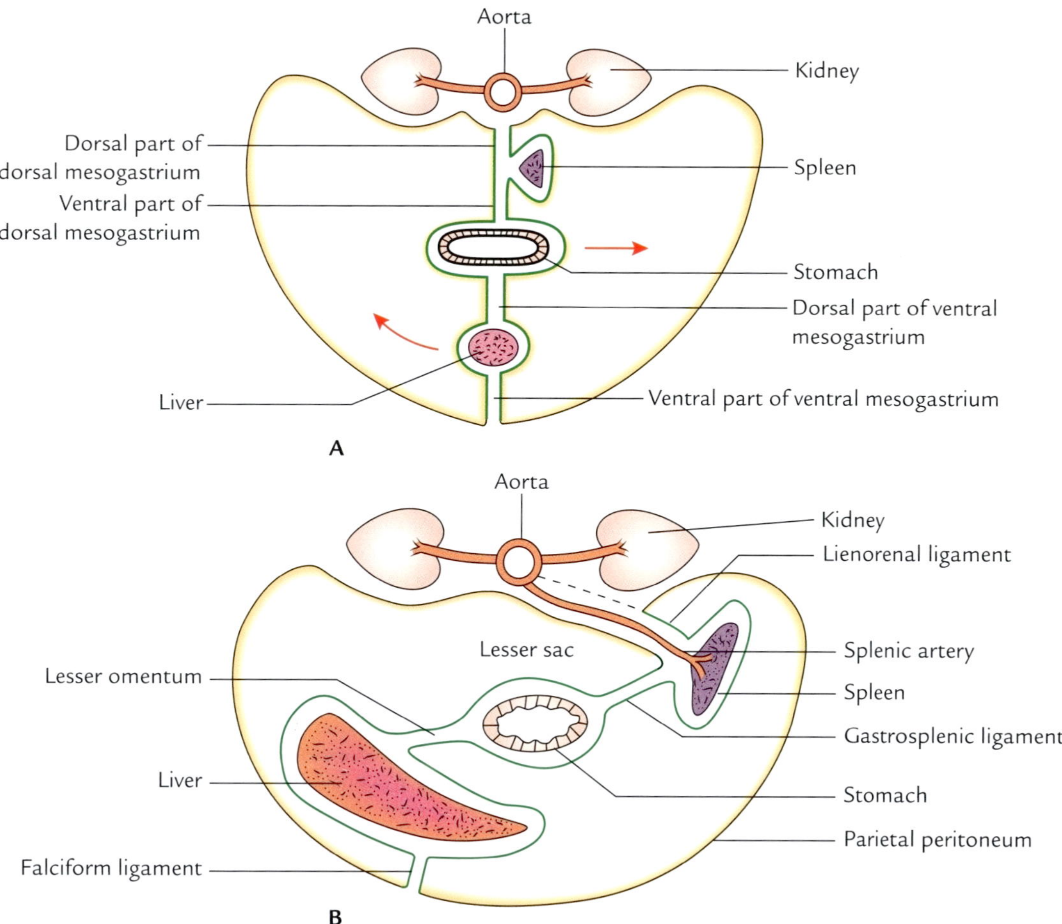

Fig. 18.12 Transverse sections through developed foregut showing ventral and dorsal mesogastria and their derivatives. (A) Early stage. (B) Late stage. Note the formation of lesser sac.

> **CLINICAL CORRELATION**
>
> **Congenital hypertrophic pyloric stenosis:** It occurs due to hypertrophy of circular muscle layer at pylorus. It causes narrowing of pylorus, converting it into probe-admitting channel **(probe patency)**. This causes consequent obstruction to passage of food through pylorus.
>
> The newborn appears normal at birth, but 2–3 h after feeding there is **forceful progressive projectile vomiting** and epigastrium shows distension of the stomach. The vomit does not contain bile. Clinically, it presents as an enlargement of the abdomen with a palpable mass in right hypochondriac region with visible peristalsis. The condition can be surgically corrected. For details, see *Anatomy of Abdomen and Lower Limb* by Dr Vishram Singh.

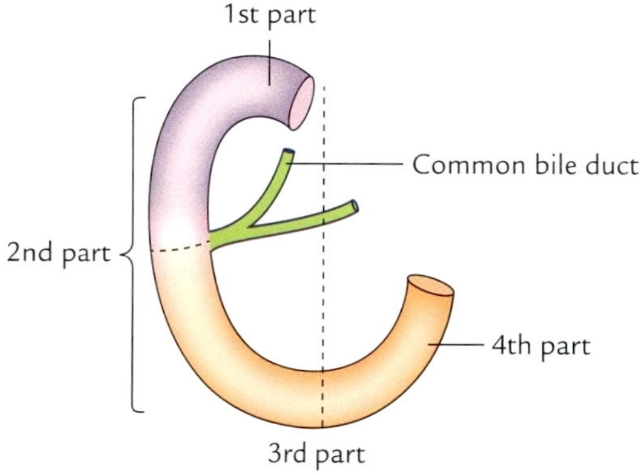

Fig. 18.13 Development of duodenum. Note that the first part and second part up to the opening of common bile duct is derived from foregut (violet color). The second part of the duodenum (distal to opening of common bile duct) along with third and fourth parts is derived from midgut.

Duodenum

The duodenum develops from two sources (dual origin): (a) proximal half is derived from foregut and (b) distal half is derived from midgut. The details are as follows:

(a) The first and second part of duodenum up to the opening of common bile duct develop from foregut, and (b) the second part of the duodenum below the opening of common bile duct along with third and fourth part develop from midgut (Fig. 18.13).

The developing duodenum forms a loop that is attached to posterior abdominal wall by a mesentery

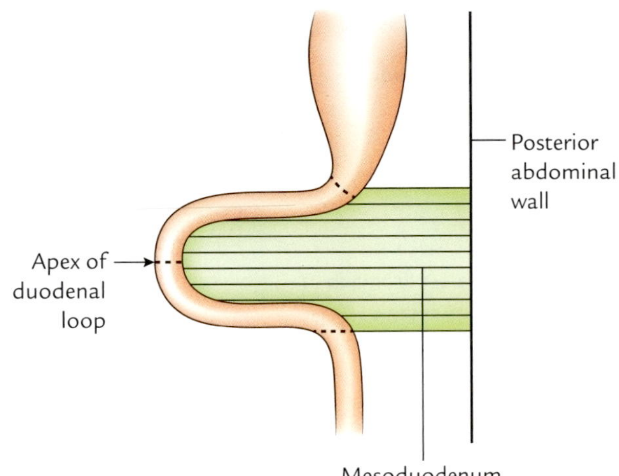

Fig. 18.14 Duodenal loop formed from parts of foregut and midgut. Note the mesoduodenum extending between duodenal loop and posterior abdominal wall.

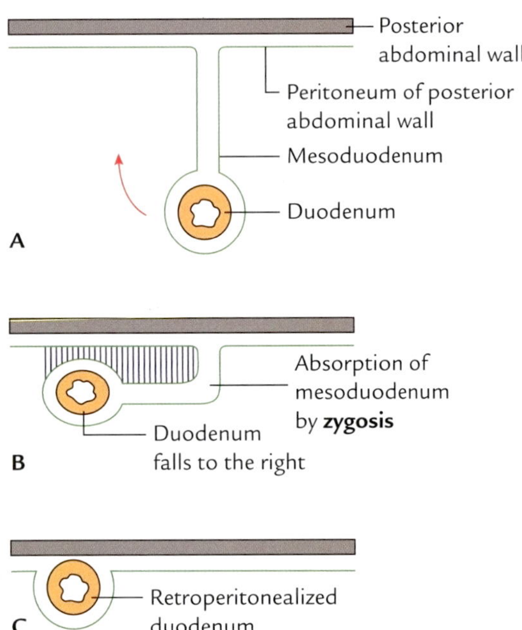

Fig. 18.15 Retroperitonealization of the duodenum by **zygosis**.

called **mesoduodenum** (Fig. 18.14). The loop is present in the sagittal plane; its apex is at the junction of foregut and midgut. The clockwise rotation of the stomach to the left makes the duodenal loop to fall on the right side. Its mesentery (mesoduodenum) is absorbed by zygosis and becomes retroperitoneal (Fig. 18.15).

However, the mesoduodenum persists in relation to a small portion of duodenum adjoining pylorus. This part is seen as a triangular shadow – the **duodenal cap** in barium meal X-ray abdomen.

Initially, development of the lumen of the duodenum is obliterated by the proliferation of endodermal cells. Later on, cells in the lumen disintegrate and the duodenum gets recanalized.

N.B. The proximal half of duodenum, i.e., up to the opening of common bile duct, develops from foregut, and hence it is supplied by artery of the foregut – the **celiac trunk**.

The distal half of duodenum develops from the midgut, and hence it is supplied by artery of the midgut – the superior mesenteric artery.

CLINICAL CORRELATION

1. ***Duodenal atresia:*** It occurs due to failure of recanalization of the duodenum. The duodenal atresia nearly always occurs just distal to opening of hepatopancreatic ampulla, but occasionally involves third part of the duodenum. Clinically, in infants with duodenal atresia vomiting begins a few hours after birth. The vomit almost always contains bile (*bilious emesis*). The *double bubble sign* seen in abdomen X-ray or ultrasound indicates duodenal atresia.
2. ***Duodenal stenosis:*** It occurs because of incomplete recanalization of the duodenum. The cells in lumen disintegrate only in small central part producing a narrow lumen. Duodenal stenosis commonly affects third and fourth parts of the duodenum. Duodenal stenosis produces partial obstruction.
3. ***Duodenal diverticula:*** They are seen along the inner border of the second and third part of the duodenum.

DEVELOPMENT OF MIDGUT DERIVATIVES AN 52.6

The midgut elongates to form a **U-shaped primary intestinal loop**. This U-shaped loop is suspended from posterior abdominal wall by a short mesentery, and at its apex it communicates with the **yolk sac** through narrow **vitelline duct/vitellointestinal duct/yolk stalk.** (In adults, the midgut extends from just distal to opening of common bile duct in the duodenum to junction between the proximal two-third and distal one-third of the transverse colon.)

The *superior mesenteric artery*, the artery of midgut, runs posteroanteriorly through the middle of the mesentery of the midgut loop. The superior mesenteric artery divides the midgut loop into two segments:

1. Prearterial (proximal) segment
2. Postarterial (distal) segment

The **prearterial segment** is cranial and the **postarterial segment** is caudal. The postarterial segment near the apex of midgut loop develops a small conical diverticulum – the **cecal bud** at its antimesenteric border (Fig. 18.16).

Derivatives of Midgut

The **prearterial segment** of midgut loop gives rise to

1. Distal half of duodenum below the ampulla of Vater
2. Jejunum
3. Ileum, except its terminal part

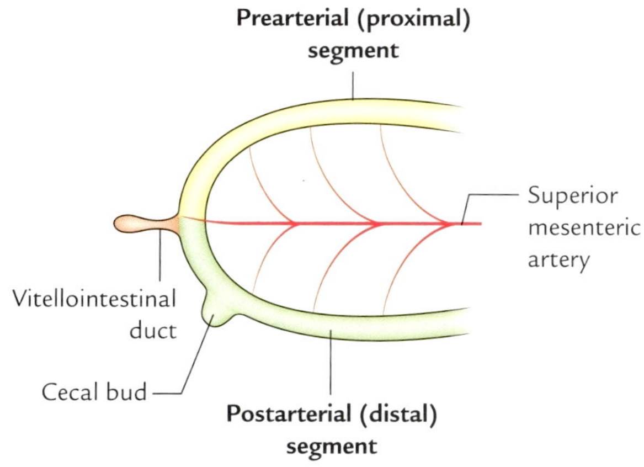

Fig. 18.16 Midgut loop.

The **postarterial segment** of midgut loop gives rise to

1. Terminal part of ileum
2. Cecum
3. Appendix
4. Ascending colon
5. Proximal (right) two-third of the transverse colon

N.B. All parts derived from **midgut** are supplied by superior mesenteric artery.

The exact sources of development of different adult derivatives of the midgut are given in Table 18.2.

Physiological Umbilical Hernia (i.e., Herniation of Midgut Loop)

During the 3rd week of IUL, the midgut loop elongates rapidly, particularly its prearterial segment. As a result of rapid growth of midgut loop and enlargement of liver at the same time, the abdominal cavity temporarily becomes too small to accommodate all the loops of midgut (i.e., intestine). Consequently, *during the 6th week of IUL, the loops of midgut (intestine) herniate through umbilical opening* (i.e., go outside the abdominal cavity) to enter into remains of extraembryonic coelom (in the proximal part of umbilical cord). This herniation of intestinal loops through umbilical opening is called **physiological umbilical hernia.**

Table 18.2 Source of development of adult derivatives of midgut

Adult Structure	Source of Development
Distal Half of duodenum	Prearterial segment of midgut loop
Jejunum	Prearterial segment of midgut loop
Ileum	• Prearterial segment of midgut loop • Small postarterial segment of midgut loop proximal to the cecal bud
Cecum and appendix	Cecal bud of postarterial segment of midgut loop
Ascending colon and proximal two-third of transverse colon	Postarterial segment of midgut loop beyond the cecal bud

Reduction of Physiological Umbilical Hernia (Rotation of Midgut Loop [Syn. Rotation of Gut]; Fig. 18.17)

The midgut loop begins to enter into abdominal cavity during 10th week of IUL, following regression in size of developing liver and mesonephric kidneys, supplemented by the enlargement of abdominal cavity.

Rotation of midgut occurs when herniated intestinal loops return back to the abdominal cavity. This helps not only in return of herniated loops back into the abdominal cavity but also in establishing definitive relationships of various parts of the intestine. Therefore, students must clearly understand the steps of rotation.

The herniated loops of midgut begin to return into the abdominal cavity at the end of the ***3rd month of IUL.***

- Before rotation, the **prearterial segment** of midgut loop, **superior mesenteric artery**, and **postarterial segment of midgut loop** lie in the same vertical (sagittal) plane from above to downward (Fig. 18.16).

Stages of rotation

The stages of rotation of the gut are as follows:

First stage of rotation

1. While within the umbilical cord, the prearterial segment of midgut loop undergoes *90° anticlockwise rotation around the superior mesenteric artery*. As a result (as seen from the front), the **prearterial segment** comes to the right and the **postarterial segment** goes to the left in a horizontal plane. Now **the prearterial segment of midgut loop elongates extensively and forms coils of jejunum and ileum**, which lie on the right side of superior mesenteric artery, outside the abdominal cavity.

Second stage of rotation

2. For these coils of jejunum and ileum to return to the abdominal cavity, the midgut loop undergoes *second 90° anticlockwise rotation* so that coils of jejunum and ileum (derived from prearterial segment) pass

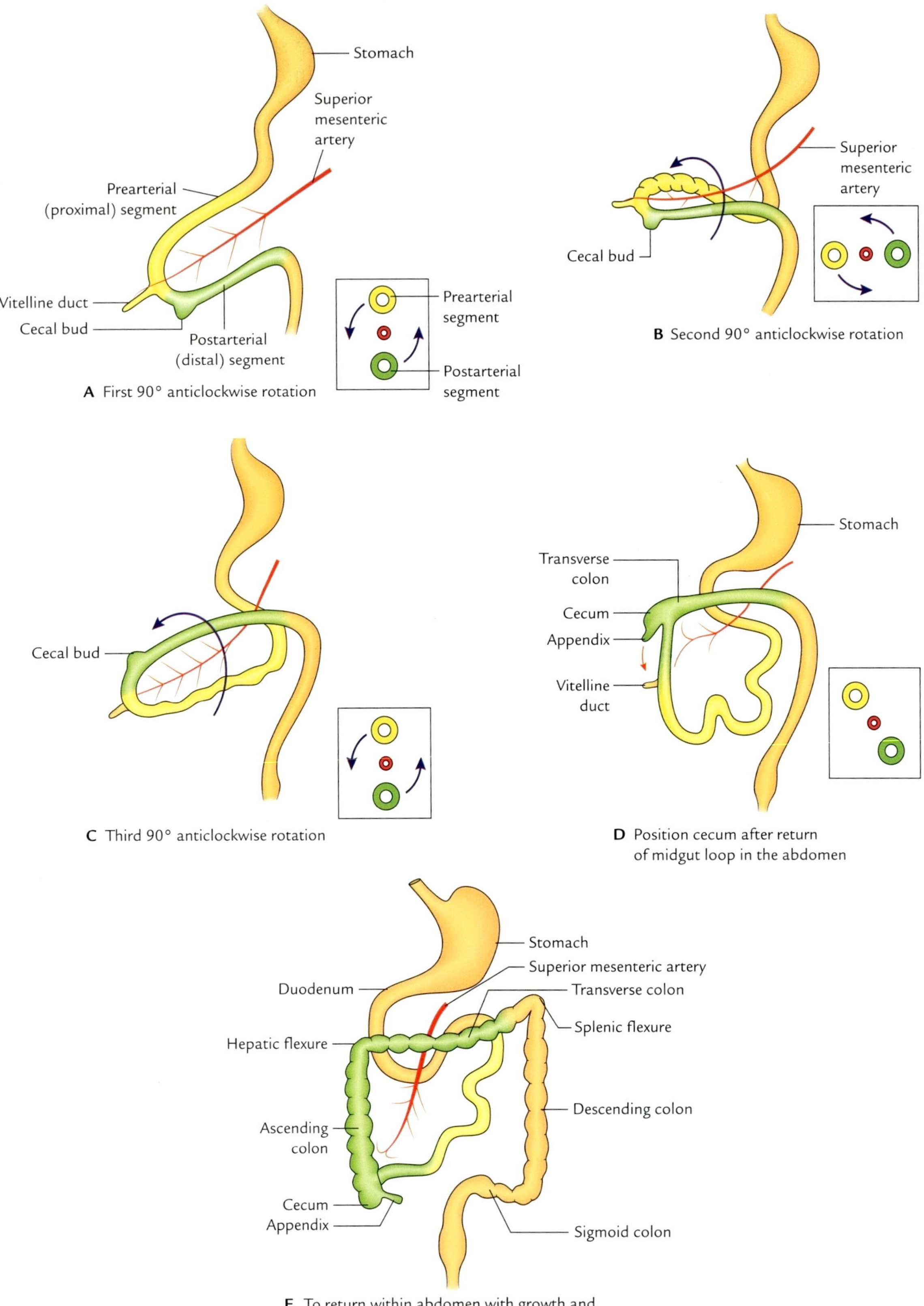

Fig. 18.17 Stages of rotation of midgut loop as seen in left side view. (A) Primitive loop before rotation. (B) Anticlockwise 90° rotation of midgut loop while it is in the extraembryonic coelom in the umbilical cord. (C) Anticlockwise 180° rotation of midgut loop as it is withdrawn into the abdominal cavity. (D) Subhepatic cecum, descent takes place later. (E) Intestinal loops in final position. The figures in the insets on the right side of each figure show orientation of prearterial and postarterial segments of midgut loop during its different stages of rotation.

behind the superior mesenteric artery. As a result, the duodenum goes behind the superior mesenteric artery.

Third stage of rotation

3. Lastly when the postarterial segment returns to the abdominal cavity, it undergoes **third 90° anticlockwise rotation**. As a result, **cecum and an appendix that develop from cecal bud now come to lie on the right side just below the liver** (Fig. 18.17D). *The orientation of pre- and postarterial segments of midgut loop at different phases of rotation (three 90° anticlockwise rotations) is shown in* Fig. 18.17 on the right side of each diagram.

Further growth

The ascending colon is not visible at this stage. The ascending colon is formed when cecum descends to right iliac fossa. The transverse and descending colons also get defined. The transverse colon lies anterior to superior mesenteric artery.

The development of the cecum and appendix is described in detail in the following text.

Development of Cecum and Appendix (Fig. 18.18)

The cecum and appendix develop from cecal bud – a conical dilatation that appears in the postarterial segment of the midgut loop near its apex (i.e., site of attachment of vitelline duct) in the 6th week.

The proximal part of the bud grows rapidly and forms cecum, while its distal part remains narrow to form the appendix.

Change in Shape of Cecum and Appendix

The growth of the cecum after birth leads to a change in its shape and change in position of attachment of the appendix.

At birth, the cecum is conical in shape and vermiform appendix is attached at its apex. Later, cecal growth results in formation of two **saccule** – one on either side.

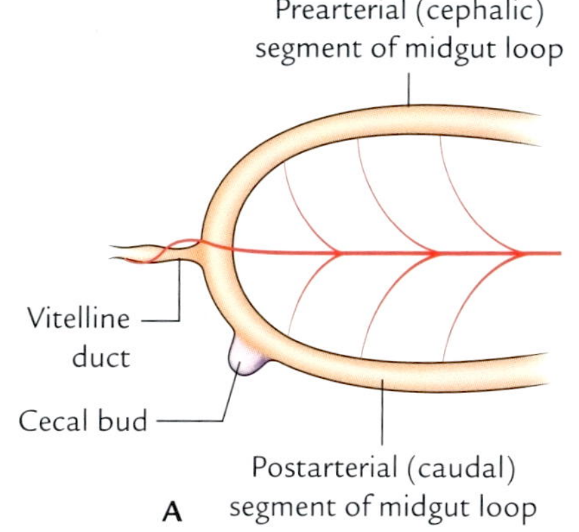

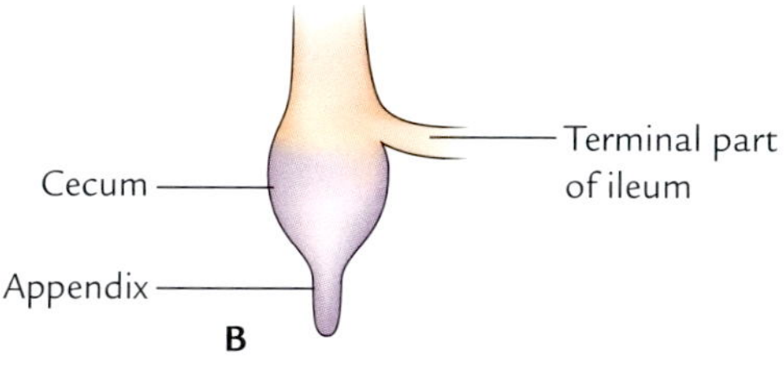

Fig. 18.18 Development of cecum.

The **right saccule** grows faster than the left. As a result, the apex of the cecum and the base of the appendix are pushed toward left, nearer to ileocecal junction. For this reason in adults, the base of the appendix is attached to posteromedial wall of the cecum, near the ileocecal junction.

On the basis of shape of the cecum and site of attachment of appendix, the cecum is classified into following four types (Fig. 18.19):

1. Conical (fetal) type (2%)
2. Infantile (quadrate) type (3%)
3. Normal type (80%–90%)
4. Exaggerated type (4%–5%)

For details, see *Anatomy of Abdomen and Lower Limb* by Dr Vishram Singh.

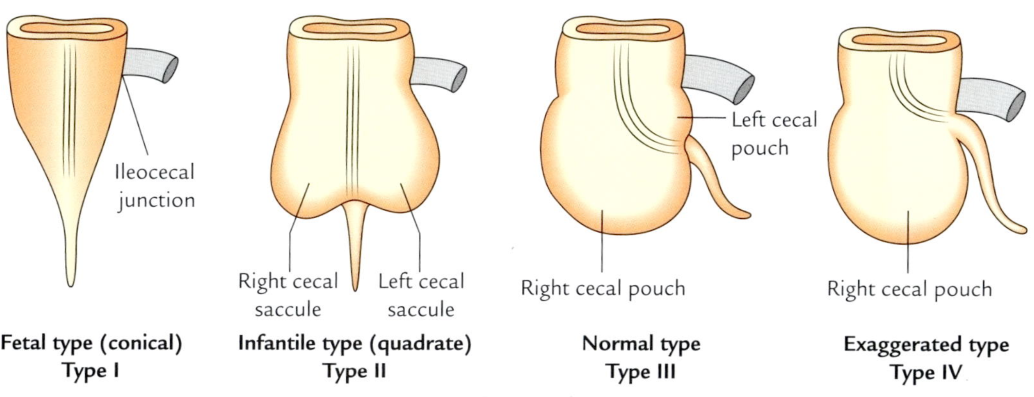

Fig. 18.19 Types of cecum.

CLINICAL CORRELATION

1. ***Exomphalos or omphalocele*** (Fig. 18.20): This anomaly results from failure of coils of the small intestine to return into abdominal cavity from their physiological herniation into extraembryonic coelom during 6th–10th week of IUL. It occurs in 2.5/10,000 births and could be associated with cardiac and neural tube defects.
   Clinically, it presents as a rounded mass protruding from the umbilicus. This mass contains coils of the small intestine and is covered by a transparent amniotic membrane.
2. ***Congenital umbilical hernia:*** In this anomaly, there is herniation of abdominal viscera through the weak umbilical opening (poorly closed umbilicus). Clinically, it presents as a protrusion in the linea alba. The contents are covered with peritoneum, subcutaneous tissue, and skin. This hernia can be reduced by pushing the intestines back into the abdominal cavity through the umbilical opening. The size of hernia increases during crying, coughing, and straining because of increased abdominal pressure.

N.B. The congenital umbilical hernia gets reduced on its own within 2–3 years of life. Therefore, child is subject to surgery only when the hernia stays up to age of 2–3 years.

The differences between the omphalocele and congenital umbilical hernia are given as follows:

Omphalocele	Congenital Umbilical Hernia
• Herniation of bowel loops occurs through umbilical opening as a normal event of development (physiological herniation) but fails to return to abdominal cavity later	• Herniation of bowel loops occurs through weak umbilical opening (i.e., occurs when umbilicus fails to close properly)
• Covered by Wharton's jelly, and amnion	• Covered by peritoneum, subcutaneous tissue, and skin
• Has genetic basis	• Has no genetic basis
• Has bad prognosis (mortality rate 25%)	• Has a good prognosis

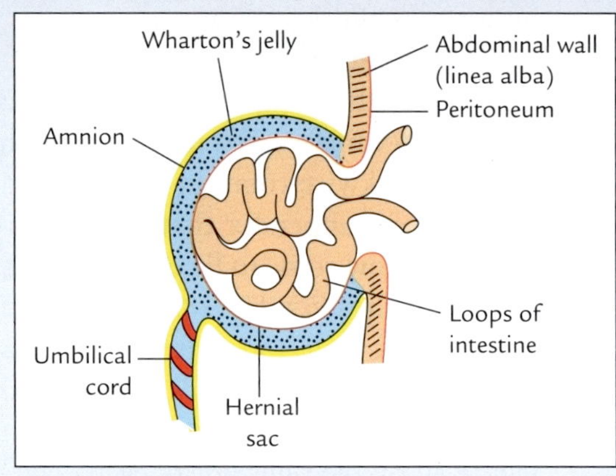

Fig. 18.20 Exomphalos/omphalocele.

3. ***Gastroschisis:*** In this anomaly, there is a linear defect in anterior abdominal wall through which abdominal contents herniate out. It occurs lateral to the umbilicus, usually on to the right.
   This defect is produced when lateral folds of embryo fail to fuse with each other around connecting stalk.
4. ***Anomalies of vitellointestinal duct:*** Vitellointestinal duct connects the apex of midgut loop to yolk sac. Normally, it disappears completely. The failure to disappear completely or in part will produce following anomalies of vitellointestinal duct:
   (a) *Meckel's diverticulum* (Fig. 18.21): A small persistent proximal part of vitellointestinal duct close to midgut (ileum) persists and forms the Meckel's diverticulum. It may be connected to the umbilicus by a fibrous cord (the obliterated remaining part of vitellointestinal duct).
   Characteristic features:
   - Arises from antimesenteric border of ileum
   - Is about *2 inches (5 cm) in length*
   - Is present about *2 feet (60 cm) proximal to ileocecal junction*
   - Occurs in about *2% of people*
   - Contain 2 types of ectopic tissues, gastric mucosa or pancreatic tissue
   - Presents clinical symptoms usually at the age of *2 years*

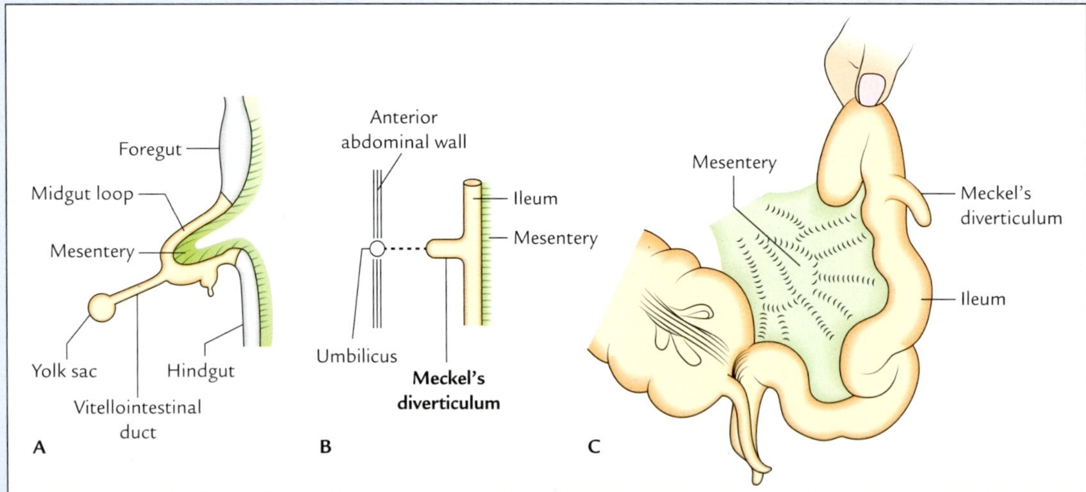

Fig. 18.21 Meckel's diverticulum. (A) Vitellointestinal duct connecting midgut loop with the yolk sac. (B) Meckel's diverticulum (schematic representation). (C) Meckel's diverticulum as seen during surgery.

N.B.

- There might be ulceration.
- Meckel's diverticulum may cause intestinal obstruction.

(b) *Umbilical sinus* (Fig. 18.22A): It occurs when part of vitellointestinal duct close to umbilicus persists, i.e., fails to close. The sinus communicates with the umbilicus.

(c) *Vitelline (umbilical) fistula* (Fig. 18.22B): It occurs when vitellointestinal duct fails to obliterate along its entire extent. This fistula communicates with ileum at one end and opens to exterior at the umbilicus at the other end.
Clinically, the ileal contents may be discharged through the umbilicus.

(d) Vitelline cyst (Fig. 18.22C): When small middle part of vitellointestinal duct persists (i.e., fails to obliterate), it forms cyst.

5. ***Anomalies due to errors of rotation of midgut loop***

(a) *Nonrotation:* In this anomaly, the midgut loop fails to rotate. The caudal or postarterial segment returns first in the abdominal cavity. Hence, large intestine occupies the left side of the abdominal cavity, while the small intestine derived from prearterial segment returns later and occupies the right side of the abdominal cavity (Fig. 18.23A).

(b) *Partial rotation:* In this anomaly, first 180° of rotation takes place normally but last 90° of rotation does not take place. As a result, cecum and appendix, instead of being on the right side of the abdominal cavity, are located just below pylorus of stomach.

(c) *Reversed rotation:* In this anomaly, the midgut loop rotates clockwise instead of anticlockwise. In this condition, transverse colon passes behind duodenum and lies behind the superior mesenteric artery (Fig. 13.23B).

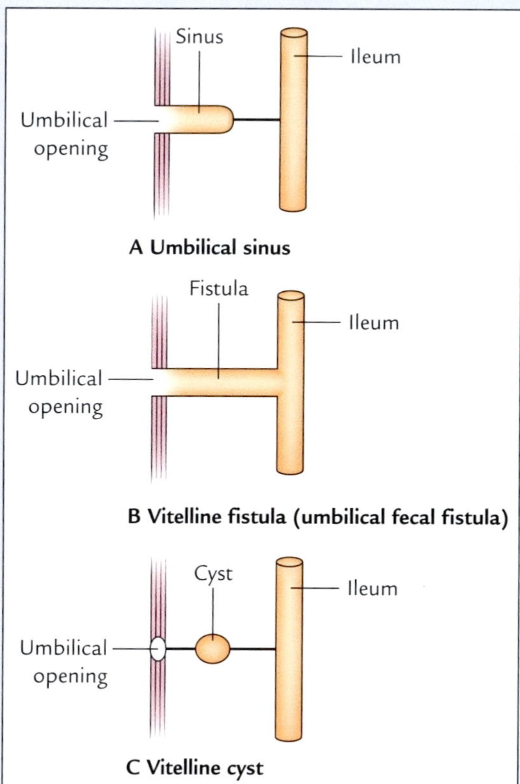

Fig. 18.22 Anomalies of vitellointestinal duct. (A) Umbilical sinus. (B) Umbilical fistula. (C) Vitelline cyst.

6. ***Subhepatic cecum and appendix (undescended cecum and appendix):*** The cecum develops from a **cecum bud** – a small conical dilatation that appears in the caudal segment of midgut loop near its apex at about the 6th week of IUL.

When the caudal segment of midgut loop returns to the abdominal cavity, cecum comes to lie below liver (**subhepatic position**).

As the postarterial segment of midgut loop elongates to form ascending colon, the cecum and appendix acquire a definitive position in the right iliac fossa.

But if ascending colon does not form or remains too short, the cecum does not descend and remains permanently below the liver leading to congenital anomaly called **subhepatic cecum** and **appendix** (Fig. 13.24).

In cases of subhepatic cecum and appendix, the inflammation of appendix (**appendicitis**) would cause tenderness in right hypochondrium that may lead to mistaken diagnosis of **cholecystitis** (inflammation of gallbladder).

N.B. Sometimes, the cecum may descend only partially in the lumbar region or may descend too much to reach in the pelvic region.

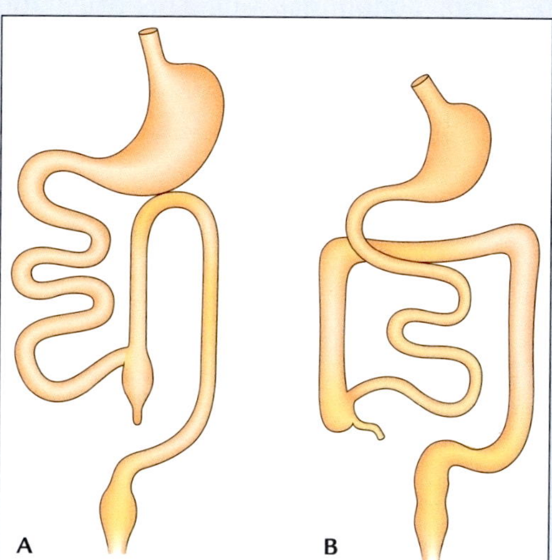

Fig. 18.23 Anomalies due to errors of rotation of gut. (A) Location of colon on the left half of the abdomen and small coils of the small intestine on the right side of abdomen due to nonrotation. (B) Location of transverse colon behind the duodenum due to reversed rotation.

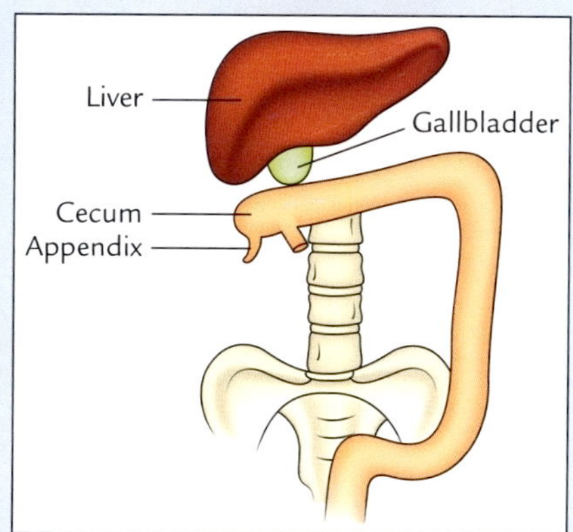

Fig. 18.24 Subhepatic cecum and appendix.

Fixation of Midgut Derivatives

The midgut loop has a dorsal mesentery (**mesentery proper**) that is attached to posterior abdominal wall in midline. As coils of small intestine return to the abdominal cavity, the line of attachment of its mesentery shifts and lies obliquely from *duodenojejunal flexure* to *ileocecal junction*. It undergoes profound changes with rotation. When the caudal (postarterial) limb of the loop moves to the right side of the abdominal cavity, the dorsal mesentery twists around **superior mesenteric artery**.

The **ascending colon** has a short mesentery at first, but as the ascending colon elongates its mesentery fuses with parietal peritoneum and the ascending colon becomes retroperitoneal by **zygosis**.

The transverse colon retains its mesentery, the attachment of which runs transversely from right to left on the posterior abdominal wall. This orientation of the **transverse mesocolon** can be explained by the last 90° rotation of midgut loop when postarterial segment returns to the abdominal cavity.

DEVELOPMENT OF HINDGUT DERIVATIVES AN 52.6

The hindgut gives rise to following parts of the gastrointestinal tract:

1. Left one-third of transverse colon
2. Descending colon
3. Sigmoid colon
4. Rectum
5. Upper part of the anal canal

Development of Transverse Colon

The right two-third of transverse colon develops from the postarterial segment of the midgut loop, while the left one-third of transverse colon develops from the hindgut. For this reason, the right two-third of transverse colon is supplied by superior mesenteric artery (the artery of midgut) and left one-third of transverse colon is supplied by the inferior mesenteric artery (the artery of hindgut).

Development of Descending Colon

It develops from hindgut.

Development of Sigmoid Colon

It also develops from hindgut.

Development of Rectum (Fig. 18.25)

The terminal dilated part of the hindgut distal to allantois is called **cloaca**. It is divided into two parts by urorectal septum: (a) a broad ventral part called **primitive urogenital sinus** and (b) a narrow dorsal part is called **primitive rectum**.

The **urogenital sinus** gives rise to the urinary bladder and urethra, while the primitive rectum gives rise to the rectum and upper part of the anal canal.

Development of Anal Canal (Fig. 18.26)

The anal canal develops from two sources: (a) hindgut and (b) proctodeum. The details are as follows:

The upper half of the anal canal is **endodermal in origin** and develops from primitive rectum.

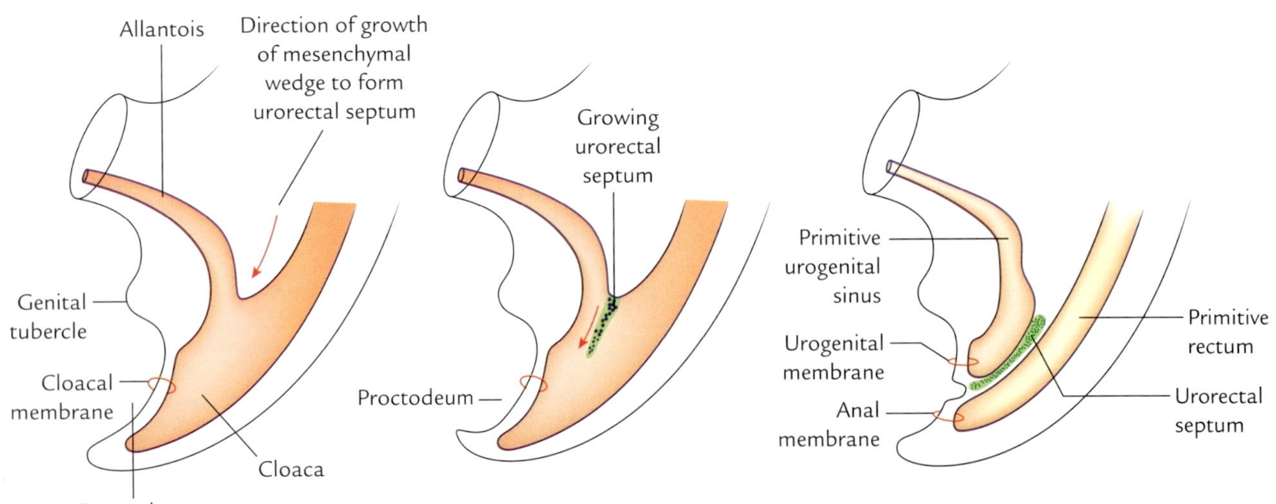

Fig. 18.25 Successive stages of formation of urorectal septum, which divides the cloaca into anterior part (the primitive urogenital sinus) and posterior part (the primitive rectum).

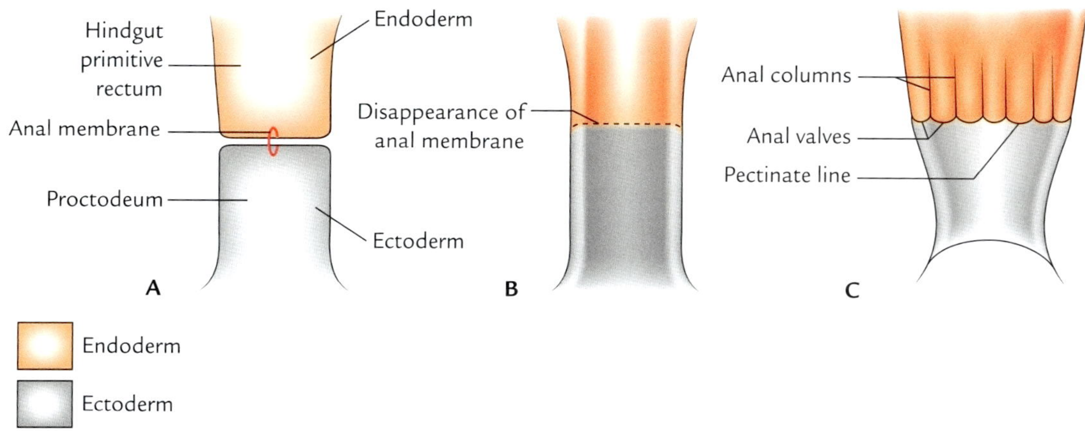

Fig. 18.26 Development of the anal canal.

The **lower half of the anal canal is ectodermal in origin** and develops from **anal pit** called **proctodeum.**

Initially, the two parts are separated from each other by **anal membrane.** Later at the end of 7th week, this membrane ruptures and the two parts communicate with each other. The site of anal membrane is represented by **pectinate line** in adults.

The main differences between upper and lower halves of the anal canal regarding their development, arterial supply, venous drainage, and nerve supply are given in Table 18.3.

Table 18.3 Differences between the upper and lower halves of the anal canal

	Upper Half of Anal Canal	Lower Half of Anal Canal
Development	Primitive rectum (endodermal in origin)	Proctodeum/anal pit (ectodermal in origin)
Arterial supply	Superior rectal artery	Inferior rectal artery
Venous drainage	Superior rectal vein (portal vein)	Inferior rectal vein (systemic veins)
Nerve supply	Autonomic	Somatic

CLINICAL CORRELATION

1 ***Congenital megacolon (Hirschsprung disease,*** Fig. 18.27): In this anomaly, a segment of the colon is dilated. However, it is the segment distal to dilatation that is abnormal. In this abnormal segment, autonomic parasympathetic ganglia are absent in the myenteric plexus. As a result, there is no peristalsis in this segment. Since contents of colon cannot pass through this segment, the segment proximal to it grossly dilates.

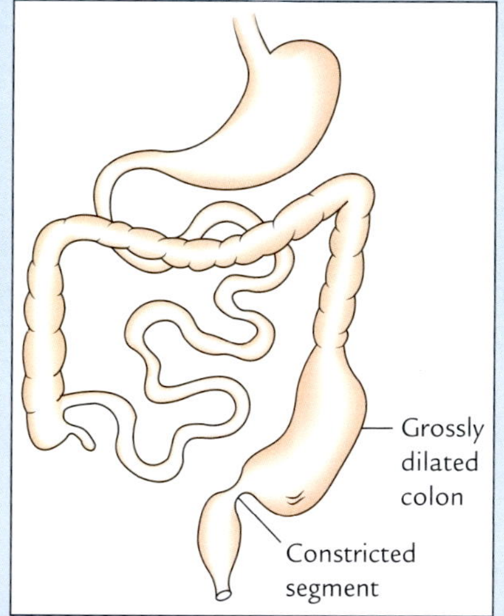

Fig. 18.27 Congenital megacolon (Hirschsprung disease).

It occurs in 1 in 5000 newborns.

This anomaly is produced due to failure of migration of **neural crest cells** in the wall of the affected segment of the colon. This anomaly is commonly seen in the sigmoid colon or rectum. Clinically, it presents as (a) loss of peristalsis, (b) fecal retention, and (c) abdominal distension.

N.B. The newborns with aganglionic congenital megacolon may fail to pass **meconium** in first 24–48 h after birth.

2. ***Imperforate anus:*** It is a clinical condition in which the lower part of gut (GIT) fails to communicate with exterior.

The various types of imperforated ani are as follows (Fig. 18.28):

(a) The rectum and anal canal develop normally, but anal membrane fails to breakdown. The anal membrane bulges out with accumulated contents proximal to it. This is a minor form of imperforated anus and can be corrected by excision of the anal membrane.

(b) The proctodeum remains a solid mass of ectodermal cells, and there is a big gap between this and the upper part of the anal canal.

Continued

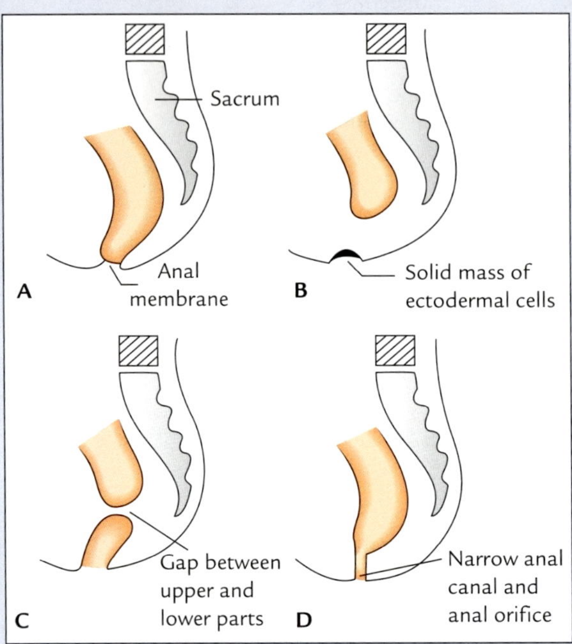

Fig. 18.28 Various types of imperforated anus. (A) Persistence of anal membrane. (B) Failure of anal pit to develop. (C) Upper and lower parts of rectum separated by a gap. (D) Stenosis of the anal canal.

(c) The upper and lower parts of the anal canal remain separated by a gap.

(d) The anal canal is stenosed. In this condition, anal canal and anal orifice are extremely narrow. It occurs when urorectal septum deviates dorsally as it reaches cloacal membrane.

3. ***Rectal fistulae*** **(Fig. 18.29):** The rectal fistulae are frequently seen in association with the imperforated anus. The common types of rectal fistulae are (a) rectovaginal fistula, (b) rectovesical fistula, and (c) rectourethral fistula. The rectal fistulae are usually associated with rectal atresia.

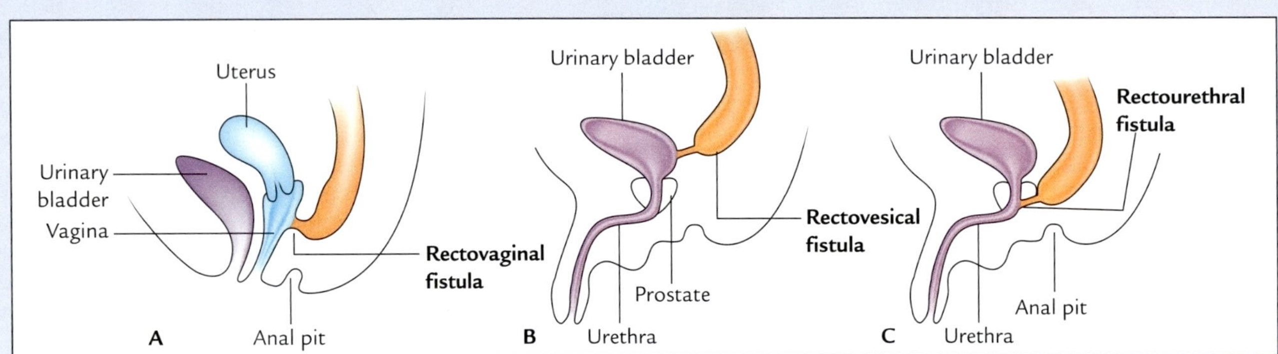

Fig. 18.29 Rectal fistulae. (A) Rectovaginal fistula. (B) Rectovesical fistula. (C) Rectourethral fistula. Note that rectal fistulae are associated with rectal atresia.

FIXATION OF MESENTERY OF THE GUT AS A WHOLE

Initially all parts of small and large intestine have mesentery through which they are suspended from the posterior abdominal wall. But once the rotation of the gut is complete, the mesenteries of (a) duodenum (except first inch of its first part), (b) ascending colon, (c) descending colon, and (d) rectum fuse with parietal peritoneum lining the posterior abdominal wall and undergo zygosis. As a result, these structures become **retroperitoneal**. The original mesentery of intestine now persists as (a) mesentery of the small intestine (**mesentery proper**), (b) mesentery of transverse colon (**transverse mesocolon**), (c) mesentery of the sigmoid colon (**sigmoid mesocolon**), and (d) mesentery of the appendix (**mesoappendix**) (Fig. 18.30).

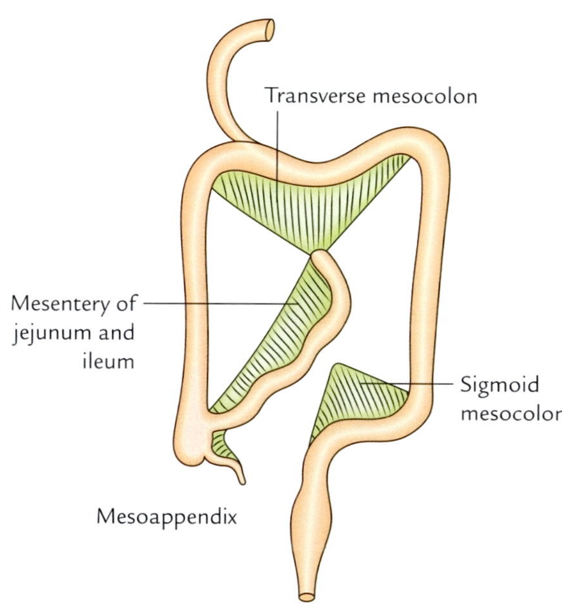

Fig. 18.30 Fate of dorsal mesentery of midgut and hindgut.

CLINICAL CORRELATION

1. ***Congenital anomalies due to errors of fixation of the gut***
   (a) The parts of intestine that normally become retroperitoneal may retain mesentery. As a result, they become highly mobile due to hypermotility – a portion of intestine twists along with its blood vessels on the axis of mesentery. Consequently, the blood supply is compromised. This condition is called **volvulus**. If volvulus is not corrected timely, it may cause an ischemic necrosis of part of the intestine involved.
   (b) The parts of intestine that normally retain their mesentery may be fixed particularly with any other organ by abnormal adhesions of peritoneum.
2. ***Situs inversus:*** In this condition, all the abdominal and thoracic viscera present on one side go to the opposite side, i.e., they are laterally transposed. Examples are as follows:
   (a) Appendix and duodenum lie on the left side
   (b) Stomach lies on the right side
   (c) Right atrium lies on the left side
   (d) Superior and inferior venae cavae lie on the left side

GESTATIONAL AGE OF KEY DEVELOPMENTAL EVENTS

Developmental Event	Gestational Age
➤ Primitive gut forms during	4th week
➤ Primordium of stomach (fusiform dilation of foregut)	4th week
➤ Development of duodenum	4th week
➤ Physiological umbilical hernia occurs during	6th week
➤ Appearance of cecal bud	6th week
➤ Obliteration of vitellointestinal duct occurs by	10th week
➤ Cloacal membrane rupture at the end of	7th week

GOLDEN FACTS TO REMEMBER

➤ **Most important confirmatory signs of esophageal atresia**	Continuous pouring of saliva from mouth
➤ **Commonest congenital anomaly of intestine**	Meckel's diverticulum
➤ **Most important role of rotation of gut**	(a) Helps in the retraction of herniated loops of intestine back into the abdominal cavity (b) Helps in establishing definitive relationships of various parts of the intestine
➤ **Total anticlockwise rotation of midgut loop during its return to abdominal cavity**	270°
➤ **Most anorectal anomalies result from**	Abnormal partitioning of the cloaca by urorectal septum
➤ **Perineal body is formed by**	Tip of urorectal septum
➤ **Meconium**	Earliest stool passed after birth
➤ **Situs inversus**	Horizontal transcription of thoracic and abdominal viscera

CLINICAL PROBLEM SOLVING

PROBLEMS

1. **The left vagus nerve innervates the anterior surface of the stomach and the right vagus nerve innervates the posterior surface of the stomach**. Give the **embryological basis**.
2. A female baby started vomiting few hours after her birth. On physical examination, a marked distention in epigastric region was noted. The vomitus contained bile; the radiograph of the abdomen revealed gas in the stomach and proximal half of duodenum. What is the most probable diagnosis? Give its embryological basis.
3. Umbilicus of a newborn infant was swollen, and there was a persistent discharge (mucus and feces) from the umbilicus. The fluoroscopy using radiopaque oil revealed a fistulous tract that was communicating with distal part of the ileum. What is this sinus tract called? Give its embryological basis.
4. A newborn was born with a shiny mass of about the size of an orange that was protruding from the umbilicus. The mass was covered by a thin, transparent membrane. After exposure to air, the transparent membrane lost its shiny appearance. What is the most probable diagnosis? Give its embryological basis.
5. What are congenital anomalies of foregut, midgut, and hindgut? AN 52.6

SOLUTIONS

1. Initially left and right vagus nerves innervate the left and right sides of the stomach, respectively. Following 90° clockwise rotation of stomach along its longitudinal axis, the left and right sides of stomach become the anterior and posterior surfaces of the stomach, respectively. As a result, left and right vagus nerves supply the anterior and posterior surfaces of the stomach, respectively.
2. The most probable diagnosis is **duodenal atresia**. It usually affects the second part of duodenum distal to the opening of bile duct. The duodenal atresia (obstruction) results from incomplete recanalization of lumen of the duodenum during the 8th week of intrauterine life (IUL).

   The obstruction causes bilious vomiting as the obstruction is distal to the opening of bile duct. The obstruction also causes distension of the stomach and proximal duodenum because fetus swallows amniotic fluid and subsequently newborn baby swallows air. This leads to distension in epigastric region.

N.B. Duodenal atresia is common in infants with Down syndrome (trisomy 21).

3. The vitellointestinal duct (omphaloenteric tract) normally completely obliterates by the 10th week of IUL. In about 2% of cases, a remnant of vitellointestinal duct persists as a small diverticulum called **Meckel's diverticulum**. In the present case, the entire vitellointestinal duct persisted and formed vitellointestinal fistula.
4. This is a congenital anomaly called **exomphalos (omphalocele)**. It occurs when intestine fails to return to the abdominal cavity during the 10th week of IUL. The transparent membrane covering is derived from amnion. Once this membrane is exposed to air, it rapidly loses its shiny appearance. It becomes thicker and gets covered with an opaque fibrinous exudate. The students often confuse exomphalos with congenital umbilical hernia (for details, see p. 198).
5.
   - The **common congenital anomalies of foregut** are esophageal atresia or stenosis, pyloric stenosis, hepatobiliary malformations, and annular pancreas.
   - The **common anomalies of midgut** are Meckel's diverticulum and umbilical hernia.
   - The **common anomalies of hindgut** are Hirschsprung disease, anorectal anomalies, and imperforated anus.

19 Major Digestive Glands (Salivary Glands, Liver, and Pancreas) and Spleen

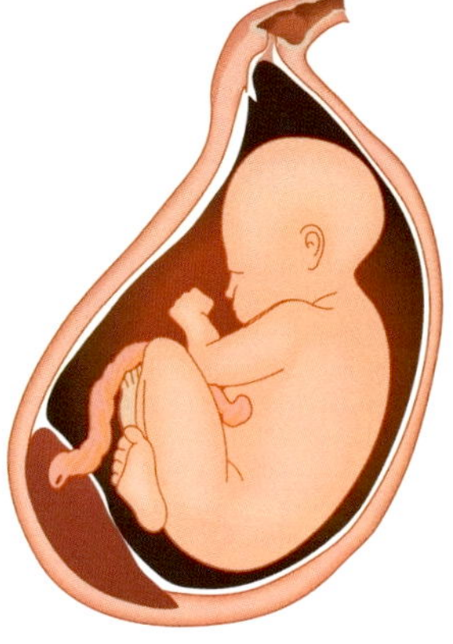

LEARNING OBJECTIVES

After studying this chapter, the student should be able to:

- Describe the development of liver in brief.
- Write short notes on Riedel's lobe and Caroli disease.
- Describe the development of extrahepatic biliary apparatus, and discuss the associated common congenital anomalies.
- Describe the development of pancreas in brief with special focus on the development of its main and accessory ducts.
- Give the embryological basis of (a) annular pancreas and (b) accessory spleens.

OVERVIEW

The major glands associated with digestive system are salivary glands, liver, and pancreas. All these glands develop from endodermal lining of gut except parotid gland, which develops from ectodermal lining of the oral cavity. Ducts of these glands open into different parts of the digestive tract. Although the **spleen** is not a gland of the digestive tract, it is described here because of its close association with the digestive tract. Note that the spleen develops between two layers of dorsal mesogastrium.

SALIVARY GLANDS

There are three pairs of major salivary glands: (a) *parotid*, (b) *submandibular*, and (c) *sublingual*. The salivary glands are described in detail in Chapter 17.

LIVER

OVERVIEW

Liver, the largest gland in the body, which in addition to other functions produce bile. The bile from liver is poured into duodenum through extrahepatic biliary apparatus. The liver develops from following three sources:

1. **Parenchyma of the liver and extrahepatic biliary apparatus**-from **endodermal hepatic bud of foregut.**
2. **Fibrous stroma of the liver** from **mesenchyme of septum transversum.**
3. **Sinusoids of liver** from absorbed and broken vitelline and umbilical veins within the septum transversum.

The liver develops from an **endodermal hepatic bud** that arises from ventral aspect of the distal part of foregut, just at its junction with the midgut in the middle of 3rd week of IUL (Fig. 19.1).

The hepatic bud grows into the ventral mesogastrium and through it into the **septum transversum.** The bud soon divides into two parts: a large cranial part called **pars hepatica** and a small caudal part called **pars cystica.** The pars hepatica forms the **liver**, while pars cystica forms the **gallbladder** and **cystic duct**. The part of bud proximal to pars cystica forms **common bile duct (CBD).**

The pars hepatica further divides into right and left portions that form right and left lobes of the liver respectively. Initially, both lobes of the liver are of equal size.

As the right and left portions of the pars hepatica enlarge, they extend into the septum transversum. The cells arising from *these form interlacing hepatic cords* or *cords of hepatocytes*. In this process, **vitelline and umbilical veins** present within the septum transversum get absorbed and broken to form the **liver sinusoids** (Fig. 19.2). The cells of hepatic cords later become radially arranged in hepatic lobules. The **bile canaliculi** and **ductules** are formed in liver parenchyma and establish connections with extrahepatic bile ducts secondarily at a later stage (Fig. 19.3). Because of rapid enlargement, liver occupies major portion of the abdominal cavity forcing the coils of the gut to herniate through umbilicus (physiological hernia). The oxygen-rich blood supply and proliferation of hemopoietic tissue are responsible for the massive enlargement of the liver.

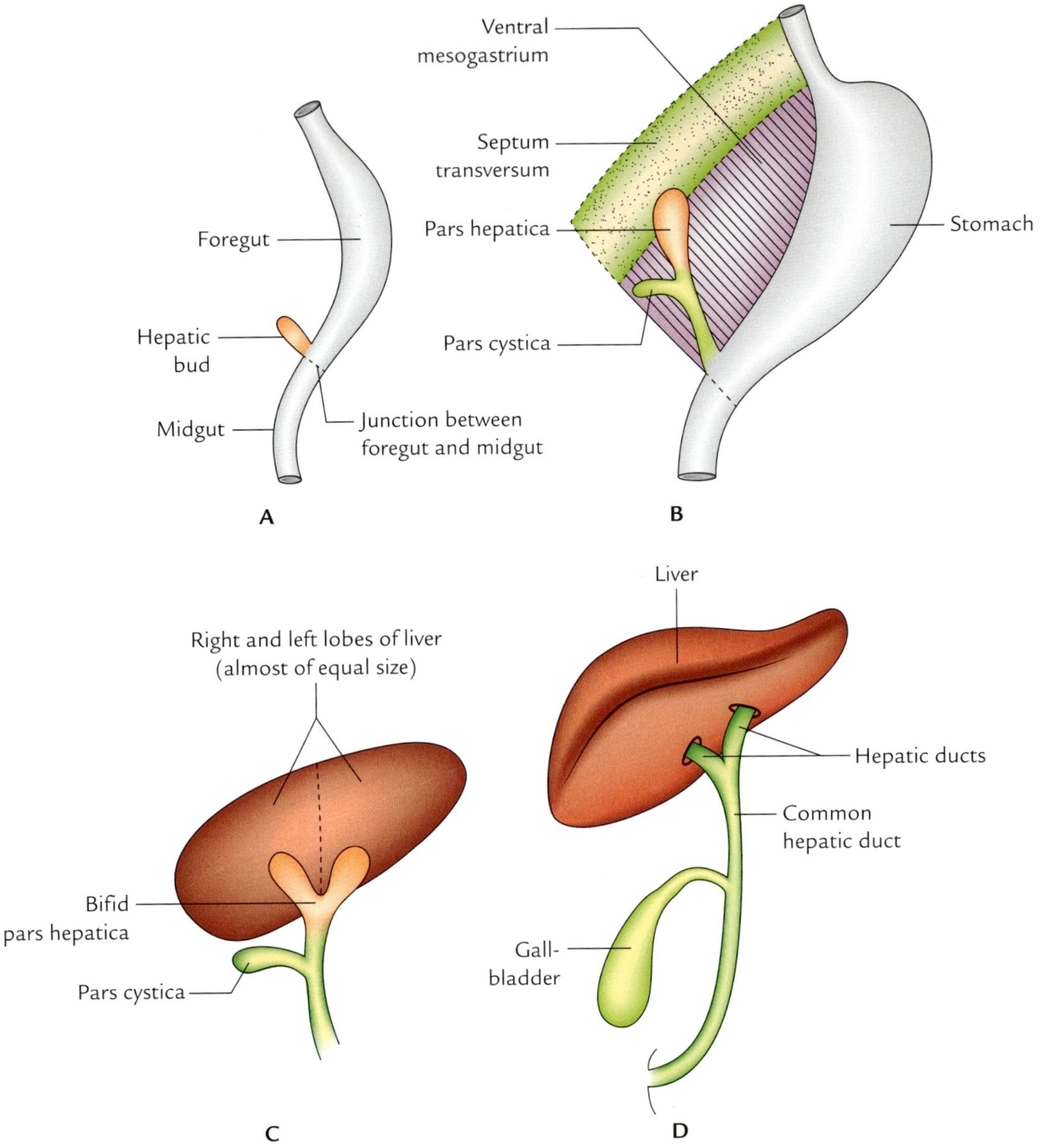

Fig. 19.1 Successive stages of the development of the liver. (A) Hepatic bud arising from foregut at its junction with the midgut. (B) Growth of hepatic bud toward septum transversum through ventral mesogastrium. Note the subdivision of hepatic bud into pars hepatica and pars cystica. (C) Division of pars hepatica into right and left portions. (D) Fully formed liver and gallbladder along with their ducts.

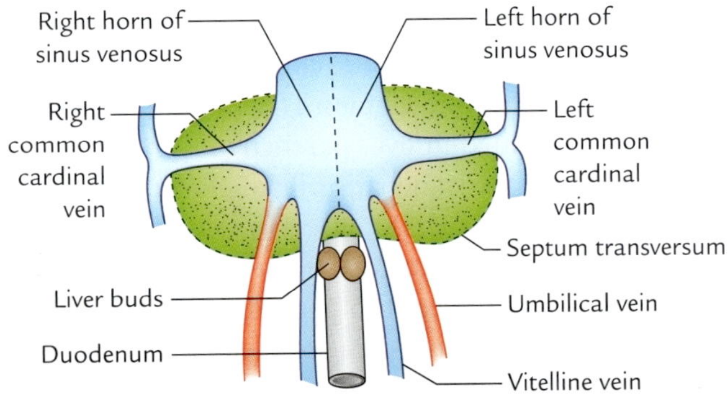

Fig. 19.2 Umbilical and vitelline veins passing through the septum transversum to enter the sinus venosus.

Adult derivatives of various components of liver from embryonic structures are given in Table 19.1.

N.B.

- Liver is an important center of **hemopoiesis** (i.e., blood formation). The hemopoiesis begins in the liver at about the 6th week of intrauterine life (IUL) and continue almost till birth. Later, the hemopoietic function of the liver is taken over by the spleen and bone marrow.
- Weight of liver:
  (a) In 10th week = 10% of total body weight (due to hemopoietic function).
  (b) At birth = 55% of total body weight.
- The hepatocytes start secreting bile at about 12th week (3rd month) of IUL. The bile enters intestine and imparts a dark green color to first stools (meconium) passed by newborns.

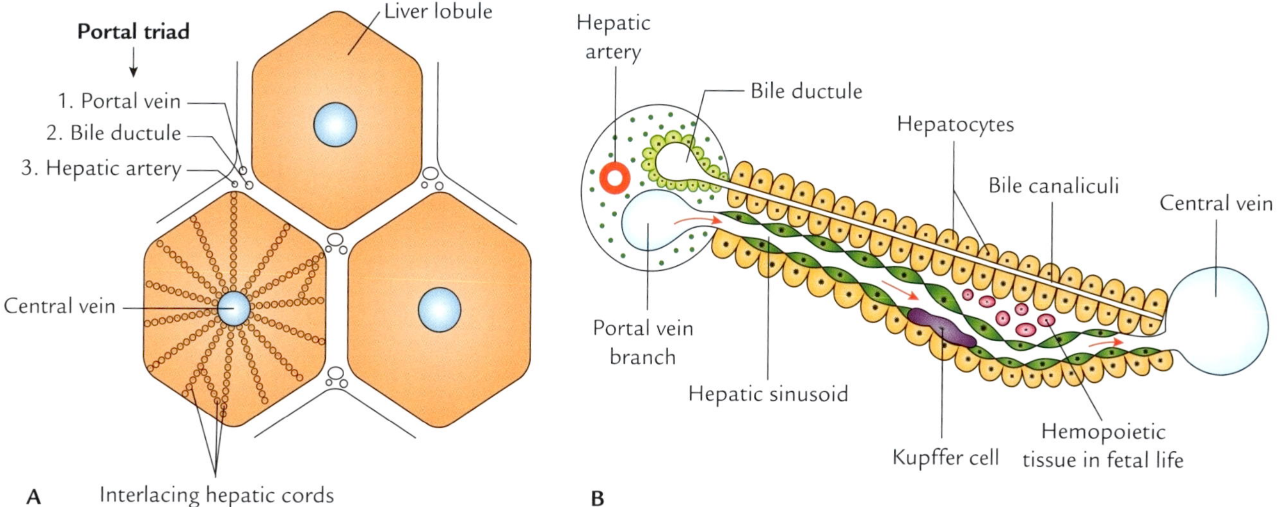

Fig. 19.3 Histological components of developing liver. (A) Arrangement of hepatic cords. Note that they radiate from central vein toward periphery. (B) Location of bile canaliculi and bile ductule (derivatives of hepatic bud), liver sinusoids (derivatives of vitelline and umbilical veins), and hemopoietic tissue (derivative of septum transversum).

Table 19.1 Source of development of various components of the liver

Embryonic Structure	Adult Derivatives
• Hepatic bud	Liver parenchyma Bile canaliculi and bile ductules
• Vitelline and umbilical veins within septum transversum	Liver sinusoids
• Septum transversum (mesodermal in origin)	• Connective tissue stroma of the liver including Glisson capsule (fibrous capsule of the liver) • Peritoneal coverings of liver • Kupffer cells • Hemopoietic cells • Blood vessels of liver

CLINICAL CORRELATION

Congenital anomalies of the liver

1. ***Riedel's lobe:*** It is a tongue-like extension from the right lobe of the liver (Fig. 19.4). It develops as an extension of normal hepatic tissue from the inferior margin of the right lobe of the liver.
2. ***Polycystic disease of the liver:*** The biliary tree within the liver (i.e., bile canaliculi and bile ductules) normally connects them with the extrahepatic bile ducts. Failure of union of some of these ducts may cause the formation of cysts within the liver. The polycystic disease of liver is usually associated with cystic disease of kidney and pancreas.
3. ***Intrahepatic biliary atresia:*** It is a *very serious anomaly.* The intrahepatic biliary atresia cannot be subjected to surgical correction. As a result, there are only two options for parents: (a) to go for liver transplant of the child or (b) to let the child die.
4. ***Caroli disease:*** It is characterized by *congenital dilatation of intrahepatic biliary tree,* which may lead to the formation of *sepsis, stone,* and even *carcinoma.*

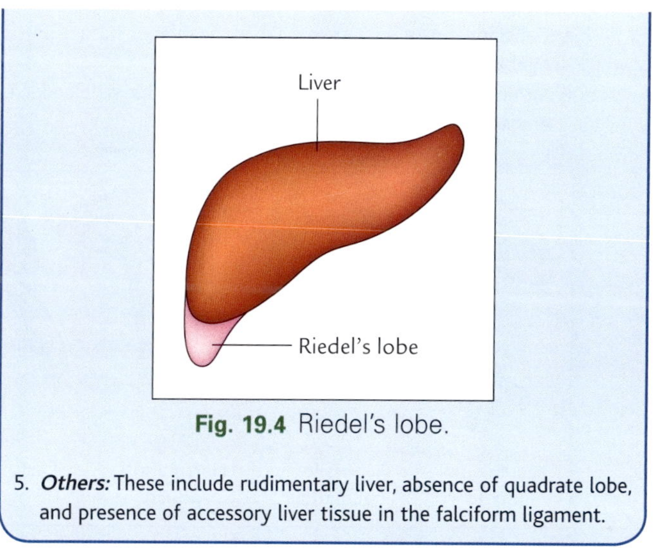

Fig. 19.4 Riedel's lobe.

5. ***Others:*** These include rudimentary liver, absence of quadrate lobe, and presence of accessory liver tissue in the falciform ligament.

Development of Extrahepatic Biliary Apparatus

The **gallbladder** and **cystic duct** develop from **pars cystica**. The bifid pars hepatica forms common hepatic duct, right and left hepatic ducts. (Within the liver parenchyma, right and left hepatic ducts branch repeatedly, acquire lumen and form intrahepatic biliary passages.) The part of hepatic bud proximal to the pars cystica forms *CBD*. Initially, the CBD/bile duct opens on the ventral aspect of developing duodenum. However, as the duodenum grows and rotates, the opening of CBD is carried to dorsomedial aspect of the duodenum along with ventral pancreatic bud.

N.B. Initially, the extrahepatic biliary apparatus is occluded with epithelial cells, but later it is recanalized by way of vacuolation resulting from degeneration of the cells.

CLINICAL CORRELATION

Anomalies of the extrahepatic biliary apparatus: The anomalies of the extrahepatic biliary apparatus are very common.

1. ***Anomalies of gallbladder*** (Fig. 19.5)
   (a) *Agenesis of gallbladder (absence of gallbladder):* If the pars cystica from the hepatic bud fails to develop, the gallbladder and cystic duct will not develop.
   (b) *Absence of the cystic duct:* It occurs when entire growth of cells of the hepatic bud form gallbladder. In such a case, the gallbladder drains directly into the CBD. It is called **sessile gallbladder**.
   (c) *Anomalies of shape*
   - *Phrygian cap:* It occurs when fundus of the gallbladder folds on itself to form a cap-like structure – the *Phrygian cap*. It can simulate a mass of liver during hepatobiliary imaging.
   - *Hartmann's pouch:* It is a pouch formed when the posteromedial wall of the neck (infundibulum) of gallbladder projects downward. This pouch may be adherent to the cystic duct or even to the CBD. The gallstone is usually lodged in this pouch.
   - *Septate gallbladder and double gallbladder:* In humans, the gallbladder may be partially or completely subdivided by a septum. On the other hand, in some cases gallbladder may be partially or completely duplicated.

   (d) *Anomalies of the positions*
   - Gallbladder may lie transversally on the inferior surface of the right or left lobe of the liver.
   - *Intrahepatic gallbladder:* In this condition, the gallbladder is embedded within the substance of the liver.
   - *Floating gallbladder:* In this condition, the gallbladder is completely surrounded by peritoneum and attached to the liver by a fold of peritoneum (mesentery).

2. ***Anomalies of extrahepatic biliary ducts*** (Fig. 19.6): These anomalies occur due to failure of recanalization of these ducts. Some common anomalies of extrahepatic biliary ducts are as follows:
   (a) *Atresia of ducts*
   - Atresia of bile duct
   - Atresia of entire extrahepatic biliary duct system
   - Atresia of common hepatic duct
   - Atresia of hepatic ducts

N.B. The atresia of the bile duct manifests as persistent progressive jaundice of newborn and may be associated with the absence of the *ampulla of Vater.*

   (b) *Accessory ducts*
   - *Small accessory bile ducts* may open directly from the liver into the gallbladder. In this case, there may be leakage of bile into the peritoneal cavity after cholecystectomy if they are not recognized at the time of surgery.
   - *Choledochal cyst* rarely develops due to an area of weakness in the wall of bile duct. It may contain up to 2 L of bile and thus may compress the bile duct to produce an **obstructive jaundice**.
   - *Moynihan hump:* In this condition, the hepatic artery lies in front of the common bile duct forming a caterpillar-like loop.

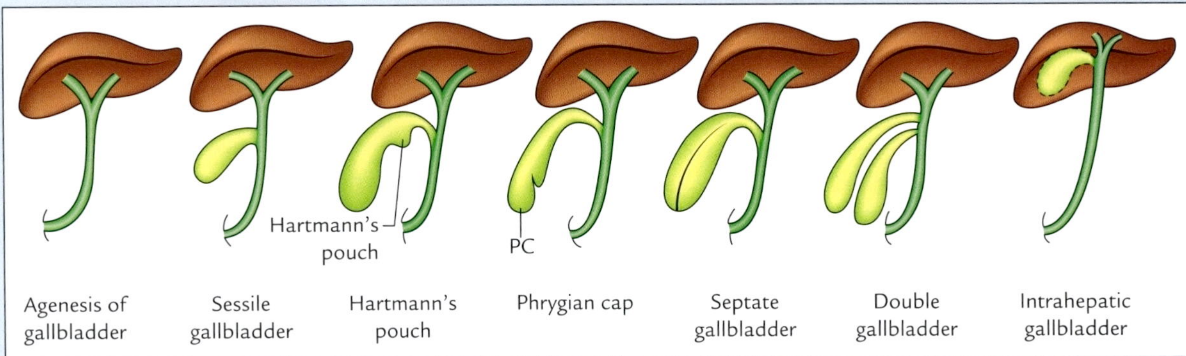

Fig. 19.5 Some common congenital anomalies of the gallbladder. PC, phrygian cap.

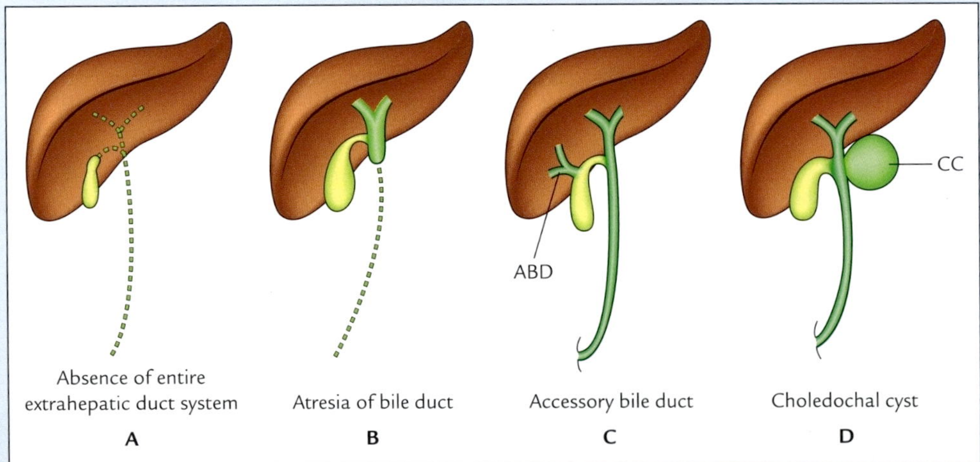

Fig. 19.6 Some congenital anomalies of the extrahepatic biliary ducts. (A and B) Atresia. (C and D) Accessory bile ducts. CC, choledochal cyst.

DEVELOPMENT OF PANCREAS (FIG. 19.7)

OVERVIEW

The pancreas develops from two endodermal pancreatic buds that arise from junction of foregut and midgut. The **dorsal bud** forms the upper part of the head, neck, body, and tail of the pancreas, while **ventral bud** forms the lower part of the head and uncinate process. Thus, most of the pancreas is formed by the larger dorsal bud. The main pancreatic duct is formed by the distal three-fourth of the duct of dorsal bud and proximal one-fourth of the duct of the ventral bud. The accessory pancreatic duct is formed by proximal one-fourth of the duct of dorsal pancreatic bud.

First the **dorsal pancreatic bud** arises from dorsal wall, foregut at the end of 3rd week of IUL, a short distance above the **ventral bud.** It grows between two layers of the dorsal mesentery of duodenum (also called mesoduodenum). A little later, the **ventral pancreatic bud** arises from ventral wall of foregut at its junction with the foregut in common with/or close to the primitive bile duct and grows between the two layers of ventral mesentery (Fig. 19.8).

When the duodenum rotates to right and becomes C shaped, the ventral pancreatic bud is on the right and the dorsal pancreatic bud is on the left of the duodenum. With rapid growth of right duodenal wall, the ventral pancreatic bud shifts from right to left and lies just below the dorsal pancreatic bud.

The dorsal and ventral pancreatic buds grow in size and fuse with each other to form the pancreas. The *dorsal pancreatic bud* forms the upper part of head, neck, body, and tail of the pancreas, while *ventral pancreatic*

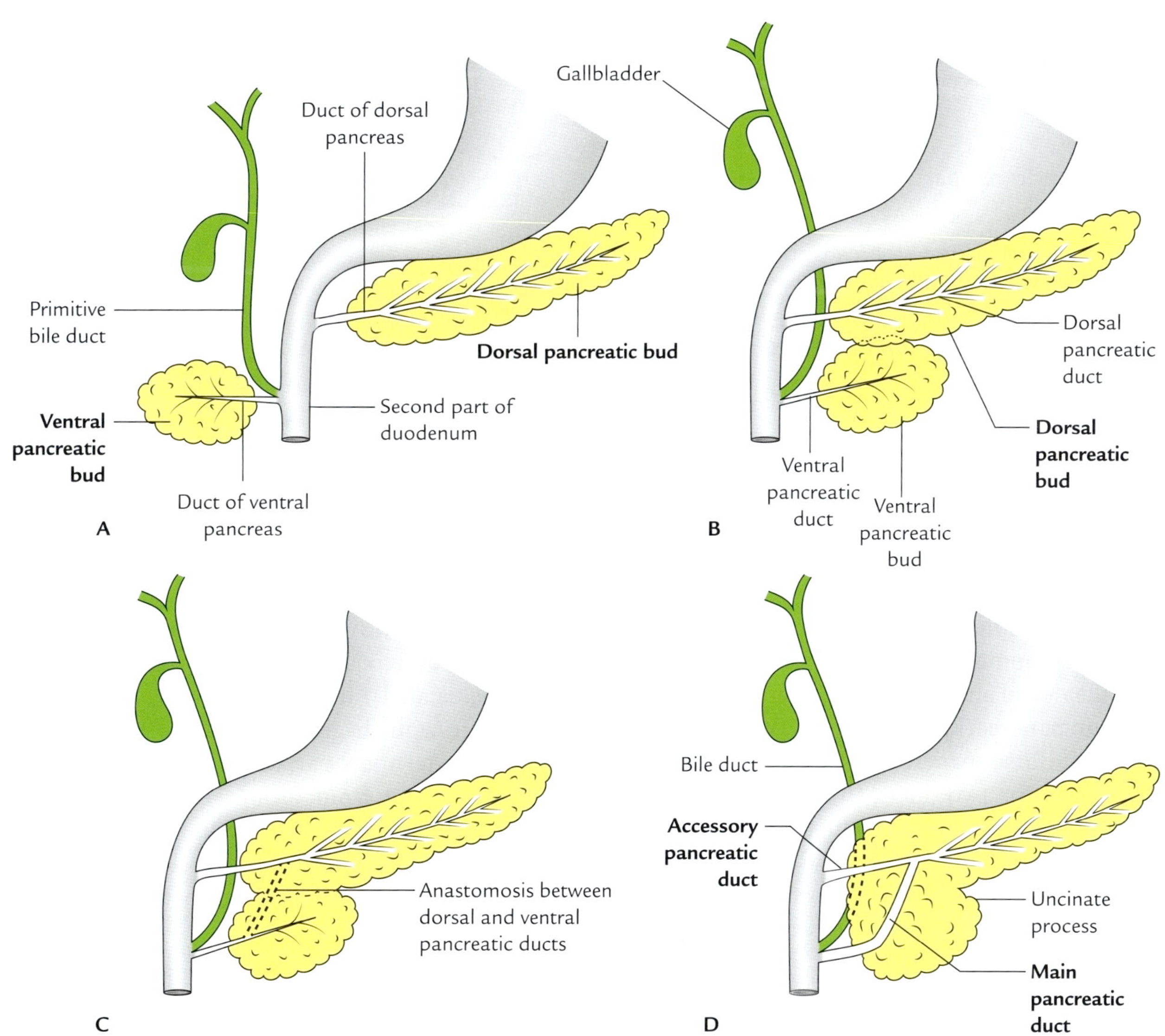

Fig. 19.7 Development of pancreas and its ducts.

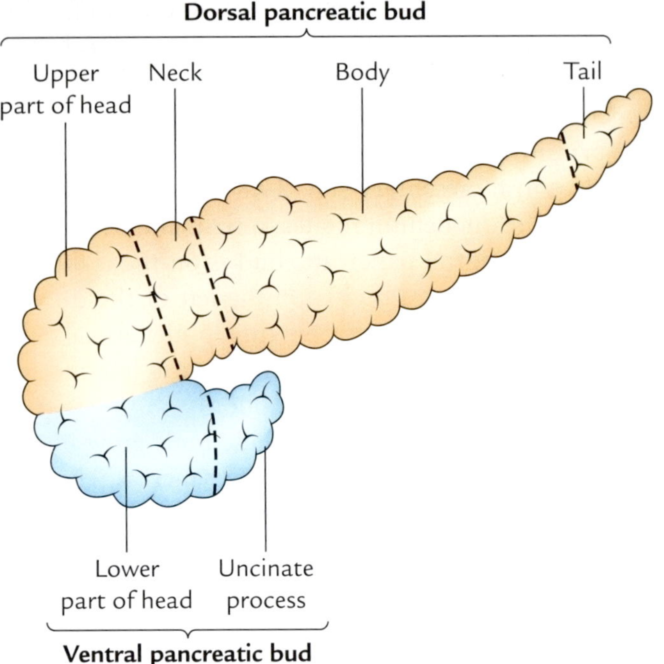

Fig. 19.8 Derivation of various parts of pancreas from dorsal and ventral pancreatic buds.

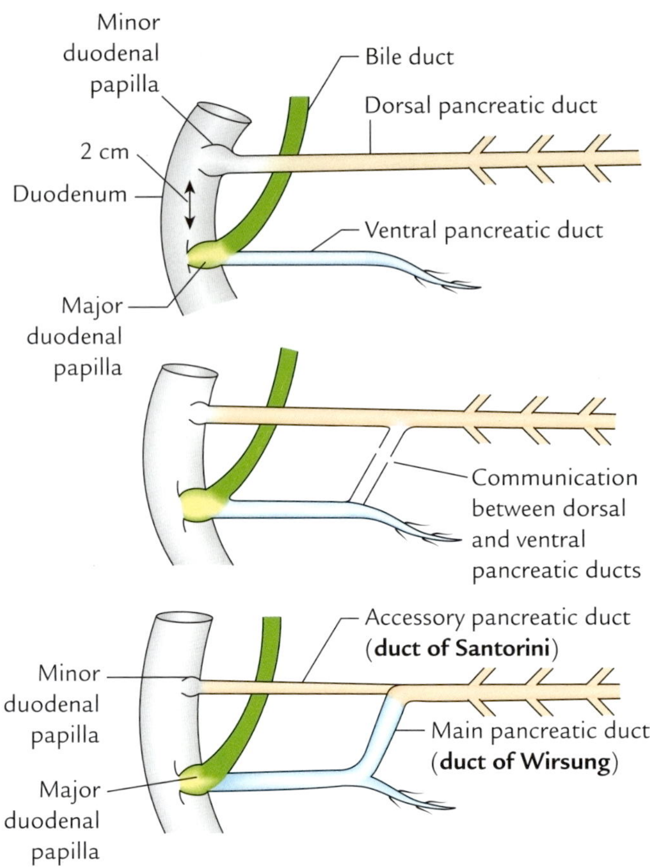

Fig. 19.9 Schematic diagram showing the development of main and accessory pancreatic ducts.

bud forms the lower part of the head and uncinate process of pancreas.

N.B. At first, the ventral pancreatic bud forms a bilobed structure that subsequently fuses to form a single mass.

Development of Ducts of the Pancreas (Fig. 19.9)

Initially, two parts of the pancreas are derived from two pancreatic buds, i.e., dorsal and ventral pancreatic buds have separate ducts called **dorsal and ventral pancreatic ducts** that open separately into the duodenum. Opening of dorsal pancreatic duct is about 2 cm proximal to opening of the ventral pancreatic duct. The ventral pancreatic duct opens in common with the bile duct derived from the hepatic bud.

Now communication (anastomosis) develops between the dorsal and ventral pancreatic ducts.

The **main pancreatic duct** (**duct of Wirsung**) develops from (a) dorsal pancreatic duct, distal to anastomosis between the two ducts, (b) anastomosis (communication) between the two ducts, and (c) ventral pancreatic duct proximal to the anastomosis. From its development, it is clear that the main pancreatic duct that opens in the duodenum is common with the bile duct at the major duodenal papilla. The proximal part of the dorsal pancreatic duct may persist as **accessory pancreatic duct** (**duct of Santorini**) that opens in the duodenum at **minor duodenal papilla** located about 2 cm proximal to major duodenal papilla.

N.B. In about 10% of people, the dorsal and ventral pancreatic ducts fail to fuse and original two ducts persist.

Histogenesis of Pancreas

Parenchyma of the pancreas is derived from endoderm of the pancreatic buds.

The pancreatic buds branch out in surrounding mesoderm and form various ducts (such as intralobular [intercalated], interlobular, and main duct). The pancreatic acini begin to develop from cell clusters around the terminal parts of the ducts. **Islets of Langerhans** develop from groups of cells that separate from the duct system. The capsule covering the gland, septa, and other connective tissue elements of the pancreas with blood vessels develop from surrounding mesoderm.

N.B. The β-cells of islets of Langerhans start secreting insulin by 10th week of IUL. The α-cells, which secrete somatostatin, develop prior to the insulin-secreting β-cells.

CLINICAL CORRELATION

Anomalies of pancreas

1. ***Annular pancreas*** (Fig. 19.10): In this condition, the pancreatic tissue completely surrounds second part of the duodenum causing its obstruction. This anomaly is produced as follows: The bifid ventral pancreatic bud fails to fuse to form a single mass. The two lobes (right and left) of the ventral pancreatic bud grow and migrate in opposite directions around the second part of the duodenum and form a **collar of pancreatic tissue** before it fuses with dorsal pancreatic bud. Thus, duodenum gets completely surrounded by the pancreatic tissue that may cause *duodenal obstruction.*

   Clinical features

   (a) Vomiting may start a few hours after birth.

   (b) *Radiograph* of abdomen reveals *double bubble appearance.* It is associated with duodenal stenosis. It indicates gas in the stomach and dilated part of the duodenum proximal to the site of obstruction.

   Early surgical intervention to relieve the obstruction is necessary. The surgical procedure consists of duodenojejunostomy and not cutting of the pancreatic collar.

2. ***Divided pancreas*** (Fig. 19.11): It occurs when the dorsal and ventral pancreatic buds fail to fuse with each other to form a single pancreas. As a result, the two parts of pancreas derived from dorsal and ventral buds remain separate from each other and drain through separate dorsal and ventral pancreatic ducts into the duodenum.

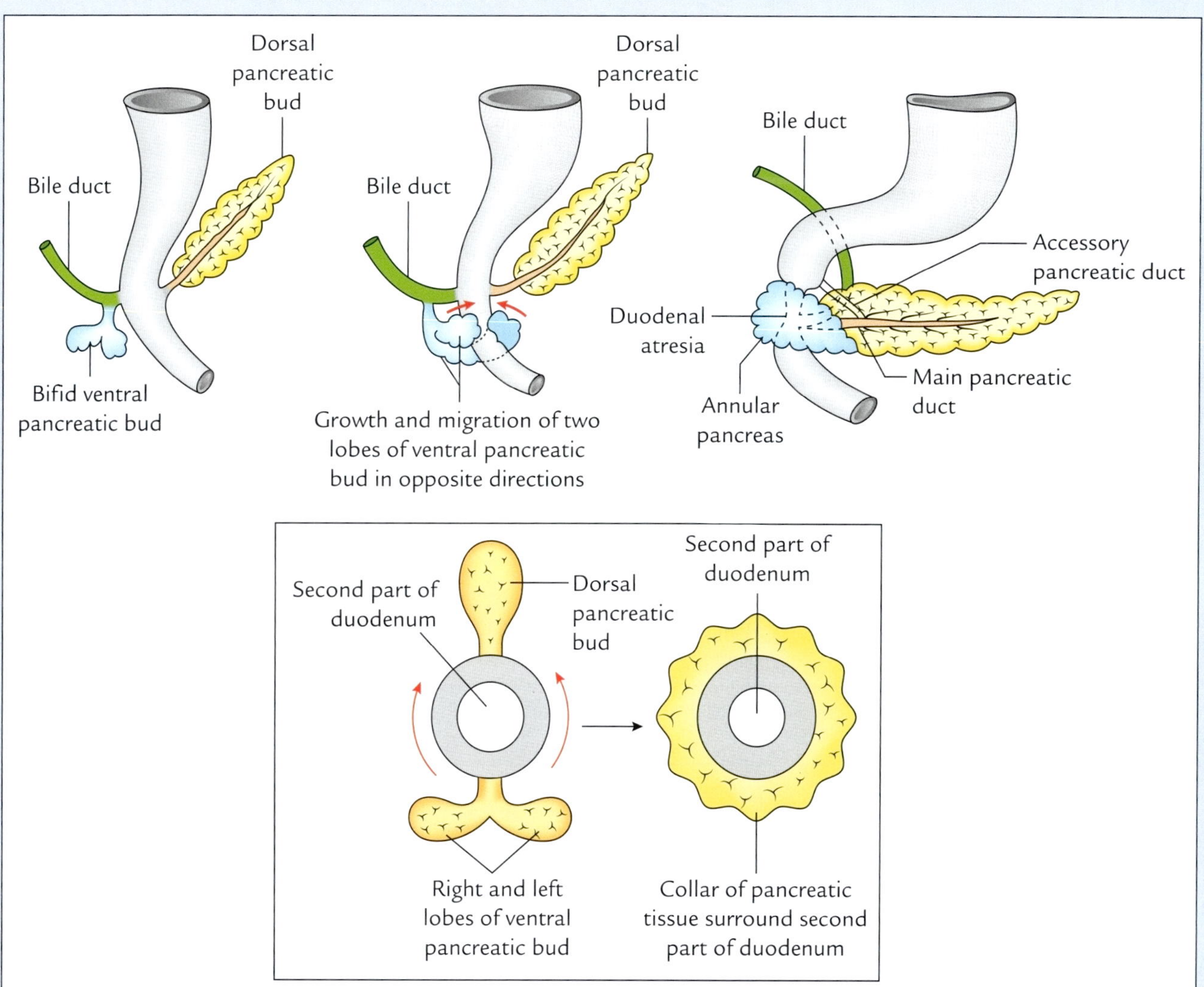

Fig. 19.10 Formation of annular pancreas. Figure in the inset is a highly schematic diagram showing the formation of collar of pancreatic tissue around second part of the duodenum.

Continued

3. ***Accessory (ectopic) pancreatic tissue:*** In this condition, small masses/nodules of pancreatic tissue are located at the following sites:
   (a) Wall of duodenum
   (b) Meckel's diverticulum
   (c) Gallbladder
   (d) Lower end of esophagus
   (e) Wall of stomach

   Ectopic pancreatic tissue may present with obstruction, bleeding, etc.
4. ***Inversion of pancreatic ducts*** (Fig. 19.12): In this condition, the main pancreatic duct is formed by duct of the dorsal pancreatic bud and opens on the *minor duodenal papilla.* It drains most of the pancreatic tissue. The duct of ventral pancreatic bud develops poorly and opens on *major duodenal papilla.*

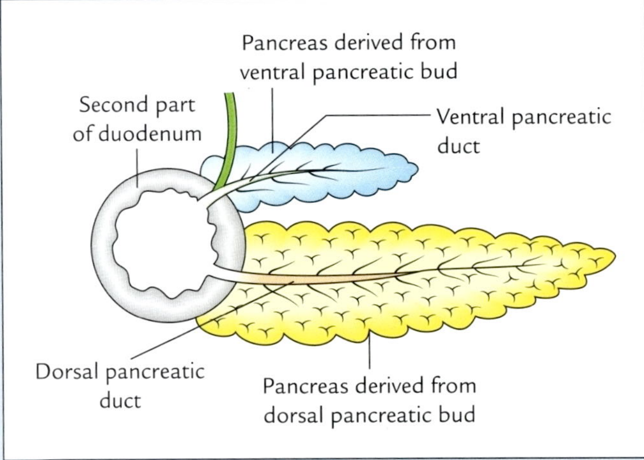

Fig. 19.11 Divided pancreas.

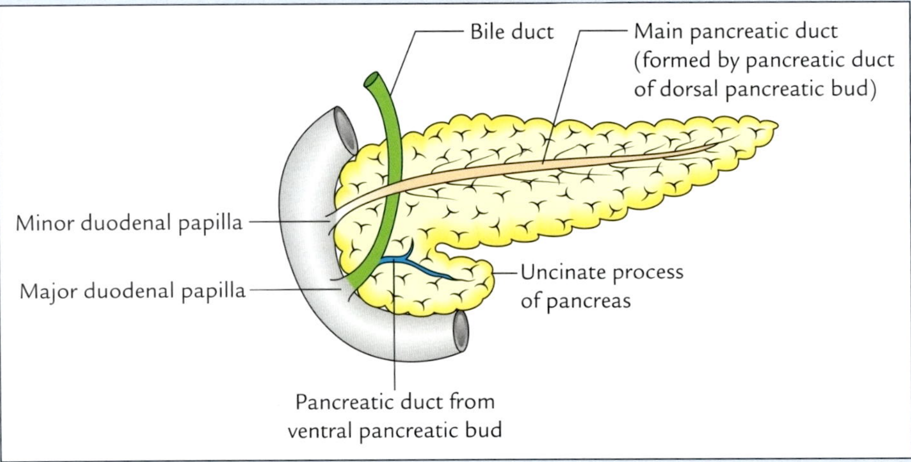

Fig. 19.12 Inversion of pancreatic duct.

DEVELOPMENT OF SPLEEN

The spleen is mesodermal in origin. It is a vascular lymphoid organ and begins to develop during 5th week from mass of mesenchymal cells located between the two layers of the dorsal mesogastrium in close relation to stomach.

The mesenchymal cells lying between the two layers of dorsal mesogastrium condense to form a number of small mesenchymal masses (called lobules of splenic tissue/**spleniculi**) that latter fuse to form a single mesenchymal mass (**splenic mass**), which projects from under cover of left layer of the mesogastrium. It is important to note that although the spleen begins to develop during the 5th week, it acquires its characteristic shape only in the early fetal life.

The development of the spleen in the dorsal mesogastrium divides the latter into two parts: (a) part that extends between hilum of the spleen and greater curvature of the stomach is called **gastrosplenic ligament**, while (b) the part of dorsal mesogastrium that extends between the spleen and left kidney on the posterior abdominal wall is called **splenorenal ligament/lienorenal ligament**.

The spleen is lobulated in the fetus but lobules generally disappear before birth.

N.B. The presence of splenic notches on the anterior (superior) border of adult spleen indicates lobulated origin of the spleen. They represent the remnants of grooves that separated the fetal lobules.

Histogenesis of Spleen

All elements of the spleen are derived from mesoderm. The mesodermal cells form capsule, septa, and connective tissue network including reticular fibers. The primordium of splenic tissue forms branching cords and isolated free cells. Some of the free cells form lymphoblasts, while the others differentiate into hemopoietic cells.

The process of blood formation in spleen begins in early embryonic life and continues during fetal life but stops after birth. The production of lymphocytes, however, continues in the postnatal period.

CLINICAL CORRELATION

Anomalies of spleen

1. ***Accessory spleen (spleniculi):*** These are accessory nodules of splenic tissue (supernumerary spleens) less than 2 cm in diameter and may be found at many sites such as *hilum of spleen, gastrosplenic ligament, lienorenal ligament, in the tail of the pancreas, along the splenic artery, greater omentum (rarely)*, etc.

   The clinical importance of accessory spleens is that they may undergo hypertrophy after splenectomy and may be responsible for symptoms of disease for which the splenectomy was done.
2. ***Lobulated spleen*** (Fig. 19.13): It is persistence of fetal spleen, which is formed due to fusion of a number of small lobules of splenic tissue (spleniculi).

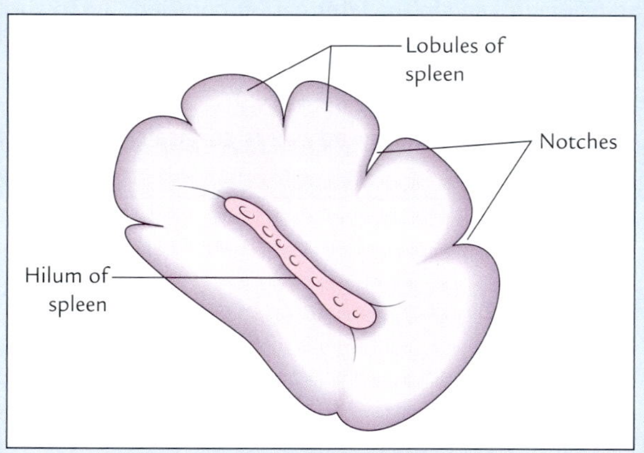

Fig. 19.13 Lobulated spleen.

GESTATIONAL AGE OF KEY DEVELOPMENTAL EVENTS

Developmental Event	Gestational Age
➤ Hepatic bud appears in the middle of	3rd week
➤ Hemopoiesis begins in liver at about	6th week
➤ Pancreatic buds develop at the end of	3rd week
➤ Dorsal and ventral pancreatic buds fuse during	7th week
➤ Islets of Langerhans develop in the	3rd week
➤ Insulin secretion begins at about	10th week
➤ Secretion of bile by hepatocytes begins at about	12th week
➤ Development of spleen begins during	5th week

GOLDEN FACTS TO REMEMBER

➤ **Most common site of the accessory pancreatic tissue**	Mucosa of the stomach and Meckel's diverticulum
➤ **Annular pancreas**	Pancreatic tissue forming a collar around the second part of the duodenum
➤ **Most fatal congenital anomaly of the liver**	Intrahepatic biliary atresia
➤ **Spleniculi**	Accessory spleens less than 2 cm in diameter
➤ **Most common source of aberrant right hepatic artery**	Superior mesenteric artery
➤ **Most common source of aberrant left hepatic artery**	Left gastric artery
➤ **Main pancreatic duct is formed by**	Distal part of dorsal pancreatic duct and entire ventral pancreatic duct

CLINICAL PROBLEM SOLVING

PROBLEMS

1. **In adults, the left lobe of the liver is smaller than the right lobe.** Why? Give its embryological basis.
2. **Give the embryological basis of presence of notches on the superior/anterior border of the spleen.**
3. **Give the embryological basis of Riedel's lobe** and discuss its clinical significance.
4. **What is Phrygian cap?** Give the embryological basis of Phrygian cap.
5. **What is the embryological basis of extensive enlargement of liver in the intrauterine life?** Give reasons for the proportionately large size of the liver in early postnatal life.
6. Intrahepatic biliary atresia has a very poor prognosis as compared to extrahepatic biliary atresia. Why?

SOLUTIONS

1. In early development, both the lobes of liver (right and left) are of equal size. After the 9th week of intrauterine life (IUL), the growth rate of left lobe of the liver regresses and some of its hepatocytes degenerate due to reduced nutritional and oxygen supply to this part of the liver. Such degeneration may be complete at the left end of the left lobe so as to leave only a fibrous appendage at the left extremity of the liver called **appendix of liver**. (Also see answer to Clinical Problem No. 5.)
2. The spleen develops by condensation of mesenchymal cells between two layers of dorsal mesogastrium. At first, small lobules of splenic tissue are formed by condensation of mesenchymal cells lying between the two layers of the dorsal mesogastrium. Later, the lobules of splenic tissue fuse together to form the spleen.

   The notches on superior (anterior) border of adult spleen are a reflection of lobular origin of the spleen.
3. The Riedel's lobe is a tongue-like downward extension of right lobe of the liver. It develops as an extension of normal hepatic tissue from inferior margin of the liver, usually from the right lobe.

   Its clinical significance is that it may be mistaken for an abnormal abdominal mass.

N.B. Rarely, there may be an anomalous extension of the hepatic tissue through the diaphragm into chest.

4. It is a folded fundus of gallbladder. It may occur due to failure of canalization of the fundus of the gallbladder. This anomaly is so named because the folded fundus of gallbladder looks like a cap worn by people of **Phrygia** – an ancient country of Asia Minor.
5. During the early phase of development, liver is far more highly vascularized than rest of the gut. As a result, liver parenchyma gets abundant oxygenated blood, which stimulates its extensive growth. Moreover, fetal liver is hemopoietic in function. At 3 months of gestation, the liver almost fills abdominal cavity and its left lobe is nearly as large as right. When the hemopoietic function of the liver is taken over by the spleen and bone marrow, the left lobe undergoes some regression and becomes smaller than the right.
   - In the early part of development, the liver forms about 10% of body weight, and in the later part, it comes down to about 5% of body weight.
   - The hemopoietic function of the liver is sufficiently diminished during last 2 months of pregnancy.
6. The extrahepatic biliary atresia is surgically correctible, whereas the intrahepatic biliary atresia is surgically untreatable. Therefore, the intrahepatic biliary atresia has a very poor prognosis.

20 Respiratory System

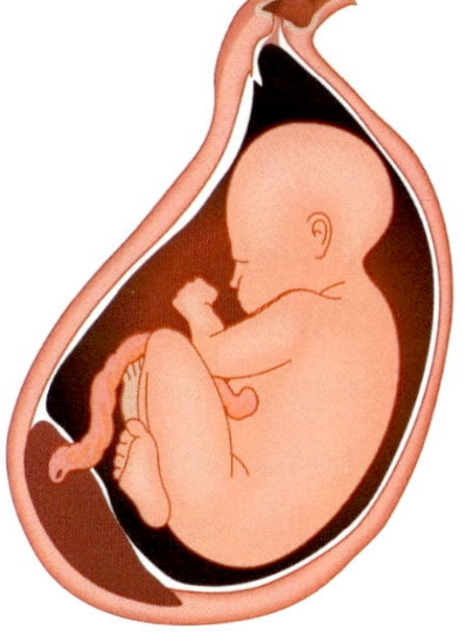

LEARNING OBJECTIVES

After studying this chapter, the students should be able to:

- Describe the development of various components of respiratory tract.
- Describe the development of lung and pleura AN 25.2
- Describe the embryological basis of tracheoesophageal fistula. AN 25.5
- Describe the various stages of maturation of lung.
- Write short notes on (a) medicolegal importance of a newborn lung, (b) respiratory distress syndrome/hyaline membrane disease, and (c) azygos lobe of the lung.

OVERVIEW

The respiratory tract is divided into two parts: **upper respiratory tract** (URT) and **lower respiratory tract** (LRT).

- The URT consists of nose, nasopharynx, and oropharynx.
- The LRT consists of larynx, trachea, principal bronchi, intrapulmonary bronchi, and lungs.

The development of various components of URT is described separately in other chapters. This chapter discusses development of the LRT, which is conventionally termed **development of the respiratory system** by embryologists.

DEVELOPMENT OF RESPIRATORY SYSTEM

The respiratory system is endodermal in origin. *It develops from a median diverticulum of foregut called* **respiratory diverticulum** when embryo is about 4 weeks old (Fig. 20.1). Therefore, lining epithelium of larynx, trachea, bronchi, and lungs is derived from endoderm. The cartilages, muscles, and connective tissue components of the respiratory system develop from **splanchnic mesoderm** surrounding the foregut.

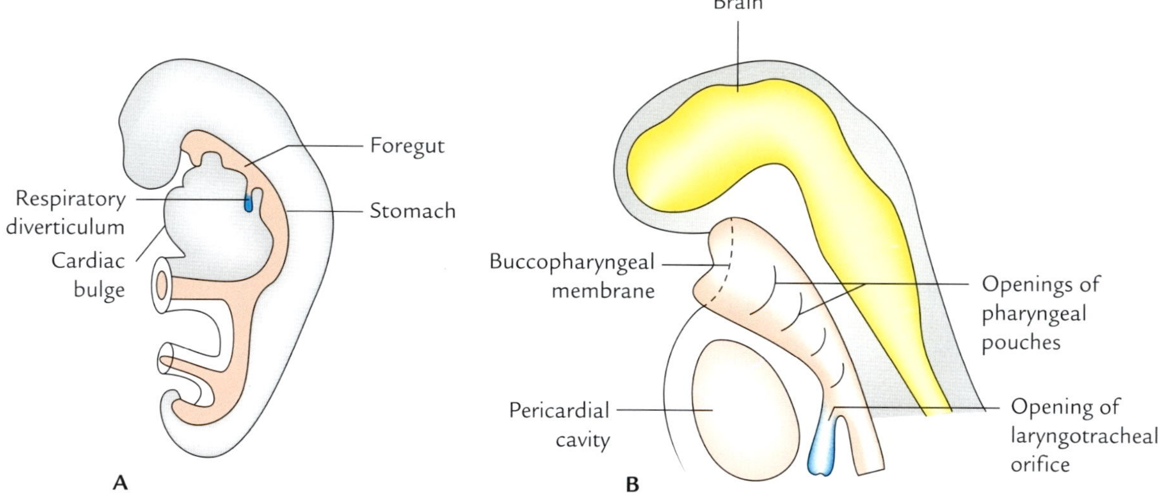

Fig. 20.1 Site of development of respiratory diverticulum as seen in embryo. (A) A 25-day-old embryo. Note the relationship of diverticulum to stomach. (B) Sagittal section of 5-week-old embryo showing openings of pharyngeal pouches and laryngotracheal orifice.

Development of Respiratory (Laryngotracheal) Diverticulum

The respiratory diverticulum develops as an outgrowth from ventral aspect of the cranial part of foregut.

This diverticulum is first seen as a midline groove (**laryngotracheal groove**) in the endodermal lining of floor of primitive pharynx just caudal to hypobranchial eminence (to be very precise *epiglottal swelling*) during the 4th week of the intrauterine life (IUL) (Fig. 20.2). The groove is flanked by sixth pharyngeal arches. The groove deepens to form a longitudinal diverticulum called **laryngotracheal diverticulum** (Fig. 20.3).

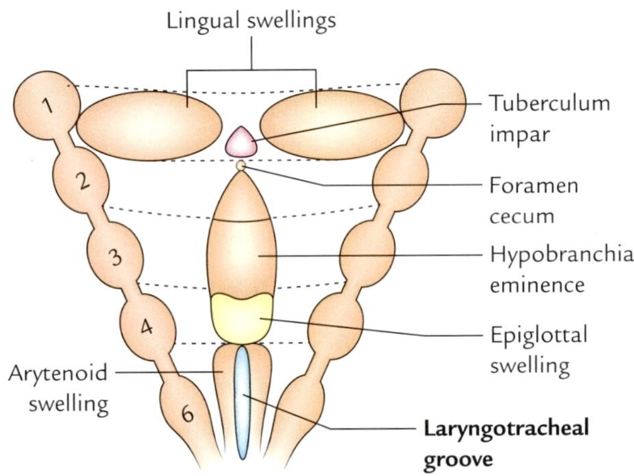

Fig. 20.2 Formation of laryngotracheal groove.

The distal part of this diverticulum is separated from the esophagus by development of **tracheoesophageal septum,** whereas its cranial part continues to communicate with the pharynx. This communication with pharynx forms **laryngeal inlet**.

Separation of Tracheobronchial Diverticulum from Esophagus

The **tracheoesophageal septum** develops from two lateral folds – the **tracheoesophageal folds** that grow medially and fuse with each other in the midline to form this septum.

The laryngotracheal diverticulum grows downward to enter thorax, where it becomes bifid to form **two** (right and left) **bronchial/lung buds**.

The part of diverticulum proximal to bifurcation forms the larynx and trachea, whereas the bronchial buds form the bronchi and lung parenchyma.

Each lung bud invaginates into **pericardioperitoneal canal**. The right and left pericardioperitoneal canals form the right and left pleural cavities, respectively.

Development of Individual Parts of the Respiratory System

Larynx

The larynx develops from the cranial-most part of **laryngotracheal diverticulum**. The communication

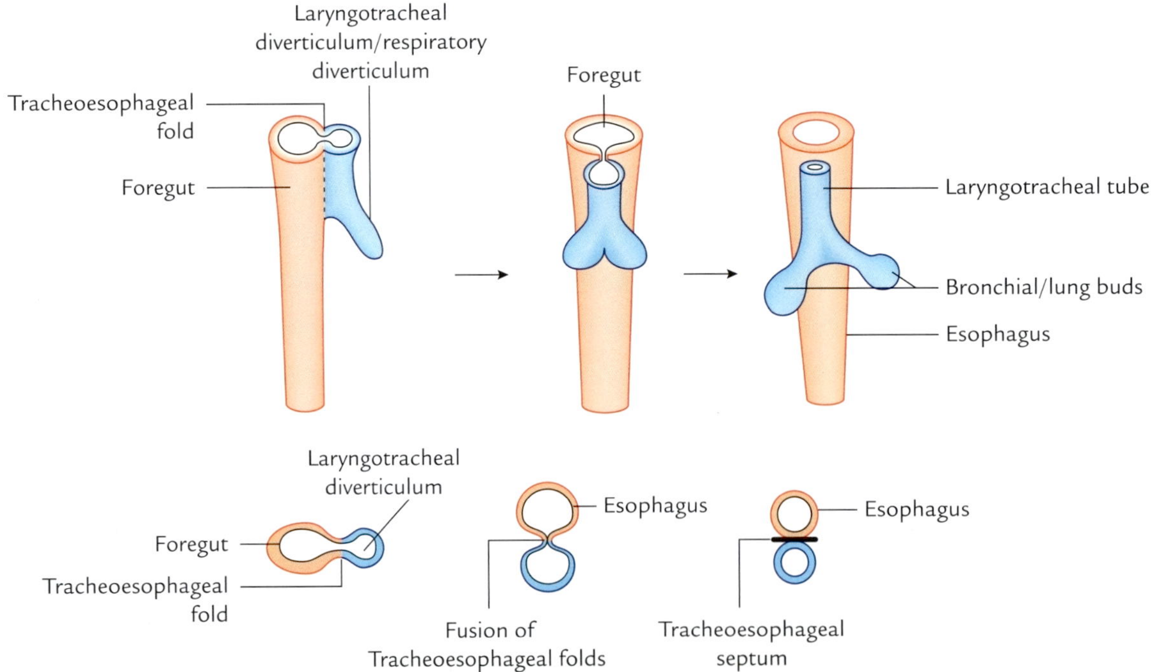

Fig. 20.3 Successive stages in the development of respiratory diverticulum. Figures below are transverse section of the above figures to show the formation of tracheoesophageal septum and appreciate how it separates foregut into trachea and esophagus.

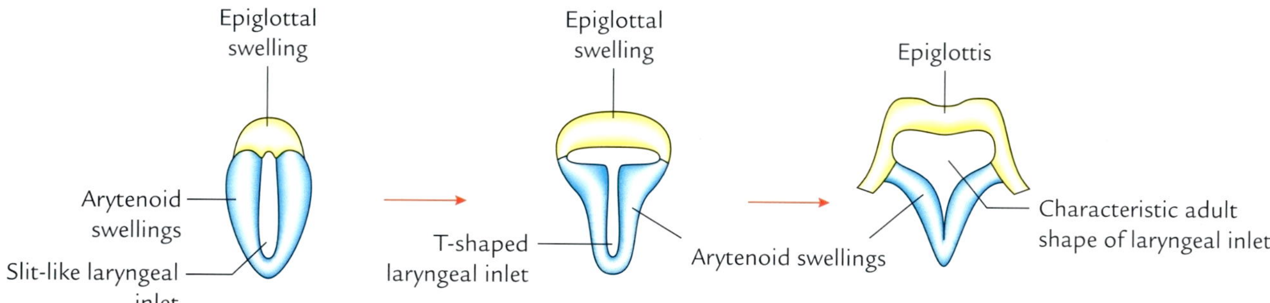

Fig. 20.4 Change in shape of laryngeal inlet during development of larynx.

between the laryngotracheal diverticulum and primitive pharynx persists as a **laryngeal inlet**. The mesenchyme (of fourth and sixth pharyngeal arches) surrounding the laryngeal orifice proliferates. As a result, the slit-like laryngeal orifice becomes T shaped. Subsequently, mesenchyme of fourth and sixth pharyngeal arches forms thyroid, cricoid, and arytenoids cartilages, and laryngeal orifice acquires a characteristic adult shape (Fig. 20.4). The lining epithelium of larynx develops from endoderm of the cranial end of laryngotracheal diverticulum. At first, the endodermal cells proliferate and completely obliterate the lumen of larynx. Later on, the cells obliterating the lumen breakdown and recanalization of larynx takes place. During recanalization, the endodermal cells form two pairs of folds: an upper pair of **vestibular folds** and a lower pair of **vocal folds,** which extend anteroposteriorly in the lumen of the larynx and give rise to **false and true vocal cords,** respectively. A pair of lateral recesses bound by these folds is called **laryngeal ventricles.**

All the cartilages of the larynx (e.g., thyroid, cricoid, arytenoids, and cuneiform), except **epiglottis,** develop from mesenchyme of fourth and sixth pharyngeal arch, which is derived from neural crest cells. The epiglottis develops from the caudal part of **hypobranchial eminence.**

The muscles of the larynx develop from the mesoderm of fourth and sixth pharyngeal arches. Therefore, these muscles are supplied by nerve of the fourth arch (**superior laryngeal nerve**) and nerve of the sixth arch (**recurrent laryngeal nerve**).

CLINICAL CORRELATION

Anomalies of Larynx

1. **Laryngeal atresia and stenosis:** This rare anomaly of larynx results from failure of recanalization of the larynx that leads to obstruction of the upper respiratory tract (also called *congenital high airway obstruction syndrome*) due to narrowing of some sites. Most commonly, the atresia (blockage) and stenosis (narrowing) are seen at the level of vocal folds.
2. **Laryngeal web:** In this anomaly, membranous, web-like tissue is present in the laryngeal lumen, usually at the level of vocal folds, which may partially obstruct the airway. This web-like tissue is derived from endodermal cells that fail to break out during recanalization of larynx.

Trachea

The trachea develops from part of the laryngotracheal diverticulum (respiratory diverticulum), which lies between the larynx and point of division of the diverticulum into **bronchial buds.** The endoderm of laryngotracheal diverticulum forms the lining epithelium and glands of the trachea. The cartilage, muscle, and connective tissue of trachea develop from surrounding splanchnopleuric intraembryonic mesoderm surrounding laryngotracheal groove.

N.B. Trachea is separated from the esophagus by a tracheoesophageal septum (see p. 216).

CLINICAL CORRELATION

Anomalies of trachea

1. **Tracheoesophageal fistula (TEF):** It is an abnormal communication between the trachea and esophagus. This anomaly is often associated with *esophageal atresia*. It occurs in 1/3000–4500 births.

   The TEF occurs due to defective development of *tracheoesophageal septum*. The tracheoesophageal folds fail to fuse with each other in a small segment, producing an abnormal communication between the trachea and esophagus – the TEF.

   The various types of TEF are as follows (Fig. 20.5):

   (a) **Upper part of the esophagus ends in a blind pouch and its lower part communicates with the trachea (85%–90%)** (Fig. 20.5A). This is most common variety.
   Clinical features: See p. 190 and Fig. 18.7).

Continued

(b) As type (a) but the tracheoesophageal communication/canal is replaced by a fibrous cord (Fig. 20.5B).
(c) Both upper and lower parts of the esophagus communicate with the trachea by a common narrow canal. It is called H-shaped TEF (4%) (Fig. 20.5C).
(d) Upper part of the esophagus communicates with the trachea and lower end forms a blind pouch (Fig. 20.5D).
(e) Both upper and lower parts of the esophagus communicate with the trachea separately (Fig. 20.5E).

When milk or fluid is given to newborn infants with TEF, it causes coughing and choking because milk or fluid enters into the respiratory tract. It may also lead to lung infection (pneumonia).

2. **Tracheal stenosis (narrowing of trachea):** It is rare and occurs due to anterior deviation of the tracheoesophageal septum.
3. **Tracheal atresia (tracheal obstruction):** It occurs due to the presence of a web of tissue within tracheal lumen. This tissue is derived from proliferation of endodermal cells.
4. **Tracheal bronchus and tracheal lobe:** Sometimes, the trachea presents a diverticulum that may either end blindly (blind bronchus) or supply a lobe of lung called *tracheal lobe*, which is not a normal part of the lung. Sometimes, it may replace a normal terminal bronchus, namely, apical bronchus of upper lobe of lung (Fig. 20.6).

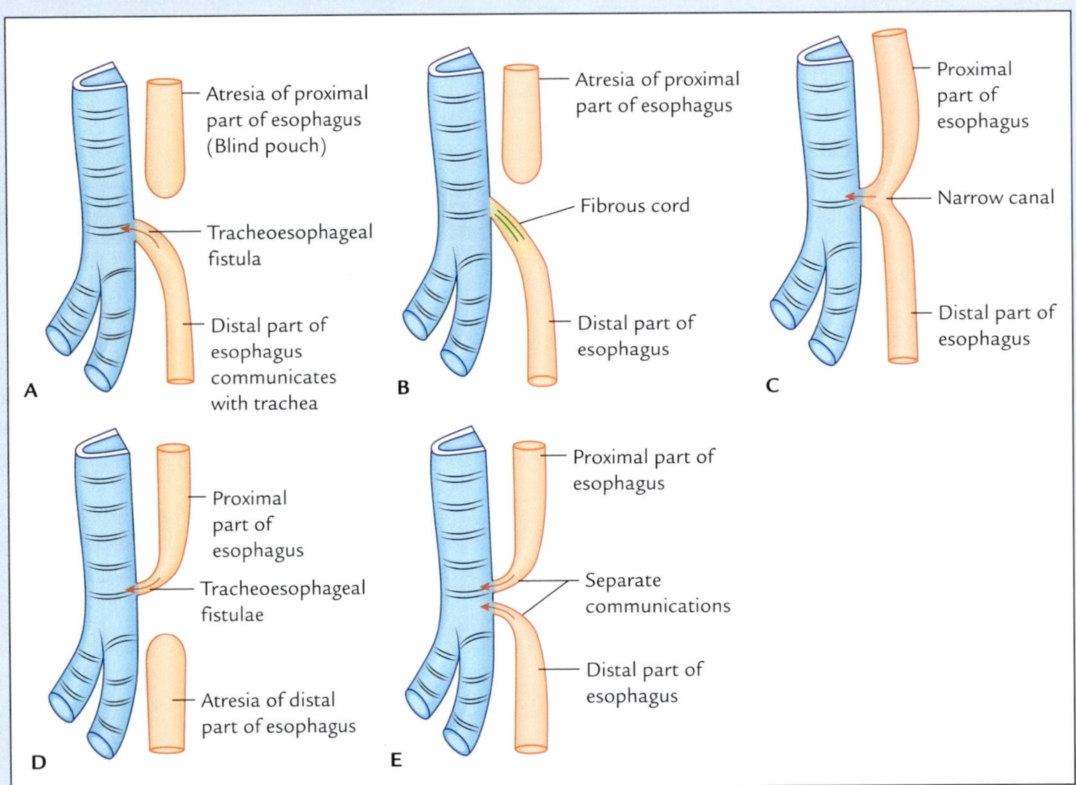

Fig. 20.5 Types of tracheoesophageal fistulae. (A) Atresia of the upper part of the esophagus and lower part communicating with trachea (commonest type of tracheoesophageal fistula). (B) Atresia of the esophagus and connection between the distal part of esophagus and trachea by a fibrous cord. (C) Both proximal and distal parts of esophagus connected to the trachea by a narrow canal. (D) Atresia of distal part of esophagus and connection between the proximal part of esophagus and trachea. (E) Separate communications of proximal and distal parts of esophagus to the trachea.

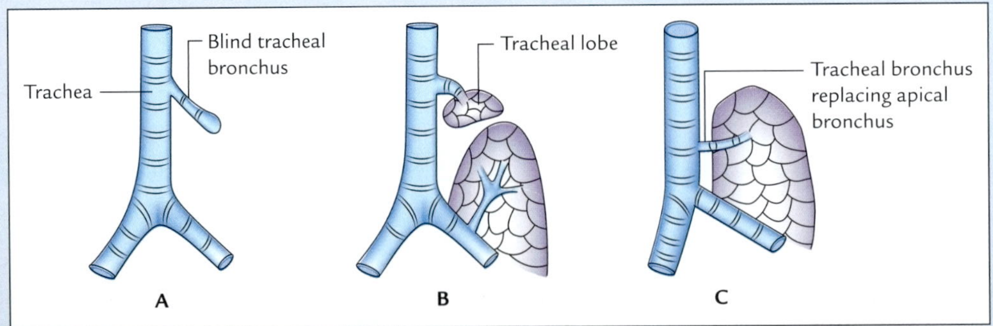

Fig. 20.6 Accessory bronchi arising from trachea. (A) Blind tracheal bronchus. (B) Tracheal bronchus supplying an accessory lobe of lung. (C) Tracheal bronchus replacing apical bronchus.

Development of Lung and Pleura (Fig. 20.7)

The lung basically consists of *bronchial tree, lung parenchyma, and a little amount of connective tissue stroma.*

During 5th week of IUL, the laryngotracheal (respiratory) diverticulum divides into two **bronchial buds.** Each bronchial bud develops into a **principal bronchus**, thus forming **right and left principal bronchi.** The right principal bronchus is slightly larger than the left and oriented more in line with the trachea. The left principal bronchus comes to lie more transversely than the right. This embryonic relationship persists in the adult life, and therefore foreign body is more likely to enter into the right principal bronchus.

The principal bronchi subdivide into **secondary bronchi**, which further divide and subdivide to form **lobar** and **segmental bronchi**, respectively.

Thus, the **right principal bronchus gives rise to three lobar bronchi: upper, middle, and lower**, which supply the upper, middle, and lower lobes of the right lung.

On the left side, the left **principal bronchus** gives rise to **two lobar bronchi (upper and lower)** that supply the superior and inferior lobes of the left lung, respectively. The lobes are separated from each other by fissures.

Each lobar bronchus divides into 10 segmental bronchi for each lung by the 7th week of IUL. Each segmental bronchus with its surrounding mass of mesenchyme forms the **bronchopulmonary segment**. Therefore, each lung consists of 10 bronchopulmonary segments.

By the end of 6th month, about 17 generations of bronchial subdivisions are formed. About six to seven divisions of bronchial tree form after birth.

Thus, divisions and subdivisions of each segmental bronchus form the distal part of the bronchial tree consisting of **bronchioles, respiratory bronchioles, alveolar ducts,** and **alveoli.**

The ***respiratory bronchioles, alveolar ducts, and alveoli together form parenchyma of lung***, which is involved in the transfer of gases between blood within capillaries and air in the alveoli.

The **endoderm** of respiratory diverticulum gives rise to **lining epithelium of the bronchial tree.** All other elements in the wall of the bronchial tree such as cartilages, smooth muscles, and connective tissue are derived from surrounding splanchnic mesoderm. The splanchnic mesoderm also forms the connective tissue and capillaries of the lung.

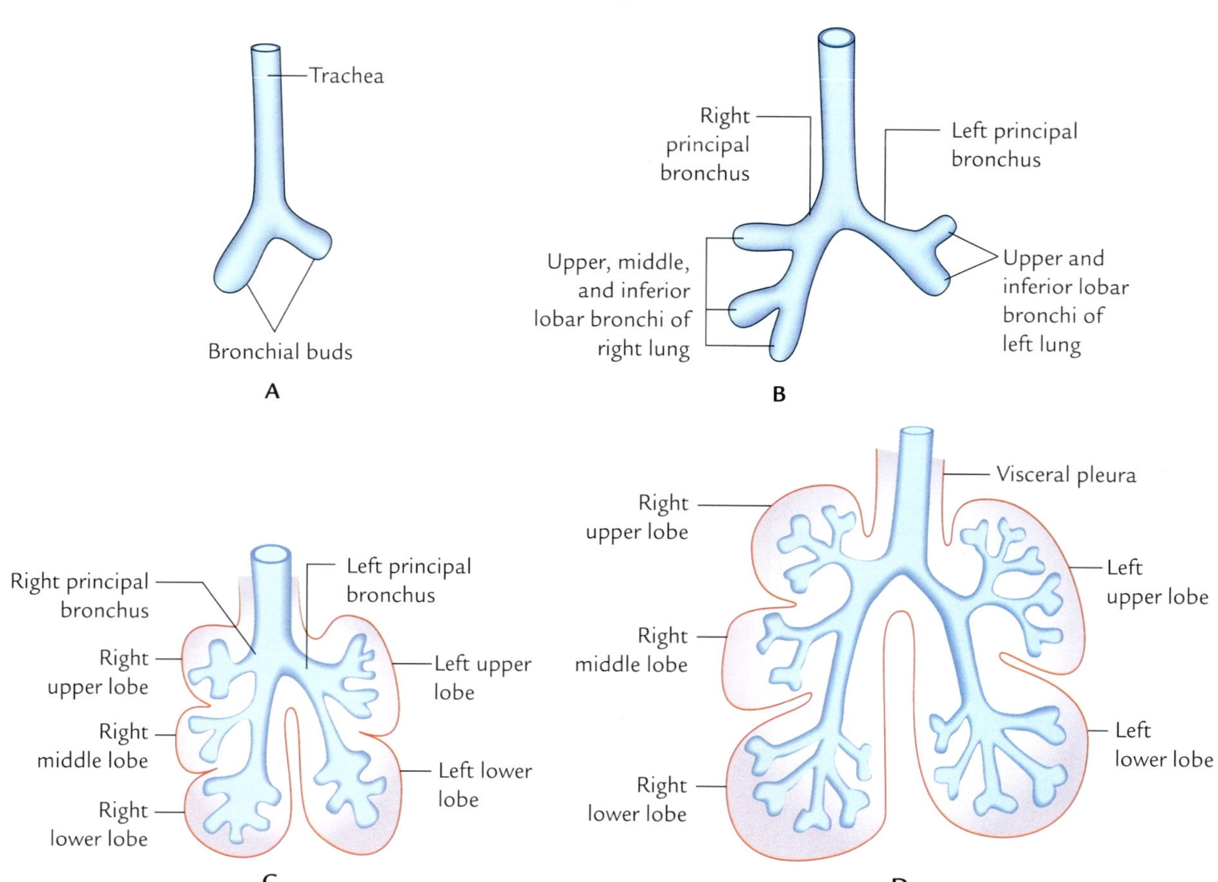

Fig. 20.7 Successive stages in the development of bronchi and lungs: (A) At 4 weeks, (B) at 5 weeks, (C) at 6 weeks, and (D) at 8 weeks.

The lung parenchyma developing from bronchi is separated from each other by mesoderm. The mesoderm also forms the connective tissue basis of the lung and pleura lining its surface. Because pleura lines the surface of each lobe separately, the lobes become separated by the **fissures.**

N.B. The bifurcation of the trachea at the time of birth lies opposite to T4 vertebra.

Development of Pleura

The **pleural cavity** develops from **pericardioperitoneal canals of coelomic cavity**.

The lung buds arising from tracheal part of laryngotracheal diverticulum invaginate the pleuroperitoneal canals (primitive pleural cavities) and grow to gradually fill them to form **definitive pleural cavity.**

Thus, the pleural cavity consists of two layers: a **visceral pleura** and a **parietal pleura**. The visceral pleura lines the lung, while the parietal pleura lines the thoracic wall. The two layers are separated from each other by a slit-like pleural cavity.

The visceral pleura develops from splanchnopleuric mesoderm, hence supplied by autonomic nerves, while parietal pleura develops from somatopleuric mesoderm, hence supplied by somatic nerves. For details, see p. 230.

Maturation of the Lungs

Maturation of the lungs is divided into four stages/periods (Fig. 20.8): **pseudoglandular stage, canalicular stage, terminal sac stage**, and **alveolar stage**.

1. **Pseudoglandular stage/period (5–16 weeks):** During this period, histologically the appearance of the lung resembles a developing exocrine gland. The divisions of bronchi have reached up to terminal bronchioles (i.e., all major elements of the lung are formed), but respiratory elements (e.g., respiratory bronchioles and alveoli) that are involved in respiration are not formed. Hence, **fetus born during this period cannot survive.**
2. **Canalicular stage (16–26 weeks):** During this stage, lumen of terminal bronchioles dilate and there is a further subdivision of terminal bronchioles into respiratory bronchioles. The respiratory bronchioles divide into alveolar ducts. Few terminal sacs (primitive alveoli) may also be formed at the ends of respiratory

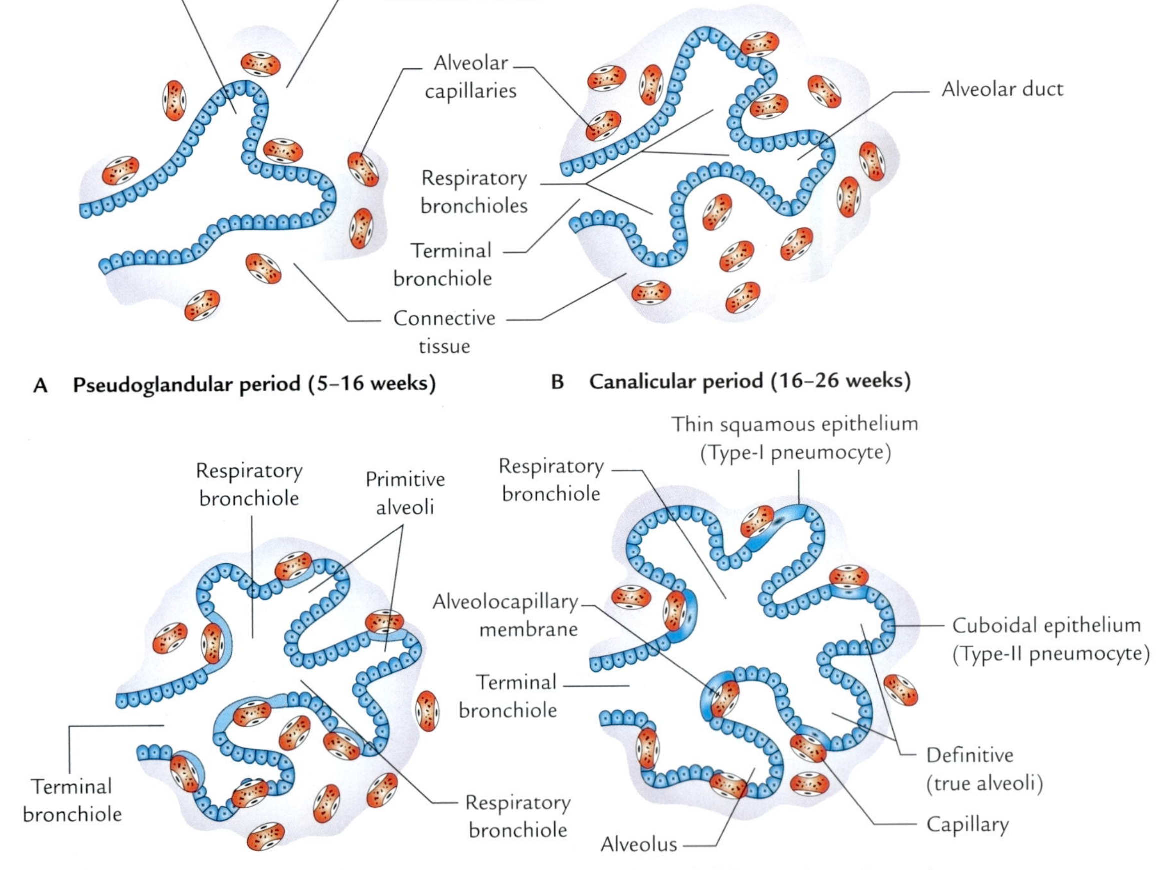

Fig. 20.8 Schematic diagrams showing stages of lung maturation.

Table 20.1 Stages of maturation of lungs

Stage	Period	Development Changes
Pseudoglandular stage	5–16 weeks	• Bronchial tree is formed up to terminal bronchioles • Elements of the bronchial tree involved in respiration (e.g., respiratory bronchioles, alveolar ducts, and alveoli) are not formed • Respiration is not possible at this stage; hence, **fetuses born at this stage cannot survive**
Canalicular stage	16–26 weeks	• Respiratory bronchioles and alveolar ducts are formed • Few alveolar sacs are also formed • Lung tissue is well vascularized • **Fetuses born at the end of this stage can survive if given intensive care**
Terminal sac (saccular) stage	26 weeks to birth	• Large number of terminal sacs (primitive alveoli) develop • Capillaries bulge into developing sacs • Intimate contact develops between epithelium of sac and endothelium of capillary to permit adequate exchange of gases for survival of fetus, if born prematurely; **fetuses born at this stage survive**
Alveolar stage	8 months to 8 years	• Formation of definitive (true) alveoli with an increase in their number • Type II pneumocytes produce a sufficient amount of surfactant • Free exchange of gases begins across the respiratory membrane/alveolocapillary membrane (blood–air barrier) formed by epithelium of alveoli and endothelium of capillaries • Independent and parallel pulmonary and systemic circulations are established

bronchioles. The **fetus born toward the end of this period may survive if given intensive care.**

The main thing that happens in this stage is that the lung tissue is well vascularized.

3. **Terminal sac stage (26 weeks to birth):** During this period, a large number of terminal sacs (primitive alveoli) develop. The capillaries also proliferate and form a plexus around the terminal sacs. The walls (epithelium) of terminal sacs become very thin and capillaries bulge into these sacs. The intimate contact between epithelial and endothelial cells establishes the **blood–air barrier**, which permits adequate exchange of gases for survival of the fetus if born prematurely. Terminal sacs are mainly lined by endodermal squamous cells called **type I alveolar epithelial cells (type I pneumocytes)** across which gaseous exchange takes place. Scattered among the squamous epithelial cells (type I pneumocytes), a few rounded **type II alveolar epithelial cells** (type II pneumocytes) are also present. The type II pneumocytes secrete **surfactant** and their number gradually increases toward the full-term. There is also an increase in number of lymphatic capillaries.
4. **Alveolar stage (8 months to 8 years):** In this stage, the terminal sacs and respiratory bronchioles divide and form the alveolar ducts; at the end of alveolar ducts, the **definitive (true) alveoli are formed.** The formation of mature (true) alveoli continues even after birth till the age of about 8 years.

The true alveoli that are formed have extremely thin wall and are lined by type I and type II pneumocytes. The **type II pneumocytes produce a sufficient amount of surfactant** for survival. The capillaries also proliferate and vascularize the newly formed alveoli. A number of alveoli reach the adult level by the 8th year.

N.B.

- The characteristic mature alveoli do not form until after birth.
- About 95% of mature alveoli develop after birth.

The stages of lung maturation are summarized in Table 20.1.

FETAL BREATHING MOVEMENTS

The real-time ultrasonography has revealed that fetal breathing movements (FBMs) start before birth. They occur intermittently and exert sufficient force to cause aspiration of amniotic fluid in the lungs. The FBMs are essential for the normal lung development and increase as the time of delivery approaches.

N.B. Before birth, the fetus undergoes breathing exercises for several months.

At birth, the lungs are approximately half filled with the fluid, which is derived from amniotic fluid and tracheal glands.

Aeration of lungs at birth rapidly replaces the intra-alveolar fluid by the air.

This fluid from the lungs is cleared by following three routes:

1. Through the mouth and nose by pressure on the fetus's thoracic wall during vaginal delivery
2. Through pulmonary arteries, veins, and capillaries
3. Through lymphatics

N.B. Three important factors essential for normal lung development are (a) adequate thoracic space to allow lung growth, (b) fetal breathing movements, and (c) an adequate volume of amniotic fluid.

CLINICAL CORRELATION

1. ***Medicolegal importance of the newborn lung:*** The lungs of a newborn infant *born alive* always contain some air within them; hence, they float in water and crepitate on pressure. The lungs of a newborn infant *born dead* (*stillborn*) are firm and sink when placed in water because they contain fluid, not air. For this reason, it is firm and does not crepitate on pressure.

   This fact is of medicolegal importance because it tells whether the newborn infant was born alive or born dead (stillborn).
2. ***Respiratory distress syndrome (RDS):*** This clinical condition affects about 2% of live newborn infants. As the name suggests, infants born with this condition develop rapid, labored breathing shortly after birth. This condition is common in premature infants. The most common cause of RDS is deficiency of surfactant.

   In this disease, alveoli of lungs are often filled with fluid having high protein content, which resembles glassy hyaline membrane. Hence, RDS is also known as **hyaline membrane disease.**

   The hyaline membrane disease accounts for about 20% of deaths among newborn infants.

   Corticosteroids (glucocorticoids) and thyroxine, which are involved in lung maturation and production of surfactant, may be used therapeutically. The baby should be supported by oxygen therapy, maintaining continuous positive airway pressure (CPAP).
3. ***Congenital anomalies of the lung***
   (a) **Agenesis (nondevelopment) of the lung:** It is a rare condition and occurs if one of the bronchial buds fails to develop. Agenesis of both the lungs is still rare. The unilateral agenesis of the lung is compatible with life.
   (b) **Hypoplasia of lungs:** In this condition, the lungs are small and underdeveloped. It usually occurs due to *congenital diaphragmatic hernia* (*CDH*) in which abdominal contents herniate into thorax and the lung is unable to develop normally because it gets compressed by abdominal viscera. The lung hypoplasia is characterized by a markedly reduced lung volume and hypertrophy of smooth muscle of pulmonary arteries.
   (c) **Abnormal lobes of lungs** (Fig. 20.9): In this condition, sometimes the right lung may consist of two lobes instead of three or the left lung may consist of three lobes instead of two. These anomalies occur due to abnormal division of principal bronchi into lobar bronchi, and are associated with anomalies of lung fissures. These anomalies are not clinically significant.

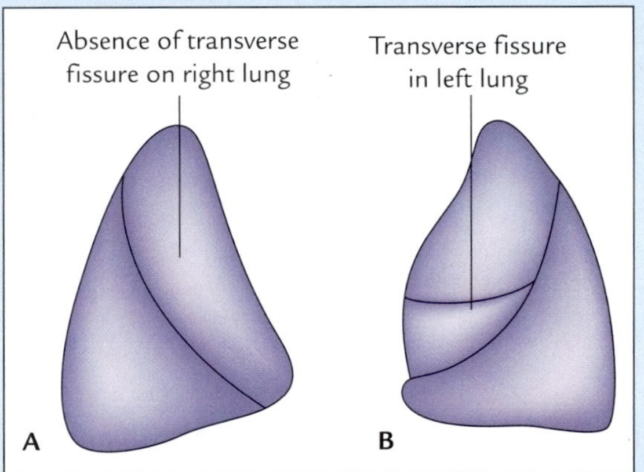

Fig. 20.9 Abnormal lobes of the lungs: (A) Right lung with two lobes due to the absence of transverse fissure and (B) left lung with three lobes due to the presence of the transverse fissure.

   (d) **Azygos lobe of the lung (lobe of Wrisberg)** (Fig. 20.10): It is a portion of upper lobe of the right lung that lies medial to *arch of the azygos vein.* The azygos vein lies in floor of vertical fissure lined by pulmonary pleura. The azygos lobe is found in the right lung because azygos vein itself is on the right side. **Azygos lobe is the commonest accessory lobe of the lung.** It is considered as a normal anatomical variation of right lung present in 0.1% cases. For details, see *Clinical and Surgical Anatomy* by Dr Vishram Singh.
   (e) **Ectopic lung lobes** (Fig. 20.11): They arise from trachea or esophagus. These lobes probably form additional respiratory buds of the trachea and foregut that develop independently of main respiratory system.
   (f) **Congenital polycystic lung:** Multiple cysts are formed in the lung due to abnormal dilatation of terminal bronchioles. These cysts are small and multiple, giving the lung a **honeycomb appearance**, which can be seen in the radiograph. Because these cysts usually drain poorly, they frequently cause chronic infections. For this reason, congenital polycystic lung is clinically most important.

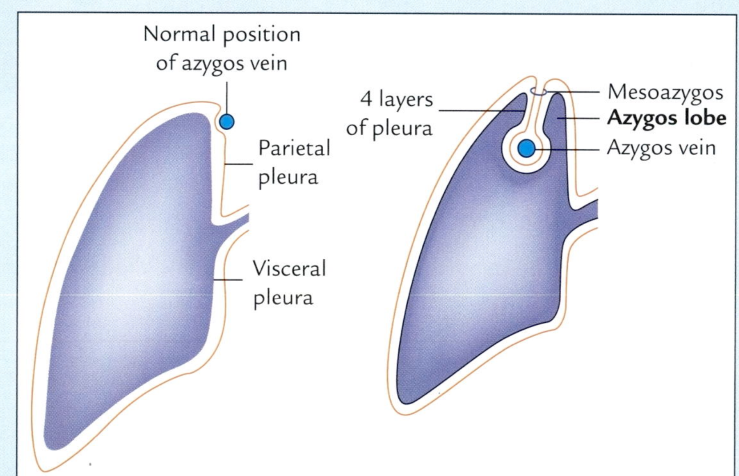

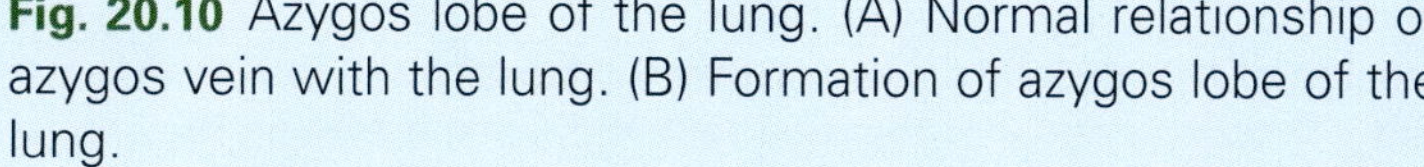
Fig. 20.10 Azygos lobe of the lung. (A) Normal relationship of azygos vein with the lung. (B) Formation of azygos lobe of the lung.

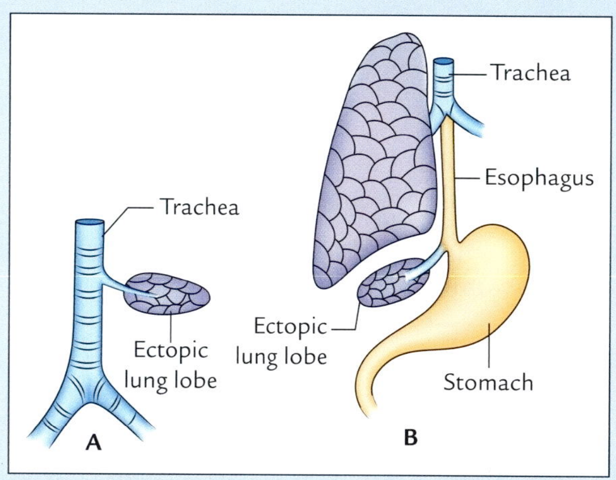

Fig. 20.11 Ectopic lung lobes. (A) Arising from trachea. (B) Arising from esophagus.

GESTATIONAL AGE OF KEY DEVELOPMENTAL EVENTS

Developmental Event	Gestational Age
➢ Respiratory diverticulum appears during	4th week of IUL
➢ Tracheoesophageal septum develops by the end of	5th week of IUL
➢ Maturation of lungs begins during	5th–6th week of IUL
➢ Maturation of lungs (formation of definitive alveoli) takes place during	8 months to 8 years
➢ Breathing movements occur	Before birth
➢ Respiration occurs	At birth

GOLDEN FACTS TO REMEMBER

➢ **All the cartilages of larynx develop from neural crest cells in the mesenchyme of fourth and sixth pharyngeal arches *except***	Epiglottis, which develops from caudal part of the hypopharyngeal/hypobranchial eminence
➢ **Commonest type of tracheoesophageal fistula**	One in which the upper part of esophagus ends in a blind pouch and lower end of esophagus communicates with the trachea
➢ **Commonest accessory lobe of the lung**	Azygos lobe
➢ **Production of surfactant begins by**	20th week of IUL
➢ **Most of mature (true) alveoli are formed**	After birth
➢ **Most common cause of respiratory distress syndrome**	Deficiency of surfactant
➢ **Most important congenital anomaly of the lung (clinically)**	Congenital polycystic lung

CLINICAL PROBLEM SOLVING

PROBLEMS

1. **An obstetrician observed continuous choking and coughing in a newborn boy.** A pediatrician was called for expert opinion and management of the case. **He noted that the infant's mouth was full of saliva**, and **he had difficulty in breathing.** The pediatrician tried to pass a catheter through the esophagus into the stomach, but he failed to do so. A **radiograph revealed the presence of air in the stomach.** What is the most likely diagnosis? Give its embryological basis.
2. **A premature infant has labored breathing immediately after birth. The baby soon became cyanotic and died. What is the most likely diagnosis?** Give its embryological basis.
3. A newborn baby was born with **tracheoesophageal fistula (TEF).** What is the most common type of TEF? Give the embryological basis of TEF.
4. **Babies born after 7 months of gestation usually survive. Why?**
5. **Babies born at 6 months of gestation develop respiratory distress syndrome and die.** Give its embryological basis.
6. **What is surfactant**? How does it reduce the surface tension of the alveoli to prevent their collapse?
7. Which therapy is used during pregnancy for prevention of respiratory distress syndrome (RDS) in preterm labor?
8. **Shadows of lungs in chest radiograph of a newborn infant are denser than those of adults. Why?**

SOLUTIONS

1. The most likely diagnosis is **tracheoesophageal fistula** associated with atresia of the upper part of the esophagus. The catheter could not be passed due to atresia of the esophagus. The air could enter the stomach through communication between the trachea and lower part of the esophagus (also see p. 190).
2. The most likely diagnosis is **respiratory distress syndrome.** In this disease, the lungs are underinflated and alveoli are filled with fluid. It occurs due to deficiency of surfactant produced by type II pneumocytes. By labored breathing (characterized by increased rate and depth of respiration, flaring of nostrils, and retraction of the sternum and intercostal spaces), the baby was trying to overcome respiratory problems, in which he failed, became cyanotic, and finally died.
3. **TEF** occurs due to incomplete separation of the esophagus from trachea due to incomplete development of tracheoesophageal septum. The most common type of TEF is one in which trachea communicates with the lower part of the esophagus, and upper part of esophagus ends as a blind pouch.
4. **A premature baby born after 7 months of gestation can survive** due to following two reasons:
   (a) By the 7th month of gestation, sufficient number of blood capillaries make close contact with the wall of alveolar sac to allow exchange of gases.
   (b) After 7 months of gestation, lung alveoli (type II pneumocytes) produce a sufficient amount of surfactant to reduce the surface tension of alveoli to prevent their collapse during expiration. This leads to normal lung function.
5. **A baby born before or at 6 months of gestation does not produce a sufficient amount of surfactant** to reduce surface tension in the alveoli to permit normal lung function. Consequently, alveoli collapse, baby develops respiratory distress syndrome, and usually dies.
6. The **surfactant is a complex mixture of phospholipids and proteins.** It is produced by type II pneumocytes and its production begins by 20th week of gestation.

   Before actual breathing takes place, the alveoli of the lung are filled with fluid, containing surfactant and mucus from bronchial glands. When respiration begins after birth, the fluid is cleared from the lung alveoli (see p. 221), but surfactant remains as a thin layer lining the alveoli. The surfactant prevents collapse of lung alveoli during expiration of newborn babies.
7. The **maternal glucocorticoid during pregnancy** accelerates fetal lung development and surfactant production. Based on this finding, corticosteroids (betamethasone) are now routinely used to prevent the RDS in preterm labor.
8. On chest radiograph, the lungs of a newborn infant appear denser than those of adults because **they have fewer alveoli.**

21 Body Cavities and Diaphragm

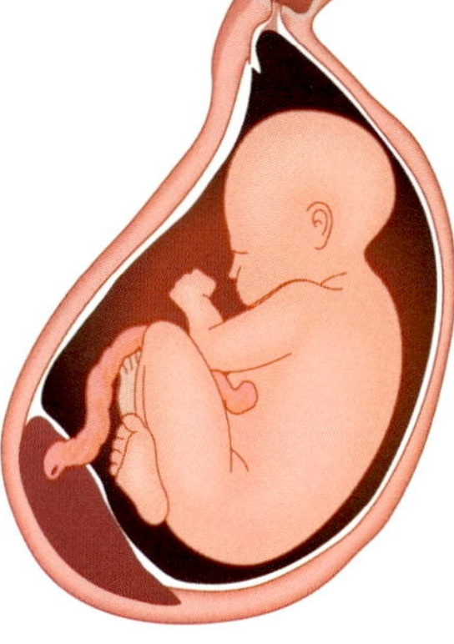

LEARNING OBJECTIVES

After studying this chapter, the student should be able to:

- Describe the formation of intraembryonic coelom. AN 79.4
- Describe in brief the formation of body cavities.
- Describe the development of diaphragm in detail and discuss the congenital anomalies associated with it. AN 52.5
- Write short notes on (a) foramen of Bochdalek, (b) congenital diaphragmatic hernia, and (c) retrosternal hernia.

OVERVIEW

There are three body cavities, viz. **pericardial**, **pleural**, and **peritoneal**. The **pericardial cavity** is related to heart, the **pleural cavity** to lungs, and the **peritoneal cavity** to abdominal viscera. All these cavities develop from intraembryonic coelom.

Initially, the intraembryonic coelom is one continuous space. Later, it is divided into three parts: pericardial, pleural, and peritoneal cavities by the development of two partitions: *paired pleuropericardial membranes* and *diaphragm*.

The two important events involved in the development of body cavities are (a) **formation of intraembryonic coelom** and (b) **partitioning of intraembryonic coelom**.

FORMATION OF INTRAEMBRYONIC COELOM

Intraembryonic coelom develops in lateral plate mesoderm. With the development of the intraembryonic coelom, the lateral plate mesoderm is split in two layers: **splanchnopleuric layer** related to endoderm and **somatopleuric layer** related to ectoderm (Fig. 21.1).

At the end of 3rd week of IUL, an intraembryonic coelom appears as a *horseshoe-shaped cavity* in the lateral plate mesoderm. Its narrow central part lies cranially in the midline behind the septum transversum and in front of prechordal plate. It represents the future **pericardial cavity**. Its right and left lateral parts represent the future **peritoneal cavities**. The canals that connect the pericardial and peritoneal cavities are called **pericardioperitoneal canals.** They represent the future **pleural cavities** (Fig. 21.2A). Later, the two primitive peritoneal cavities fuse to form a single **peritoneal cavity** (Fig. 21.2B).

After folding of embryo, the pericardial cavity lies ventrally and the two **pericardioperitoneal canals** pass on either side of the foregut (Fig. 21.3). The two lung buds arising from foregut invaginate the pericardioperitoneal canals. With the growth and enlargement of lung buds, these canals also expand and form the **pleural cavities**.

N.B. The intraembryonic coelom provides room for organs to develop and move about.

PARTITIONING OF THE INTRAEMBRYONIC COELOM

To form the definitive pericardial, pleural, and peritoneal cavities from a single intraembryonic coelom, three partitions develop. These are as follows:

- Paired pleuropericardial membranes
- Diaphragm

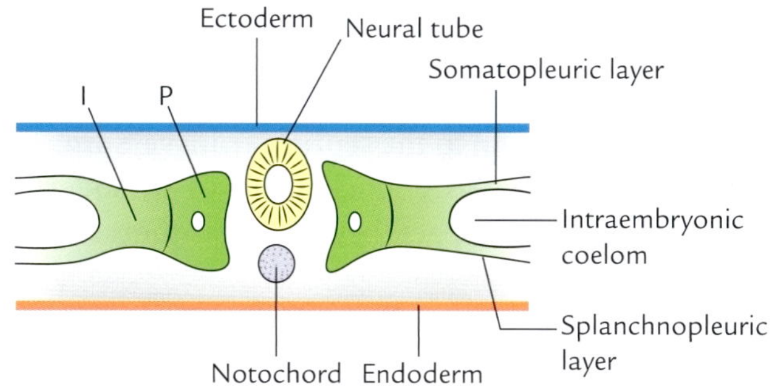

Fig. 21.1 Splitting of lateral plate mesoderm by intraembryonic coelom (P, paraxial mesoderm; I, intermediate mesoderm).

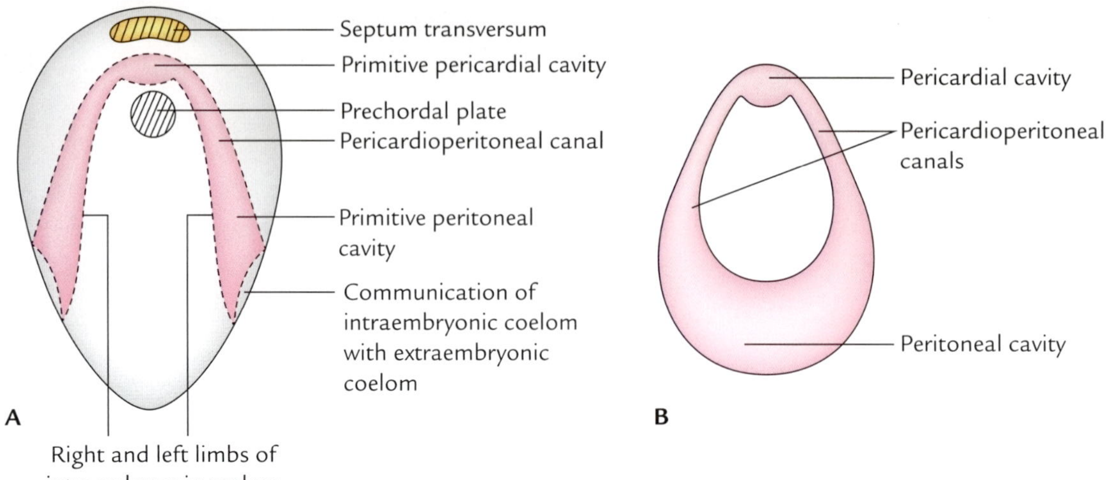

Fig. 21.2 Horseshoe-shaped primitive intraembryonic coelom. (A) Subdivisions of intraembryonic coelom. (B) Fusion of two primitive peritoneal cavities to form single horseshoe-shaped peritoneal cavity.

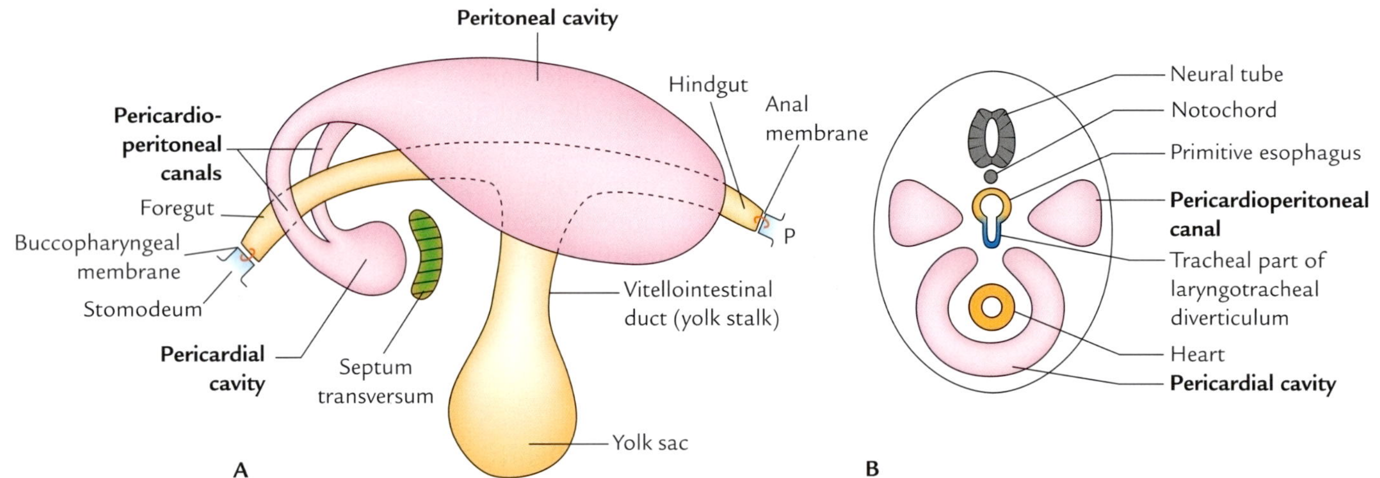

Fig. 21.3 Parts of intraembryonic coelom in relation to the gut. (A) Lateral view. (B) Transverse section of an embryo showing the relationship of pericardioperitoneal canals in relation to the tracheal part of the laryngotracheal diverticulum. P, proctodeum.

Development of Pleuropericardial Membranes (Fig. 21.4)

Each pleuroperitoneal canal lies lateral to the **primitive esophagus** and dorsal to the **septum transversum**. The septum transversum is a thick plate of mesodermal tissue that occupies space between the thoracic and abdominal cavities.

A partition forms in each pericardioperitoneal canal that separates the pericardial cavity from the peritoneal cavity.

With the growth of lung bud into the pericardioperitoneal canal, a pair of membranous ridges are produced in the lateral wall of this canal. These are as follows:

1. A cranial ridge called **pleuropericardial fold** above the developing lung
2. A caudal ridge called **pleuroperitoneal fold** below the lung bud

The pleuropericardial folds separate the pericardial cavity from the pleural cavities as they enlarge. Gradually, the folds become membranous and form the **pleuropericardial membranes**.

As the pleuroperitoneal fold enlarges, it projects into the pericardioperitoneal canal. Gradually, the fold

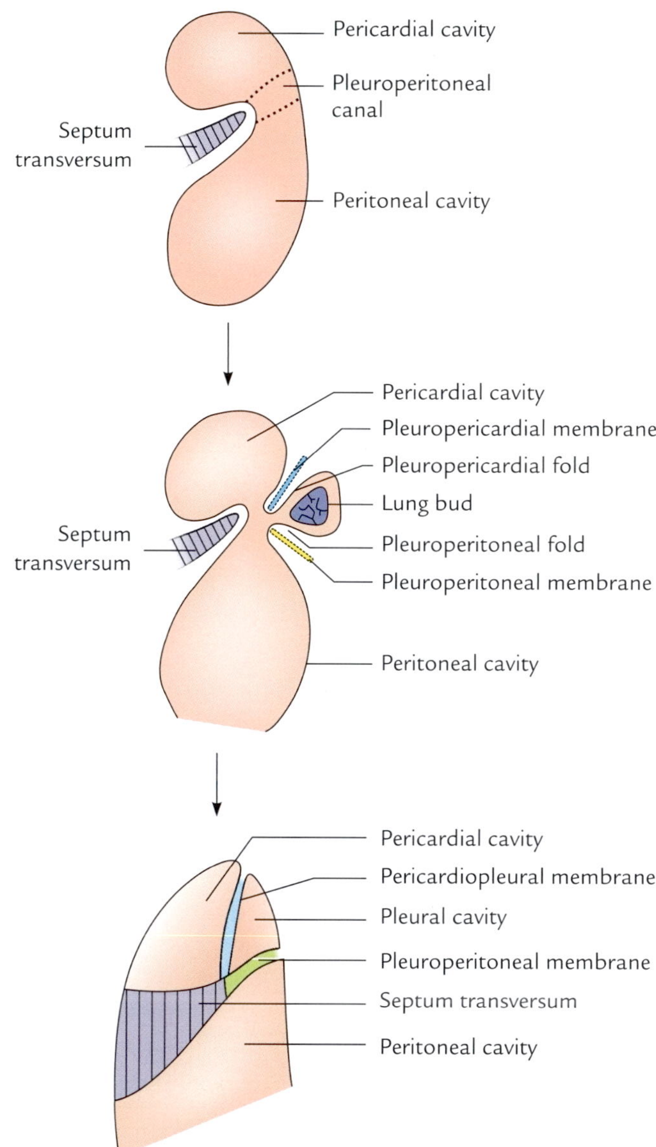

Fig. 21.4 Formation of the pleural cavity from pleuroperitoneal canal and its separation from pericardial and peritoneal cavities by the formation of pleuropericardial and pleuroperitoneal membranes.

becomes membranous and forms the **pleuroperitoneal membrane**.

Development of the Diaphragm (Figs 21.5 and 21.6)

AN 52.5

The diaphragm is a dome-shaped musculotendinous partition between thoracic and abdominal cavities. The pericardial and pleural cavities lie above the diaphragm, while the peritoneal cavity lies below the diaphragm.

The diaphragm is a composite structure that develops from the following four embryonic components:

1. Septum transversum
2. Paired pleuroperitoneal membranes
3. Dorsal mesentery of esophagus
4. Mesoderm of body wall

N.B. Several genes on the long arm of chromosome 15 (15q) play a critical role in the development of the diaphragm.

1. The **septum transversum** lies between pericardial and peritoneal cavities. Dorsal to it lies esophagus with its surrounding mesoderm and mesentery (**dorsal mesentery of esophagus**). On each side, dorsolateral to septum transversum, pleural and peritoneal cavities communicate with each other through **pleuroperitoneal canals.**

   The liver develops in the caudal part of septum transversum. The cranial part of septum transversum forms the central tendon of diaphragm.
2. The **pleuroperitoneal membranes** develop and close the pleuroperitoneal canals. They fuse with the dorsal mesentery of the esophagus and the septum transversum. The pleuroperitoneal membranes not only form a large portion of early fetal diaphragm but also represent only small portion of the diaphragm in the newborn.
3. The **dorsal mesentery of the esophagus** is invaded by myoblasts and forms **crura of the diaphragm.**
4. On each side, the developing pleural cavity (pleuroperitoneal canal) burrows into the lateral body wall and splits it into two layers: external and internal (Fig. 21.6).
   (a) The external layer forms the definitive body wall.
   (b) The internal layer forms the peripheral parts of the diaphragm external to the parts derived from the pleuroperitoneal membranes.

The development of the diaphragm is summarized in Table 21.1.

Nerve Supply of Diaphragm

Initially (i.e., during the 4th week of IUL), the septum transversum lies in the cervical region opposite third, fourth, and fifth cervical somites and is supplied by corresponding cervical spinal segments (i.e., C3, C4, and C5).

The **phrenic nerve** (root value C3, C4, and C5) reaches the diaphragm through pleuropericardial folds. Later (i.e., by the 6th week of IUL), the diaphragm descends caudally to its definitive position – the thoracoabdominal junction opposite T7–T12 spinal segments. The descent of diaphragm occurs due to elongation of neck, descent of heart, and expansion of pleural cavities. When the diaphragm descends, it carries its nerve

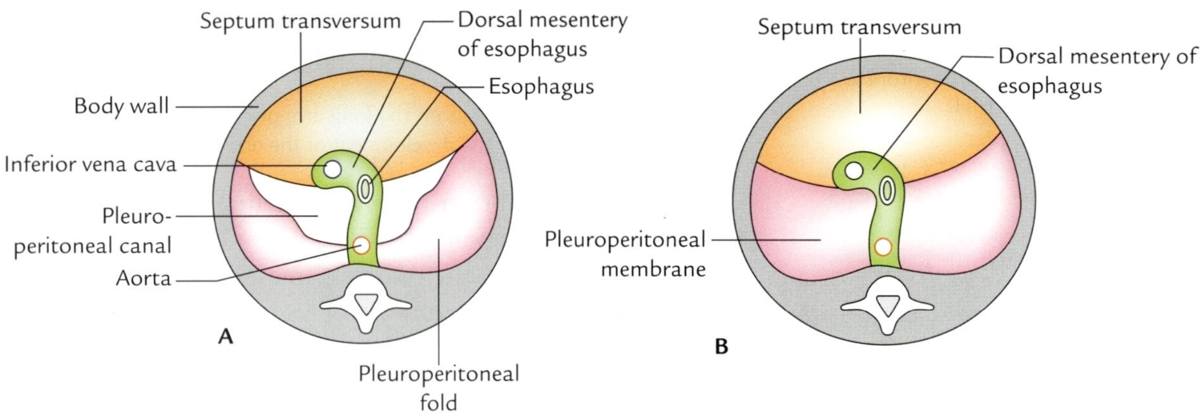

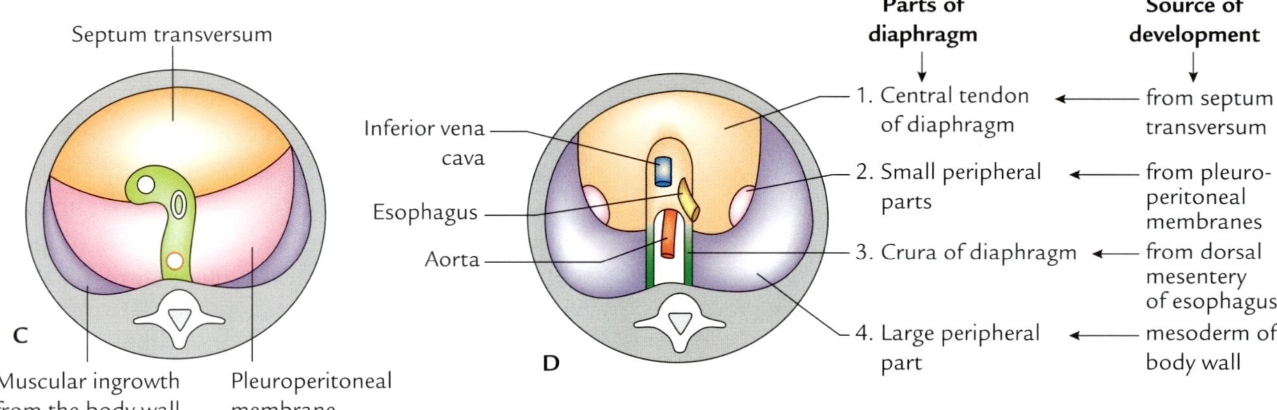

Fig. 21.5 (A–D) Successive stages of the development of the diaphragm.

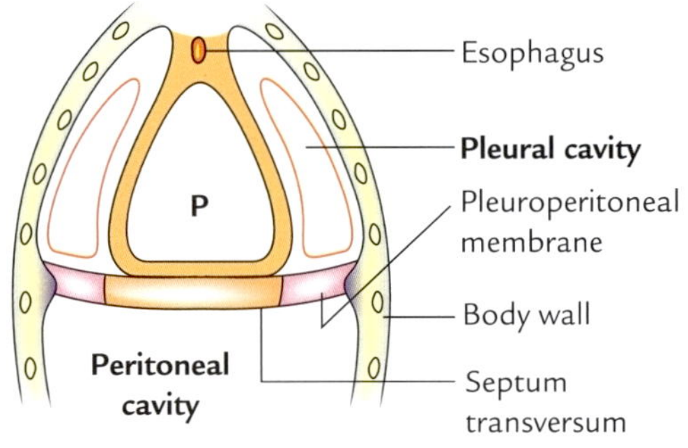

Fig. 21.6 Splitting of lateral body wall by developing pleural cavities. P, pericardial cavity.

Table 21.1 Development of diaphragm

Parts of Diaphragm	Embryonic Structures
Central tendon of diaphragm	From septum transversum
Small peripheral part of diaphragm	From pleuroperitoneal membranes
Crura of diaphragm	From dorsal mesentery of esophagus
Large peripheral parts of diaphragm external to parts derived from pleuroperitoneal membranes	From mesoderm of the body wall

supply with it; hence, the diaphragm is supplied by the phrenic nerve.

Since the peripheral parts of the diaphragm develop from the lateral body wall, it receives its sensory innervation from lower intercostal nerves.

N.B. **Position of septum transversum:** During the 4th week, the septum transversum lies opposite to cervical somites (C3, C4, and C5), and by the 6th week, it lies at the level of thoracic somites (T7–T12).

CLINICAL CORRELATION

Congenital anomalies of the diaphragm

1. ***Congenital diaphragmatic hernia (CDH):*** It is the herniation of abdominal contents into the pleural cavity through a large gap/defect present in posterolateral part of diaphragm, most commonly on the left side (Fig. 21.7).

   This defect (also called **foramen of Bochdalek**) occurs due to defective development of **pleuroperitoneal membrane** or failure of fusion of pleuroperitoneal membrane with other elements of the diaphragm.

   When the abdominal contents like intestines, stomach, and/or spleen herniate in the thorax, they compress the developing lungs and cause hypoplasia (Fig. 21.8).

   The diaphragmatic hernia is more common on the left side probably because right pleuroperitoneal canal closes earlier than the left one.

   Clinical features

   Three cardinal signs of CDH are as follows:
   - Breathlessness
   - Cyanosis
   - Unusually flat abdomen

   The death in CDH commonly occurs due to respiratory distress and cyanosis.

2. ***Congenital hiatus hernia (CHH):*** It is a herniation of part of fetal stomach through an excessively large esophageal hiatus in the diaphragm, through which esophagus and vagus nerves pass.

   CHH is uncommon, but the congenitally enlarged esophageal hiatus may be a predisposing factor for **acquired hiatal hernia**.
3. ***Retrosternal hernia*** (**parasternal hernia**): In this condition, there is a large gap in sternocostal part of the diaphragm between the sternal and costal slips of diaphragm (**foramen of Morgagni**) through which the intestines may herniate into the pericardial cavity or conversely a part of heart may herniate into the epigastric region.
4. ***Eventration of diaphragm:*** In this condition, musculature in one-half of the diaphragm remains thin and membranous. As a result, it balloons out in the thorax forming a diaphragmatic pouch because of upward displacement of abdominal viscera akin to CDH.

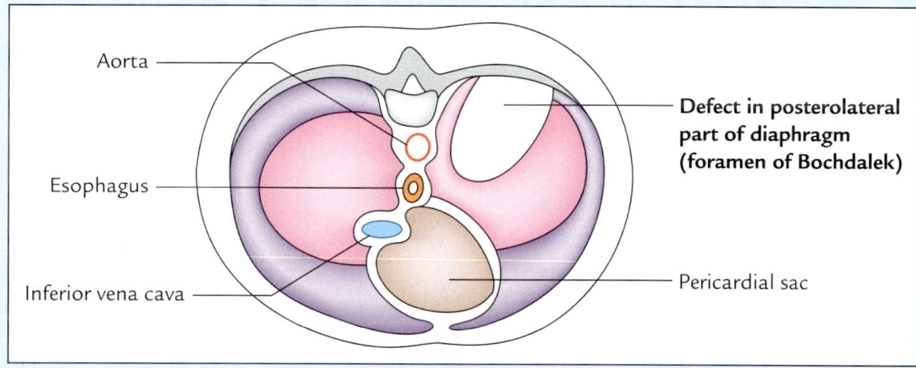

Fig. 21.7 Defect in the posterolateral part of the diaphragm.

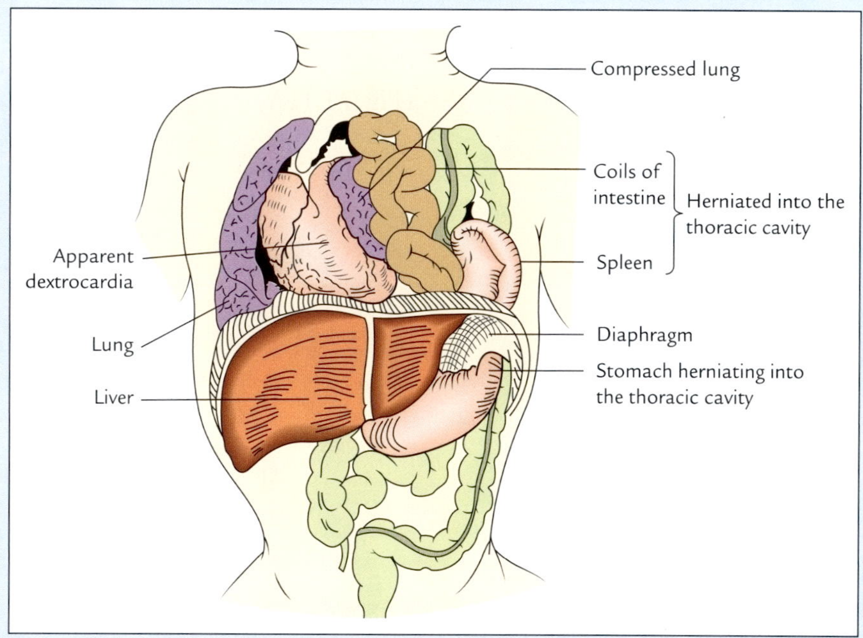

Fig. 21.8 Congenital diaphragmatic hernia (CDH).

FURTHER DETAILS OF BODY CAVITIES

Further details of the three body cavities and associated structures are discussed in the following text.

Development of Pericardial Cavity

The pericardial cavity develops from *narrow midline portion of intraembryonic coelom which lies in front of prechordal plate near the cranial end of embryonic disk.* The heart develops from splanchnopleuric mesoderm forming floor of this narrow part of coelom.

The primitive pericardial cavity bulges ventrally between the stomodeum (cranially) and the septum transversum (caudally). The primitive heart tube lies dorsal to the pericardial cavity. The development of the pericardial cavity is closely related to the development of the heart; hence, it is described in detail in Chapter 22.

Development of Pleural Cavities

Right and left pleural cavities develop from *right and left pericardioperitoneal canals.*

The pleural cavities at first lie dorsolateral to the pericardial cavity and communicate with it by pericardiopleural canals. As the pleural cavities enlarge and heart descends, the *pleuropericardial membranes* derived from *pleuropericardial folds* project into the pleuropericardial canals and ultimately separate the pleural cavities from pericardial cavity. The lung buds arise from tracheal part of the laryngotracheal diverticulum and invaginate the primitive pleural cavities to form the definitive pleural cavities (Fig. 21.9).

Each pleural cavity communicates caudally with peritoneal cavity by a wide **pleuroperitoneal canal.** Later on, this communication is closed by pleuroperitoneal membrane.

N.B. It is important to note that with the expansion of the pleural cavity, the mesoderm of the body wall splits into two parts: (a) an outer part that forms the thoracic wall and (b) an inner part that lies over the pericardial cavity and is called **pleuropericardial membrane.** The phrenic nerve runs through this membrane (Fig. 21.10). Later, the pleuropericardial membrane forms the fibrous pericardium. This provides the embryological basis of **course of the phrenic nerve** over fibrous pericardium.

Development of Peritoneal Cavity

Peritoneal cavity is the largest of the three body cavities. During lateral folding of embryo, the distal parts of the lateral limbs of the horseshoe-shaped intraembryonic coelom come closer to each other and fuse to form a single large peritoneal cavity. The peritoneal cavity is connected with the extraembryonic coelom at the umbilicus. The peritoneal cavity loses its connection with the extraembryonic coelom during the 10th week of IUL following return of midgut loop into the abdomen from the umbilicus. The **splanchnopleuric intraembryonic mesoderm** in addition to forming the wall of the gut also differentiates into a layer of mesothelial cells – the **mesothelium** – which lines the peritoneal cavity. It is called the **visceral layer of peritoneum**; the **parietal layer of peritoneum** lines the body wall. The line of reflection of parietal peritoneum to visceral peritoneum forms the **mesentery of various organs.**

Mesentery

The mesentery is a double-layered fold of visceral peritoneum that connects the primitive gut with the body wall and conveys nerves and vessels to it.

Transiently, the dorsal and ventral mesenteries divide the peritoneal cavity into right and left halves (Fig. 21.11A).

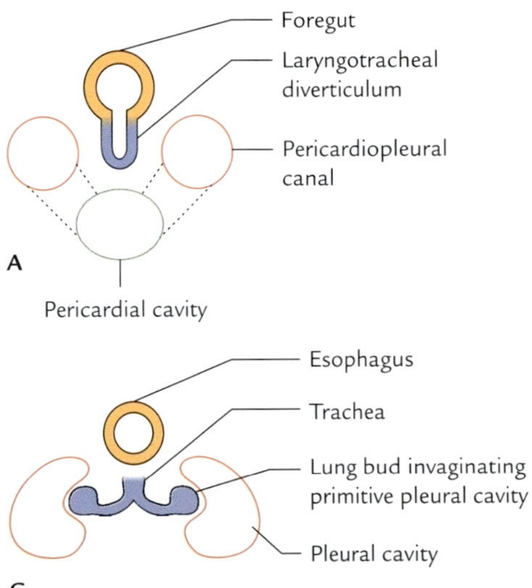

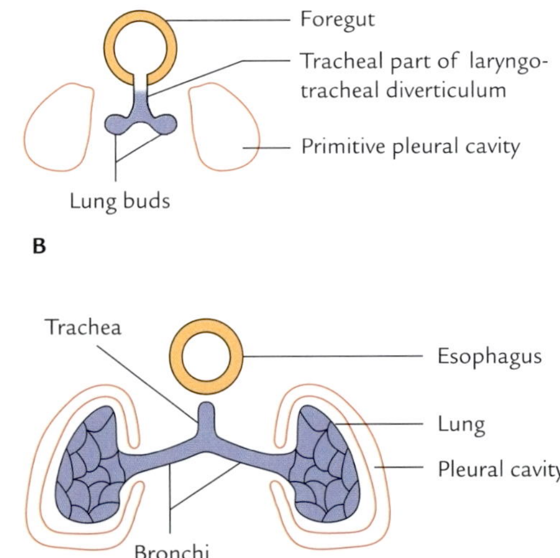

Fig. 21.9 Development of pleural cavities. Note the invagination of pericardioperitoneal canals by the lung buds to form pleural cavities.

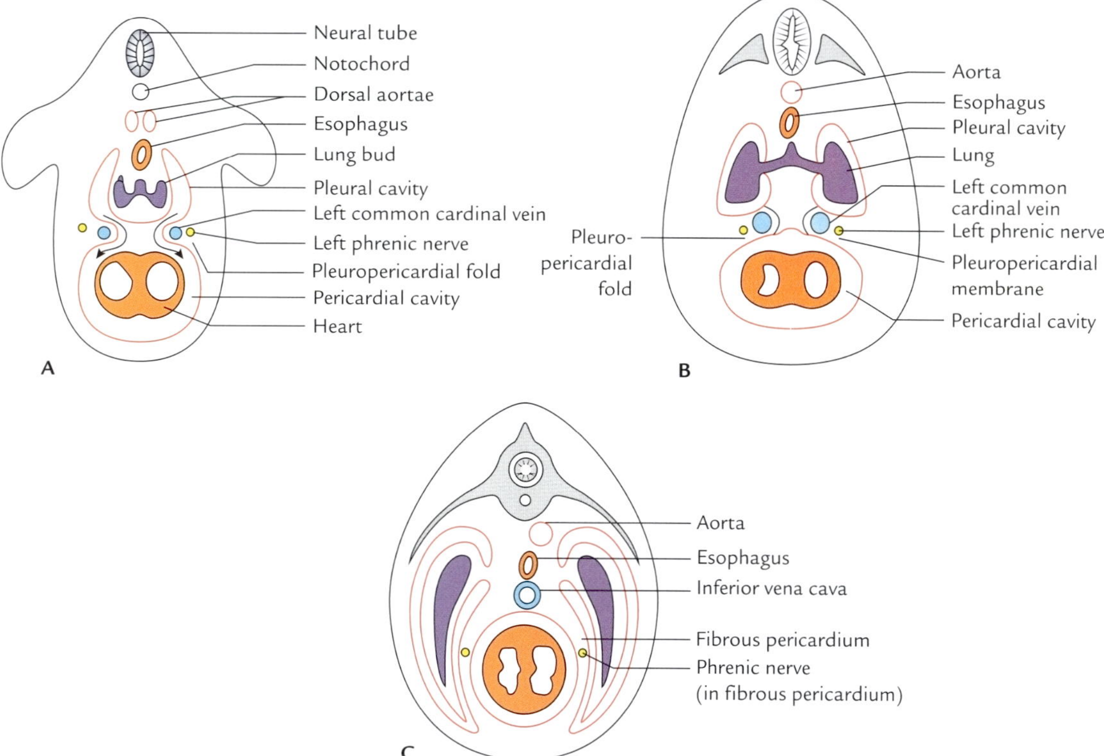

Fig. 21.10 Transverse section through embryo's cranial to septum transversum. (A) Position of pleuropericardial canals and pleuropericardial folds. (B) Development of pleural cavities due to growth of lungs and formation of pleuropericardial membrane. (C) Fusion of pleuropericardial membranes. Note the position of phrenic nerve in the fibrous pericardium.

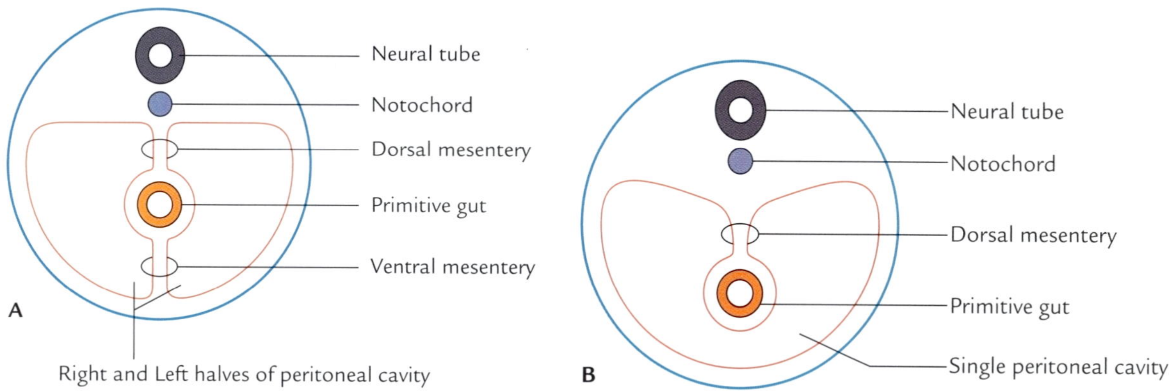

Fig. 21.11 Mesentery of the primitive gut. (A) Right and left halves of peritoneal cavity. (B) Single peritoneal cavity.

The ventral mesentery soon disappears, except where it is attached to the distal part of the foregut (which forms stomach and proximal part of the duodenum). As a result, the peritoneal cavity now becomes a single continuous space (Fig. 21.11B).

Development of Lesser Sac

The lesser sac is a part of the peritoneal cavity that lies behind the stomach and lesser omentum. It communicates with the peritoneal cavity through a small opening called **epiploic foramen** (*foramen of Winslow*).

Development of lesser sac is closely related to the development of the stomach and infolding of greater omentum. It involves following three distinct processes of peritoneum to occur (Fig 21.12).

First process

Two small cavities appear in thick dorsal mesogastrium – the **right and left pneumoenteric recesses** (Fig. 21.12).

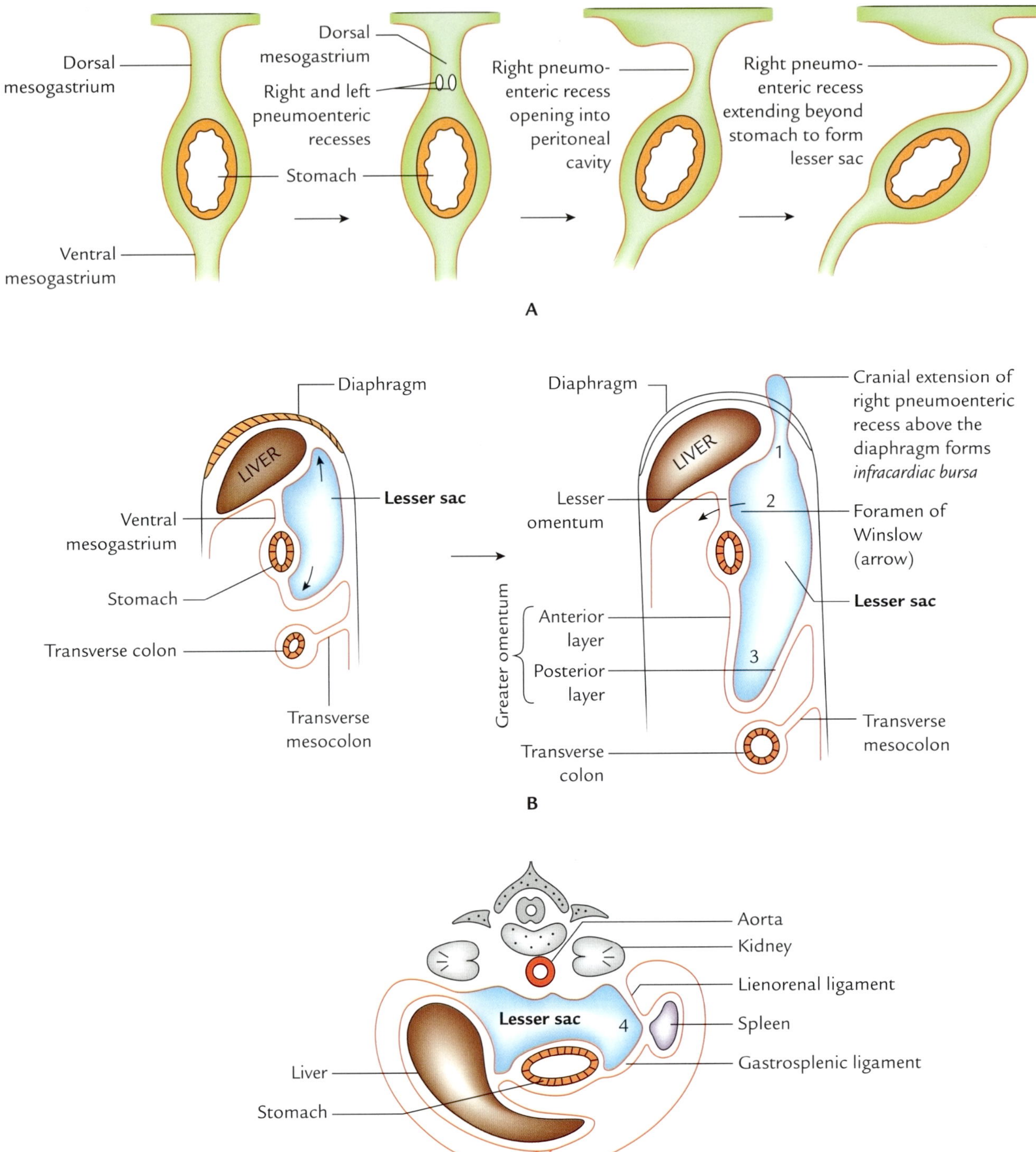

Fig. 21.12 Development of the lesser sac. (A) First process: Formation of pneumoenteric recesses. (B) Second process: Formation of lesser sac and most of its recesses. (C) Third process: Formation of splenic recess. 1. superior recess, 2. vestibule of lesser sac, 3. inferior sac, 4. splenic recess.

Table 21.2 Parts of lesser sac derived from various embryonic sources

Part of Lesser Sac	Source of Development
Vestibule	Part of peritoneal cavity that comes to lie behind the ventral mesogastrium (now lesser omentum)
Superior recess	Cranial extension of right pneumoenteric recess below diaphragm
Inferior recess	Cavity formed by elongation and folding of greater omentum on itself
Splenic recess	Part of right pneumoenteric recess extending to the left between gastrosplenic and lienorenal ligaments

The **left pneumoenteric recess** disappears. The right pneumoenteric recess enlarges and extends to the left to open into the peritoneal cavity.

The right pneumoenteric recess also extends cranially behind the liver and by the side of esophagus to form the **superior recess of lesser sac**. With the development of diaphragm, the part of superior recess above the diaphragm becomes detached and forms the **infracardiac bursa.**

N.B. Part of cranial extension of right pneumoenteric recess below the diaphragm forms **infracardiac recess**.

Second process

When the right pneumoenteric recess extends to the left, there occurs a counterclockwise rotation of the stomach around the longitudinal axis. As a result, the ventral mesogastrium shifts to the right (**lesser omentum**), dorsal mesogastrium shifts to the left, left surface becomes anterior, and right surface becomes posterior. Because of this rotation, the part of the peritoneal cavity now lies behind the stomach and lesser omentum; it forms the **vestibule of lesser sac**, which is continuous on the left side with the small part of lesser sac developed from **right pneumoenteric recess**.

Third process

With the development of spleen in dorsal mesogastrium attached to the fundus of stomach, dorsal mesogastrium is divided into **gastrosplenic and lienorenal ligaments**. These ligaments now form the left boundary of the lesser sac. The part of lesser sac enclosed between these two ligaments forms the **splenic recess of the lesser sac**. Dorsal mesogastrium attached to greater curvature of stomach below the fundus elongates and forms a large fold of peritoneum – **the greater omentum.** The cavity enclosed between the layers of greater omentum forms the third part of the lesser sac – the **inferior recess of the lesser sac.**

On the right side, the lesser sac opens into greater sac through an opening called **foramen epiploicum** (**foramen of Winslow**), which lies behind right free margin of lesser omentum.

The parts of lesser sac derived from various sources are summarized in Table 21.2.

GESTATIONAL AGE OF KEY DEVELOPMENTAL EVENTS

Developmental Event	Gestational Age
➢ Intraembryonic coelom (horseshoe-shaped cavity) appears at the end of	3rd week
➢ Septum transversum forms incomplete partition between pericardial and abdominal cavities during	4th week
➢ Diaphragm descends to the thoracic level during	6th week
➢ Pleuroperitoneal membranes separate the pleural cavities from peritoneal cavity during	6th week

GOLDEN FACTS TO REMEMBER

➢ **Largest serous cavity in the body**	Peritoneal cavity
➢ **Primordium of central tendon of diaphragm**	Septum transversum
➢ **Most common cause of pulmonary hypoplasia**	Congenital diaphragmatic hernia (CDH)
➢ **Chromosomal region involved in CDH**	Chromosome 15q26
➢ **Four embryonic components of diaphragm**	(a) Septum transversum, (b) pleuroperitoneal membranes, (c) dorsal mesentery of esophagus, and (d) muscular ingrowth from lateral body walls
➢ **Commonest congenital hernia of diaphragm**	Bochdalek hernia/congenital posterolateral hernia of diaphragm (CDH)

CLINICAL PROBLEM SOLVING

PROBLEMS

1. The **most of diaphragm is innervated by the phrenic nerves derived from C3, C4, and C5 spinal segments** providing motor and sensory innervation to it, **except the peripheral parts that are innervated by the lower intercostal nerves (T7–T11 spinal segments) providing only sensory innervation. Give the embryological basis.**
2. **Give the embryological basis of intimate relationship of phrenic nerve with the fibrous pericardium.**
3. **A newborn infant developed severe respiratory distress and cyanosis. On physical examination, the infant's abdomen was unusually flat and intestinal peristaltic movements were heard over the left side of the thorax. What is the most likely provisional diagnosis and tell whether this ailment can be detected prenatally? Give the embryological basis of this ailment.**
4. An ultrasonography of newborn infant revealed the presence of intestine in the pericardial cavity. **Name the congenital defect that may cause herniation of intestine into the pericardial cavity**. Give the embryological basis of this defect.

SOLUTIONS

1. The diaphragm is innervated by phrenic nerves (C3, C4, and C5) **because diaphragm develops in the cervical region opposite C3, C4, and C5 spinal segments.** When the diaphragm descends in the thoracic region, it carries its nerve supply (phrenic nerves) with it.

   The lateral parts of diaphragm develop from lateral thoracic wall opposite T7–T12 spinal segments, and hence it receives its sensory innervation from the lower thoracic spinal (intercostal) nerves.
2. Because of the expansion (burrowing) of primitive pleural cavity (pleuroperitoneal canal) into the lateral body wall, the mesoderm of lateral thoracic wall splits into two parts: lateral and medial. The lateral part forms the thoracic wall, while the medial part forms the pleuropericardial membrane. The **phrenic nerve** runs through this membrane, which later forms the fibrous pericardium. This provides the embryological basis of intimate relationship of phrenic nerve with the fibrous pericardium.
3. The most likely diagnosis is **congenital diaphragmatic hernia** (CDH). In this condition, the abdominal viscera, i.e., loops of small intestine, herniate through a defect in the posterolateral part of the diaphragm (usually on the left side) into the thoracic cavity. This causes compression and hypoplasia of lungs, especially the left one and consequent severe respiratory distress and cyanosis.

   The defect in the diaphragm causing CDH can be detected prenatally by ultrasonography. The ultrasonography reveals characteristic air- and/or fluid-filled spaces indicating loops of the small intestine in the left hemithorax.
4. The congenital defect in this condition is enlarged **sternocostal hiatus (foramen of Morgagni)** between the sternal and adjoining costal slips of origin of diaphragm. This defect leads either to herniation of intestine into the pericardial sac or displacement of heart into the superior part of the peritoneal cavity. The defect occurs if the sternal and costal slips of the diaphragm are poorly developed or fail to develop.

N.B. Radiologists often note the fatty herniation through the sternocostal hiatus, but it is of no clinical relevance.

22 Development of Heart

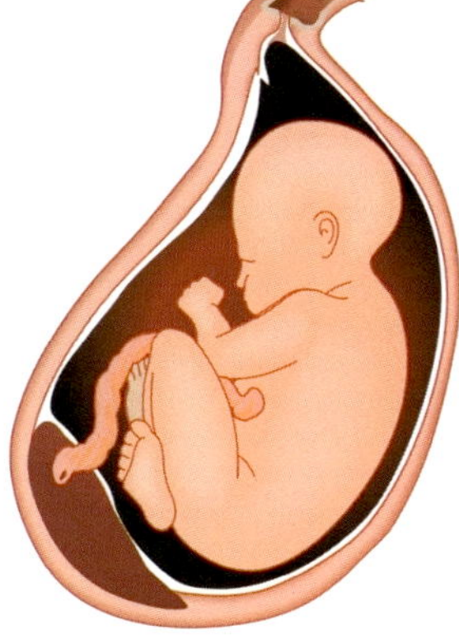

LEARNING OBJECTIVES

After studying this chapter, the student should be able to:

- Describe the development of heart. AN 25.2
- Give a brief account about the formation of heart tube.
- Describe the subdivisions of heart tube and enumerate their derivatives.
- Write short notes on (a) dextrocardia, and (b) transposition of great vessels. AN 25.5
- Give a brief account of (a) formation of interatrial septum and (b) formation of interventricular septum.
- Give the embryological basis of (a) atrial septal defects, (b) ventricular septal defect, and (c) Fallot tetralogy. AN 25.4
- Write short notes on (a) foramen ovale and (b) ectopia cordis.

OVERVIEW

The cardiovascular system is the first major system of the body to develop and start functioning (develops by the end of 3rd week) to meet the nutritional needs of the embryo.

The heart is mesodermal in origin. It develops from **primitive heart tube**, which forms from mesenchyme in the **cardiogenic area of the embryo**. This tube forms the **endocardium** of the heart. The splanchnic mesoderm surrounding the primitive heart tube forms **myocardium** and **epicardium**.

The heart starts functioning at the end of the 3rd week of intrauterine life (IUL), i.e., on day 22. The blood flow begins during the 4th week of IUL and can be visualized by Doppler ultrasonography.

N.B. **Cardiogenic area** (Fig. 22.1 A): It is an area at the cranial end of trilaminar embryonic disk between the septum transversum and prechordal plate. The part of intraembryonic coelom lying in this area forms **pericardial cavity** and the splanchnopleuric mesoderm underneath the pericardial cavity forms the heart tube.

The progenitor heart cells develop from epiblast lying immediately adjacent to the cranial part of primitive streak.

From here, they migrate into splanchnic layer of lateral plate of mesoderm. From where they migrate cranial to prechordal plate/oropharyngeal membrane and caudal to septum transversum into splanchnic layer of mesoderm forming the floor of pericardial cavity to form cells of **primary heart field (PHF; Fig. 22.1B).** The cells of PHF are induced by underlying endoderm to form mesenchymal cells of horseshoe-shaped **cardiogenic area.**

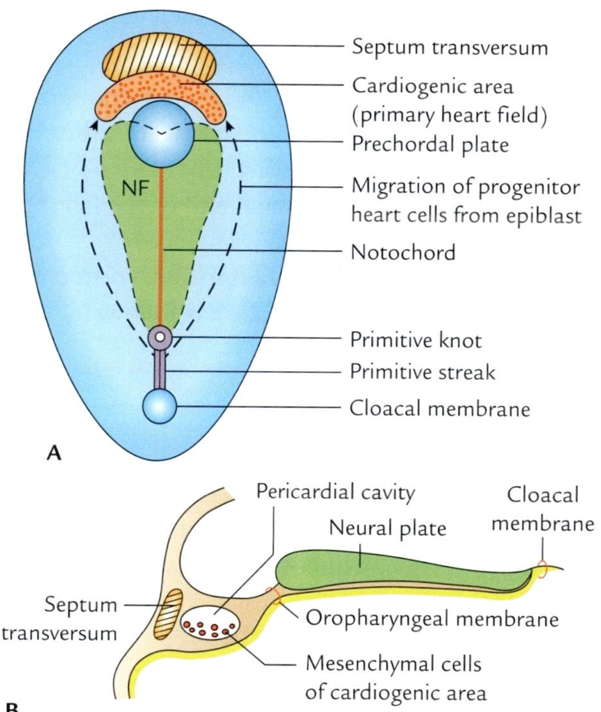

Fig. 22.1 Location of cardiogenic area. (A) Dorsal view of embryo. (B) Craniocaudal section of embryo. NF, neural fold.

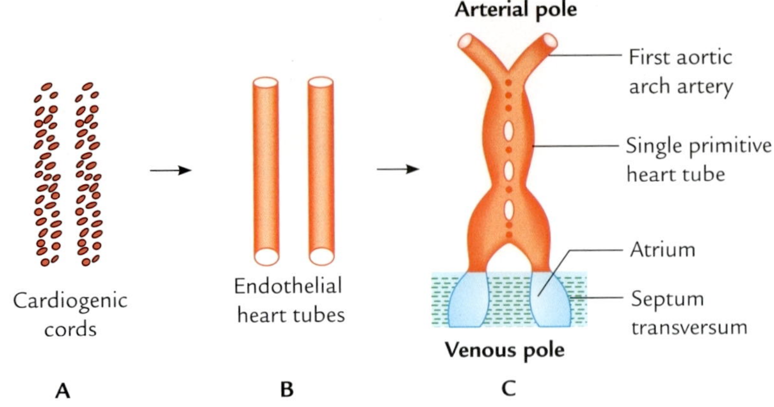

Fig. 22.2 Formation of the heart tube: Fusion of the endothelial heart tubes.

DEVELOPMENT OF HEART

AN25.2

Formation of Heart Tube and Its Subdivisions

The mesenchymal cells in the cardiogenic area are located ventral to the developing pericardial cavity. These cells condense to form two angioblastic cords called **cardiogenic cords** (Fig. 22.2A). These cords get canalized to form **two endothelial heart tubes** in the 3rd week of IUL (Fig. 22.2B).

These tubes fuse with each other in a craniocaudal direction to form a **single primitive heart tube.** However, the caudal ends of two heart tubes fail to fuse with each other. As a result, the caudal end of the heart tube remains bifurcated (Fig. 22.2C).

The **heart tube forms five dilatations.** From cranial-to-caudal end, these are (Fig. 22.3) as follows:

1. Truncus arteriosus
2. Bulbus cordis
3. Primitive ventricle
4. Primitive atrium
5. Sinus venosus

The truncus arteriosus is the arterial end of the primitive heart tube, while sinus venosus is the venous end of this tube.

Since the fusion of the heart tube is partial in the region of sinus venosus, it consists of a central part that communicates with the primitive atrium and right and left horns of sinus venosus that represent unfused caudal parts of the two heart tubes.

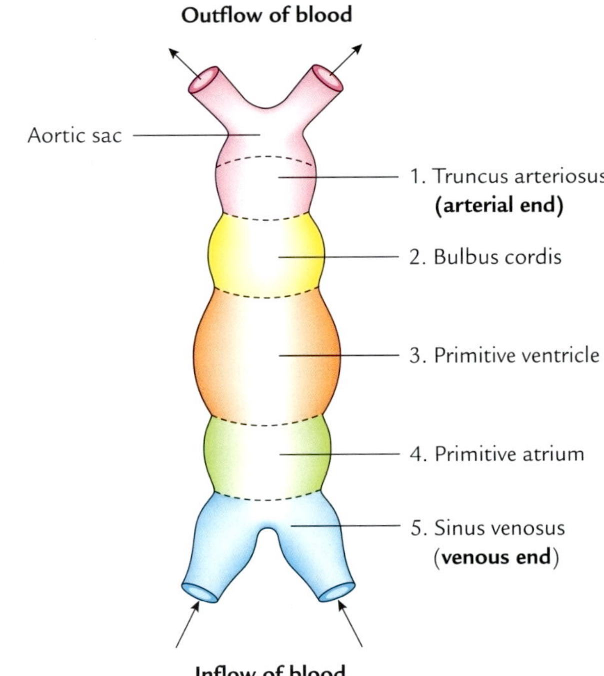

Fig. 22.3 Five embryonic dilatations (subdivisions) of the heart tube.

Arterial and Venous Ends of the Heart Tube

Arterial End

The truncus arteriosus represents the arterial end of the heart (vide supra). Cranially, it is continuous with aortic sac having right and left horns. From each horn of aortic sac, the **first pharyngeal arch artery** arises and passes backward on the lateral side of the foregut to become continuous with the **respective dorsal aorta** (Fig. 22.4A).

Venous End

The sinus venosus represents the venous end of the heart (vide supra). Each horn of sinus venosus receives three primitive veins: (a) *vitelline vein* from the yolk sac, (b) *umbilical vein* from the placenta, and (c) *common cardinal vein* from the body wall (Fig. 22.4B).

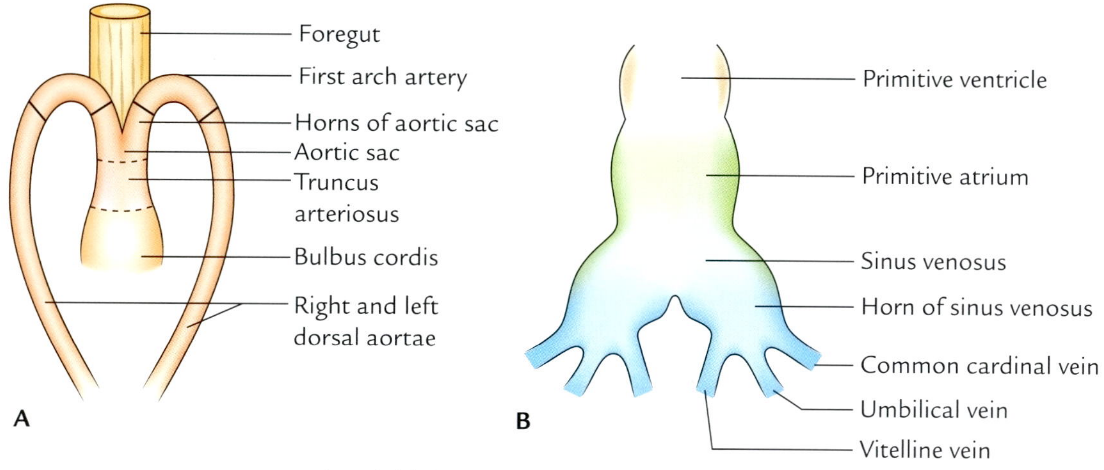

Fig. 22.4 Arterial (A) and venous (B) ends of the heart tube.

Fate of Various Dilatations of the Heart Tube

1. The **central part and right horn of sinus venosus** are absorbed into the primitive atrium to form the smooth part of the right atrium. The **left horn of sinus venosus** forms part of coronary sinus that opens into the smooth part of the right atrium.
2. **Primitive atrium** is partitioned to form rough part of right and left atria.
3. **Primitive ventricle and bulbus cordis** are partitioned to form the right and left ventricles.
   (a) The *primitive ventricle* forms the rough inflowing part of the right and left ventricles.
   (b) The *bulbus cordis* forms the smooth outflowing part of the right and left ventricles.
4. **Truncus arteriosus** is partitioned to form the ascending aorta and pulmonary trunk.

The fate of embryonic dilatations of the primitive heart tube is summarized in Table 22.1.

N.B. The smooth part of the left atrium is formed by the incorporation of pulmonary veins into the left atrium.

Table 22.1 Fate of the embryonic dilatations of the primitive heart tube

Embryonic Dilatation	Adult Derivatives
1. Truncus arteriosus	• Ascending aorta • Pulmonary trunk
2. Bulbus cordis	• Smooth upper part of the right ventricle (**conus arteriosus**) • Smooth upper part of the left ventricle (**aortic vestibule**)
3. Primitive ventricle	• Trabeculated part of the right ventricle • Trabeculated part of the left ventricle
4. Primitive atrium	• Trabeculated part of the right atrium • Trabeculated part of the left atrium
5. Sinus venosus	
a. Right horn	• Smooth part of the right atrium (**sinus venarum**)
b. Left horn	• Coronary sinus • Oblique vein of the left atrium

Position of Heart Tube in Relation to Pericardial Cavity

Before the formation of the head fold, the endothelial heart tube lies in the floor of the pericardial cavity caudal to septum transversum. After the formation of the head fold, the pericardial cavity and heart tube come to lie ventral to the foregut and cranial to the septum transversum, with heart tube lying on the roof of the pericardial cavity.

N.B. During formation of head fold, the pericardial cavity and heart tube undergo 220° rotation; as a result, the heart tube comes to lie on the roof of the pericardial cavity (Fig. 22.5).

Formation of Cardiac Wall

The cardiac wall is made up of three layers. From inside to outside, these are

1. Endocardium
2. Myocardium
3. Epicardium

These layers develop as follows (Fig. 22.6):

- **Endocardium**, from the wall of endothelial heart tube

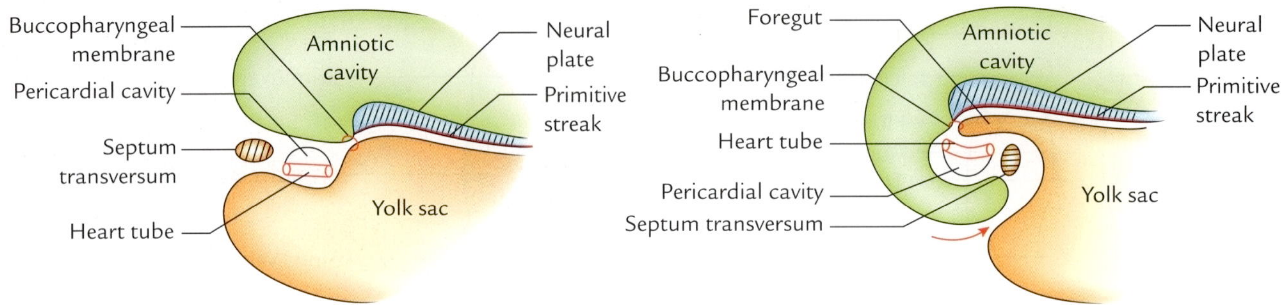

Fig. 22.5 Changing positions of the pericardial cavity and heart tube following the formation of head fold.

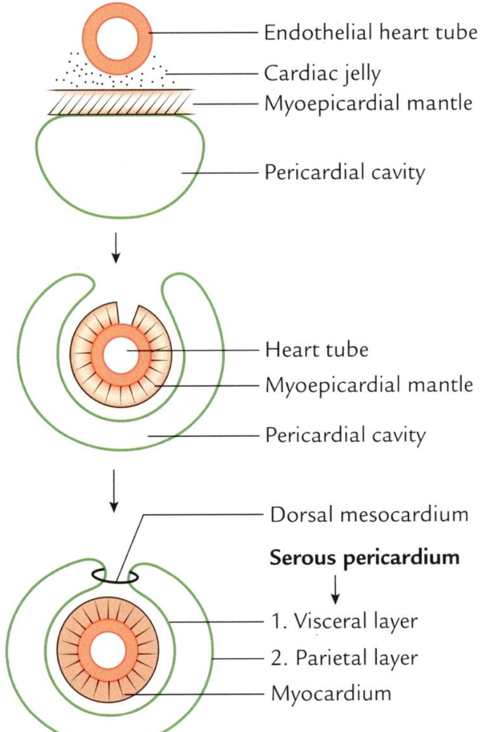

Fig. 22.6 Schematic diagram showing the development of cardiac wall.

- **Myocardium**, from splanchnopleuric mesoderm (myocardial mantle)
- **Epicardium**, from outer cell layer of primitive cardiac tube

N.B. According to recent theory, epicardium develops from proepicardial cells derived from coelomic epithelium.

The detailed description of three layers of myocardium is as follows:

The splanchnopleuric mesoderm on dorsal aspect of the pericardial cavity proliferates and becomes thick to form **myoepicardial mantle**, which invests the front and sides of endothelial heart tube. At this stage, the heart tube is separated from myoepicardial mantle (primordial myocardium) by a cellular gelatinous connective tissue called **cardiac jelly**, which is an acellular matrix secreted by developing myocardium. Subsequently, it is replaced by the myocardium.

- The **endothelial heart tube** forms the **endocardium** of the heart.
- The **myoepicardial mantle** forms the **myocardium.**
- The **proepicardial cells** form the **epicardium.**

Acquisition of External Adult Form of the Heart (Figs 22.7 and 22.8)

The sacculated primitive heart tube acquires adult form of the heart as follows:

1. As the development progresses, the sacculated heart tube, particularly bulbus cordis and primitive ventricle, grows rapidly in a limited space dorsal to the pericardial cavity. Since the arterial and venous ends of the heart tube are fixed, it gradually invaginates into the pericardial cavity in a "U"-shaped manner, thus forming a **cardiac loop**. This cardiac loop mainly involves **bulbus cordis** forming **cephalic limb of the loop** and primitive ventricle forming the **caudal limb of the loop**. Hence, this loop is also called **bulboventricular loop.**
2. Initially, the bulboventricular loop is suspended from the dorsal wall of the pericardial sac by a mesentery called **dorsal mesocardium**, but the central part of this mesentery soon degenerates forming a communication between the right and left sides of the pericardial cavity – the **transverse pericardial sinus.**
3. As the transverse pericardial sinus forms, the bulboventricular loop lies free in the pericardial cavity, but the primitive atrium and sinus venosus lie outside the pericardial cavity embedded in the septum transversum.
4. As the primitive atrium and sinus venosus get freed from the septum transversum, they enter the pericardial

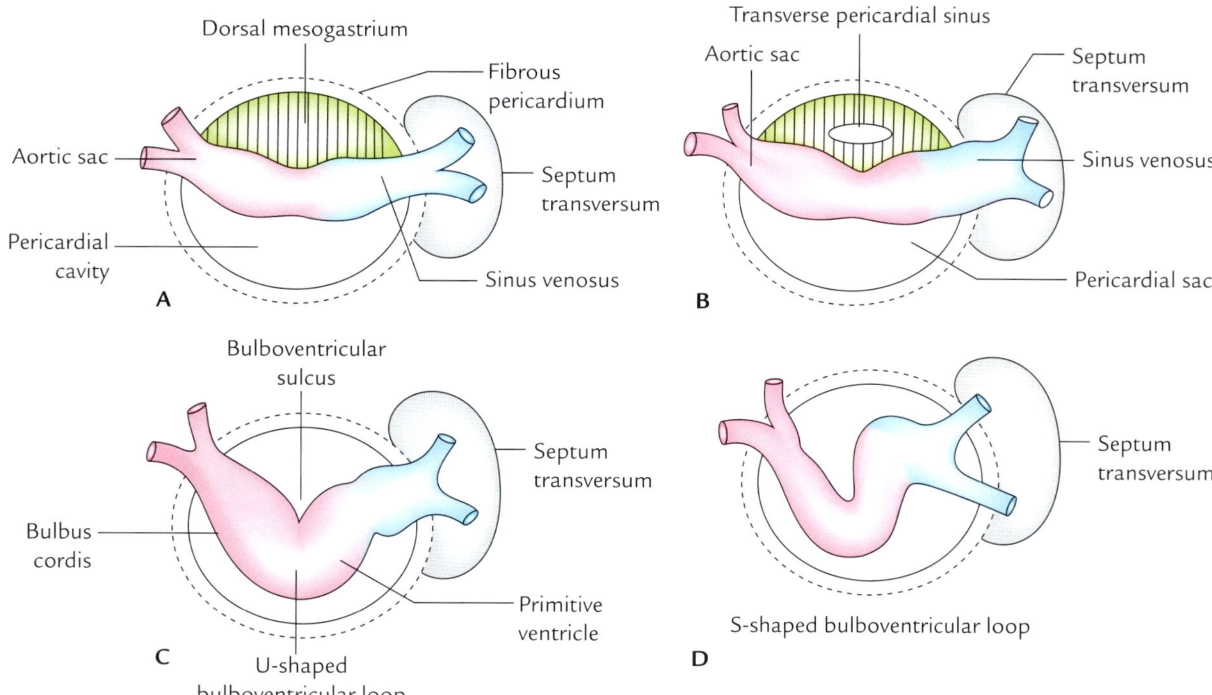

Fig. 22.7 Invagination and bending of the heart tube within pericardial cavity.

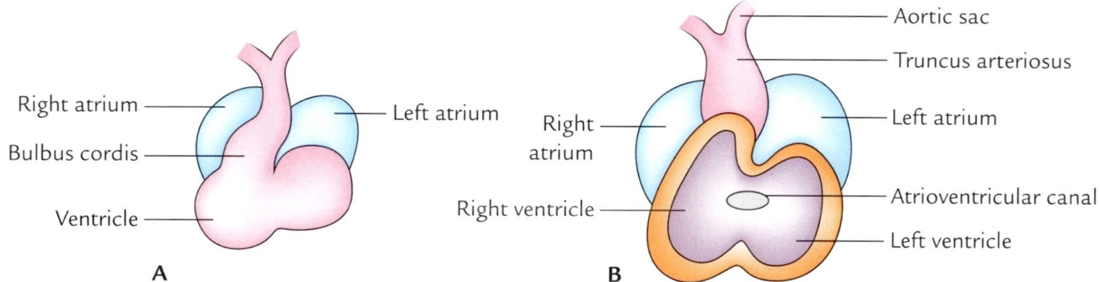

Fig. 22.8 (A) Establishment of the external form of the heart. (B) The interiors of developing ventricles are shown on the right.

cavity and occupy position posterosuperior to the ventricle. The heart tube now becomes S shaped.

5. The bulboventricular sulcus disappears, and bulbus cordis and primitive ventricle together form a common chamber.
6. The atrial chamber that lies behind and above truncus arteriosus expands, and with this its parts come to project forward on either side of truncus arteriosus as auricles.

CLINICAL CORRELATION

1. ***Dextrocardia*** (Fig. 22.9): In this rare condition, the heart points toward the right side instead of usual left side of thoracic wall (L. Dexter = right; G. Kardia = heart). Further, all the chambers of the heart and associated blood vessels are reversed as a mirror image, i.e., all the structures that normally lie on to the right side are on to the left side as a mirror image of their normal configuration. Dextrocardia occurs if the heart tube bends to the left instead of the right, the heart is displaced to the right, and there is transposition. It occurs in 1 out of 700 individuals. It may be an isolated condition or associated with **situs inversus** (transposition of abdominal viscera). **The dextrocardia is the most common positional anomaly of the heart.** AN 25.5
2. ***Ectopia cordis*** (Fig. 22.10): It is a rare condition in which the heart lies exposed on the surface of the thorax. It occurs due to nonunion of two sternal plates of developing sternum. Death occurs in most of the cases during the first few days of the birth.

Continued

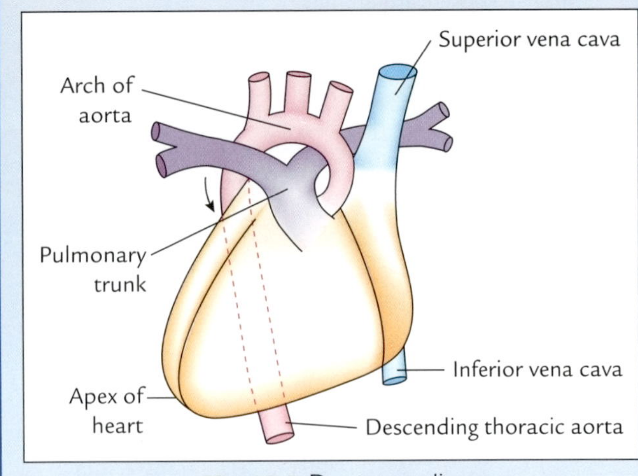

Fig. 22.9 Dextrocardia.

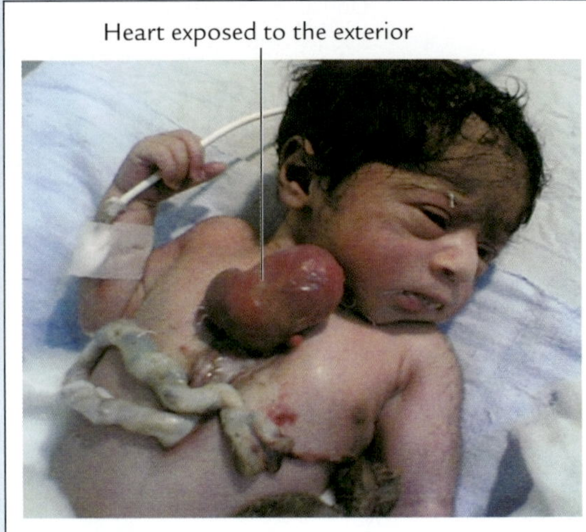

Fig. 22.10 A newborn baby with ectopia cordis. (*Source:* Courtesy of Dr Basant Kumar, Assistant Professor, Department of Pediatric Surgery, SGPGIMS, Lucknow.)

Development of Various Chambers of the Heart

The primitive heart tube has a single lumen. This lumen is partitioned into four definitive chambers by the formation of following four septa:

1. Atrioventricular (AV) septum
2. Interatrial septum
3. Interventricular (IV) septum
4. Aorticopulmonary septum

In addition to the formation of septa, other embryological events such as regression and absorption of sinus venosus into the right atrium and absorption of pulmonary veins into the left atrium also help in the formation of definitive chambers of the heart.

Formation of Atrioventricular Septum (Fig. 22.11)

The AV septum divides the AV canal into right and left AV canals (partitioning of AV canal). The AV septum is formed by the fusion of AV cushions as follows:

Two thickenings appear – one on dorsal wall and one on ventral wall of AV canal. These are called **AV cushions or endocardial cushions**. These cushions grow toward each other and fuse together to form **AV septum** (also called **septum intermedium**) that divides the AV canal into right and left AV canals (vide supra).

Formation of Interatrial Septum (Fig. 22.12)

The interatrial septum divides the primitive atrium into the right and left atria.

It is formed by two septa – *septum primum* and *septum secundum.*

At the end of 4th week, the septum primum starts developing from the roof of the primitive atrial chamber a little to the left of the opening of sinus venosus. It is crescent shaped and is present in an oblique plane. It grows downward toward **septum intermedium**

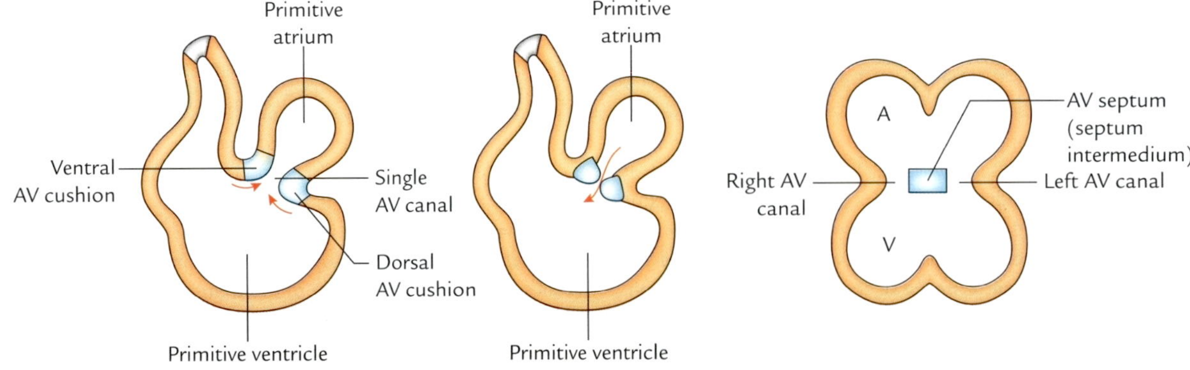

Fig. 22.11 Development of atrioventricular (AV) septum. A, atrium; V, ventricle.

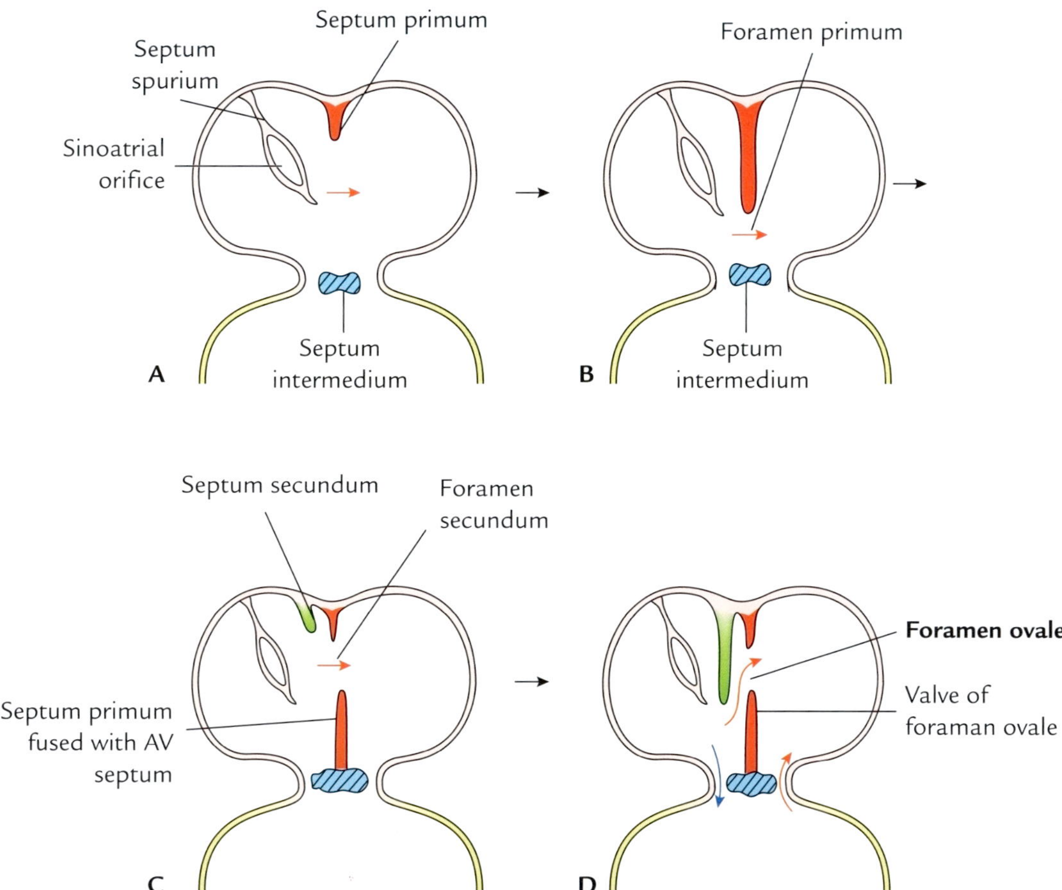

Fig. 22.12 Development of interatrial septum. Red arrows indicate the passage of oxygenated blood. Blue arrow indicates passage of poorly oxygenated blood.

(AV septum). The gap between the lower edge of septum primum and septum intermedium is called **foramen primum**.

As **septum primum** fuses with AV septum (septum intermedium), the upper part of septum primum breaks down. The foramen thus formed is called **foramen secundum** (**ostium secundum**).

A second crescent-shaped septum now arises from the roof of primitive atrial chamber immediately to the right of septum primum. It is called **septum secundum**.

The septum secundum grows downward toward septum intermedium. It overlaps the foramen secundum. The right and left atria now communicate with each other through an oblique valvular passage between the upper margin of septum primum and the lower margin of septum secundum. This passage is called **foramen ovale**.

The interatrial septum is thus formed by two septa: (a) septum primum that forms the lower part of interatrial septum and (b) septum secundum that forms the upper part of interatrial septum.

(i) Functional Mechanism of Foramen Ovale

The foramen ovale acts like one-way valve from right to left. Septum primum is thin and mobile like a flap, while septum secundum (crista dividens) is thick, firm, and immobile. When blood accumulates in the right atrium, it pushes the septum primum toward left and foramen ovale opens and blood flows from the right atrium to the left atrium. When the blood flows from the right to the left atrium, the thin flap of septum primum moves away and there is no obstruction to the blood flow. But after birth, the left atrium receives blood from lungs and pressure within it becomes greater than that in the right atrium. As the pressure of blood in the left atrium increases, it pushes the septum primum to the right. It comes in opposition with septum secundum and foramen ovale is closed (physiological closure); thus, the blood is prevented from flowing from the left atrium to the right atrium.

N.B. In adults, the **fossa ovalis** represents the **septum primum**, and **annulus fossa ovalis** represents the lower free edge of the septum secundum.

CLINICAL CORRELATION

AN25.4

Atrial septal defects (ASDs) (Fig. 22.13): In this condition, there is a defect in interatrial septum, which results in the communication between right and left atrium. It occurs in 6.4/10,000 births with a female-to-male ratio of 2:1. In this condition, there is a mixing of oxygenated and deoxygenated blood, thereby giving rise to symptoms like cyanosis and breathlessness.

The different types of ASDs are as follows (Fig. 22.13):

1. ***Septum primum defect:*** The **septum primum** fails to reach the **septum intermedium**. As a result, *persistent foramen primum* persists.
2. ***Septum secundum defect:*** It occurs if the septum secundum does not grow downward adequately to overlap the septum primum or the septum primum may undergo *excessive resorption*, because of which septum secundum fails to overlap the septum primum. As a result, foramen secundum remains large and unclosed – *ostium secundum defect*. This results in patent foramen ovale. It is the most significant ASD (Fig. 22.13B).
3. ***Patent (persistent) foramen ovale (probe patency of foramen ovale*** [Fig. 22.13C]): The oblique passage between septum primum and septum secundum is closed functionally but remains patent anatomically so that a probe can be passed through it.

N.B. The ASD is most common congenital anomaly of the atria. If the ASD is small, the clinical symptoms may be delayed up to the 30 years of age.

4. ***Premature (prenatal) closure of foramen ovale:*** In this condition, the closure of foramen ovale occurs during prenatal life. This results in the massive hypertrophy of the right side of the heart and underdevelopment of the left side of the heart.
5. ***Cor triloculare biventriculare/common atrium:*** In this condition, there is a complete absence of the interatrial septum, and this results in three-chambered heart. It is the most serious congenital anomaly of the atria and is always associated with other defects of the heart.

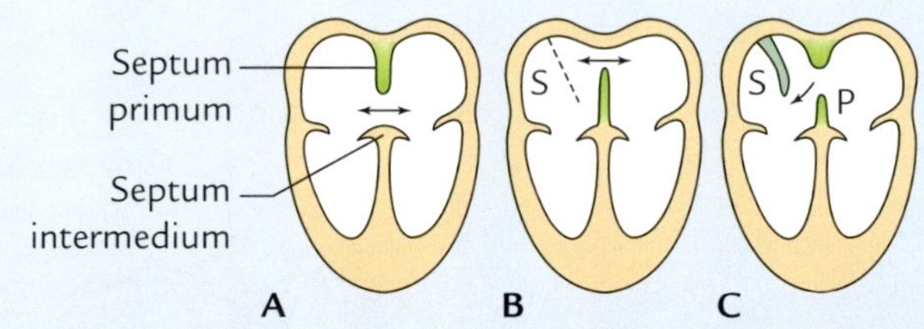

Fig. 22.13 Types of atrial septal defects: (A) septum primum defect; (B) septum secundum defect; and (C) patent foramen ovale. S, septum secundum; P, septum primum.

(ii) Fate of Sinus Venosus

Regression of Sinus Venosus (Fig. 22.14) The sinus venosus consists of a small transverse part called body and two horns – right and left. Initially, sinus venosus and primitive atrium are in open communication with each other. This communication (sinoatrial [SA] orifice) is transverse and located in the middle of posterior aspect of the atrial chamber and its two horns are of equal size. Because of left to right shunts developing between the primitive veins, most of blood is drained

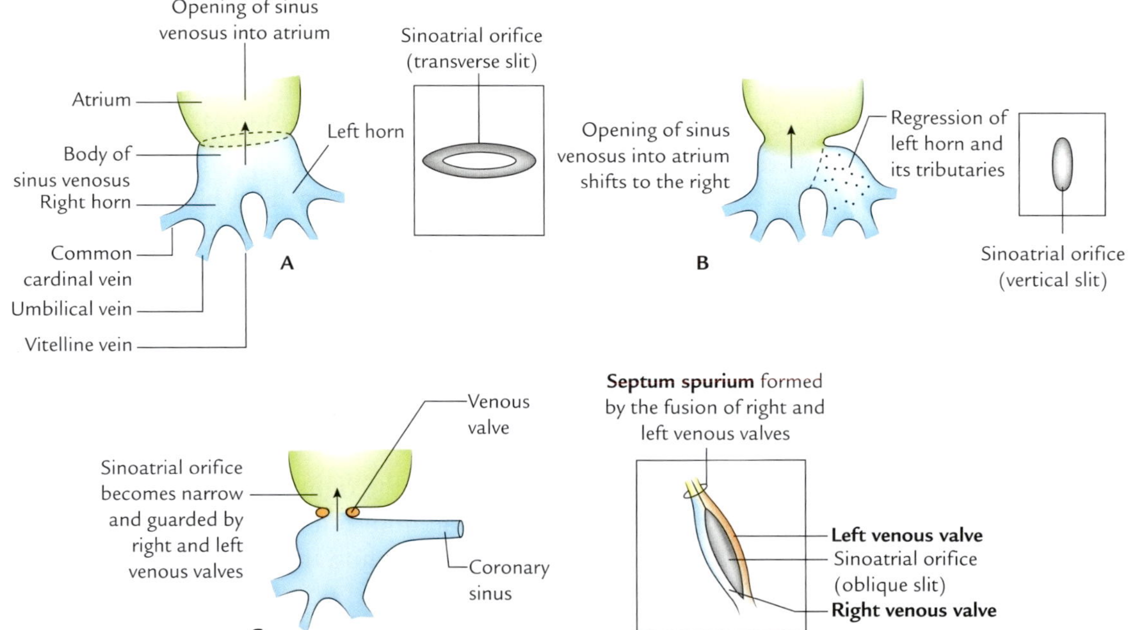

Fig. 22.14 Regression of sinus venosus. The changes in shape of sinusoidal orifice are shown in the insets on the right side. (A) Transverse slit. (B) Vertical slit. (C) Oblique slit.

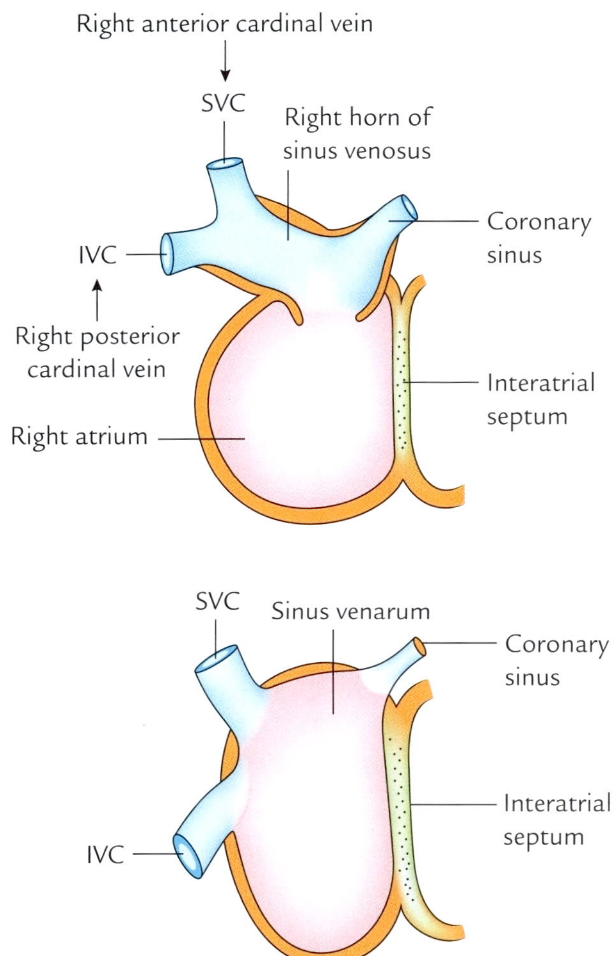

Fig. 22.15 Absorption of sinus venosus into the right atrium. SVC, superior vena cava; IVC, inferior vena cava.

into the right horn of sinus venosus, which therefore increases in size whereas the left horn becomes smaller. Because of these changes, opening of sinus venosus in atrium shifts to right and becomes vertical. It is guarded by two distinct lips – the **right and left venous valves**. The upper ends of two valves fuse to form **septum spurium**.

The right horn of sinus venosus receives all the venous blood through superior and inferior venae cavae and the left horn becomes **coronary sinus**.

Absorption of Sinus Venosus Into the Right Atrium (Fig. 22.15) After the formation of interatrial septum, the right horn and body of sinus venosus are absorbed into the right atrium so that superior vena cava (SVC), inferior vena cava (IVC), and coronary sinus (regressed left horn) now open in the right atrium.

With the absorption of sinus venosus in the right atrium, the right and left venous valves separate from each other.

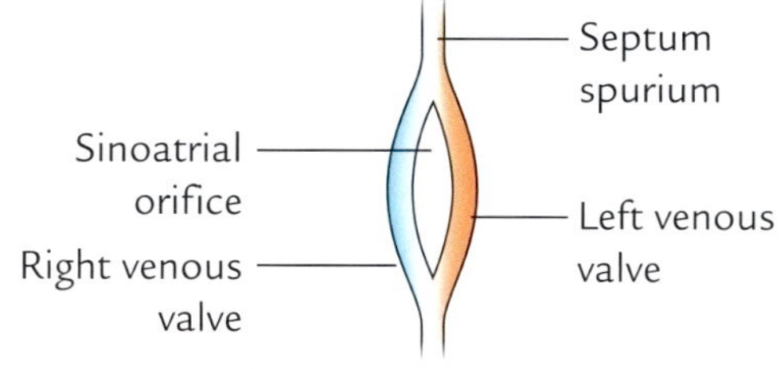

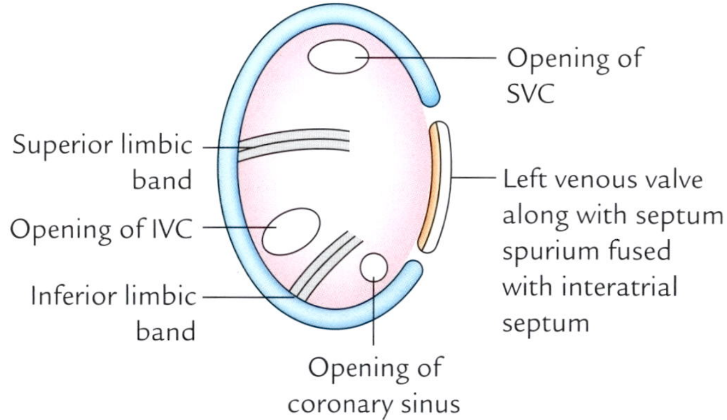

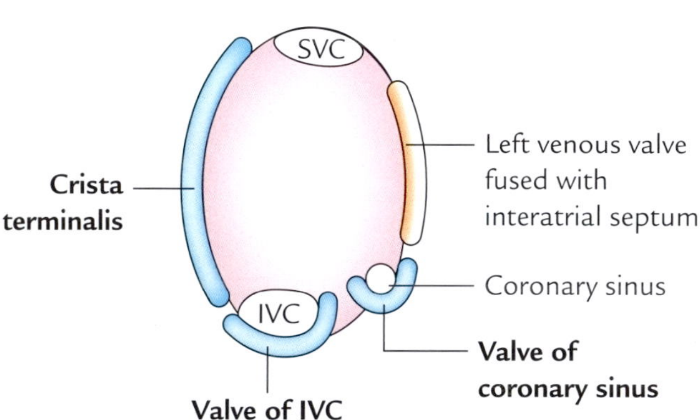

Fig. 22.16 Fate of right and left venous valves.

(iii) Fate of Left and Right Venous Valves (Fig. 22.16)

The left venous valve along with septum spurium fuses with the interatrial septum.

The right venous valve is greatly stretched out and becomes subdivided into three parts with formation of two muscular bands – the **superior and inferior limbic bands**. The three parts of right venous valves from above to downward form (a) **crista terminalis**, (b) **valve of IVC**, and (c) **valve of coronary sinus**.

(iv) Absorption of Pulmonary Veins Into the Left Atrium

Most of the left atrial wall is smooth because it is formed by the incorporation of primordial pulmonary vein.

The primordial **pulmonary vein** develops as an outgrowth of the dorsal atrial wall, just to the left of the **septum primum**.

Initially, a single large pulmonary vein opens into the left atrium when traced upward. It divides into right and left pulmonary vein. Each of the right and left pulmonary vein further divides into two branches before entering the corresponding lung. In this way, four pulmonary veins (two on each side) are formed (Fig. 22.17). Gradually, as the atrium expands, primordial pulmonary vein and its main branches and parts of four pulmonary veins nearest to the atrium are absorbed into the atrium. As a result, four separate pulmonary veins, two from each lung, come to open into the left atrium (Fig. 22.18).

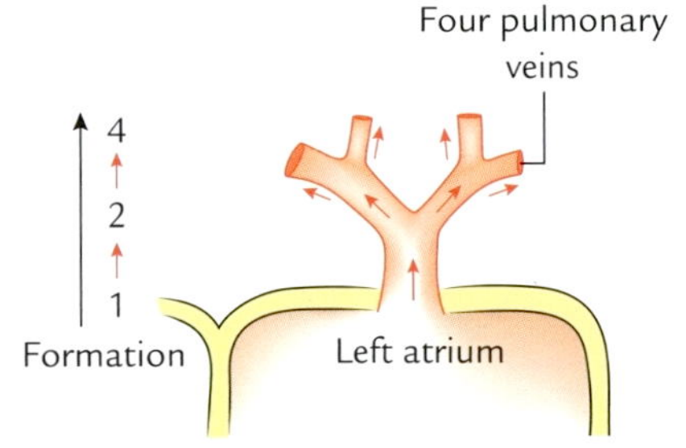

Fig. 22.17 Formation of pulmonary veins.

N.B. The left auricle is derived from primitive atrium; hence, its internal surface is rough and trabeculated.

The large, posterior, smooth part of the left atrium is derived from absorbed pulmonary veins, while the small, rough, anterior part is derived from primitive atrium (atrium proper).

The embryonic structures forming different components of right and left atria of adult heart are given in Table 22.2.

Formation of Interventricular Septum

The IV septum consists of three parts. From inferior to superior, these are (a) **muscular part**, (b) **bulbar part**,

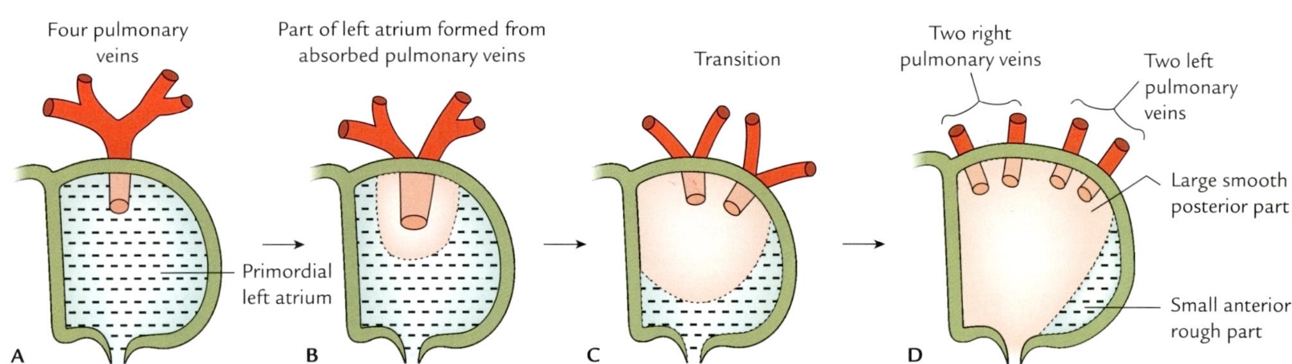

Fig. 22.18 Absorption of pulmonary veins into the left atrium. RPV, right pulmonary vein; LPV, left pulmonary vein.

Table 22.2 Adult components of the right and left atria and their embryonic source of development

Adult Component	Embryonic Sources of Development
Right Atrium	
• Rough trabeculated part (atrium proper) in front of crista terminalis • Right auricle	Primitive atrium (right half)
• Smooth part behind crista terminalis (sinus venarum)	Sinus venosus
• Crista terminalis valve of IVC and valve of coronary sinus	From right venous valve
• Most ventral smooth part	Right half of AV canal
Left Atrium	
• Posterior smooth part between the openings of pulmo-nary veins	Absorption of pulmonary veins near the atria
• Anterior rough part and left auricle	Left half of primitive atrium
• Most ventral smooth part	Left half of the AV canal

and (c) **membranous part** (Fig. 22.19). These three parts develop from three different sources (Fig. 22.20).

1. **Muscular part develops from the floor of the ventricle:** A median muscular ridge grows upward from the floor of primitive ventricle (near its apex) and reaches almost up to the AV cushions. It forms the muscular part of the IV septum. It is present in the oblique plane and its upper margin is concave.
2. **Bulbar part develops from right and left bulbar ridges:** From the conical part of common ventricular chamber, the two ridges (i.e., *right and left bulbar ridges*) develop in the distal part of bulbus cordis. They grow and approach each other to fuse together to form the *bulbar part of the IV septum.* The gap between the upper margin of muscular septum and lower margin of bulbar septum is called *IV foramen.*
3. **Membranous part develops as follows:** The gap between the upper edge of the muscular part of the IV septum and the lower end of the bulbar part of IV septum is filled by proliferation of tissue from the right side of the AV cushions and from the right and left bulbar ridges. Thus, the membranous part of IV septum is derived from three sources: right bulbar ridge, left bulbar ridge, and AV cushions. Formation of membranous part closes the IV foramen.

N.B. Once the right and left ventricles are formed, the proximal part of the bulbus cordis becomes incorporated into the right ventricle as the **conus arteriosus or infundibulum** and into the left ventricle as the **aortic vestibule**. The embryonic source of development of different components of adult right and left ventricles is summarized in Table 22.3.

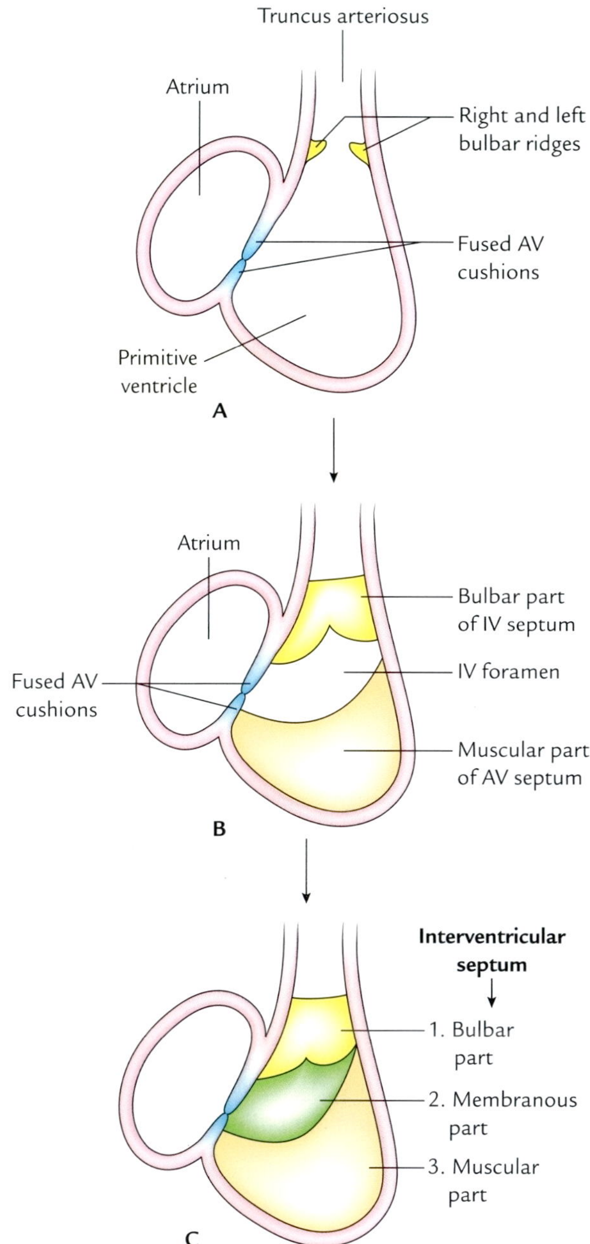

Fig. 22.20 Development of interventricular septum.

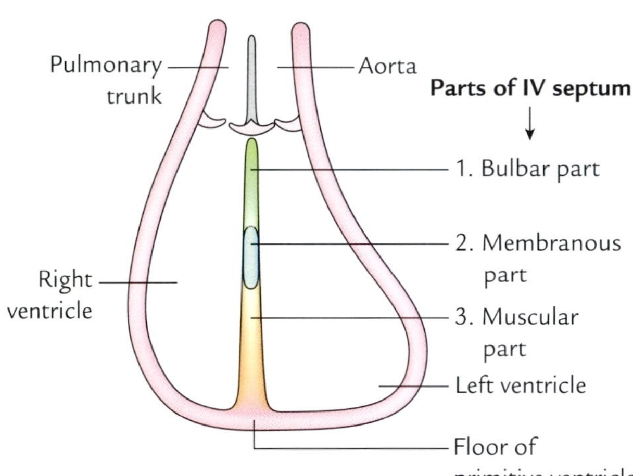

Fig. 22.19 Components of the interventricular (IV) septum.

Table 22.3 Adult components of the right and left ventricles and their embryonic source of development

Adult Component	Embryonic Source of Development
Right Ventricle	
• Inflowing rough part	• Primitive ventricle
• Outflowing smooth part (infundibulum)	• Bulbus cordis
Left Ventricle	
• Inflowing rough part	• Primitive ventricle
• Outflowing smooth part (aortic vestibule)	• Bulbus cordis

CLINICAL CORRELATION

1. ***Ventricular septal defect (VSD),*** Fig. 22.21: It is the most common congenital anomaly of the heart. This defect is most common in the membranous part of the IV septum. It is caused by failure of fusion of right and left bulbar ridges with the AV cushions, which form the membranous part of the IV septum. Thus, there occurs a defect in the IV septum which results in communication between right and left ventricles. Blood flows from the left to the right ventricle. As a result of left-to-right shunting of blood, the output from the left ventricle is reduced. Consequently, the patient complaints of excessive fatigue on exertion. Rarely, the defect may be present in muscular part of the IV septum. AN 25.4
2. ***Fallot tetralogy (tetralogy of Fallot*** [Fig. 22.22]): This condition occurs due to combination of four cardiac anomalies, namely, (a) pulmonary stenosis, (b) overriding aorta (i.e., displacement of aortic orifice to the right to override the IV septum), (c) IV septal defect, and (d) hypertrophy of the right ventricle. The resultant right-to-left shunting of blood leads to cyanosis. *The Fallot tetralogy is the commonest congenital cyanotic heart disease.* AN 25.5

   Clinical features:
   1. **Cyanosis,** i.e., blue-tinged skin, lips and nail bed, due to low level of oxygen – poor supply of blood to rest of the body.
   2. **Early fatigability** – child acquires a **typical squatting posture** after a short play.
   3. **Shortness of breath.**
   4. **Paroxysmal hypercyanotic attacks.**

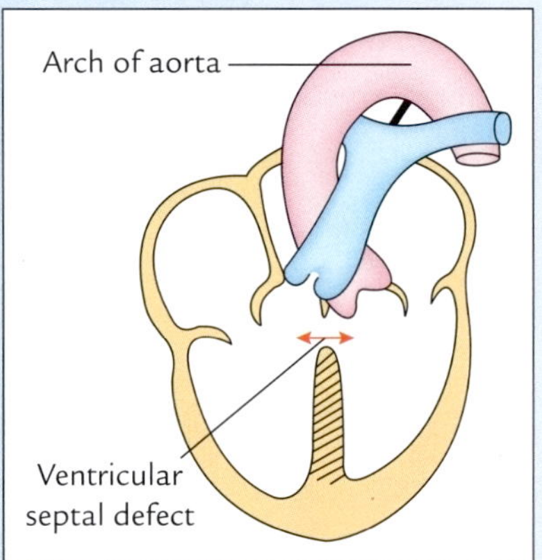

Fig. 22.21 Ventricular septal defect.

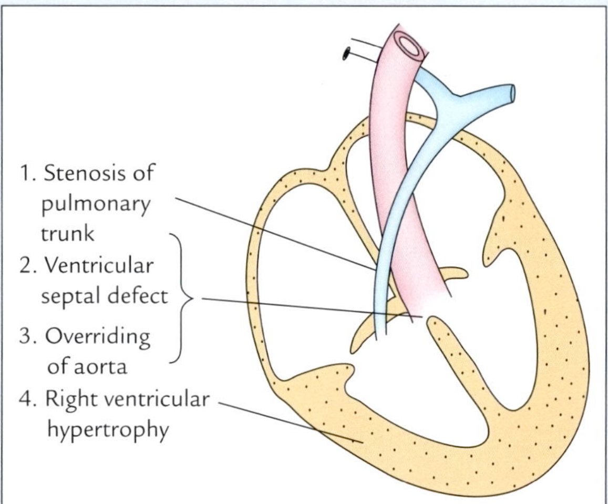

Fig. 22.22 Fallot tetralogy.

Formation of Aorticopulmonary Septum (Fig. 22.23)

The aorticopulmonary septum is a **spiral septum** that divides the truncus arteriosus into the **aorta** and **pulmonary trunk**. It develops from two truncal ridges. The truncal ridges develop due to proliferation of mesenchymal cells derived from neural crest cells that migrate in the walls of truncus arteriosus near the conus. The truncal ridges grow and fuse with each other to form the **spiral septum** close to the conical part of the ventricle. Because the pulmonary trunk and aorta are separated from each other by a septum that is spiral, the relationship of the pulmonary trunk and aorta with each other differs in the lower, middle, and upper parts. The details are as follows:

1. **In the lower part:** The *spiral septum* and *bulbar septum* are in the same plane and continuous with each other close to the ventricle. The spiral septum here is in the coronal plane. As a result, the pulmonary trunk is in front and ascending aorta is posterior.
2. **In the middle part:** The spiral septum is in the sagittal plane so that pulmonary trunk and ascending aorta are situated side-by-side, with aorta being on right side and pulmonary trunk on left side.
3. **In the upper part:** The spiral septum is again in the coronal plane but the aorta lies anteriorly and pulmonary trunk lies posteriorly.

CLINICAL CORRELATION

Anomalies of truncus arteriosus

1. ***Persistent truncus arteriosus:*** In this anomaly, spiral septum (aorticopulmonary septum) fails to develop. Pulmonary arteries and aorta arise from a common vessel. AN 25.5
2. ***Defect in the development of spiral septum*** results in communication between ascending aorta and pulmonary trunk.
3. ***Transposition of great vessels*** (Fig. 22.24): In this anomaly, the ascending aorta arises from the right ventricle and the pulmonary trunk arises from the left ventricle. It occurs due to nonspiral development of aorticopulmonary septum. AN 25.5

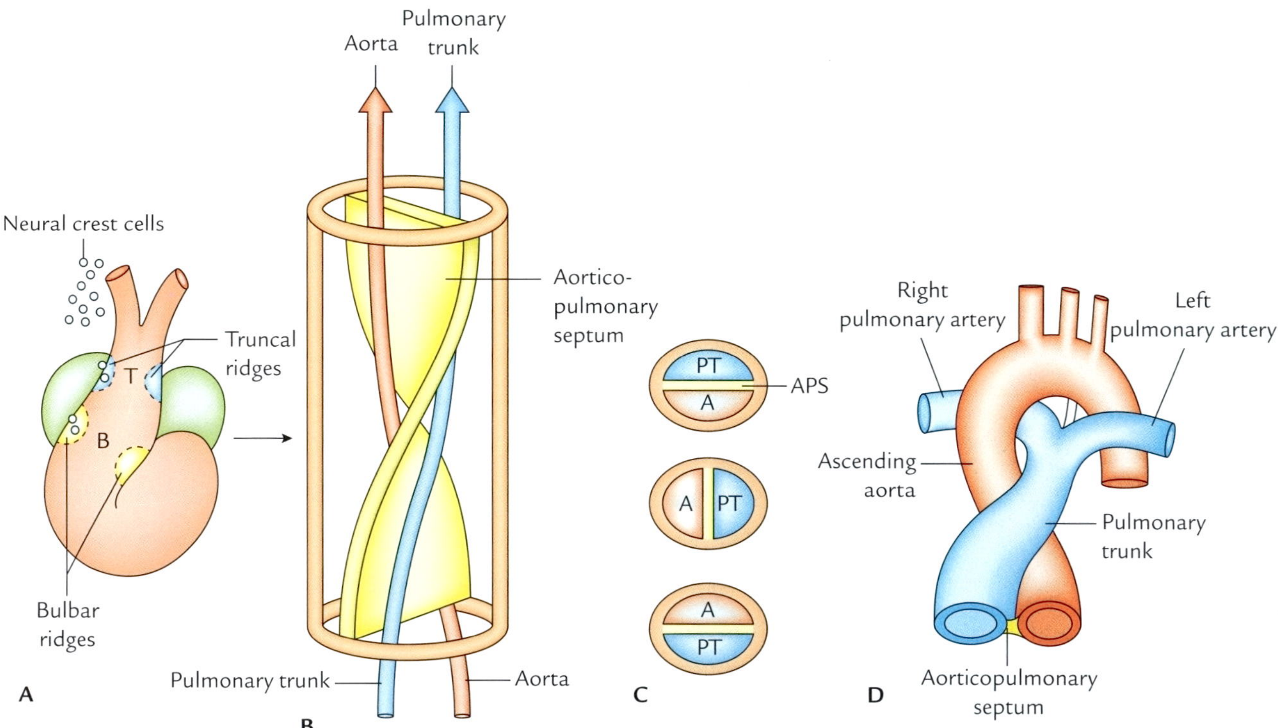

Fig. 22.23 Formation of aorticopulmonary septum. (A) Partitioning of truncus arteriosus and bulbus cordis involves migration of neural crest cells from truncal and bulbar ridges. (B) Aorticopulmonary septum develops in a spiral fashion. (C) Sections through the newly formed A and PT showing the position of aorticopulmonary septum in upper, middle, and lower parts. (D) Adult gross anatomical relationship between ascending aorta and pulmonary trunk. A, aorta; T, truncus arteriosus; B, bulbus cordis; PT, pulmonary trunk; APS, aorticopulmonary septum.

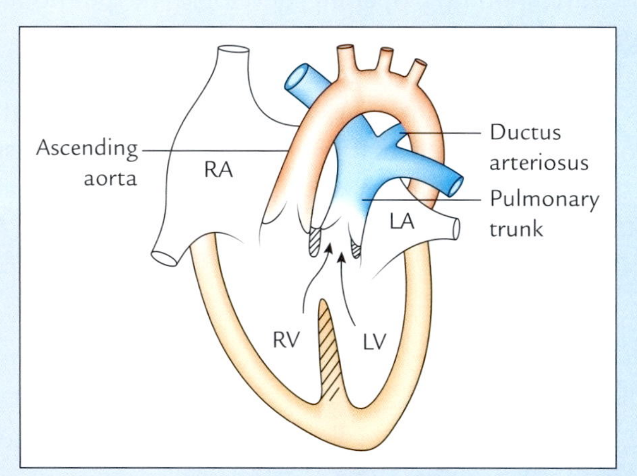

Fig. 22.24 Transposition of great vessels. RA, right atrium; LA, left atrium; RV, right ventricle; LV, left ventricle.

N.B. The errors in formation of spiral septum are caused by abnormal migration of neural crest cells in truncal ridges of truncus arteriosus.

Development of Valves of the Heart

Atrioventricular Valves

(v) Tricuspid Valve (Fig. 22.25)

Tricuspid valve is present between the right atrium and right ventricle, and guards the right AV canal. In the AV canal, subendocardial mesenchyme proliferates and forms three swellings (anterior, posterior, and septal) that project in the AV canal. The swellings enlarge and meet each other in the lumen. But the free margins of these swellings do not fuse with each other. When the bloodstream starts flowing, the mesenchymal tissue degenerates and is replaced by connective tissue. The ventricular surface of these swellings is hollowed and cusps are formed. There are three cusps – the anterior, posterior, and septal – and consists of connective tissue covered by endocardium. The free margin ventricular surfaces of these valves are connected to thick trabeculae in the wall of the ventricle (the **papillary muscles**) by thin tendinous cords (the **chordae tendineae**) much like the cords attaching to a parachute.

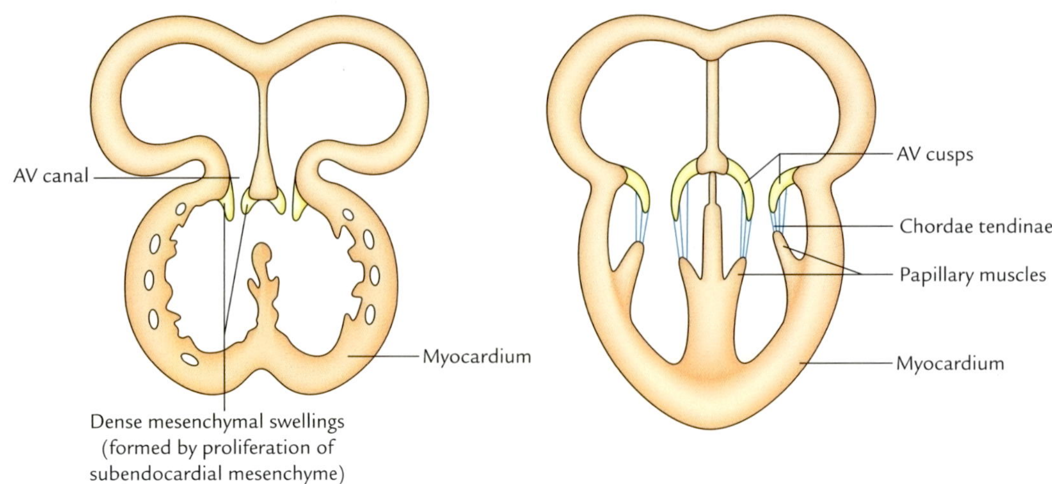

Fig. 22.25 Formation of atrioventricular valves.

(vi) Mitral Valve

Mitral valve is present between the left atrium and left ventricle, and guards the left AV canal. It develops by the proliferation of subendocardial mesenchyme forming two swellings: anterior and posterior in the same way as the tricuspid valve. There are only two cusps in left AV valve (anterior and posterior) that are obliquely placed. It is also called **bicuspid valve**.

N.B. The left AV valve is called **mitral valve** due to valve's resemblance to a bishop's miter (headdress).

> **CLINICAL CORRELATION**
>
> **Tricuspid atresia:** In this condition, there is complete agenesis of tricuspid valves. It is caused by an insufficient amount of tissue in AV cushion for the formation of tricuspid valve.
>
> Tricuspid atresias are always associated with (a) patent foramen ovale, (b) VSD, (c) underdeveloped right ventricle, and (d) hypertrophy of the left ventricle.
>
> N.B. The blood reaches the right ventricle through patent foramen ovale and IV foramen.

Pulmonary and Aortic Valves (Fig. 22.26)

Pulmonary and aortic valves develop from endocardial cushions that are formed at the junction of truncus arteriosus and conus. The two endocardial cushions develop in the right and left wall. Simultaneously, two more cushions, anterior and posterior, appear. The truncus arteriosus now has four cushions: anterior (A), posterior (P), right (R), and left (L). With the separation of aortic and pulmonary openings by aorticopulmonary septum, the right and left cushions divide into two parts. One part goes to aortic opening and the other part goes to pulmonary opening. Now each opening has three cushions from which three cusps of the corresponding opening develop. The pulmonary opening is first ventral to the aortic opening.

Now the heart undergoes partial rotation to the left. As a result, the pulmonary opening comes to lie anterior and to the left of the aortic opening; and cusps acquire their definitive relationship, i.e., pulmonary trunk has one posterior (L) and two anterior (R and A)

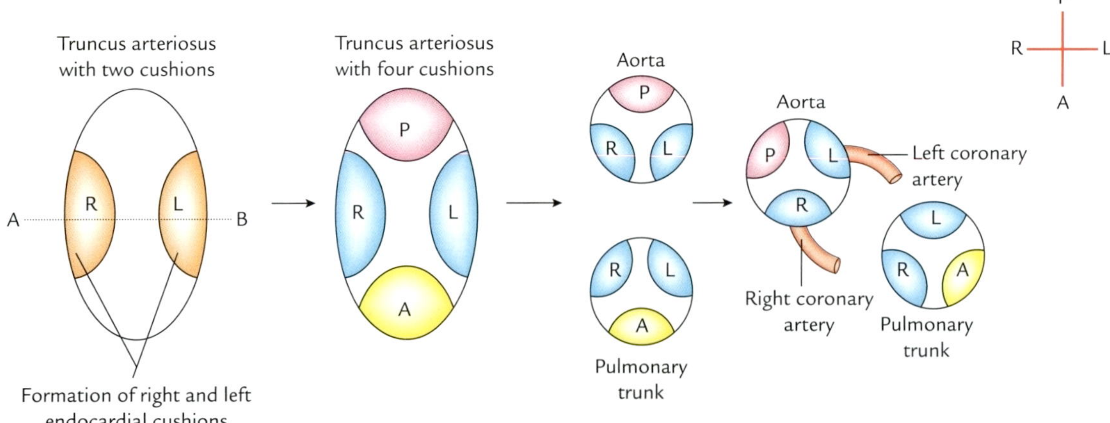

Fig. 22.26 Formation of pulmonary and aortic valves.

cusps; and aorta has one anterior (R) and two posterior (P and L) cusps.

N.B. Embryologically, the pulmonary valve has right, left, and anterior cusps, whereas the aortic valve has right, left, and posterior cusps. This terminology is in accordance with the origin of coronary arteries as the right coronary artery arises from the right aortic sinus superior to the right cusp of the aortic valve, and the left coronary artery arises from the left aortic sinus superior to the left cusp of the aortic valve. The posterior cusp and sinus do not give rise to the coronary artery, and hence it is referred as noncoronary cusp.

Development of the Conducting System of the Heart

The **conducting system of the heart** consists of four components:

1. SA node (pacemaker of the heart)
2. AV node
3. Bundle of His
4. Purkinje fibers

SA node: SA node develops during the 5th week of IUL. Initially, it is located in the right wall of the sinus venosus, but when the sinus venosus is incorporated (absorbed) into the right atrium, it comes to lie in the wall of the right atrium near the opening of the SVC.

AV node and AV bundle of His: These are derived from cells in the left wall of the sinus venosus and AV canal. After incorporation of sinus venosus into the right atrium (vide supra), these cells come to lie on the base of interatrial septum just anterior to the opening of coronary sinus. Here, these cells form **AV node and AV bundle of His.**

Purkinje fibers: The fibers arising from AV bundle pass from atrium into the ventricle and split into **right and left bundle branches**. The branches from these bundles are distributed throughout the ventricular myocardium and are termed *Purkinje fibers*.

N.B. The SA node, AV node, and AV bundle are richly innervated by autonomic nerve fibers; however, the conducting system is well developed before these nerve fibers enter the heart. The conducting system is made up of specialized cardiomyocytes and normally it is the only pathway that initiates impulses and conducts them rapidly throughout the heart. Thus, contraction of cardiac muscle is **myogenic** and not **neurogenic**.

Formation of Pericardium

The pericardium consists of two components: (a) serous pericardium and (b) fibrous pericardium. The serous pericardium consists of two layers: (a) visceral layer and (b) parietal layer.

Embryological Source of Development

- Visceral layer of serous pericardium is derived from splanchnopleuric mesoderm lining the dorsal side of the pericardial cavity.
- Parietal layer of serous pericardium and fibrous pericardium is derived from somatopleuric mesoderm lining the ventral side of the pericardial cavity.

Mode of Formation of Two Layers of Serous Pericardium and Fibrous Pericardium (Figs 22.27 and 22.28)

1. The pericardial cavity is derived from the part of intraembryonic coelom that lies in the midline cranial to prechordal plate.
2. Following the formation of head fold, the pericardial cavity comes to lie on the ventral aspect of the foregut.
3. The splanchnopleuric mesoderm on the dorsal aspect of the pericardial cavity forms myoepicardial mantle.
4. The heart tube invaginates the pericardial cavity from the dorsal aspect; hence, it gets completely covered by myoepicardial mantle and a layer of the pericardial cavity. The myoepicardial mantle forms the myocardium and the layer of the pericardial cavity applied to it forms the visceral layer of the pericardium (also called epicardium).
5. Initially, the heart tube becomes suspended within the pericardial cavity by a double-layered fold of the layer of the pericardial cavity called **dorsal mesocardium.**

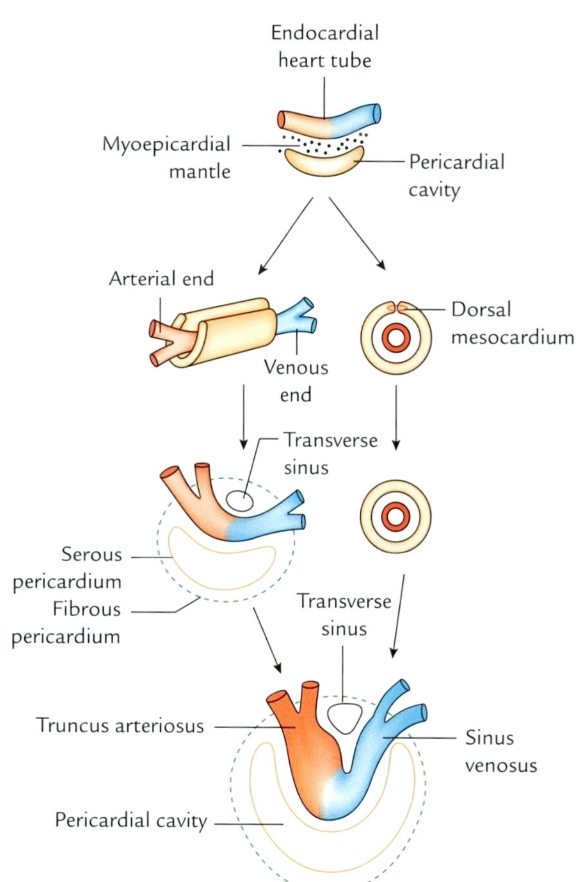

Fig. 22.27 Formation of serous and fibrous pericardia.

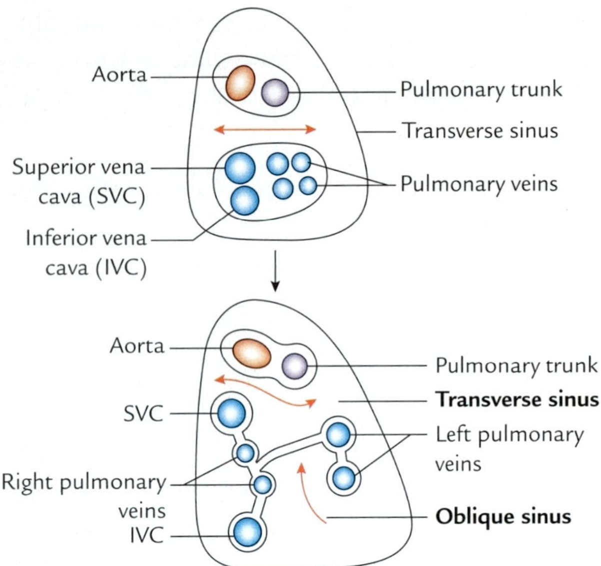

Fig. 22.28 Formation of transverse and oblique sinuses of the pericardium.

6. With the folding of the heart tube, the arterial and venous ends come close. The dorsal mesogastrium disappears to form **transverse sinus of pericardium**. Now the parietal and visceral layers of serous pericardium become continuous with each other at the arterial and venous ends of the heart tube, i.e., serous pericardium gets arranged into two tubes: one enclosing the aorta and pulmonary trunk and the other enclosing the SVC, IVC, and four pulmonary veins. The two tubes are separated by the transverse sinus of pericardium.

   The definitive reflections of the pericardium in accordance with the rearrangement of SVC, IVC, and pulmonary veins at the venous end lead to the formation of an isolated pouch of pericardium called **oblique sinus of the pericardium**.

GESTATIONAL AGE OF KEY DEVELOPMENTAL EVENTS

Developmental Event	Gestational Age
➤ Heart tubes are formed in	3rd week
➤ Vitelline, umbilical, and common cardinal veins drain into tubular heart in	4th week
➤ Heart begins to beat	End of 3rd week (day 22)
➤ Major septa of heart formed by the end of	5th week
➤ Conducting system of heart is formed during	5th week

GOLDEN FACTS TO REMEMBER

➤ **First system to function in embryo**	Cardiovascular system
➤ **First organ of the body to start functioning**	Heart (begins to beat at the end of 3rd week of IUL)
➤ **Most common positional anomaly of the heart**	Dextrocardia
➤ **Most common congenital anomaly of atria**	Atrial septal defect
➤ **Most severe atrial septal defect**	Cor triloculare, i.e., three-chambered heart due to complete absence of interatrial septum
➤ **Most common congenital anomaly of the heart**	Ventricular septal defect
➤ **Heart is most susceptible to teratogens**	Between 3rd and 6th weeks
➤ **Most common congenital cyanotic heart disease**	Fallot tetralogy
➤ **First sign of development of heart**	Appearance of paired angioblastic/cardiogenic cords
➤ **Main venous system of embryo is derived from**	Cardinal veins
➤ **Genetic basis of heart defects**	Mutation in NKX-5 gene

CLINICAL PROBLEM SOLVING

PROBLEMS

1. **Enumerate the different sources of nutritional supply to the developing embryo from 1st to 3rd week.**
2. A mother took her 7-year-old son to a pediatrician and complained that her child complains of excessive fatigue on exertion. After thorough investigations, the pediatrician detected a cardiac defect in the child and told his mother that your son is suffering from a defect in the heart that is a very common birth defect of heart in children. Answer the following questions:
   - What is the **most common congenital defect of the heart**?
   - What is its incidence?
   - Discuss the blood flow in this defect and explain the cause of excessive fatigue on exertion.
3. A full-term male infant, on the first day itself, presented generalized cyanosis. A chest radiograph (PA view) revealed slightly enlarged heart with a narrow base and increased pulmonary vascular markings. A probable diagnosis of **complete transposition of the great blood vessels** was made. Give the embryological basis of this anomaly and explain how the infant was able to survive after birth with such a severe anomaly.
4. **Retinoic acid (vitamin A), which is very effective in treating acne** (a common ailment in young women), **should not be given/prescribed to the pregnant women.** Why?

SOLUTIONS

1. Sources of nutritional supply to the developing embryo from 1st to 3rd week are as follows:
   (a) *During 1st week* (before implantation) by cytoplasm (i.e., cytoplasmic nutrients of oocyte).
   (b) *During 2nd week* by decidua.
   (c) *During 3rd week* by placenta (uteroplacental circulation).
2. **Ventricular septal defect (VSD)** is the most common congenital cardiac defect. It occurs in about 25% of the children. In this condition, an opening between the right and left ventricles exists. Initially, this defect allows **left-to-right shunting** of blood through the IV foramen due to increased left ventricular pressure. The child complains of excessive fatigue on exertion due to shunting of blood from left to right. Later, pulmonary hypertension causes marked proliferation of tunica intima and tunica media of pulmonary arteries and arterioles, thus narrowing their lumen.

   Consequently, the pulmonary resistance becomes higher than the systemic resistance and leads to right-to-left shunting of blood causing **cyanosis**. At this stage, the condition is called **Eisenmenger complex**.
3. **The transposition of the great blood vessels is caused by abnormal migration of neural crest cells in the wall of truncus arteriosus.** The migration of these cells is such that there is nonspiral development of AV septum (also see Clinical Correlation on p. 246). The infant was able to survive after birth because this anomaly is often associated with patent ductus arteriosus, ASD, and/or VSD that allows mixing of blood between two circulations.

N.B. The complete transposition of the great blood vessels is incompatible with life if there is no PDA or atrial and ventricular septal defects.

4. Retinoic acid (vitamin A) is **a potent teratogen that targets the neural crest cells, which contribute toward much of the development of face and spiral aorticopulmonary septum.** Therefore, if retinoic acid is given to pregnant women, it can cause craniofacial defects and transposition of the great blood vessels in the newborns.

23 Development of Blood Vessels and Lymphatic System

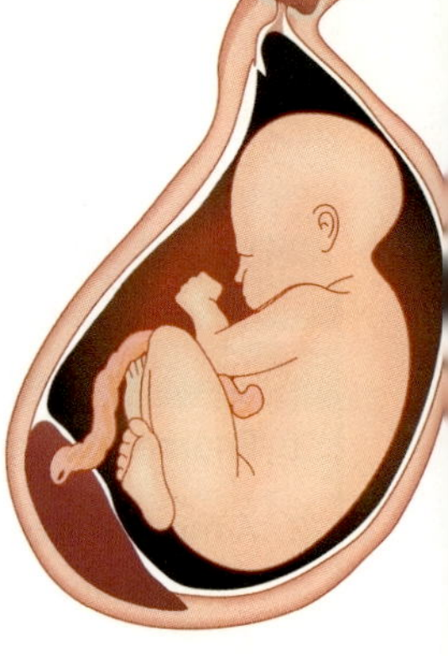

LEARNING OBJECTIVES

After studying this chapter, the student should be able to:

- Describe the development of pharyngeal arch arteries and their derivatives. AN 25.6
- Give the source of development of following arteries: (a) arch of aorta, (b) subclavian arteries, (c) pulmonary arteries, and (d) internal carotid arteries.
- Write short notes on (a) coarctation of aorta, (b) patent ductus arteriosus, and (c) dextrocardia. AN 25.5
- Describe the development of inferior vena cava and discuss the congenital anomalies associated with it.
- Describe the development of IVC, SVC, and coronary sinus. AN 25.6
- Give brief account of fetal circulation and discuss the changes in fetal circulation just after birth. AN 25.3

DEVELOPMENT OF BLOOD VESSELS

OVERVIEW

The blood vessels develop from mesenchymal cells derived from mesoderm. These are formed by two processes: *vasculogenesis* and *angiogenesis*.

1. **Vasculogenesis:** It is the process of formation of new vessels by coalescence (assembly) of angioblasts (specialized mesenchymal cells).
2. **Angiogenesis:** It is the process of formation of new vessels by budding and branching from preexisting vessels.

N.B.

- Major blood vessels of the vascular system of the body, i.e., dorsal aortae and cardinal vessels are formed by vasculogenesis, and remaining vessels are formed by angiogenesis.
- Both the processes of vasculogenesis and angiogenesis are patterned, and guided by **vascular endothelial growth factor (VEGF)** and other growth factors.

The details of vasculogenesis and angiogenesis are given in Fig. 23.1.

Vasculogenesis (Fig. 23.1A)

- The mesenchymal cells differentiate into angioblasts (vessel-forming cells) that aggregate to form isolated angiogenic cell clusters or cords.
- Lumen appears in these clusters and cords, and primitive blood vessels are formed.
- The angioblasts flatten to form endothelial cells that arrange themselves around cavities in clusters and cords to form the endothelial lining of the blood vessels.
- The primitive blood vessels get interconnected with each other to form a network of endothelial vascular channels – the blood vessels.
- Because of hemodynamic and genetic factors, certain channels enlarge to form blood vessels and channels connected to them form branches or tributaries, whereas other channels disappear.

Angiogenesis (Fig. 23.1B)

- Vessels sprout into the adjacent areas as endothelial buds and fuse with similar buds of other vessels.
- Finally, in this way, permanent vascular system is formed.

N.B. The primitive blood vessels cannot be distinguished structurally as arteries or veins. However, these are named according to their fate and relationship to the heart.

DEVELOPMENT OF ARTERIAL SYSTEM

The arteries of body develop from two main sources: **pharyngeal (aortic) arch arteries** and **dorsal aorta.**

The **aortic arches** give rise to the **arteries of head and neck region**.

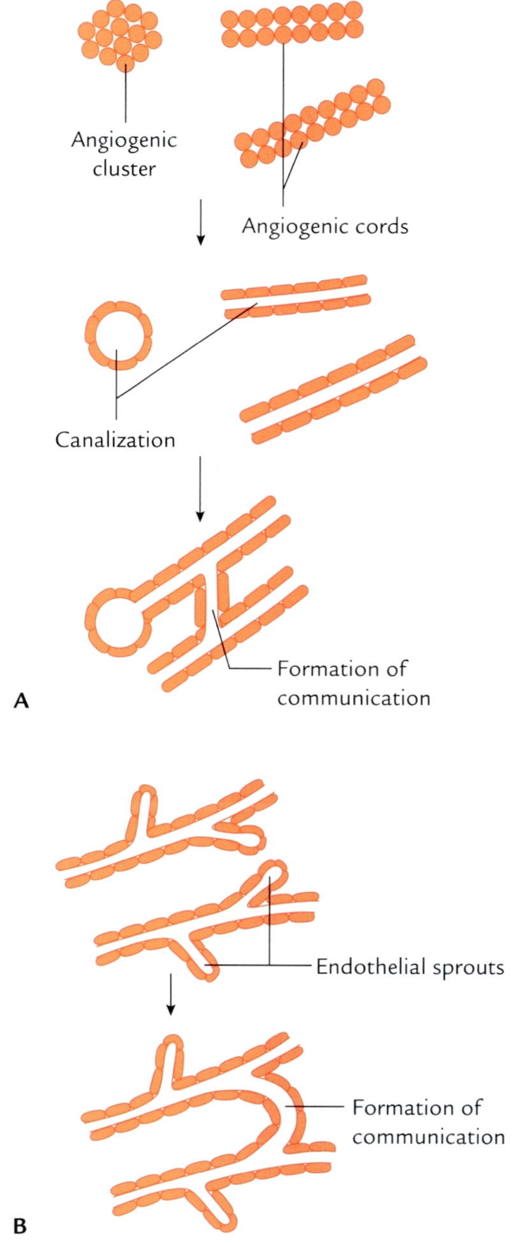

Fig. 23.1 Formation of blood vessels. (A) Vasculogenesis. (B) Angiogenesis.

The **dorsal aorta** gives rise to the **arteries of rest of the body**.

N.B. The veins of the body develop from three pairs of primitive veins, i.e., vitelline, umbilical, and cardinal (described in detail on p. 261).

The blood vessels as seen in a 26-day-old embryo are shown in Fig. 23.2.

N.B. **Circulation of blood through primitive heart** (Fig. 23.2): The blood returns to the sinus venosus through:

(a) Common cardinal veins from the embryo.
(b) Umbilical veins from developing placenta (chorionic sac).
(c) Vitelline from yolk sac (i.e., umbilical vesicle).

The blood from sinus venosus enters successively into primordial atrium and primordial ventricle. The primordial ventricle pumps the blood through bulbus cordis and truncus arteriosus into aortic sac. From here, it is distributed to the pharyngeal arch arteries. From them, it passes into the dorsal aortae for distribution to the embryo, yolk sac, and developing placenta.

Pharyngeal Arch Arteries and Their Derivatives

AN 25.6

1. First arteries to appear in a developing embryo are the **right and left primitive aortae.** These become continuous with two primitive heart tubes (Fig. 23.3).
2. Each primitive aorta is divided into three parts: ventral aorta, first aortic arch artery, and dorsal aorta as follows (Fig. 23.3, inset):
   (a) The part lying ventral to foregut is called *ventral aorta.*
   (b) The part lying dorsal to gut is called *dorsal aorta.*
   (c) The arched portion connecting the ventral and dorsal aortae lies in the first pharyngeal arch. It forms *first aortic arch artery.*

   After fusion of two primitive heart tubes, the two ventral aortae partially fuse to form *aortic sac* (Fig. 23.4).

   The unfused parts of ventral aortae form *right and left horns of the aortic sac.*

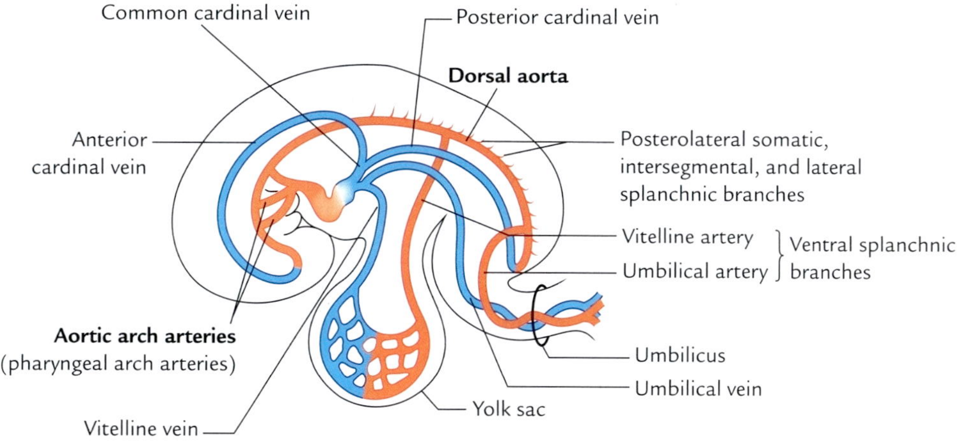

Fig. 23.2 Vessels as seen in a 26-day-old embryo.

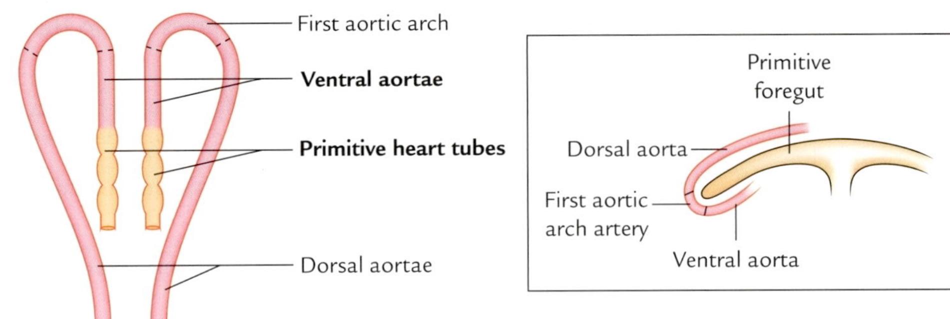

Fig. 23.3 Formation of primitive aorta. The inset shows subdivisions of the primitive aorta.

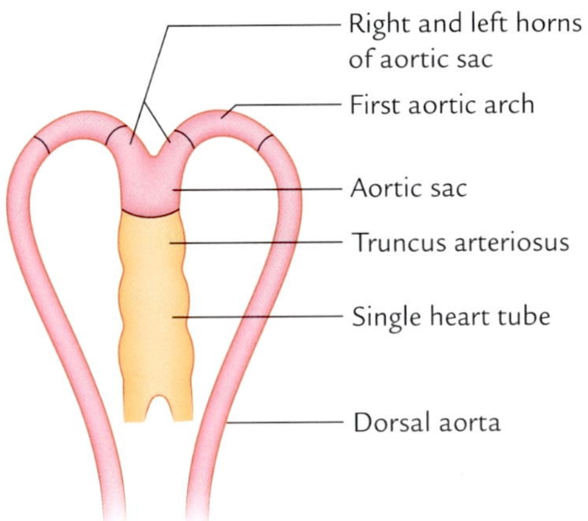

Fig. 23.4 Formation of aortic sac and its fusion with single heart tube.

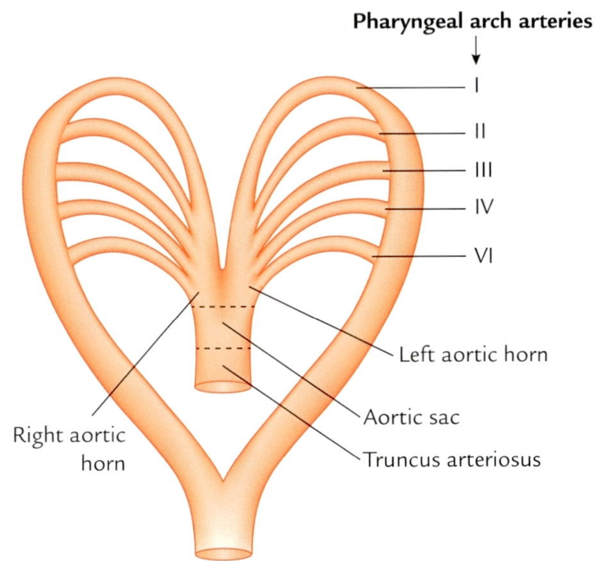

Fig. 23.5 Aortic arches (pharyngeal arch arteries).

Development of Pharyngeal (Aortic) Arch Arteries

AN 25.6

As the pharyngeal arches develop during 4th and 5th weeks, each arch is supplied by an artery – **the pharyngeal arch artery** derived from the aortic sac (i.e., aortic sac contributes a branch to each new arch as it forms). Thus, aortic sac gives rise to six pairs of aortic arch arteries. The fifth pair appears to disappear.

Hence, the five aortic arch arteries are numbered as I, II, III, IV, and VI (Fig. 23.5).

The aortic arch arteries are embedded in the mesenchyme of the pharyngeal arches and on each side connect the aortic horn with dorsal aorta of the corresponding side.

In the region of pharyngeal arches, the dorsal aortae remain paired, but caudal to this region, these fuse to form a single vessel.

N.B. Although six pairs of pharyngeal arch arteries develop, all of them are not present at the same time; for example, by the time sixth pair of pharyngeal arteries form, first two pairs of pharyngeal arteries disappear.

The derivatives of aortic arch arteries are given in Table 23.1.

Development of Main Arteries of Head, Neck, and Thorax

The major arteries of the head, neck, and thorax are derived from (a) aortic arch arteries and (b) aortic sac and its right and left horns. The details are as follows (Fig. 23.6):

- Greater part of the first arch artery disappears but its remaining part forms *maxillary artery.*
- The greater part of second arch artery disappears but its remaining part forms the *hyoid* and *stapedial arteries* in the fetal life.
- The third and fourth arch arteries open into the ventral part of aortic sac, whereas the sixth arch artery opens into the dorsal part of the aortic sac (Fig. 23.6A).

Spiral septum of truncus arteriosus extends into the aortic sac in such a way that blood from ascending aorta passes into the third and fourth arch arteries, whereas blood from the pulmonary trunk passes into the sixth arch arteries (Fig. 23.6A).

Table 23.1 Derivatives of aortic arch arteries

Arch Artery	Derivatives
First arch artery	Maxillary artery
Second arch artery	Hyaloid and stapedial arteries in fetal life only
Third arch artery	Common carotid artery, proximal part of the internal carotid artery, and external carotid artery
Fourth arch artery	• *On the left side:* Part of the arch of aorta • *On the right side:* Proximal part of the right subclavian artery
Sixth arch artery	• *On the left side:* Left pulmonary artery and ductus arteriosus • *On the right side:* Right pulmonary artery

Now further changes occur in the arterial arches to produce final fetal arterial pattern/arrangement as follows:

1. Two dorsal aortae grow cranially beyond the point of attachment of first arch arteries (Fig. 23.6B).
2. Portion of the dorsal aorta, between the entrance of third and fourth arch arteries, called **carotid duct** (**ductus caroticus**) disappears on both sides (Fig. 23.6B).
3. Right dorsal aorta below the fourth arch artery disappears.
4. Sixth arch artery on each side gives off an artery to the developing lung bud.
   (a) On the right side, "portion of the sixth arch artery beyond the artery to lung bud disappears" (Fig. 23.6C).

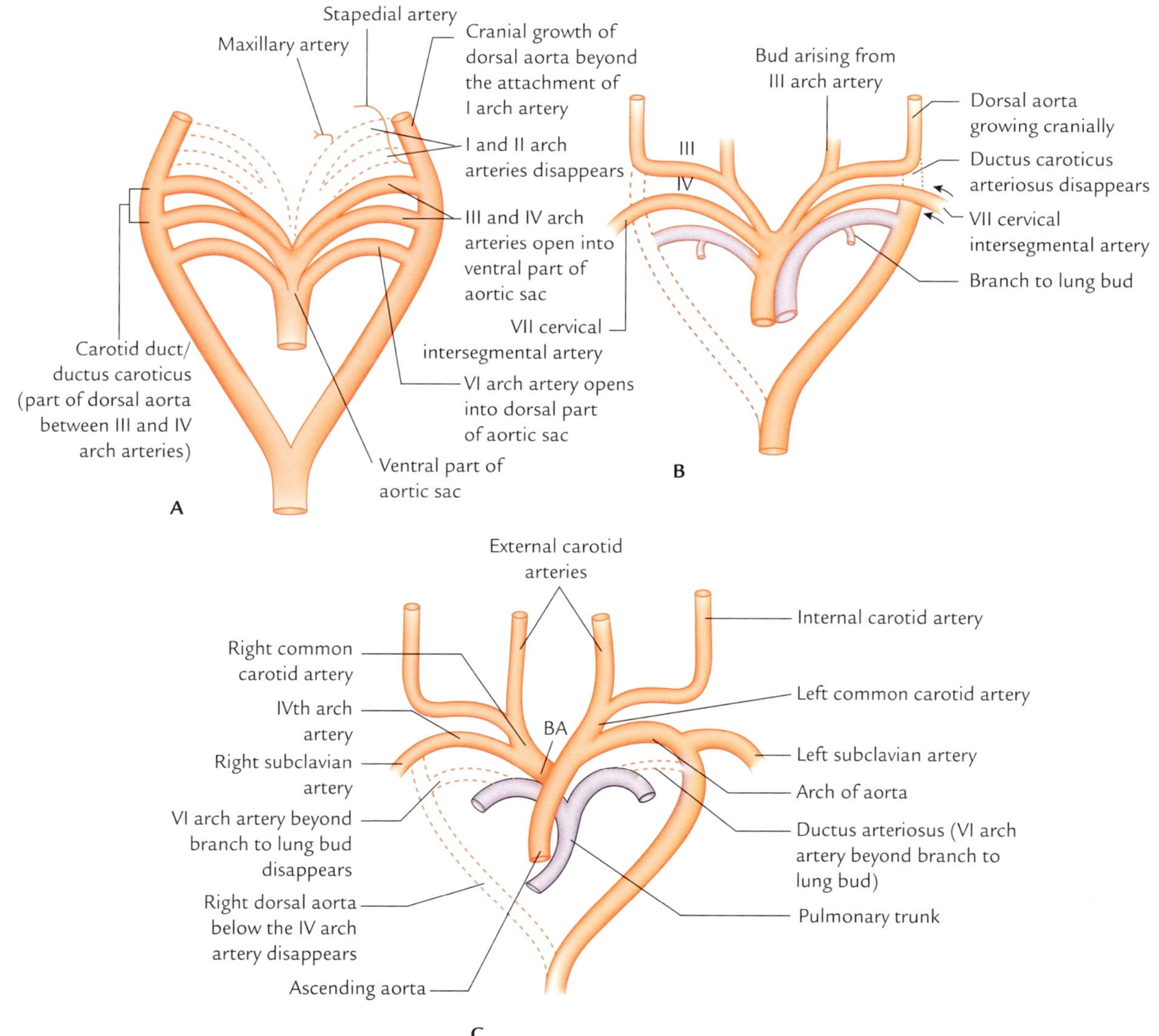

Fig. 23.6 Development of main arteries of head, neck, and thorax. (A) Extension of spiral septum into aortic sac. (B) Disappearance of ductus caroticus. (C) Formation of ductus arteriosus. BA, brachiocephalic artery.

(b) On the left side, portion of the sixth arch artery beyond the artery to lung bud remains patent and forms the **ductus arteriosus** (DA).

5. Each third arch artery gives off a bud that grows cranially to form the **external carotid artery**.
6. Seventh cervical intersegmental artery supplying upper limb bud on each side comes to be attached to the dorsal aorta at the site of attachment of the fourth arch artery.

The development of main arteries of head, neck, thorax, and upper limb is given in Table 23.2 and shown in Fig. 23.7.

N.B. On the right side, the third and fourth arch arteries arise from the right horn of aortic sac that forms brachiocephalic artery.

As a result, right common carotid artery and right subclavian artery appear as branches of the brachiocephalic artery.

Table 23.2 Source of development of main arteries

Arteries	Source of Development
Arch of aorta	(a) Aortic sac (ventral part), (b) left horn of aortic sac, and (c) left fourth arch artery
Brachiocephalic artery	Right horn of aortic sac
Right subclavian artery	(a) Proximal part from right fourth arch artery and (b) distal part from right seventh cervical intersegmental artery
Left subclavian artery	Left seventh cervical intersegmental artery
Common carotid artery	Third arch artery proximal to the external carotid artery bud
Internal carotid artery	Third arch artery distal to the external carotid bud and cranial part of dorsal aorta distal to the attachment of third arch artery
External carotid artery	Bud from third arch artery
Pulmonary arteries	Part of the sixth arch artery between pulmonary trunk and branch to lung bud on each side
Descending aorta	(a) Proximal part from left dorsal aorta distal to attachment of fourth arch artery and (b) distal part from fused dorsal aortae forming single median artery

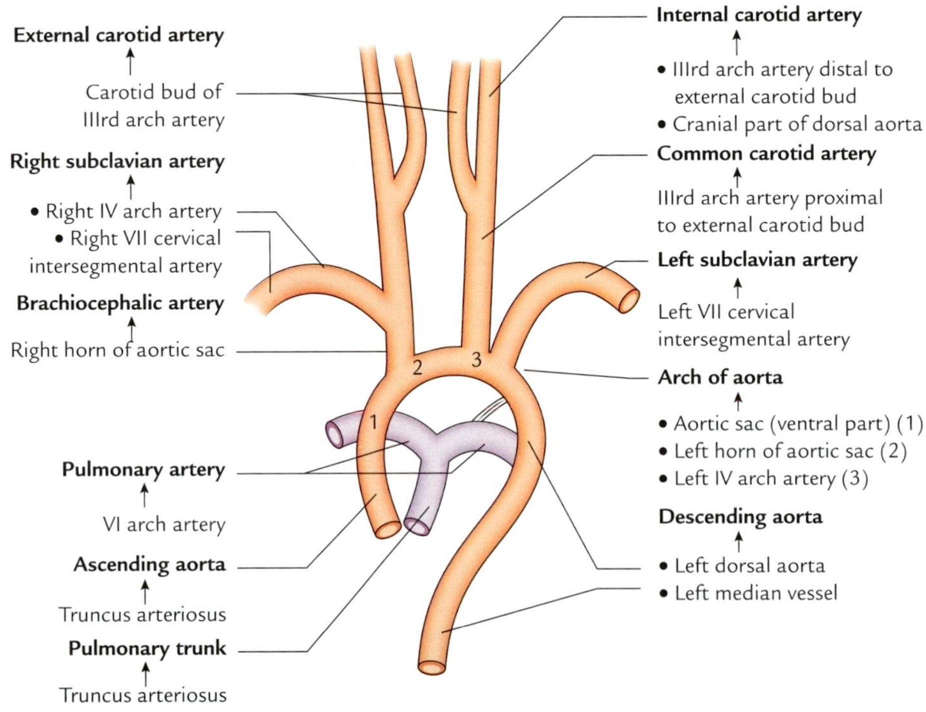

Fig. 23.7 Source of development of major arteries of head and neck, upper limb, and thorax.

CLINICAL CORRELATION

1. ***Patent ductus arteriosus** (PDA)* (Fig. 23.8) AN 25.5: It occurs when DA, a connecting channel between left pulmonary artery and the arch of aorta, fails to close. The PDA causes shunting of blood from aorta back into the pulmonary circulation. The PDA is one of the most common congenital anomalies of the great vessels occurring in 8/10,000 births, especially in premature female babies born to mothers who had suffered from *rubella infection* in the early part of pregnancy. AN 25.5

   Functional closure of the DA occurs at birth by contraction of smooth muscles of the DA. **Anatomical closure** occurs by proliferation of tunica intima of DA 1–3 months after birth. It is mediated by **bradykinin** – a substance released from the lungs, during their initial inflation.

   N.B. The **prostaglandin E** and **intrauterine asphyxia** sustain the patency of DA. Therefore, prostaglandin inhibitors (e.g., indomethacin) promote closure of the DA. The surgical treatment of PDA is limited to its ligation and resection.

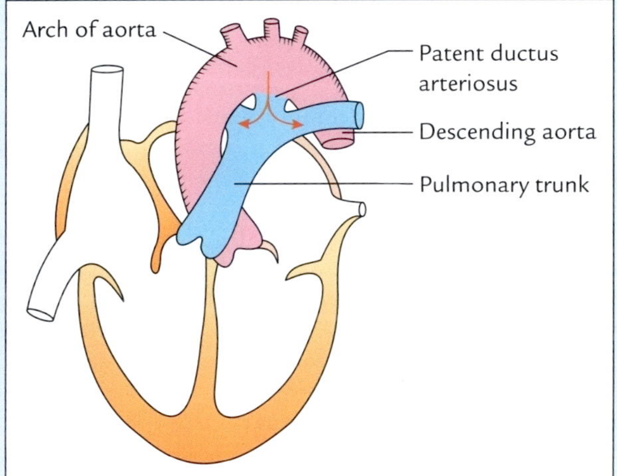

Fig. 23.8 Patent ductus arteriosus.

2. ***Coarctation of aorta*** (Fig. 23.9) AN 25.5: The coarctation means narrowing of the aorta. It occurs due to extension of the process of obliteration of DA into the aorta. The coarctation of aorta is of two types: *preductal* and *postductal.* AN 25.5
   (a) **Preductal type of coarctation of aorta:** In this type, a narrow segment of arch of aorta is proximal to entrance of the DA. The DA persists (Fig. 23.9A) in this type.
   (b) **Postductal type of coarctation of aorta** (Fig. 23.9B)**:** In this type, a narrow segment of arch of aorta is distal to the entrance of the DA. The DA usually obliterates in this type.

   N.B. The narrowing in the arch of aorta in both types is distal to the left subclavian artery. The **postductal coarctation** of aorta is more common.

   Clinically, coarctation of aorta presents as:
   - Increased blood pressure in the upper limbs, lack of femoral pulse, and a high risk of cerebral hemorrhage.
   - Collateral circulation between parts of aorta proximal and distal to narrowing involves internal thoracic, intercostal, superior epigastric, inferior epigastric, and external iliac arteries.
   - Notching of ribs.

   Dilatation of intercostal arteries causes erosion of the lower border of ribs called **notching of ribs**, which can be visualized in chest radiographs.

3. ***Abnormal origin of the right subclavian artery*** (Fig. 23.10):

   In this anomaly, the right subclavian artery arises from the descending aorta, and passes behind trachea and esophagus. The brachiocephalic artery is absent, and right common carotid artery arises directly from the arch of aorta.

   This anomaly occurs when right fourth arch artery along with part of right dorsal aorta cranial to seventh cervical intersegmental artery disappears. The part of right dorsal aorta, caudal to seventh intersegmental artery, persists and forms proximal part of the right subclavian artery; distal part is formed by seventh intersegmental artery (Fig. 23.10A). Sometimes, the right subclavian artery may arise as a last branch of the arch of aorta and runs to the right behind the esophagus and trachea.

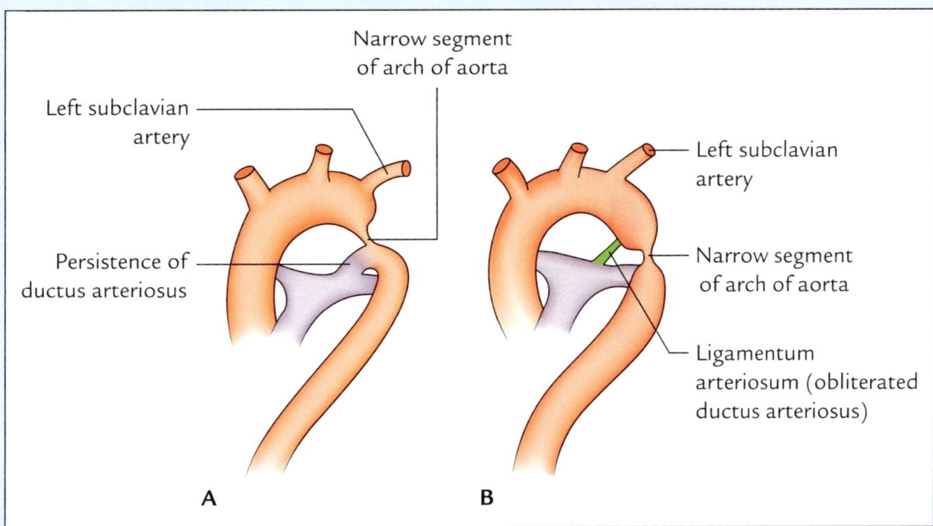

Fig. 23.9 Coarctation of aorta. (A) Preductal type. (B) Postductal type.

Continued

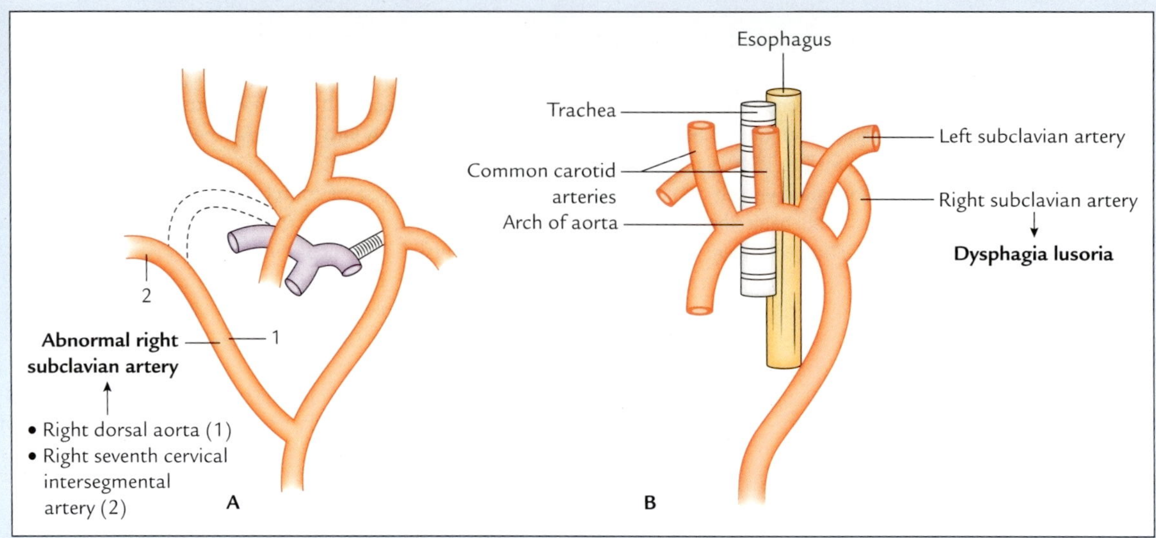

Fig. 23.10 Abnormal origin of the right subclavian artery. (A) Right fourth aortic arch and proximal portion of right dorsal aorta disappear. The right subclavian artery is formed by distal portion of right dorsal aorta and right seventh cervical intersegmental artery, and then crossing the midline behind esophagus and trachea. (B) Vascular ring around trachea and esophagus formed by right subclavian artery and aortic arch.

In this condition, a vascular ring is formed around the trachea and esophagus (right subclavian being posterior to the trachea and esophagus, and arch of aorta being anterior to them) (Fig. 23.10B). Compression of the trachea and esophagus usually does not occur as the ring is too wide. Sometimes, such an abnormal right subclavian artery may compress esophagus causing difficulty in swallowing. Clinically, this condition is termed "**dysphagia lusoria.**"

4. ***Double aortic arch*** (Fig. 23.11):

   In this anomaly, the right dorsal aorta between the origin of seventh cervical intersegmental artery and its junction with the left dorsal aorta does not disappear. As a result, there is formation of arch of the aorta on both sides. In this anomaly, the right arch of aorta passes behind the trachea and esophagus, whereas the left arch passes in front of them.

   The vascular ring thus formed between right and left aortic arches commonly causes compression of trachea and esophagus, leading to difficulty in breathing and swallowing.

5. ***Right arch of aorta:***

   This anomaly is a mirror image of the normal pattern. In this anomaly, the left dorsal aorta distal to the origin of seventh intersegmental artery disappears, whereas the right dorsal aorta persists giving rise to right aortic arch. The right pulmonary artery is connected with right arch of the aorta by the DA that subsequently forms ligamentum arteriosum. Sometimes, when the ligamentum arteriosum lies on the left side and passes below the esophagus, it may cause difficulty in swallowing.

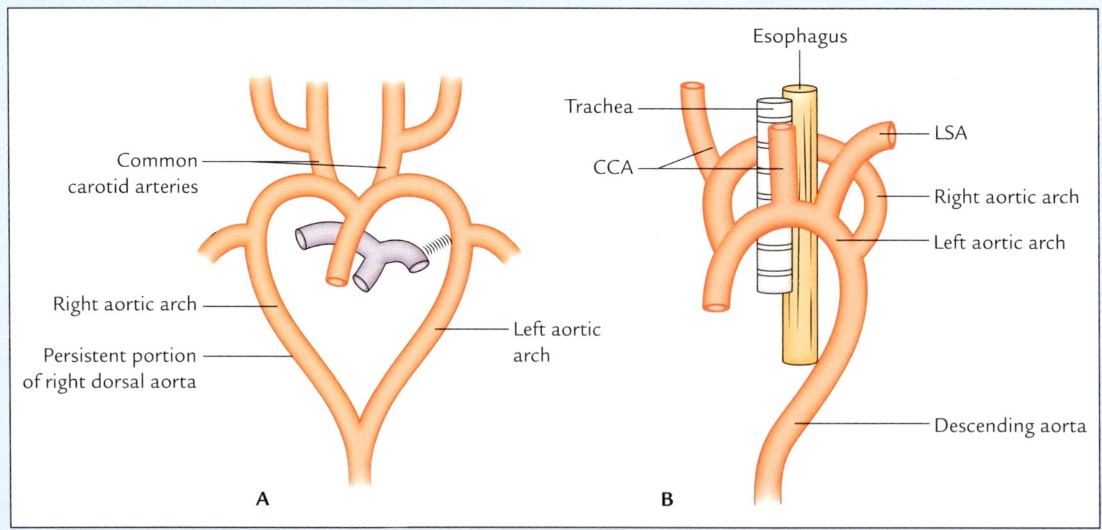

Fig. 23.11 Double aortic arch. (A) Persistence of the distal portion of right dorsal aorta. (B) Double aortic arch forming vascular ring around trachea and esophagus. CCA, common carotid arteries; LSA, left subclavian artery.

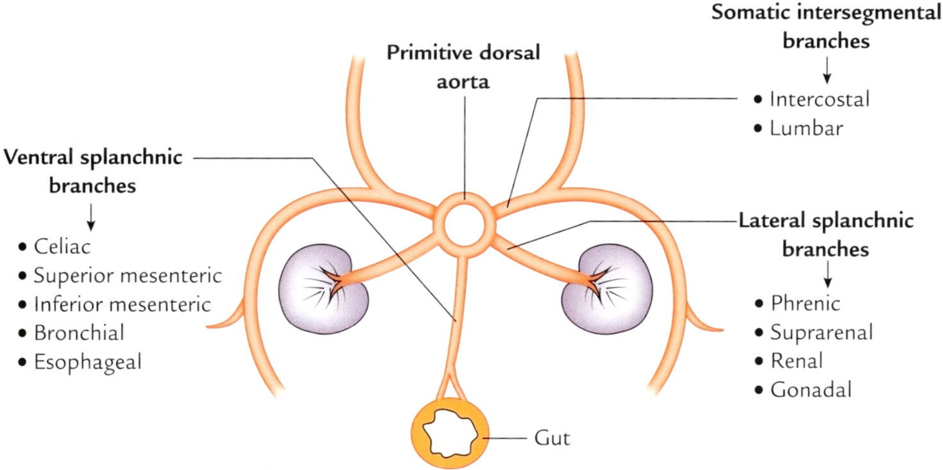

Fig. 23.12 Main branches of embryonic dorsal aorta.

Development of Other Arteries of the Body

These develop from primitive dorsal aortae. The primitive dorsal aorta gives off three sets of branches: dorsolateral (somatic intersegmental), lateral splanchnic, and ventral splanchnic (Fig. 23.12, also see Fig. 23.2).

1. The **dorsolateral (somatic intersegmental) branches** form arteries of upper and lower limbs, intercostal lumbar, and lateral sacral arteries.
2. The **lateral splanchnic branches** form phrenic, suprarenal, renal, and gonadal vessels.
3. The **ventral splanchnic branches** form *vitelline* (*celiac, superior*, and *inferior mesenteric*) and *umbilical arteries. The arteries for bronchi and esophagus also arise from ventral splanchnic branches.*

The arteries derived from the branches of the dorsal aorta are given in Table 23.3.

Table 23.3 Arteries derived from the dorsal aorta

Embryonic Structure	Adult Derivatives
Posterolateral (somatic intersegmental) branches	• Arteries of upper and lower limbs • Intercostal, lumbar, and lateral sacral arteries
Lateral splanchnic branches	• Phrenic arteries • Suprarenal arteries • Renal arteries • Gonadal (testicular and ovarian) arteries
Ventral splanchnic branches (a) Vitelline arteries	 • Celiac artery • Superior mesenteric artery • Inferior mesenteric artery
(b) Umbilical arteries	• Superior vesical arteries

Development of Umbilical Arteries (Fig. 23.13)

The two umbilical arteries (right and left) arise as *ventral splanchnic branches* of the dorsal aorta in the sacral region: Each umbilical artery develops a communication with fifth lumbar intersegmental artery. The fifth intersegmental artery becomes internal iliac artery. The part of umbilical artery between the dorsal aorta and its site of anastomosis with the fifth intersegmental artery disappears. As a result, the definitive umbilical artery arises from the internal iliac artery. The common iliac artery continues as internal iliac artery, whereas the external iliac artery sprouts from common iliac artery secondarily. In postnatal life, the proximal part of umbilical artery becomes **superior vesicle artery,** whereas its distal part becomes obliterated to form **medial umbilical ligament.**

N.B. The right and left umbilical arteries develop in the connecting stalk and then develop a connection with dorsal aorta secondarily in the sacral region.

Development of the Arteries of the Limbs

Each limb is supplied by an **axis artery** that is derived from intersegmental arteries. The axis artery runs along the central axis of the limb.

Axis Artery of the Upper Limb (Fig. 23.14)

The axis artery of the upper limb is derived from **seventh cervical intersegmental (subclavian) artery.** This artery grows distally along the ventral axial line and terminates in a palmar capillary plexus in hand. Main trunk of axis artery forms *axillary artery, brachial artery, anterior interosseous artery*, and *deep palmar arch.* The digital arteries of the hand arise from the palmar capillary plexus.

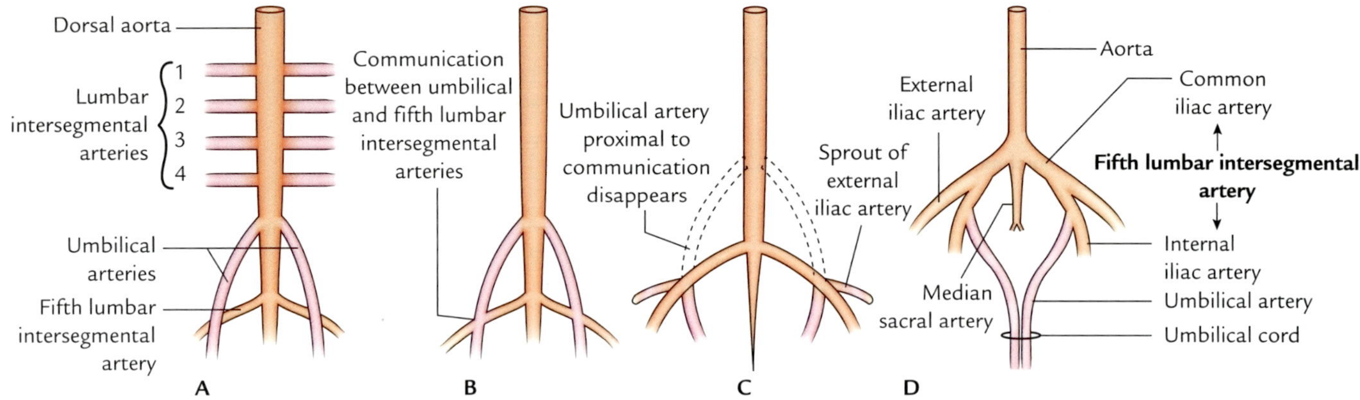

Fig. 23.13 Stages in the development of umbilical arteries.

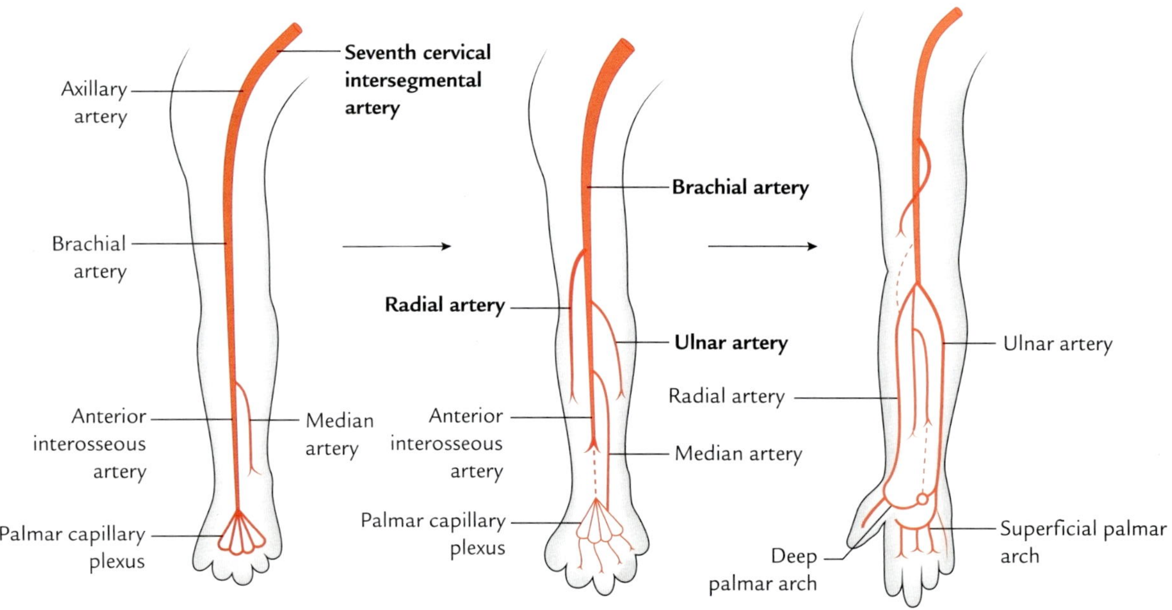

Fig. 23.14 Stages in the development of the arteries of the upper limb.

The median artery develops later from the anterior interosseous artery and grows distally to communicate with the palmar capillary plexus.

Radial and ulnar arteries develop later as sprouts of the axis artery close to bend of the elbow.

N.B. The radial artery arises somewhat proximal to the ulnar artery from the axis artery.

CLINICAL CORRELATION

The knowledge of congenital anomalies of **radial artery** is important because **nowadays it is used for cardiac catheterization** (earlier femoral artery was used for this purpose). The three common anomalies of radial artery related to its origin are as follows:

1. It may arise from the axillary artery.
2. It may arise from both axillary and brachial arteries.
3. It may arise mostly from the brachial artery and partly from the axillary artery.

Axis Artery of the Lower Limb (Fig. 23.15)

The axis artery of the lower limb is derived from **fifth lumbar intersegmental artery.**

The axis artery runs on the posterior aspect of the lower limb. It forms **inferior gluteal artery** – a small artery accompanying the sciatic nerve (called *ischiadic artery/arteria comitans nervi ischiadici*) – part of **popliteal artery** above the popliteus muscle, **distal part of peroneal artery**, and **part of plantar arch.**

The **femoral artery** appears as an entirely new vessel formed on the ventral aspect of thigh. It develops a connection with the external iliac artery above and popliteal artery below.

N.B. The external iliac artery is an offshoot of the axis artery.

The adult derivatives of axis arteries of the upper and lower limbs are given in Table 23.4.

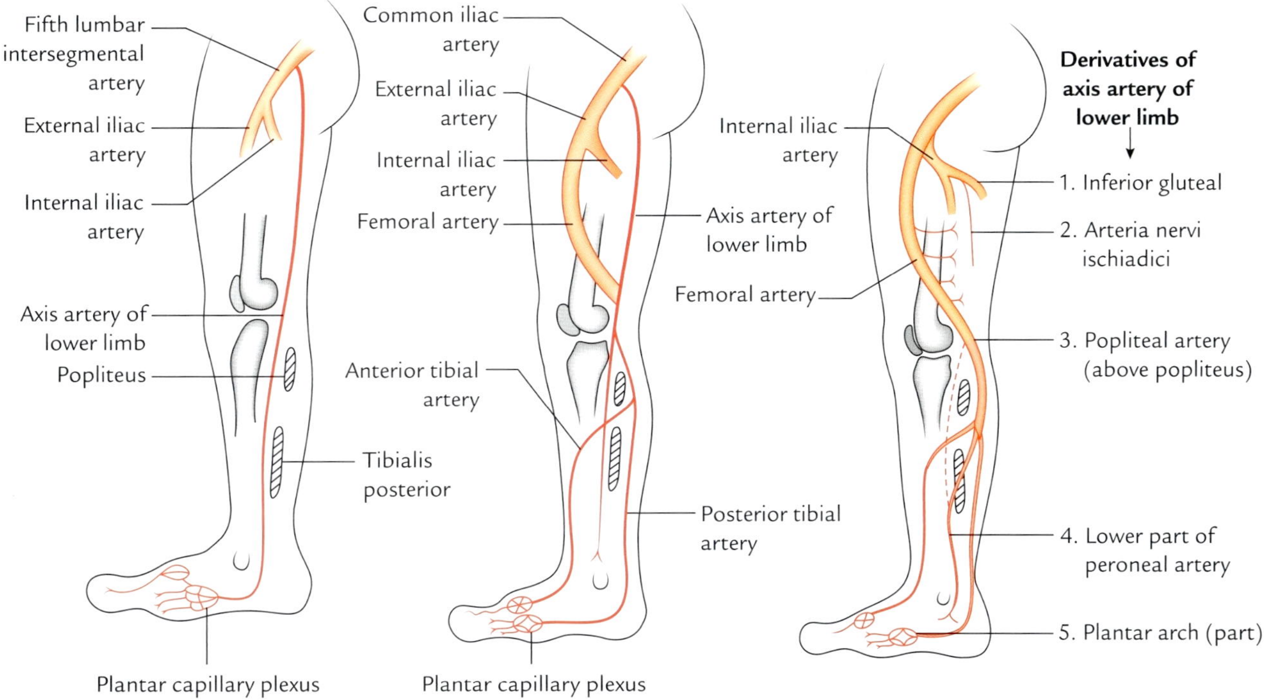

Fig. 23.15 Stages in the development of the arteries of the lower limb.

Table 23.4 Adult derivatives of axial arteries of the upper and lower limbs

Axis Artery	Adult Derivatives
Axis artery of upper limb	• Axillary artery • Brachial artery • Anterior interosseous artery • Deep palmar arch
Axis artery of lower limb	• Inferior gluteal artery • Arteria nervi ischiadici • Popliteal artery above popliteus • Lower part of peroneal artery • Some parts of plantar arch

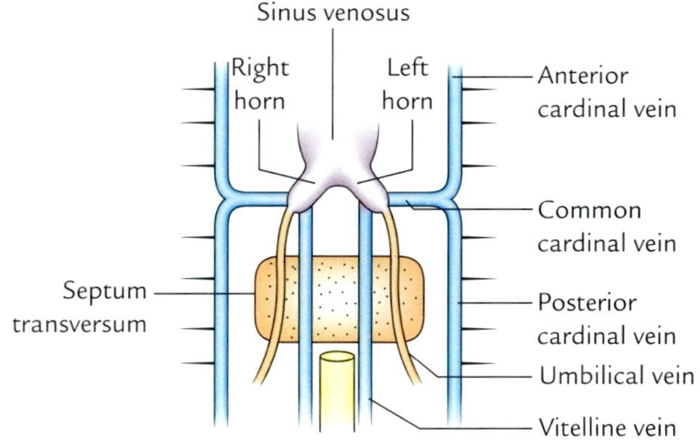

Fig. 23.16 Three sets of primitive veins.

DEVELOPMENT OF VENOUS SYSTEM

OVERVIEW

The veins of the body develop from three sets of primitive veins: vitelline, umbilical, and cardinal, which drain into sinus venosus (Fig. 23.16). These veins undergo remodeling (due to left-to-right shunting of blood to drain into the right atrium) and form adult veins.

In the 5th week of intrauterine life (IUL), three pairs of major primitive veins are seen in the developing embryo (Fig. 23.16). These are as follows:

- **Vitelline veins**, which return poorly oxygenated blood from yolk sac.
- **Umbilical veins**, which carry well-oxygenated blood from placenta.
- **Common cardinal veins**, which return poorly oxygenated blood from the body of the embryo.

N.B. Common cardinal vein on each side is formed by the union of anterior and posterior cardinal veins.

The primitive veins of embryo are classified into two groups: visceral and somatic.

Visceral Veins

There are two pairs of visceral veins in the embryo: (a) a pair of vitelline veins and (b) a pair of umbilical veins.

Vitelline Veins

The vitelline veins arise from the yolk sac. Initially, these pass from the yolk sac to the sinus venosus. When the yolk sac disappears, these veins pass on either side

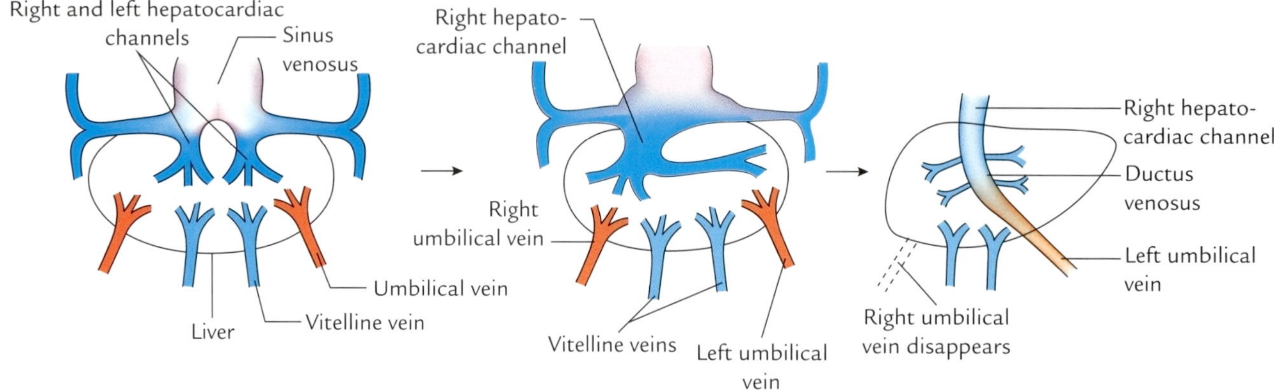

Fig. 23.17 Fate of umbilical and vitelline veins.

of duodenum to form plexus around it and open in corresponding horn of the sinus venosus. Before opening in the sinus venosus, these pass through septum transversum. These veins drain derivatives of the gut.

As liver develops in the septum transversum, portions of vitelline veins passing through the septum transversum break up by growing hepatic cords and form extensive vascular network – ***liver sinusoids***. Proximal parts of vitelline veins superior to liver sinusoids form *right and left hepatocardiac channels* (Fig. 23.17).

Umbilical Veins

Initially, there are two umbilical veins – right and left. These arise in the placenta and course through the umbilical cord to enter the fetal body through umbilicus. These carry oxygenated blood from the placenta to the fetus and open into right and left horns of the sinus venosus, respectively (Fig. 23.17).

With the development of liver in the septum transversum, the umbilical veins are absorbed and broken up within the septum transversum.

The parts of umbilical veins distal to septum transversum and the remainder of right umbilical vein disappear so that only left umbilical vein carries blood from the placenta to the liver. When there is an increase in placental circulation, to facilitate the rapid transport of blood through the liver, a large passage is formed between left umbilical vein and right hepatocardiac channel. This passage is called **ductus venosus**.

When the portal vein develops, the ductus venosus connects the left branch of portal vein to the primitive inferior vena cava (IVC) (the *right hepatocardiac channel*) and *left umbilical vein* connects with the left branch of the portal vein inside the liver.

N.B. After birth, the left umbilical vein obliterates to form *ligamentum teres hepatis* and ductus venosus obliterates to form *ligamentum venosum*.

Development of Portal Vein *(Fig. 23.18)*

The two vitelline veins lie one on either side of developing duodenum, run cranially, traverse septum transversum to finally drain into the floor of sinus venosus. The development of hepatic bud in the region of septum transversum, subdivides the vitelline veins into three parts: ***infrahepatic, intrahepatic***, and ***suprahepatic***. The ***infrahepatic parts soon get interconnected by three anastomotic channels: two ventral and one dorsal to form figure of "8" around the primitive duodenum as shown in inset on the right side of Fig. 23.18B.***

These anastomotic channels are (Fig. 23.18B) as follows:

- Proximal ventral anastomosis
- Middle dorsal anastomosis
- Distal ventral anastomosis

The superior mesenteric and splenic veins that develop independently unite with the left vitelline vein just below dorsal anastomosis.

The portal vein develops from three components:

1. Caudal part of left vitelline vein between point at which superior mesenteric and splenic vein open, and the point where dorsal anastomosis joins the left vitelline vein.
2. Middle dorsal anastomosis.
3. Part of right vitelline vein between the dorsal and proximal ventral anastomosis.

The *right branch of portal vein* develops from the part of right vitelline vein distal to proximal ventral anastomosis.

The *left branch of portal vein* develops from proximal ventral anastomosis and left vitelline vein distal to proximal ventral anastomosis.

Remaining parts of vitelline veins and distal ventral anastomosis disappear along with left hepatocardiac channel.

N.B. The development of portal vein explains that it is formed by union of superior mesenteric and splenic veins; it passes dorsally to the duodenum and divides into right and left branches that enter the liver.

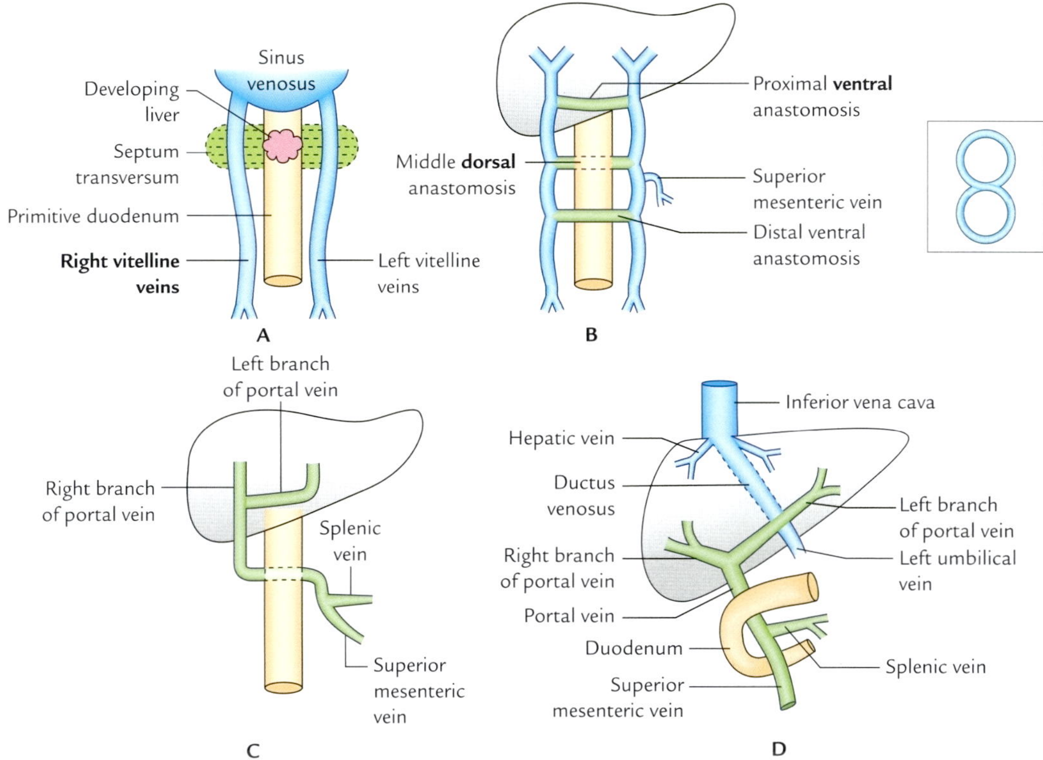

Fig. 23.18 (A–D) Development of portal vein.

Somatic Veins

There are two pairs of somatic veins in the embryo.

1. **A pair of right and left anterior cardinal veins** that drains venous blood from cranial part of the embryo.
2. **A pair of right and left posterior cardinal veins** that drains the venous blood from caudal part of the embryo.

The anterior and posterior cardinal veins on each side join to form common cardinal vein (or **duct of Cuvier**). The right and left common cardinal veins thus formed open into the right and left horns of the sinus venosus, respectively.

N.B.

- The anterior and posterior cardinal veins receive a series of intersegmental veins that drain various segments of the body.
- The intersegmental veins in the region of upper limb bud enlarge to form the *subclavian veins.*

DEVELOPMENT OF MAJOR VEINS IN THE UPPER PART OF THE BODY (FIG. 23.19) AN 25.6

OVERVIEW

- The anterior cardinal vein receives the subclavian vein that develops by enlargement of intersegmental vein in the region of upper limb bud.
- An oblique communicating channel develops and connects the two anterior cardinal veins distal to opening of the subclavian veins.

The major veins of the upper part of the body, i.e., internal jugular veins, subclavian veins, right and left brachiocephalic vein, and superior vena cava (SVC) are derived as follows:

1. **Internal jugular vein:** It develops from anterior cardinal vein cephalic to the opening of the subclavian vein.
2. **Subclavian vein:** It develops in the region of the upper limb bud by enlargement of the intersegmental veins in this region.
3. **Right brachiocephalic vein:** It develops from right anterior cardinal vein above the opening of oblique communicating channel and below the opening of the right subclavian vein.
4. **Left brachiocephalic vein:** It develops from oblique channel connecting left and right anterior cardinal veins, and left anterior cardinal vein between the opening of communicating channel (vide supra) and left subclavian vein.
5. **SVC:** Developmentally, it consists of two parts: first and second.

The *first part* develops from the right anterior cardinal vein caudal to the oblique transverse anastomosis.

The *second part* develops from the right common cardinal vein.

As the right common cardinal vein opens into the right horn of sinus venosus, the SVC at first opens

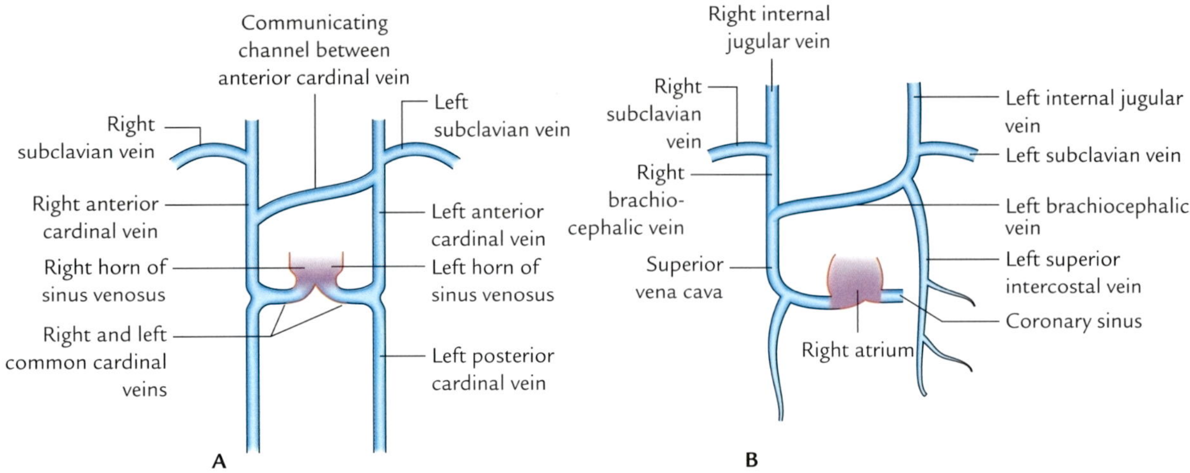

Fig. 23.19 Development of major veins of the upper part of the body.

into the right horn of sinus venosus. As and when the right horn of sinus venosus is absorbed into the right atrium, the SVC finally opens into the right atrium.

6. **Other veins:** As most of the blood is shunted from left to right, the following changes occur:
   (a) Part of the left anterior cardinal vein below the transverse anastomosis obliterates.
   (b) The most of left posterior cardinal vein also regresses. The small cranial part of left posterior cardinal vein along with regressed part of the left anterior cardinal vein caudal to transverse anastomosis forms **left superior intercostal vein.**
   (c) Coronary sinus: The coronary sinus develops from one of the two horns of sinus venosus. The left horn of sinus venosus regresses and forms **coronary sinus**. The left common cardinal vein obliterates in its lateral part and forms oblique vein of the left atrium (**oblique vein of Marshall**), whereas, its medial part contributes to the formation of coronary sinus.

   Right horn becomes part of right atrium.

External jugular veins develop as separate channels.

CLINICAL CORRELATION

Anomalies of SVC (Fig. 23.20)

1. ***Double SVC (Fig. 23.20A):*** It occurs when the anastomosis between the two anterior cardinal veins fails to form and left anterior cardinal vein persists. Thus, anterior cardinal vein on both sides develops into the SVC. *The left SVC* opens into the coronary sinus, which in turn opens into the right atrium.
2. ***Left SVC (Fig. 23.20B):*** It occurs when the anastomosis does develop between the two anterior cardinal veins, but the blood is shunted from right to left through brachiocephalic vein. As a result, the right anterior cardinal vein below the oblique transverse anastomosis regresses and the left anterior cardinal vein develops into the SVC. The left SVC opens into the coronary sinus.

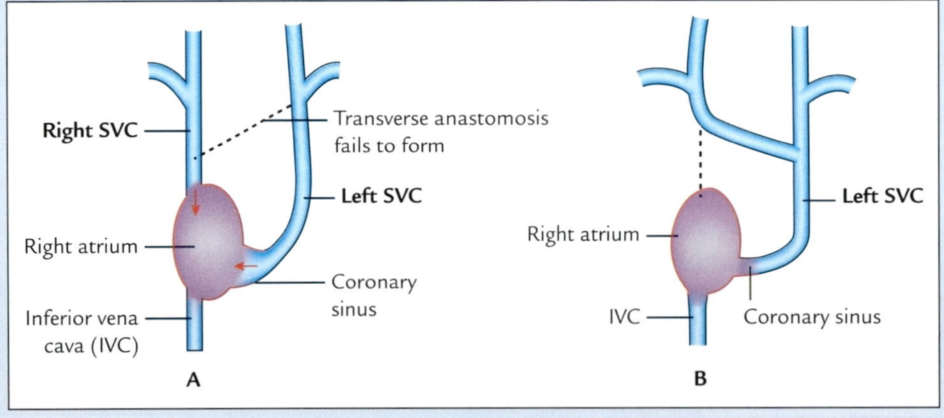

Fig. 23.20 Anomalies of the superior vena cava (SVC). (A) Double SVC. (B) Left SVC.

Development of the Veins of Abdomen

OVERVIEW

- The **posterior cardinal veins** are paired longitudinal channels that lie on the dorsolateral aspect of the mesonephros and drain the caudal part of the embryo.
- At the cranial end, it joins the anterior cardinal vein to form the common cardinal vein of the respective side.
- At the caudal ends, these receive the external iliac and internal iliac veins from the lower limb bud and the pelvis.
- There develops an anastomosis between the two posterior cardinal veins above opening of iliac veins.
- The **subcardinal veins** develop on ventromedial aspect of the mesonephros. Cranially and caudally, these communicate with the posterior cardinal veins. These receive the veins from the developing kidneys.
- At the level of renal veins, the two subcardinal veins get connected in front of the aorta by a transverse channel. The cranial part of the right subcardinal vein develops a communication with the **right hepatocardiac channel**.
- The two new longitudinal channels called **supracardinal veins** develop lateral to subcardinal veins. These communicate cranially and caudally with the posterior cardinal veins. The supracardinal veins drain the body wall by way of intercostal veins and take over functions of posterior cardinal veins.

On each side, the supracardinal vein gets connected with subcardinal vein below the transverse anastomosis between two subcardinal channels.

The **veins of the abdomen, i.e., IVC, renal veins, gonadal veins, and suprarenal veins** develop from posterior cardinal veins and related venous channels. Following shunting of blood from the left to the right, many parts of longitudinal venous channels (vide supra) disappear.

The inferior vena cava is the largest vein of the body. It drain venous blood from abdomen, pelvis, and lower limbs. Hence, discussed in detail.

Inferior Vena Cava

AN 25.6

It is the largest vein of the body and develops from six sources. From caudal to cranial, these are (Fig. 23.21) as follows:

(a) Right posterior cardinal vein (between the transverse anastomosing channel and caudal opening of the right supracardinal vein). It is termed **sacrocardinal segment of IVC** (1).

(b) Caudal part of right supracardinal vein (2).

(c) Right supracardinal–subcardinal anastomosis (3).

(d) Right subcardinal vein between (i) the supracardinal–subcardinal anastomosis and (ii) anastomotic channel connecting the right subcardinal vein with right hepatocardiac channel. It is called **renal segment of the IVC** (4).

(e) Anastomosing channel that connects the right subcardinal vein to the right hepatocardiac channel (5).

(f) Right hepatocardiac channel forms terminal segment (**hepatic segment**) of the IVC that first opens into right horn of sinus venosus, and, after the right horn is absorbed in the right atrium itself (6).

N.B. At birth, the three segments of the IVC are as follows:

- Sacrocardinal segment
- Renal segment
- Hepatic segment

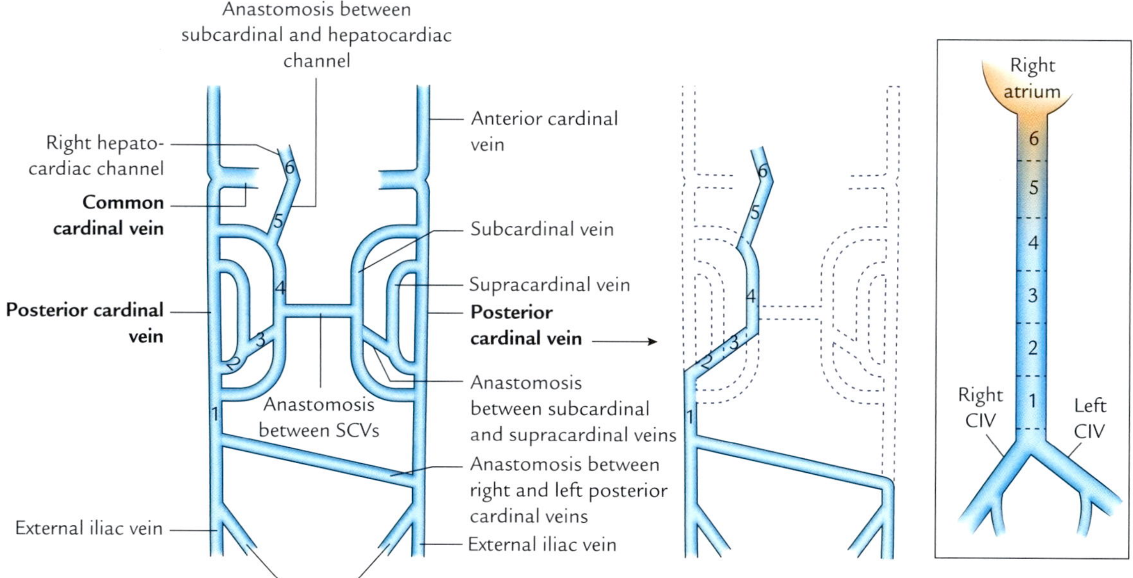

Fig. 23.21 Development of the inferior vena cava. The inset on the right shows 6 sources of development: right posterior cardinal vein (**sacrocardinal segment**) (1); supracardinal vein (2); supracardinal–subcardinal anastomosis (3); right subcardinal vein (**renal segment**) (4); anastomotic channel between subcardinal vein and right hepatocardiac channel (5); right hepatocardiac channel (hepatic segment) (6). CIV, common iliac vein; SCV, subcardinal vein.

CLINICAL CORRELATION

Anomalies of IVC (Fig. 23.22)

1. ***Double IVC (Fig. 23.22A):*** It occurs because the anastomosis between two posterior cardinal veins does not develop. Hence, the left posterior cardinal vein below the level of the renal vein develops into the IVC, whereas normal IVC develops on the right side. As a result, IVC is duplicated only below the renal veins. The left IVC opens into left renal vein.
2. ***Absence of IVC (Fig. 23.22B):*** In this condition, the anastomosing channel between right subcardinal vein and right hepatocardiac channel fails to develop. The cranial part of right subcardinal vein, which normally disappears, persists and carries the blood from the IVC to the SVC. The hepatic veins directly open into the right atrium at the site of the IVC.
3. ***Preureteric vena cava:*** In this condition, right ureter passes behind the IVC (*retrocaval ureter*). It occurs when infrarenal part of IVC develops from subcardinal vein that lies anterior to the ureter instead of supracardinal vein that lies posterior to the ureter.

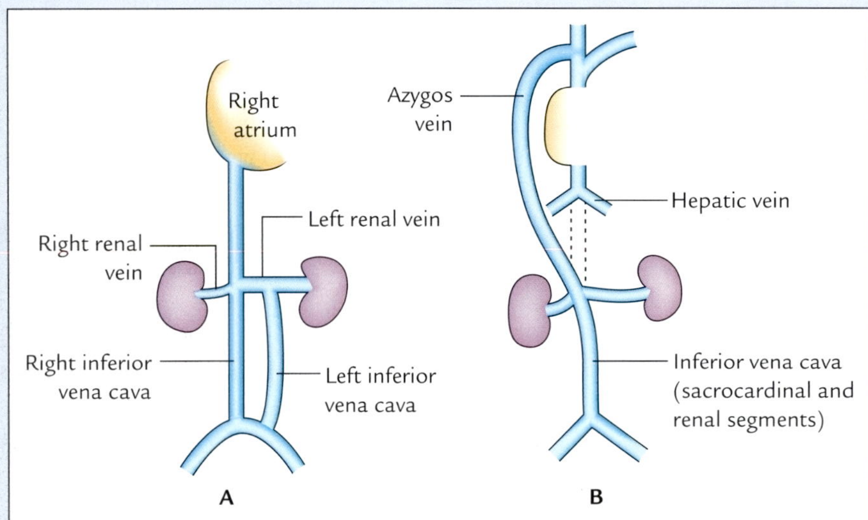

Fig. 23.22 Anomalies of the inferior vena cava. (A) Double inferior vena cava. (B) Absence of the inferior vena cava.

Other Veins of Abdomen

1. **Right common iliac vein** (Fig. 23.23): It develops from the caudal part of right posterior cardinal vein below the transverse anastomosis between the two posterior cardinal veins.
2. **Left common iliac vein** (Fig. 23.23): It develops from the transverse anastomosis between the two posterior cardinal veins and part of left posterior cardinal vein below the anastomosis.
3. **External iliac veins** (Fig. 23.23): On each side, the external iliac vein develops from one of the intersegmental veins in the region of lower limb bud. It drains the lower limb and joins the caudal end of posterior cardinal vein of the respective side.
4. **Internal iliac veins** (Fig. 23.23): The internal iliac veins drain the pelvis and join the caudal end of the posterior cardinal veins.
5. **Right renal vein** (Fig. 23.23): It develops from the vein that drains the right mesonephros. At first, it drains into the right subcardinal vein; then as this part of right subcardinal vein forms part of the IVC, it drains into the IVC.
6. **Left renal vein** (Fig. 23.23): It is longer than the right renal vein and develops from following three sources:
   (a) Mesonephric vein that drains the left mesonephros.
   (b) Part of left subcardinal vein that receives the left mesonephric vein.
   (c) Anastomotic channel between the two subcardinal veins.
7. **Suprarenal veins** (Fig. 23.23): The suprarenal veins are the remnants of parts of subcardinal veins above the anastomotic channel (intersubcardinal anastomosis).
8. **Gonadal (testicular and ovarian) veins** (Fig. 23.23): The testicular and ovarian veins are the remnants of parts of subcardinal veins below the intersubcardinal anastomosis.

This explains why right suprarenal and right gonadal veins open into the vena cava, whereas left suprarenal and left gonadal veins open into the left renal vein.

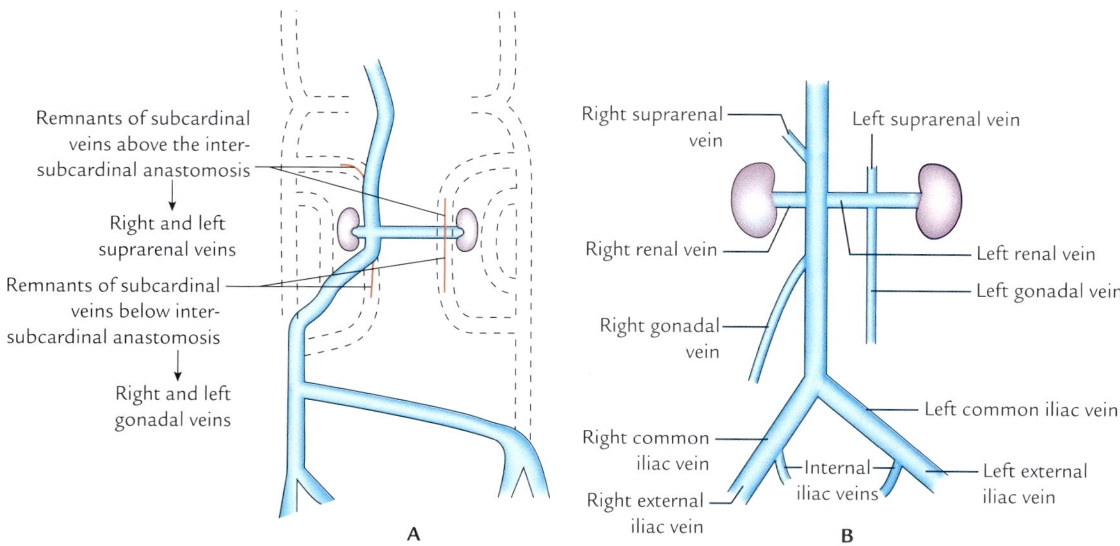

Fig. 23.23 Development of renal, suprarenal, and gonadal veins. (A) Suprarenal and gonadal veins are indicated by red lines. (B) Definitive suprarenal and gonadal veins are shown.

N.B. Major part of the right subcardinal vein forms the renal segment of the IVC (on the right side), whereas left subcardinal vein forms part of left renal vein (on the left side).

AZYGOS SYSTEM OF VEINS (FIG. 23.24)

Azygos system is located on either side of thoracic vertebral column and drain mediastinum and thoraco-abdominal wall into superior vena cava.

The azygos system of veins consists of following veins:

1. Azygos vein
2. Hemiazygos vein
3. Accessory hemiazygos vein

These veins develop as follows:

A pair of longitudinal venous channels develops one on either side – medial to sympathetic chain. These are called **veins of azygos line**. At the cranial end, these open into the **posterior cardinal veins.**

In the thoracic region, the azygos line of veins receives the intersegmental veins that later on form the intercostal veins.

The two anastomotic channels develop between the veins of right and left veins of azygos line that pass dorsal to the aorta. When most of the blood is shunted from the left to the right side, the left posterior cardinal vein regresses. The blood from the vein of left azygos line passes to the vein of right azygos line through these two anastomotic channels.

The various azygos veins are formed as follows.

Azygos Vein

It is formed caudocranially from (a) the vein of right azygos line and (b) the cranial part of posterior cardinal

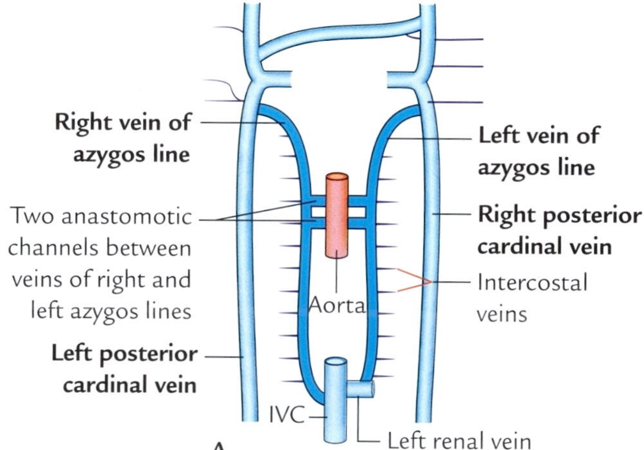

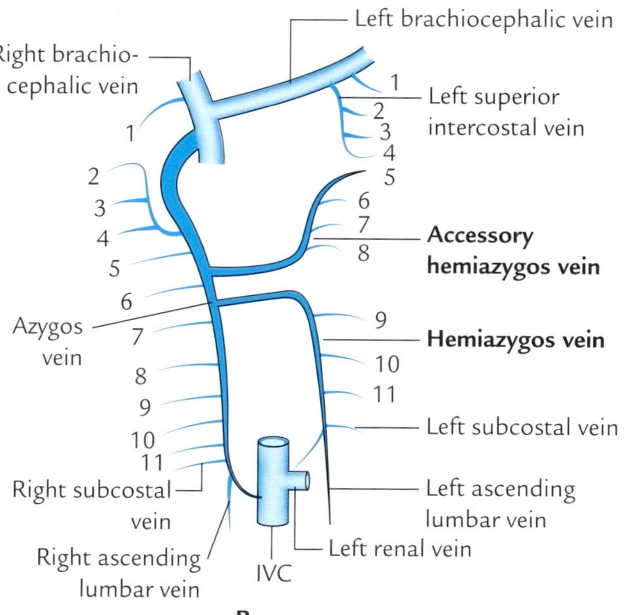

Fig. 23.24 Development of azygos system of veins.

vein. It opens into the SVC and receives the hemiazygos and accessory hemiazygos veins as its tributaries.

The vein of right azygos line communicates with right subcardinal vein, which forms part of the IVC; hence, the azygos vein communicates with IVC.

Hemiazygos Vein

It is formed from the lower part of vein of the left azygos line and the caudal postaortic anastomosis between the veins of right and left azygos lines.

N.B. The vein of left azygos line communicates below with the left subcardinal vein that forms part of left renal vein; hence, the hemiazygos vein communicates with left renal vein.

Accessory Hemiazygos Vein

It is formed by the upper part of vein of the left azygos line and cranial postaortic anastomosis between the veins of right and left azygos lines.

N.B. The cranial part of posterior cardinal vein regresses and forms the **left superior intercostals vein**. The cranial part of vein of left azygos line loses its communication with the posterior cardinal vein.

- The part of vein of left azygos line between the two anastomosing channels disappears.
- Thus, both hemiazygos and accessory hemiazygos veins drain into the azygos vein.

FETAL CIRCULATION (FIG. 23.25)

OVERVIEW

The fetal circulation is different from that of adult circulation in the following three ways:

1. Blood in the fetus is oxygenated by placenta and not by the lungs.
2. During fetal life, the lungs are collapsed; hence, the resistance to blood flow through the lung is much higher. As a result, only minimal amount of blood passes through the lungs to supply oxygen and nutrients to the lungs.
3. Portal circulation is of little significance.

In fetus (i.e., before birth), the highly oxygenated (80% saturated with O_2), nutrient-rich blood from the placenta returns to the fetus by **umbilical vein**. The umbilical vein traverses through the umbilical cord, enters the abdomen through umbilicus, and passes to the liver through falciform ligament. In the liver, the umbilical vein joins the left branch of portal vein. Here, most of blood from left umbilical vein (about 85%) bypasses the sinusoids of the liver by passing through *ductus venosus* – a channel that connects left branch of portal vein to the IVC. Only small amount of blood of left umbilical vein (about 25%) enters the liver sinusoids and mixes with the blood from the portal circulation.

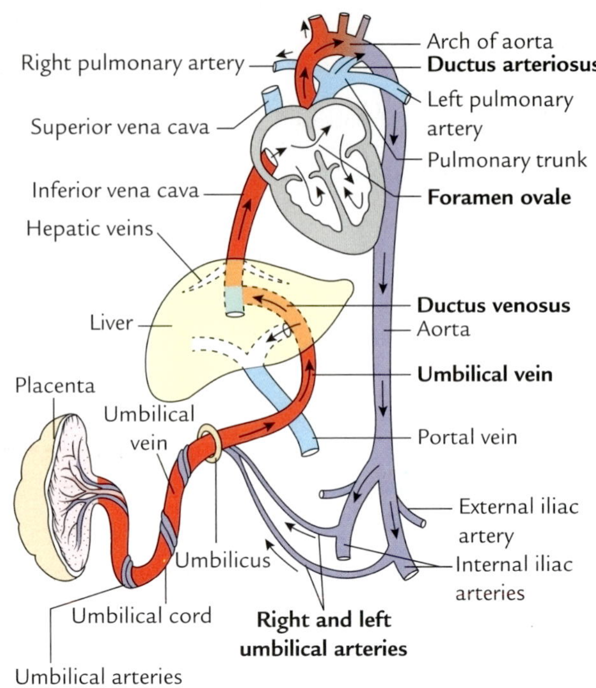

Fig. 23.25 Fetal circulation.

After a short course, the IVC opens into the right atrium. In the IVC, richly oxygenated blood mixes with the deoxygenated blood returning from the lower limbs. As this blood enters in the right atrium, it is guided by the valve of IVC toward foramen ovale. Thus, most of blood from the IVC passes through foramen ovale into the left atrium. Only small amount of blood from the IVC is prevented from doing so by the lower edge of septum secundum – the *crista dividens*. It remains in the right atrium. Here, it mixes with the deoxygenated blood from the SVC and passes to the right ventricle.

Blood from the right ventricle passes through pulmonary trunk, and right and left pulmonary arteries. But due to high resistance in pulmonary tissue during fetal life, only a small amount of blood enters the **pulmonary circulation**, and most of it passes into the aorta through the **DA** – a channel that connects the left pulmonary artery to arch of aorta.

The left atrium receives mainly oxygen-rich blood from the right atrium through the **foramen ovale.** Only a small amount of deoxygenated blood enters the left atrium from the lungs through the pulmonary veins. Blood from the left atrium passes to the left ventricle.

Blood from the left ventricle enters into the ascending aorta, which – through its three large branches (brachiocephalic artery, left common carotid artery, and left subclavian artery) – supplies oxygenated blood to the head, neck, brain, and superior extremity. Since the coronary and carotid arteries are the first branches of the aorta, the heart musculature and brain are supplied by well-oxygenated blood. Thereafter, the arch of aorta receives poorly oxygenated blood from the pulmonary trunk through the DA. Then the blood is distributed by the aorta and common iliac arteries to the lower part of the body. The lower part of the body is thus supplied with relatively less oxygenated blood as compared with the upper part of the body.

The **two umbilical arteries** arising from internal iliac branches of common iliac arteries carry deoxygenated blood, pass through umbilicus and enter the placenta through the umbilical cord. In placenta blood is oxygenated.

Changes in Fetal Circulation Just After Birth

After birth, the placenta – **fetal organ of respiration** – is separated from newborn and lungs start oxygenating the blood, i.e., respiration is established. Now, the oxygenated blood comes to the heart from the lungs. As a result, the following changes take place in fetal circulation:

1. **Umbilical vein**, as it no longer carries any blood from the placenta, obliterates and forms a fibrous ligament called *ligamentum teres hepatis.*
2. **Ductus venosus** obliterates to form a fibrous ligament called *ligamentum venosum.*
3. As the lungs are inflated and the pulmonary circulation is established, pulmonary veins bring more blood to the left atrium. Now, as the pressure of blood in the left atrium is more than that in the right atrium, the septum primum is pushed to the right and the foramen ovale is closed. At first, the closure of foramen ovale is physiological, but later on, septum primum fuses with the septum secundum and there is an anatomical closure of foramen ovale. The closed **foramen ovale** forms *fossa ovalis.*
4. DA obliterates to form a fibrous ligament called the *ligamentum arteriosum.*
5. **Umbilical arteries** (right and left) obliterate. However, their proximal parts remain open. The proximal parts of umbilical arteries form *superior vesicle arteries,* whereas their distal parts form fibrous ligaments called *medial umbilical ligaments.*

The remnants of fetal circulatory structures that remain after birth due to start of neonatal circulation are summarized in Table 23.5.

Table 23.5 Remnants of fetal circulatory structures after birth

Fetal Structure	Remnants After Birth
1. Umbilical vein	Round ligament of liver (ligamentum teres hepatis)
2. Ductus venosus	Ligamentum venosum
3. Foramen ovale	Fossa ovalis
4. Ductus arteriosus	Ligamentum arteriosum
5. Right and left umbilical arteries	• Superior vesicle arteries • Right and left medial umbilical ligaments

DEVELOPMENT OF LYMPHATIC SYSTEM

The lymphatic system is essentially a drainage system that is accessory to the venous system. Hence, it is described here.

The **lymphatic system develops at the end of the 5th week, about 1 week later to that of the cardiovascular** system. The exact development of lymph vessels is not clear but these may develop in the following two ways: (a) these may form from mesenchyme in situ or (b) these may arise as **sac-like outgrowths** from the endothelium of veins. In whatever way these develop, these connect themselves with the venous system.

CLINICAL CORRELATION

Blood transfusion through umbilical vein: The umbilical vein remains patent for a considerable time after birth; hence, it is used by pediatricians for exchange transfusions of blood during early infancy. The transfusions of blood in early infancy are often required to prevent brain damage and death of infants due to anemia caused by a condition called *erythroblastosis fetalis* (a grave hemolytic disease in newborn babies).

Development of Lymph Sacs and Lymph Vessels

The following **six primary lymph sacs** are formed during the embryonic period (Fig. 23.26):

1. **Two jugular lymph sacs** at the junction between the subclavian veins and anterior cardinal veins (future internal jugular veins).
2. **Two iliac lymph sacs** at the junction of iliac and the posterior cardinal veins.
3. **One retroperitoneal lymph sac** in the root of the mesentery on the posterior abdominal wall.
4. **One cisterna chyli** lying posterior to the retroperitoneal lymph sac.

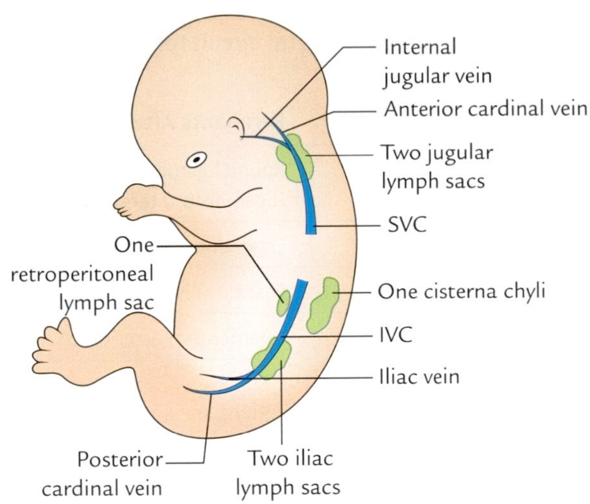

Fig. 23.26 Development of lymph sac.

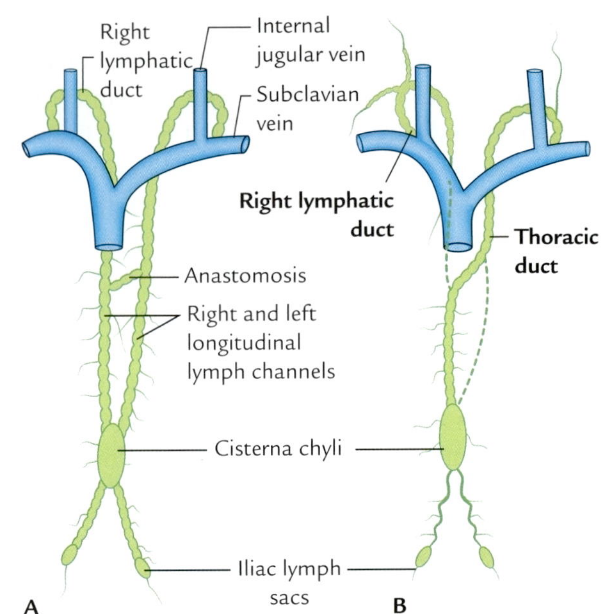

Fig. 23.27 Development of thoracic and right lymphatic ducts.

5. Numerous small lymph channels/vessels connect the lymph sacs with each other and pass along the main veins to drain lymph from limbs, body wall, head, and neck.
6. Two large lymph channels (right and left lymph channels) connect the jugular lymph sacs with the cisterna chyli. Soon large anastomosis forms between these ducts.

N.B. The lymph vessels soon connect to the lymph sacs.

Development of Thoracic Duct (Fig. 23.27)

There are three steps in the development of the **thoracic duct**:

1. **Stage I:** A network of lymph channels is formed in front of the thoracic part of the vertebral column.
2. **Stage II:** In this network of lymph channels, two large longitudinal channels appear – one left and another right with a number of cross-communications.
3. **Stage III:** Formation of cross-communication between two longitudinal channels opposite to the body of fifth thoracic vertebra takes place. Now, the right longitudinal channel below cross-communication and the left longitudinal channel above communication persist and give rise to the thoracic duct. All other channels disappear.

Thus, the ***thoracic duct is derived from the following three sources:***

(a) Caudal part of the right longitudinal lymph channel.
(b) Anastomosis between the right and left longitudinal lymph channel.
(c) Cranial portion of the left longitudinal lymph channel.

Development of Right Lymphatic Duct

It develops from the cranial portion of the right longitudinal lymph channel. Both thoracic and right lymphatic ducts open into the junction of the internal jugular and subclavian vein of the left and right side, respectively.

Development of Lymph Nodes

The lymph nodes develop from the mesenchymal cells in relation to the primary lymph sacs.

Except for the upper part of cisterna chyli, all the lymph sacs are transformed into groups of lymph nodes during early fetal life as follows:

1. Mesenchymal cells invade each lymph sac and break up its cavity into a network of lymph channels to form *lymph sinuses*.
2. Other mesenchymal cells give rise to the capsule and connective tissue network of the lymph nodes.

Development of Lymphocytes

Early on, the lymphocytes first develop from stem cells in the mesenchyme of the yolk sac and later on from the liver and spleen.

The early lymphocytes enter into bone marrow, from where these divide to form the **lymphoblasts.**

The lymphocytes that appear in the lymph nodes before birth are derived from thymus. The small lymphocytes leave the thymus to reach other lymphoid organs through circulation. Later, some mesenchymal cells of lymph nodes also differentiate into the lymphocytes.

N.B. The lymph nodules do not appear in the lymph nodes until just before and/or just after birth, as there is no exposure to foreign antigens.

Development of Spleen and Tonsils

1. **Spleen** develops from an aggregation of mesenchymal cells between the two layers of dorsal mesogastrium (for details, see p. 212).
2. **Palatine tonsil** develops from the endodermal lining of second pharyngeal pouch and underlying mesenchyme.
3. **Tubal tonsil** develops from an aggregation of the lymph nodules around the opening of pharyngotympanic tube in the nasopharynx.
4. **Pharyngeal tonsil** develops from an aggregation of the lymph nodules in the posterosuperior wall of the nasopharynx.
5. **Lingual tonsil** develops from an aggregation of the lymph nodules on dorsum of the posterior one-third of the tongue.

N.B. The lymph nodules also develop into the mucosa of gastrointestinal and respiratory tracts.

GESTATIONAL AGE OF KEY DEVELOPMENTAL EVENTS

Developmental Event	Time of Occurrence
➤ Islands of blood-forming cells (angioblastic islands) appear in	3rd week
➤ Formation of aortic arch arteries occurs during	4th week
➤ Three pairs of major primitive veins (e.g., vitelline, umbilical, and common cardinal) develop during	5th week
➤ Formation of lymphatic sacs occurs in	5th week
➤ Lymphatic system develops at the end of	5th week
➤ All the lymph sacs are present at	Birth

GOLDEN FACTS TO REMEMBER

➤ **First arteries to appear in the embryo**	Right and left primitive aortae
➤ **Most common congenital anomaly of great vessels**	Patent ductus arteriosus
➤ **Two embryonic sources that form all the arteries of the body**	(a) Pharyngeal arch arteries (b) Dorsal aorta
➤ **Fate of seventh cervical intersegmental artery**	(a) Its stem forms subclavian artery (b) Its dorsal division forms stem of vertebral artery (c) Its superolateral division forms artery of upper limb bud (d) Its ventral division forms stem of internal mammary artery
➤ **Two important radiological features seen in coarctation of aorta**	(a) Notching of the lower border of ribs (b) Double aortic knuckle
➤ **Vein of Marshall**	Oblique vein of left atrium
➤ **Coronary sinus develops from**	Left horn of sinus venosus and proximal part of left common cardinal vein
➤ **Three sources from which left renal vein forms**	(a) Mesonephric vein (b) Left subcardinal vein (c) Intersubcardinal anastomosis
➤ **Persistent caudal part of left umbilical vein represents**	Umbilical vein in umbilical cord
➤ **Umbilical veins (right and left) carry**	Well-oxygenated blood from placenta to sinus venosus
➤ **Fetal organ of respiration**	Placenta

CLINICAL PROBLEM SOLVING

PROBLEMS

1. **Why the course of recurrent laryngeal nerves differs on two sides? Give the embryological basis.**
2. **Why newborn baby develops cyanosis (i.e., face becomes blue) when he/she cries?**
3. **The blood in the umbilical vein gradually loses its high oxygen content during its course from the placenta to the fetus. Why?**

SOLUTIONS

1. The recurrent laryngeal nerves (the nerves of the sixth pharyngeal arches) initially hook around the sixth arch artery on the respective side on their way to the developing larynx (Fig. 23.28).
   (a) **On the right side** because the distal part of the sixth arch artery disappears, the *right recurrent laryngeal* nerve moves superiorly and hooks around the proximal part of the right subclavian artery (the derivative of fourth pharyngeal artery).

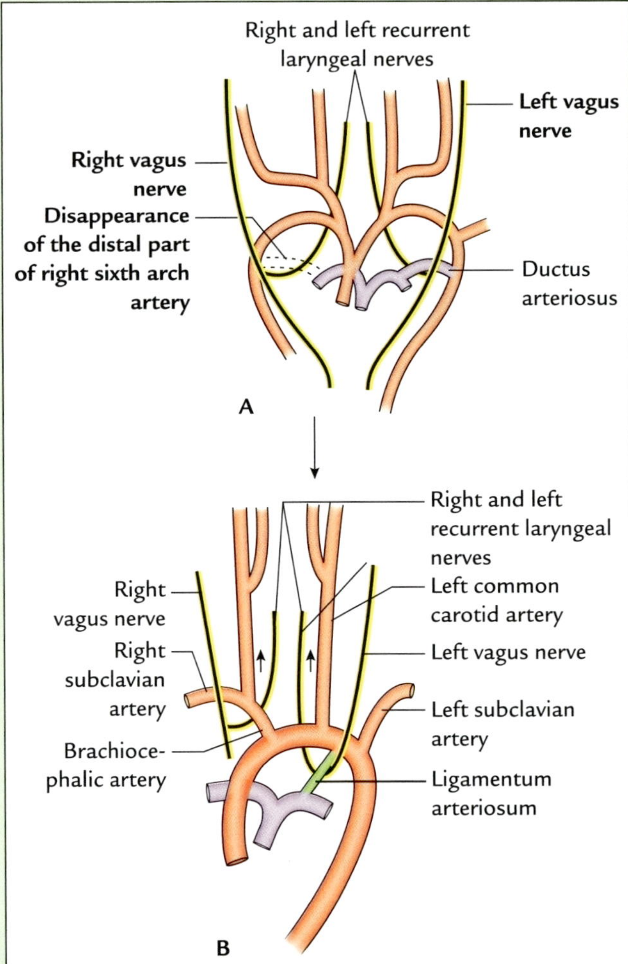

Fig. 23.28 Changing relationship of recurrent laryngeal nerves with aortic arch system. After the disappearance of the distal part of the sixth arch artery on the right side, the right recurrent laryngeal nerve hooks around the right subclavian artery. On the left side, the left recurrent laryngeal nerve remains in place and hooks around the ductus arteriosus (A) and subsequently ligamentum arteriosum (B).

(b) **On the left side**, the left recurrent nerve hooks around the distal part of sixth arch artery, which persists as DA, so it hooks around it. When DA obliterates after birth to form *ligamentum arteriosum,* the recurrent laryngeal nerve hooks around the ligamentum arteriosum and the arch of aorta (left fourth arch artery).

2. In the first few days after birth, there is only a physiological closure of the foramen ovale; hence, this closure is reversible. The crying of the baby creates a shunt from right to left, which accounts for cyanotic periods during crying in the newborn.

3. The placenta is an **organ of respiration in fetus.** The fetal blood is oxygenated in placenta. The blood leaving the placenta is about 80% saturated with oxygen. It loses its high oxygen content as it enters into the fetal circulation because it mixes with desaturated blood from the body of the fetus. The oxygenated blood from placenta gets mixed up with the deoxygenated blood from fetal body at following sites:
   (a) *Where ductus venosus opens into the IVC,* the oxygenated blood from the umbilical vein is mixed with deoxygenated blood of IVC, which it drains from lower extremities, pelvis, and kidneys.
   (b) *In the right atrium,* the blood from IVC is mixed with the blood from SVC, draining venous blood from head and upper extremities.
   (c) *In the left atrium,* the blood from IVC, which is comparatively rich in oxygen content, is mixed with the blood from the pulmonary veins, which is poor in oxygen content.
   (d) *Where DA opens in the aorta,* the blood in aorta that is comparatively rich in oxygen is mixed with the blood from the right ventricle that is poor in oxygen content.

24 Development of Urinary System

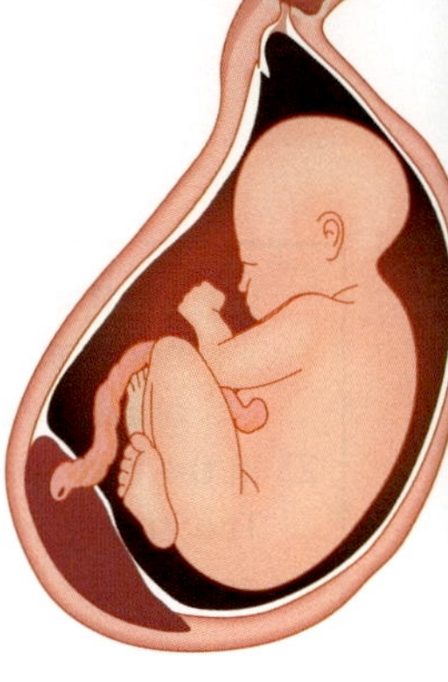

LEARNING OBJECTIVES

After studying this chapter, the student should be able to:

- Describe the development of urinary system. AN 52.7
- Describe the development of permanent kidney in brief and enumerate the common congenital anomalies associated with it.
- Describe the development of urinary bladder in brief and discuss the embryological basis of ectopia vesicae.
- Write short notes on (a) congenital polycystic kidney, (b) horseshoe kidney, (c) lobulated kidney, and (d) congenital anomalies of urachus.

OVERVIEW

The **urinary system** consists of kidneys, ureters, urinary bladder, and urethra. The urinary system develops from **intermediate mesoderm** and **primitive cloaca**. The urinary system begins to develop before the genital system. The development of human kidney repeats its evolutionary stages, i.e., **pronephros, mesonephros**, and **metanephros** in succession.

INTRODUCTION

The urinary system develops from the following two embryonic structures:

- Intermediate mesoderm
- Cloaca

Intermediate Mesoderm

The intermediate mesoderm is a longitudinal strip of intraembryonic mesoderm lying on either side of notochord between paraxial mesoderm and lateral plate mesoderm (Fig. 24.1A).

After folding of embryo, the intermediate mesoderm forms a longitudinal elevation of mesoderm along the dorsal body wall on each side of dorsal aorta/dorsal mesentery of gut. This longitudinal elevation is called **urogenital ridge** (Fig. 24.1B).

The *medial part of urogenital ridge* that gives rise to the genital system is called **genital ridge** and *lateral part of urogenital ridge* that gives rise to the urinary system is called **nephrogenic cord** (Fig. 24.1C).

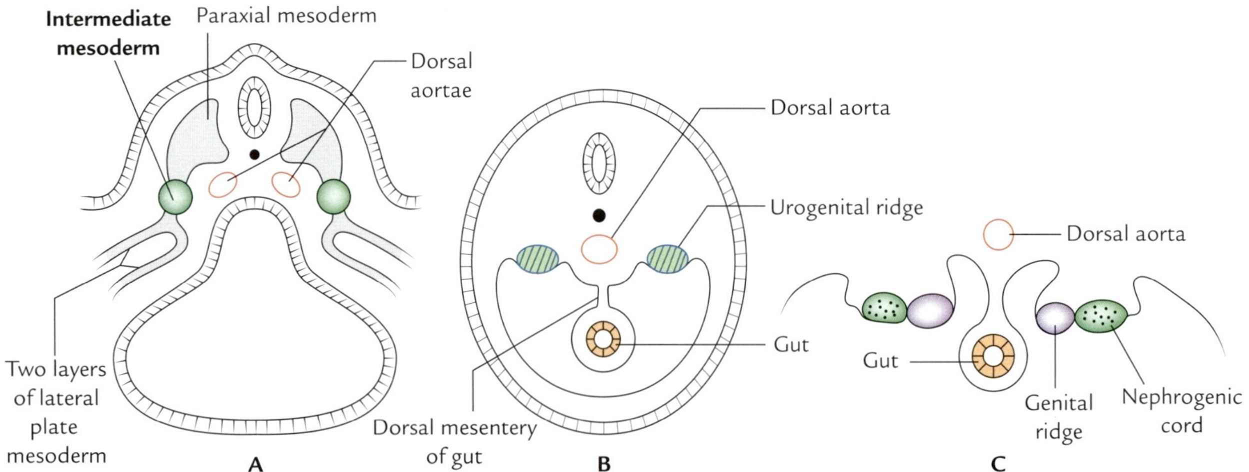

Fig. 24.1 Stages of formation of nephrogenic cord. (A) Location of intermediate mesoderm. (B) Formation of urogenital ridge. (C) Differentiation of urogenital ridge into genital ridge and nephrogenic cord.

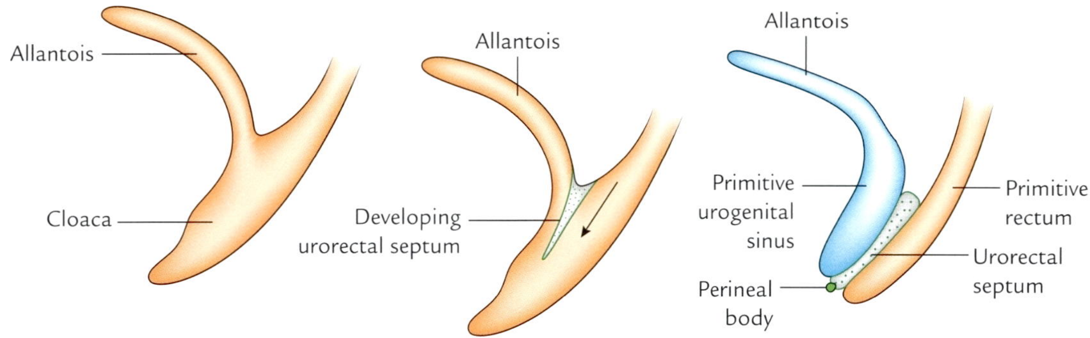

Fig. 24.2 Subdivision of the cloaca into primitive urogenital sinus and primitive rectum.

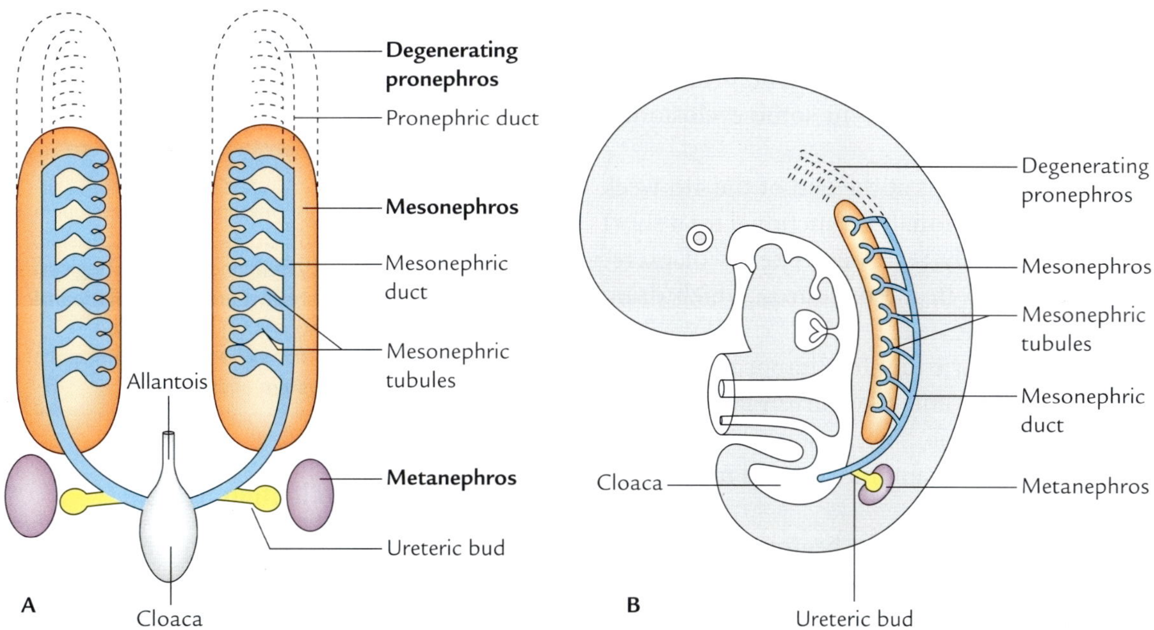

Fig. 24.3 Formation of three successive kidneys in embryo. (A) Ventral view. (B) Lateral view.

Cloaca

The part of hindgut caudal to attachment of allantois is called **cloaca.** It is divided into two parts: ventral and dorsal by a **urorectal septum** (which develops from an angle between the allantois and cloaca).

Ventral part of cloaca is called **primitive urogenital sinus** and dorsal part is called **primitive rectum** (Fig. 24.2).

Evolutionary History of Kidney

The development of kidney begins in the 4th week of intrauterine life (IUL) from intermediate (intraembryonic) mesoderm. **Nephrogenic cord** derived from intermediate mesoderm forms a longitudinal ridge on posterior abdominal wall on each side of the dorsal aorta. It extends from cervical to sacral region of the embryo. The surface of the nephrogenic cord is covered by the epithelial lining of the peritoneal cavity (coelomic cavity).

During the development of human kidney, the evolutionary history of the kidney is repeated and displays a classical example of what is called **ontogeny repeats phylogeny**.

N.B. The **evolutionary stages of the kidney** are (a) pronephros in fishes, (b) mesonephros in fishes and amphibians, and (c) metanephros in humans.

In human embryos, the **nephrogenic cord forms three sets of successive kidneys, i.e., pronephros, mesonephros, and metanephros – succeeding each other in time and space such that last to develop is retained as permanent kidney.** The details are as follows (Fig. 24.3):

1. The **pronephros** forms at the beginning of the 4th week in the *cervical region*. It is nonfunctional and completely regresses. However, its duct – the **pronephric duct** – which opens in cloaca, persists.

Table 24.1 The sequence of events of development of pronephros, mesonephros, and metanephros

Stages of Kidney	Location	Segmentation	Time of Appearance	Functional Status	Duct
Pronephros	Cervical region	Segmented	Beginning of the 4th week	Nonfunctional/disappears	Pronephric duct persists
Mesonephros	Thoracolumbar region	Segmented	End of the 4th week	Functional for a short period then disappears, except for its caudal excretory tubules	Mesonephric duct persists
Metanephros	Sacral region	Nonsegmented	Beginning of the 3rd month	Functional	Ureter

This duct is subsequently annexed by mesonephros and forms the **mesonephric duct**. The pronephros persists as permanent kidney in some cyclostomes and some teleost fishes.

2. The **mesonephros** forms at the end of the 4th week in **thoracolumbar region.** It is functional for a short period and completely regresses. A series of excretory tubules develop in mesonephros, which drain into the **mesonephric duct**.

   Most of mesonephric tubules disappear, but some of them are modified and take part in formation of **vasa efferentia of testis.** The mesonephros persists as permanent kidney in amphibians and most of the fishes.

3. The **metanephros** forms at the beginning of the 3rd month in the sacral region. It persists permanently in humans. It drains into ureter.

The sequence of events of development of pronephros, mesonephros, and metanephros are given in Table 24.1.

DEVELOPMENT OF PERMANENT KIDNEYS AND URETER

AN52.7

OVERVIEW

The **permanent kidneys** (metanephros) develop in the sacral region during 5th week of IUL. Each kidney consists of two components: (a) **excretory system** and (b) **collecting system.** Hence, it develops from two distinct sources: (a) **metanephric blastema** (metanephric mesoderm) and (b) **ureteric bud.**

The metanephros forms **excretory system** and the ureteric bud forms **collecting system** of the kidney.

Development of Collecting System

The **ureteric bud** arises from mesonephric duct and grows cranially behind the peritoneal cavity toward the metanephros. The distal end of ureteric bud becomes capped by metanephric blastema (Fig. 24.4). The growing end of ureteric bud becomes dilated like a funnel to form the **pelvis of ureter/renal pelvis.** The ureteric bud divides

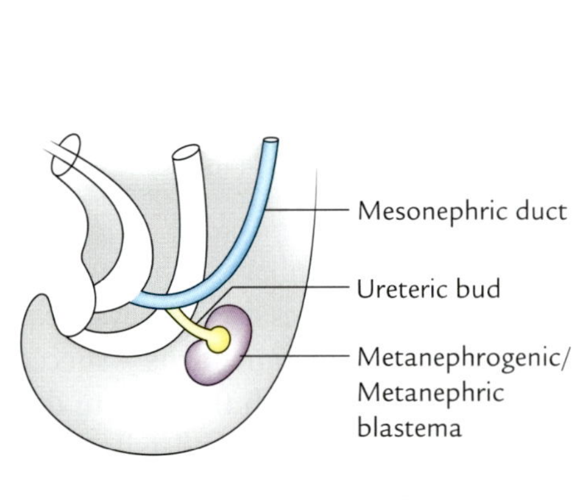

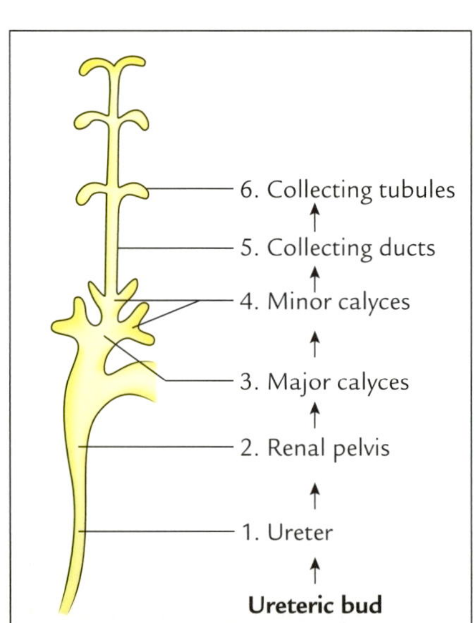

Fig. 24.4 Development of ureteric bud and metanephric blastema as seen in lateral view of embryo. The inset shows structures derived from the ureteric bud.

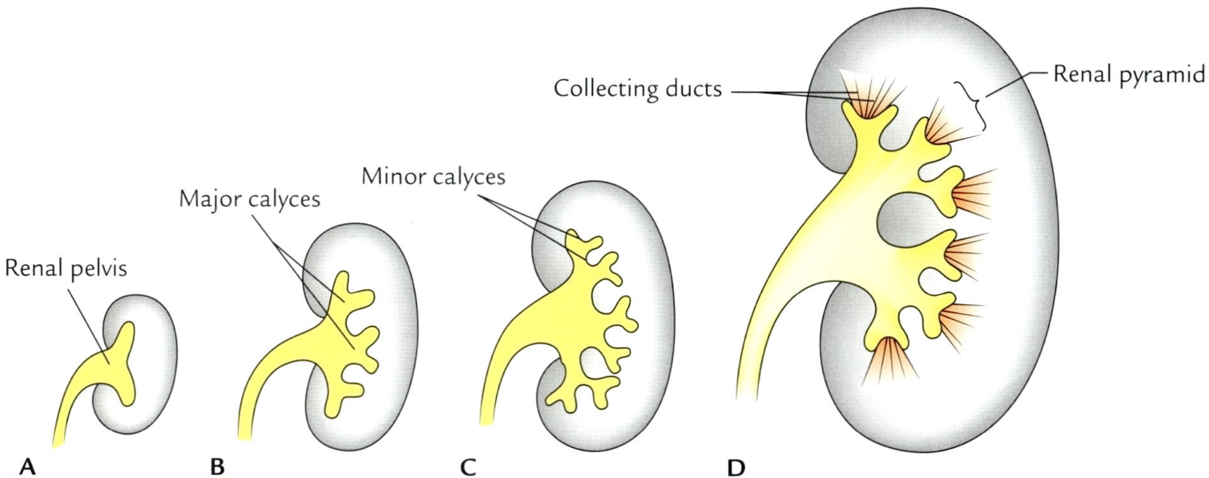

Fig. 24.5 Development of pelvicalyceal system of kidney (renal pelvis, major calyces, and minor calyces). Note pyramid contains collecting ducts that enter into the minor calyces.

dichotomously and its 13 generations form the collecting system of the kidney. The renal pelvis undergoes repeated divisions to form **major calyces, minor calyces, collecting ducts**, and **collecting tubules** (Fig. 24.4, inset).

The collecting tubules thus formed vary in number from 1 to 3 million.

The development of **pelvicalyceal system** of kidney consisting of renal pelvis, major calyces, and minor calyces is shown in Fig. 24.5.

N.B. **Structures derived from ureteric bud includes** ureter, renal pelvis, major and minor calyces, and about 1 to 3 million collecting tubules.

Development of Nephron (Fig. 24.6)

The cells of **metanephric blastema** when come in contact with each collecting tubule, these condense around it to form solid clump of cells called **metanephric cap**. Each metanephric cap is soon converted into a vesicle called **metanephric vesicle**. The metanephric vesicle first becomes a *pear-shaped vesicle*, which soon forms an *S-shaped tubule* (called **primitive renal tubule**). The proximal end of this S-shaped tubule is narrow and abuts on the collecting tubule. The distal dilated end of this tubule forms Bowman's capsule. It becomes invaginated by a tuft of capillaries to form renal glomerulus. The renal glomerulus and Bowman's capsule together form **renal corpuscle**. The primitive renal tubule eventually forms nephron (excretory unit) consisting of **renal corpuscle, proximal convoluted tubule, loop of Henle**, and **distal convoluted tubule**.

Each distal convoluted tubule joins with the collecting tubule derived from the ureteric bud to form **uriniferous tubule** (Fig. 24.6).

The development of the kidney is summarized in Flowchart 24.1. The adult derivatives of embryonic structures forming collecting and secretory systems of the kidney are summarized in Table 24.2.

N.B. The fetal kidneys are lobulated and remain in the lobulated form up to 1st year of life.

Other Developmental Events

Ascent of Kidney (Fig. 24.7)

At first, the permanent kidneys lie in the pelvis in front of **sacral region**. Later, due to differential growth of posterior abdominal wall and reduction of fetal curvature, the kidney gradually ascends to reach the definitive position – the **thoracolumbar region** – and moves farther apart (T12–L3 vertebral levels) in 9th week. The ureter elongates accordingly as the kidney ascends. The kidneys locate themselves in adult position in the 9th week of IUL.

N.B. Physiologically, the kidney ascends for two reasons: (a) It faces space crunch in smaller pelvic cavity and (b) it ascends in search for better blood supply.

Arterial Supply of the Kidney (Fig. 24.8)

The blood supply of kidney changes as it undergoes ascent. Initially, the kidney lies in the pelvis and is supplied by **median sacral artery** – *a pelvic continuation of the aorta*. As the kidney ascends, it is supplied

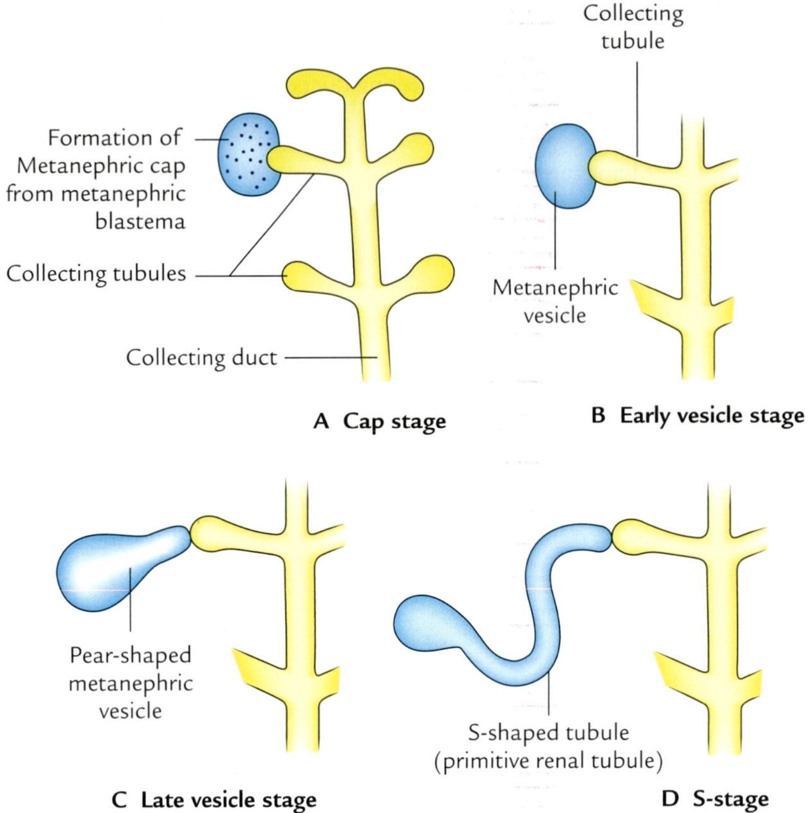

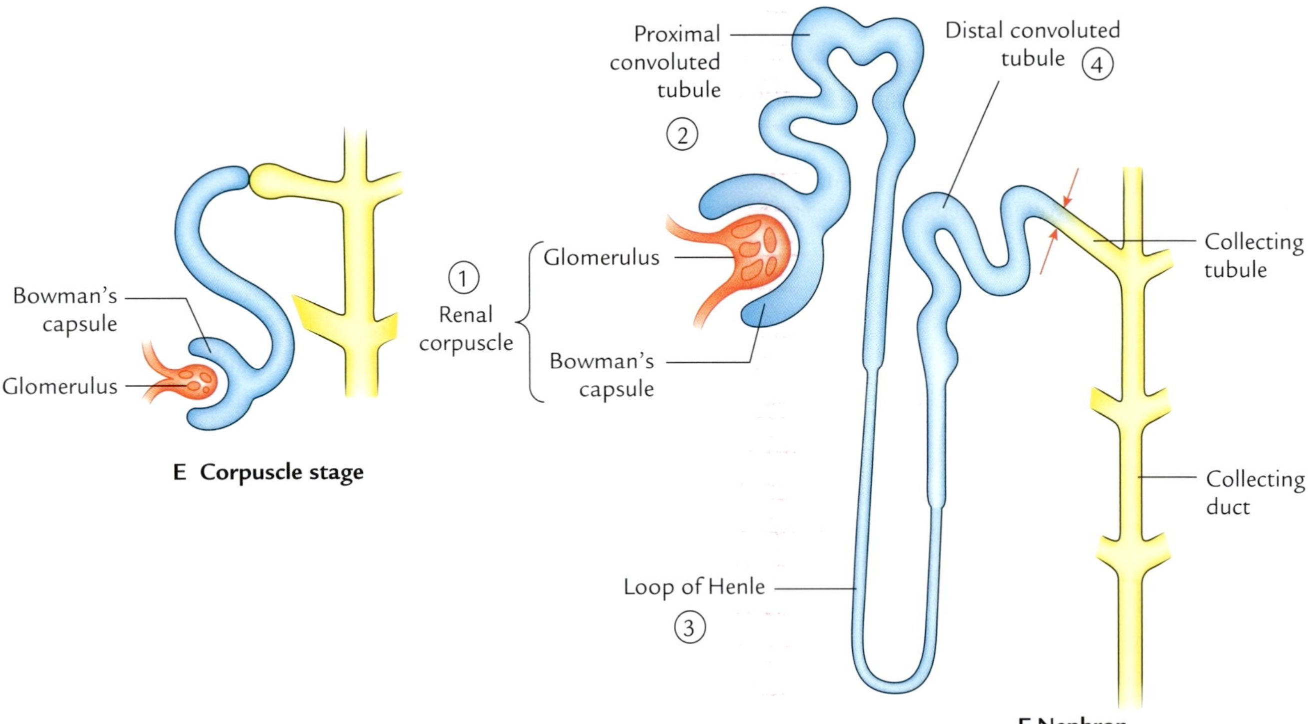

Fig. 24.6 Stages of development of nephron (excretory unit of the kidney). Note each nephron consists of: 1. Renal corpuscle, 2. Proximal convoluted tubule, 3. Loop of Henle, 4. Distal convoluted tubule. The arrows (red) indicate the place where excretory unit (blue) establishes a communication with the collecting system (yellow).

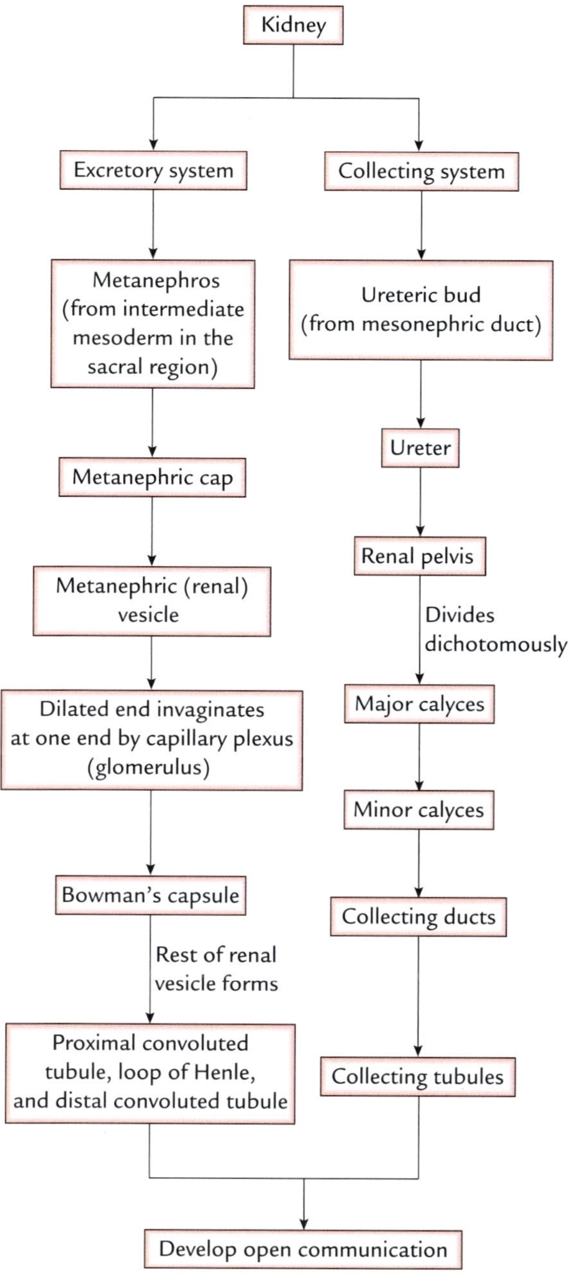

Flowchart 24.1 Development of kidney.

successively by higher lateral splanchnic branches of the aorta at successively higher levels. The kidney reaches its final position opposite the second lumbar vertebra. The **definitive renal artery** supplying the kidney arises at L2 vertebral level and represents lateral splanchnic branch of the aorta.

Rotation of the Kidneys

At first, hilum of each kidney lies/faces anteriorly. But during the ascent of the kidney, it rotates 90° medially so that hilum of each kidney now faces medially.

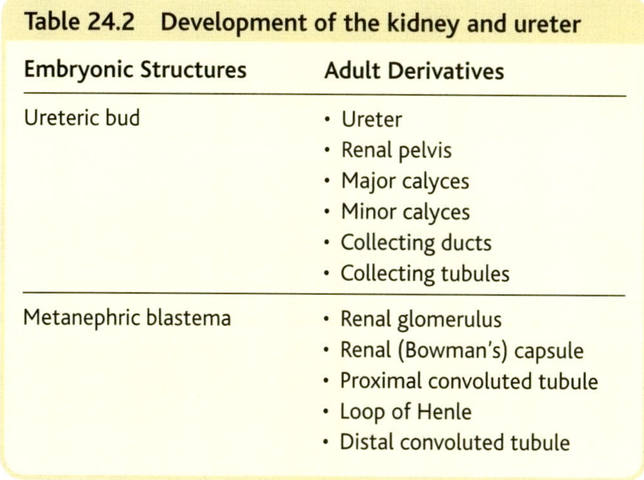

Table 24.2 Development of the kidney and ureter

Embryonic Structures	Adult Derivatives
Ureteric bud	• Ureter • Renal pelvis • Major calyces • Minor calyces • Collecting ducts • Collecting tubules
Metanephric blastema	• Renal glomerulus • Renal (Bowman's) capsule • Proximal convoluted tubule • Loop of Henle • Distal convoluted tubule

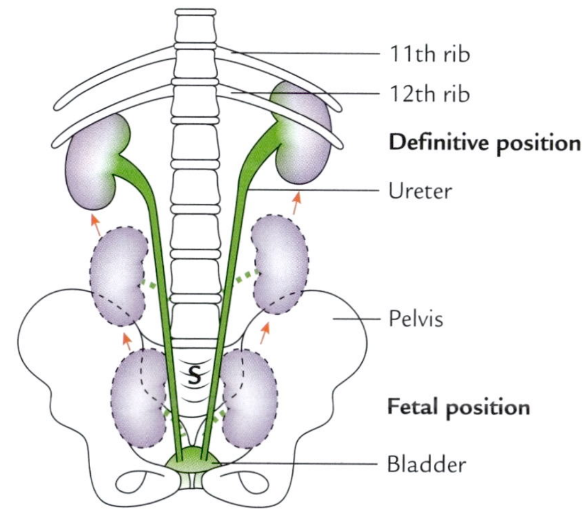

Fig. 24.7 Ascent of the kidney. S, sacrum.

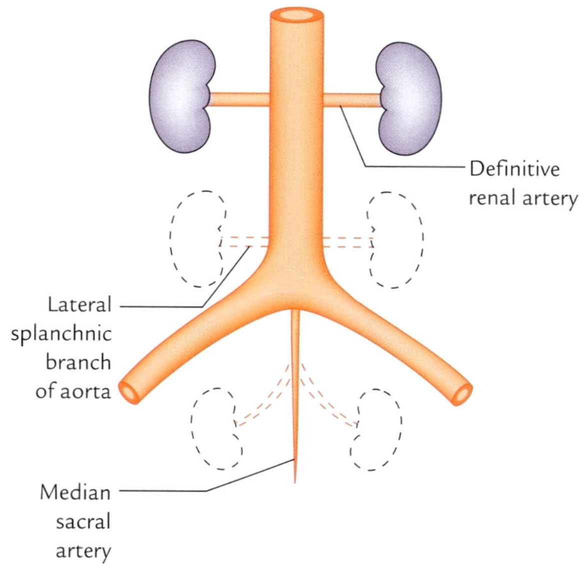

Fig. 24.8 Ascent of arterial supply of the kidney.

Functions of Kidney

The newly formed kidneys become functional in the 12th week of IUL. The urine is excreted in the amniotic sac where it mixes with the amniotic fluid. The urine-mixed amniotic fluid is swallowed by the fetus and recycled through the kidneys.

N.B. During fetal life, the kidneys are not responsible for removing waste products as it is already being excreted by the placenta.

CLINICAL CORRELATION

Congenital anomalies of kidney

1. ***Renal agenesis (absence of kidney):*** The renal agenesis occurs when ureteric bud fails to develop. It can be unilateral or bilateral. Note that the **ureteric bud induces the metanephric tissue to form metanephric blastema**.
   (a) *Unilateral renal agenesis*
   - It is relatively common (therefore, a clinician should never presume that a patient always has two kidneys).
   - It is more common in males.
   - It is asymptomatic and compatible with life because the other kidney hypertrophies to meet requirements of the body.
   - It is usually detected while carrying out investigation for some other diseases.

   (b) *Bilateral renal agenesis*
   - It is relatively uncommon.
   - It is incompatible with life and newborn infant usually dies shortly after birth, unless a suitable donor is available for a kidney transplant.
   - It causes oligohydramnios that allows the uterine wall to compress the fetus. As a result, there occurs **Potter syndrome.** The clinical features of Potter syndrome are deformed limbs, wrinkling of skin, and abnormal facial appearance.
2. ***Duplication or multiplication of the kidneys:*** More than one kidney may be present either on one or both sides. This occurs due to early division of the ureteric bud.
3. ***Congenital polycystic kidney (Fig. 24.9):*** In this condition, numerous cysts filled with urine are present in the substance of the kidney. This condition is usually bilateral. The embryological basis of congenital polycystic kidney is as follows:
   (a) Earlier it was thought that it occurs when excretory/secretory and collecting tubules fail to connect with each other.
   (b) But now it is thought that it occurs due to abnormal dilatation of different parts of the uriniferous tubules, especially the loops of Henle.
   - It is a relatively common hereditary disease and is clinically associated with cysts of the liver, pancreas, and lungs.
   - It is of two types: childhood type and adult type. The prevalence of childhood type is 1:5000 births and prevalence of adult type is 1:600 births (also see p. 277).
   - The treatment regime includes dialysis and kidney transplantation.
4. ***Horseshoe-shaped kidney (also called horseshoe kidney) (Fig. 24.10)***
   - In this condition, inferior poles of both the kidneys are fused.
   - During the ascent, the horseshoe kidney gets trapped underneath the **inferior mesenteric artery.** Hence, horseshoe kidney usually lies at the level of the lower lumbar vertebrae.
   - The ureters arise from the anterior surface of the kidney and pass in front of isthmus in a caudal direction.
   - It occurs because sometimes the kidneys are pushed so close together during their passage through the arterial fork (formed by the umbilical arteries) that their lower ends get fused.
5. ***Lobulated kidney (Fig. 24.11):*** It is persistence of normal lobulated fetal kidney. The metanephric kidney is lobulated throughout the fetal life, but this condition usually disappears during the 1st year after birth. But if it fails to do so, then it leads to lobulated kidney.

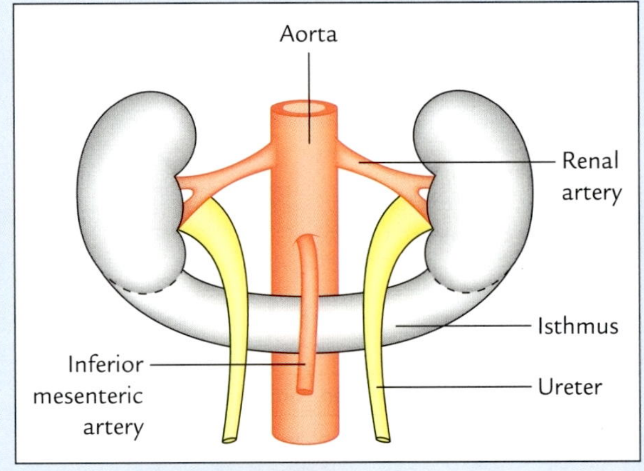

Fig. 24.10 Horseshoe kidney.

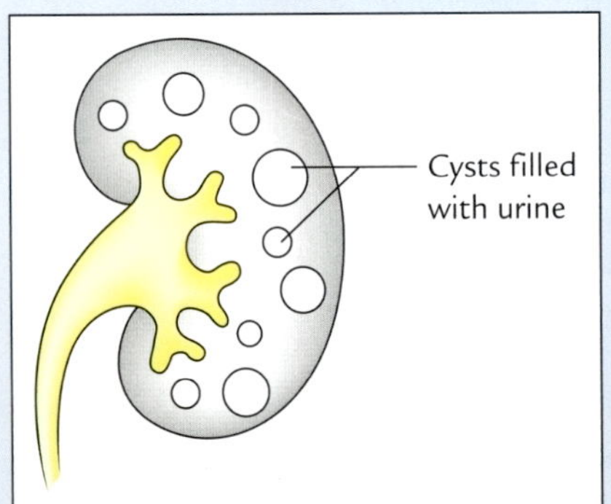

Fig. 24.9 Congenital polycystic kidney.

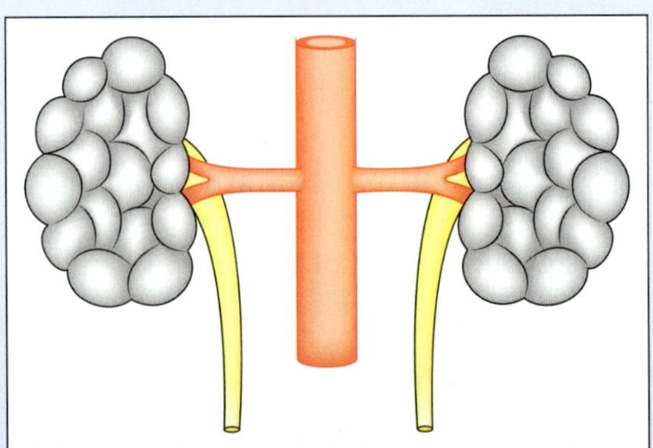

Fig. 24.11 Lobulated kidneys.

6. ***Pelvic kidney:*** In this condition, the kidney is located in the pelvis. It occurs when kidney fails to ascend. The most common cause of failure of ascent of the kidney is the presence of sickle-shaped fold of peritoneum (containing umbilical artery) that projects from lateral pelvic wall.
7. ***Pancake kidney:*** In this condition, two kidneys fuse to form a single mass that lies in midline or on one side.
8. ***Supernumerary/aberrant renal arteries (Fig. 24.12):*** These are relatively common. These represent **persistent fetal renal arteries**. The fetal renal arteries arise successively in sequence from the aorta as the kidney ascends from the pelvic to the lumbar region.

   Occurrence of aberrant arteries is clinically important because these may cross the pelviureteric junction and obstruct the outflow of urine leading to **hydronephrosis**.

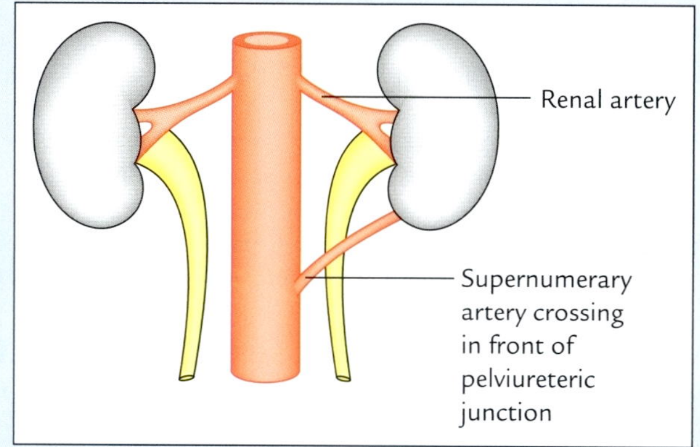

Fig. 24.12 Supernumerary/accessory renal arteries.

DEVELOPMENT OF URETER (FIG. 24.3)

The ureter develops from ureteric bud, which arises as a diverticulum from the mesonephric (Wolffian) duct just before it opens into the cloaca (vesicourethral canal).

CLINICAL CORRELATION

Congenital anomalies of ureter (Fig. 24.13)

1. ***Double renal pelvis (Fig. 24.13A):*** In this condition, upper end of ureter presents two renal pelvises: upper and lower. The *upper renal pelvis* drains the upper group of calyces, whereas the *lower renal pelvis* drains the middle and lower groups of calyces. This condition occurs due to premature division of the ureteric bud near its termination.
2. ***Bifid ureter (Fig. 24.13B):*** In this condition, the upper end of the ureter is bifid. In lower third of their course, two ureters join and open by a common orifice into the urinary bladder. Like double pelvis, this condition occurs due to premature division of the ureteric bud.
3. ***Double ureters (Fig. 24.13C):*** Duplication of the abdominal part of the ureter and renal pelvis is common. It occurs due to division of the ureteric bud, as it arises from the mesonephric duct. In such a case, one ureter crosses across its fellow and may produce a urinary obstruction.

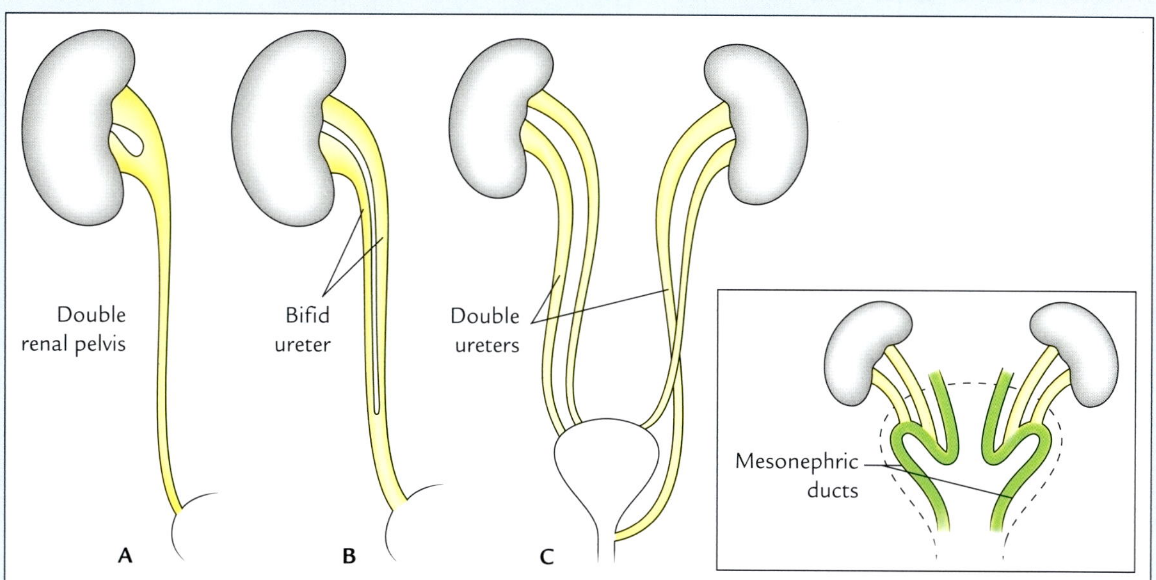

Fig. 24.13 Congenital anomalies of the ureter. (A) Double renal pelvis. (B) Bifid ureter. (C) Double ureters. The inset shows loop of formation of part of mesonephric duct.

Continued

N.B. The double pelvis and double ureters are more liable to get infected and to be the seat of calculus formation than the normal ureter.

In case of double ureters, the *lower ureter* opens in the bladder at normal site, whereas *upper ureter* migrates more caudally due to caudal shift of the terminal part of the mesonephric duct and opens in the ectopic position. This is due to the fact that the terminal part of mesonephric duct undergoes loop formation in the posterior wall of the urinary bladder (Fig. 24.13, inset).

4. ***Ectopic ureter:*** In this condition, the ureter does not open into the urinary bladder.
   (a) In males, the ectopic ureter usually opens into the neck of urinary bladder or into prostatic part of the urethra.
   (b) In females, the ectopic ureter usually opens into bladder neck, urethra, or vagina.
   (c) The *incontinence of urine* is a common complaint by patients with ectopic ureters. It occurs because urine flowing from the orifice of ectopic ureter does not enter into the urinary bladder.
   (d) An ectopic ureter occurs when the ureter is not incorporated into the trigone of the urinary bladder.

N.B. Ureters usually open into the urinary bladder when both the ureters form on one side.

5. ***Postcaval ureter:*** It occurs if right ureter ascends posterior to the inferior vena cava.

DEVELOPMENT OF URINARY BLADDER (FIG. 24.14)

The urinary bladder develops from endodermal cloaca as follows:

1. The cloaca is divided into two parts by a mesodermal **urorectal septum** during 4th to 7th week of development (see p. 275). The anterior part is called **urogenital sinus** and the posterior part is called **primitive rectum.** The tip of the urorectal septum forms **perineal body**. The cloacal membrane also divides into *anal membrane* posteriorly and *urogenital membrane* anteriorly (see Fig. 18.25).
2. The **mesonephric ducts** now open into the primitive urogenital sinus. The urogenital sinus now becomes divisible into two parts by the openings of the mesonephric ducts.

   Part above the openings of mesonephric ducts is called **vesicourethral canal** and part below the openings of mesonephric ducts is called **definitive urogenital sinus.** The definitive urogenital sinus is further divided into two parts: (a) cranial **pelvic part** and (b) caudal **phallic part** (Fig. 24.14). The subdivisions of cloaca are shown in Flowchart 24.2.

   The allantois opens at the cranial end of the vesicourethral canal.
3. The upper large part of the vesicourethral canal expands, whereas its lower part remains narrow.
4. The upper large dilated part of the vesicourethral canal forms the **urinary bladder**. It is continuous with the allantois at the apex. The allantois obliterates and forms a fibrous band called **urachus**, which extends from apex of the urinary bladder to the umbilicus. The urachus is called **median umbilical ligament** in adult.
5. The lower narrow part of vesicourethral canal forms **primitive urethra**.
6. The parts of the mesonephric ducts distal to ureteric buds are now absorbed into the wall of vesicourethral canal (Figs 24.15 and 24.16). As a result, the mesonephric ducts and ureters now open separately in the vesicourethral canal. As the kidneys ascend, the openings of ureters move upward and laterally.

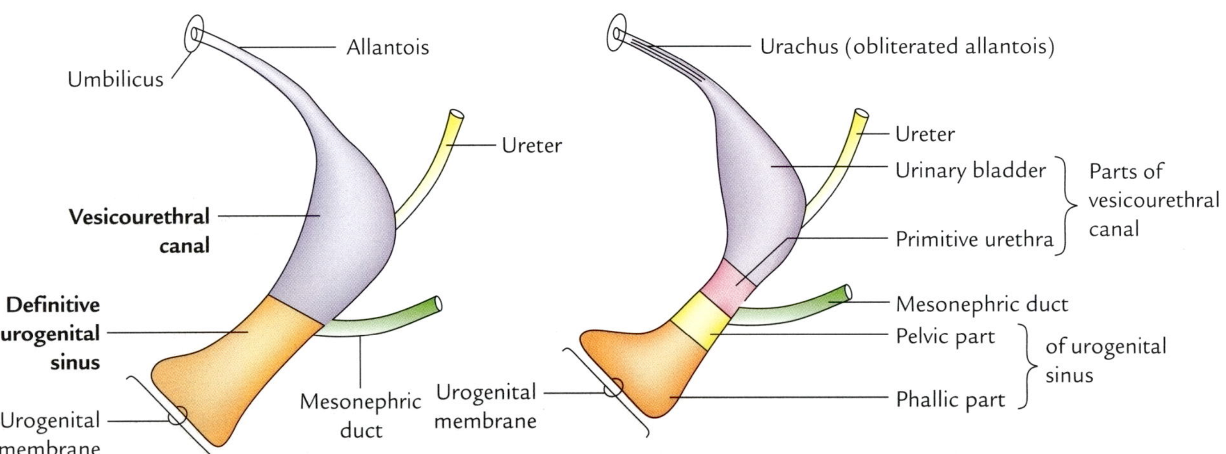

Fig. 24.14 Subdivisions of primitive urogenital sinus.

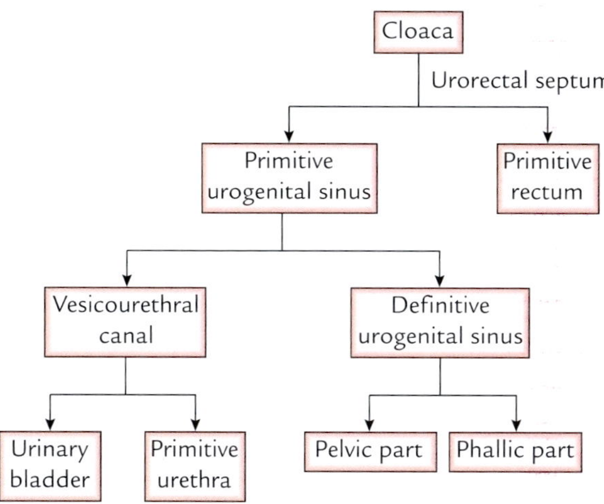

Flowchart 24.2 Subdivisions of cloaca.

Development of Trigone of Urinary Bladder (Fig. 24.16)

Initially, the ureter is formed as an outgrowth of mesonephric duct called **ureteric bud.**

1. Later on, due to absorption of mesonephric ducts into the vesicourethral canal, the mesonephric ducts and ureteric buds now have separate openings in the vesicourethral canal (primitive urinary bladder) (Fig. 24.16B).
2. At first, the openings of mesonephric ducts and ureteric buds are close together, but later the openings of ureteric buds move cranially and laterally.
3. The triangular area on the dorsal wall of vesicourethral canal between the openings of ureteric buds and mesonephric ducts is called **trigone of urinary bladder**. It is derived from absorption of the mesonephric ducts.

Development of Coats of Bladder Wall

1. The epithelial lining of whole of urinary bladder is derived from endodermal vesicourethral canal, except in the triangular area on its dorsal wall (**trigone of urinary bladder**) that is derived from mesoderm derived from the absorbed parts of the mesonephric ducts.
2. The muscular and serous coats of the urinary bladder are derived from splanchnopleuric intraembryonic mesoderm.

The adult derivatives of various embryonic structures forming urinary bladder are summarized in Table 24.3.

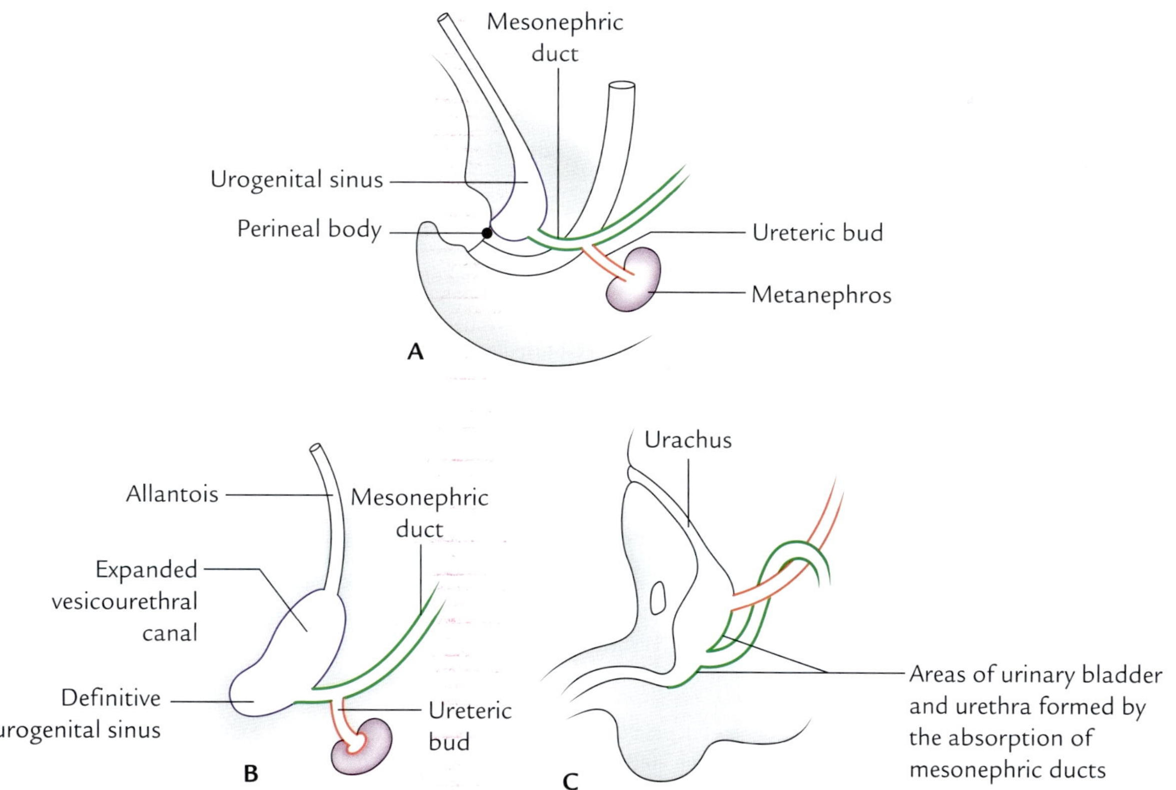

Fig. 24.15 Absorption of mesonephric ducts into the vesicourethral canal. Note parts of posterior wall of urinary bladder and urethra are formed by the absorption of mesonephric ducts.

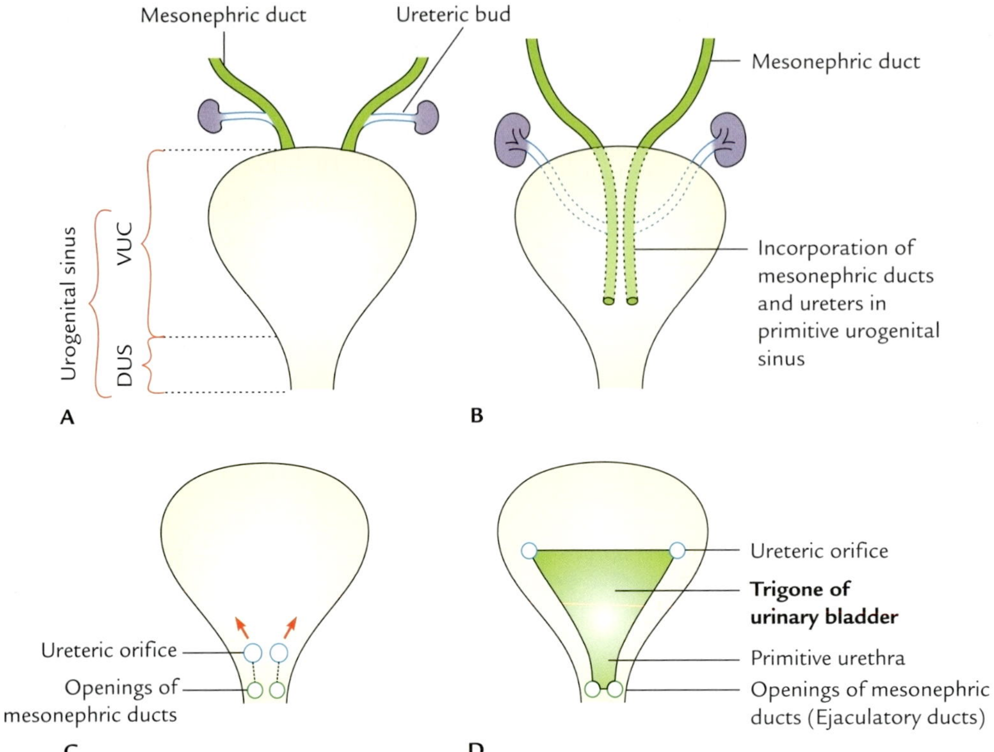

Fig. 24.16 Formation of trigone of the urinary bladder. (A) Opening of mesonephric ducts into the vesicourethral canal (VUC). (B) Absorption of mesonephric ducts into the VUC. (C) At first, openings of ureters and mesonephric ducts are close together. (D) Further absorption of ureters causes ureteric openings to shift upward and laterally. DUS, definitive urogenital sinus.

Table 24.3 Development of the urinary bladder

Embryonic Structure	Adult Derivatives
Cranial dilated part of vesicourethral canal	Endodermal epithelial lining of the whole urinary bladder except in the region of trigone
Absorption of mesonephric ducts in the dorsal wall of the vesico-urethral canal	Mesodermal epithelial lining in the region of trigone of urinary bladder
Splanchnopleuric intra-embryonic mesoderm surrounding vesicourethral canal	Muscular and serous coats of the urinary bladder
Allantois	Urachus (median umbilical ligament) and apex of urinary bladder

CLINICAL CORRELATION

1. ***Congenital anomalies of urachus:*** The urachus is adult derivative of the allantois. Normally, it obliterates to form a fibrous cord in adult called *median umbilical ligament*. Following congenital anomalies may occur in urachus (Fig. 24.17):
   (a) **Urachal sinus:** If the lumen persists in the upper part of urachus (i.e., close to the umbilicus) it is called *urachal sinus*. The urachal sinus opens at the umbilicus.
   (b) **Urachal fistula:** If the lumen persists along the entire extent of urachus, the *urachal fistula* is formed. The urachal fistula opens in the urinary bladder at one end and at the umbilicus at the other end. As a result, the urine is discharged through umbilicus.
   (c) **Urachal cyst:** If only a small part of the urachus remains patent, the secretory activity of its lining epithelium leads to the formation of a cystic dilatation called *urachal cyst*.
2. ***Exstrophy of the bladder (ectopia vesicae) (Fig. 24.18):*** In this condition, the lower median part of anterior abdominal wall and anterior wall of the urinary bladder is absent. The mucosal surface of posterior wall of the urinary bladder showing ureteric orifices is exposed to the

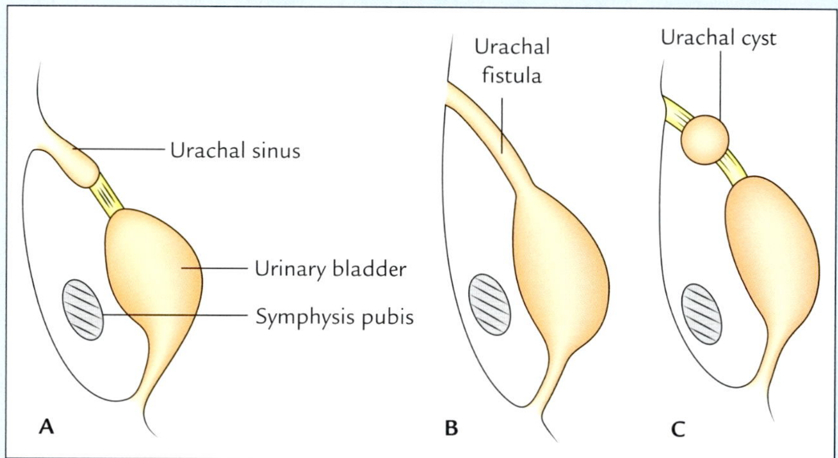

Fig. 24.17 Congenital anomalies of urachus. (A) Urachal sinus. (B) Urachal fistula. (C) Urachal cyst.

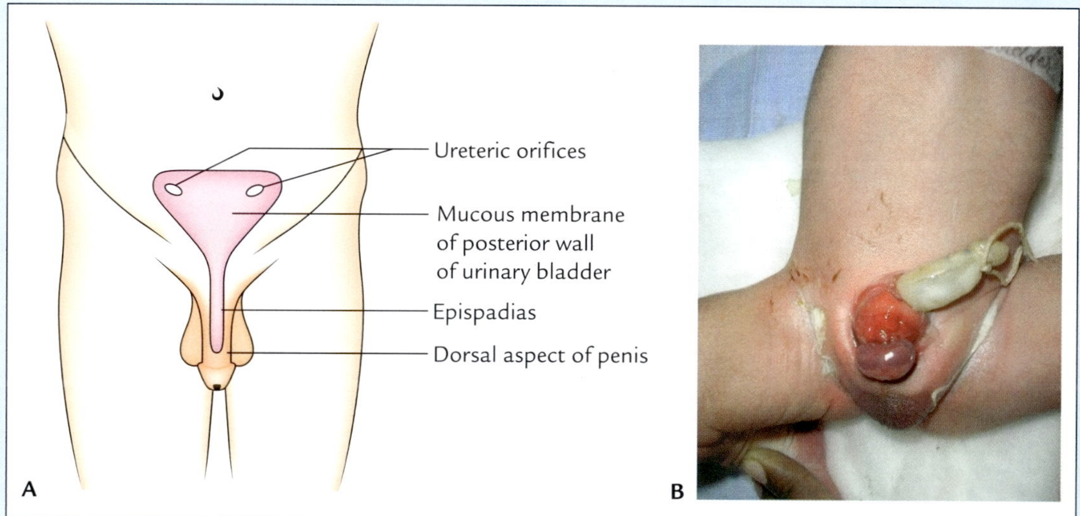

Fig. 24.18 Ectopia vesicae (exstrophy of urinary bladder). (A) Line diagram. (B) Actual clinical photograph. (*Source:* Courtesy of Dr Basant Kumar, Assistant Professor, Department of Pediatric Surgery, SGPGIMS, Lucknow.)

surface. The urine can be seen dribbling intermittently from the ureteric orifices. The epispadias is a constant feature in this condition.

This anomaly occurs due to lack of migration of mesoderm in lateral folds of the embryo in the hypogastric region. Normally, during lateral folding of embryo, the lateral folds are formed; these grow medially and fuse with each other. The mesoderm migrates in these lateral folds and forms the muscles of anterior abdominal wall.

In exstrophy of the bladder, the anterior abdominal wall muscles are not formed in the hypogastric region (between the umbilicus and genital tubercle). As a result, the surface ectoderm comes in contact with endoderm of vesicourethral canal (future urinary bladder). The ectoderm and endoderm break down and posterior wall of the urinary bladder is exposed onto the surface. The exstrophy of the bladder is rare and occurs in 1:10,000 births.

DEVELOPMENT OF URETHRA (FIG. 24.19)

The female urethra is short and its development is very simple, whereas the male urethra is long and its development is little complicated. The development of male urethra is intimately related to the development of external genital organs.

The epithelium of entire female urethra and most of the male urethra is derived from urogenital sinus.

Female Urethra (Fig. 24.19A)

Whole of the female urethra develops from narrow caudal part of the **vesicourethral canal** except a small

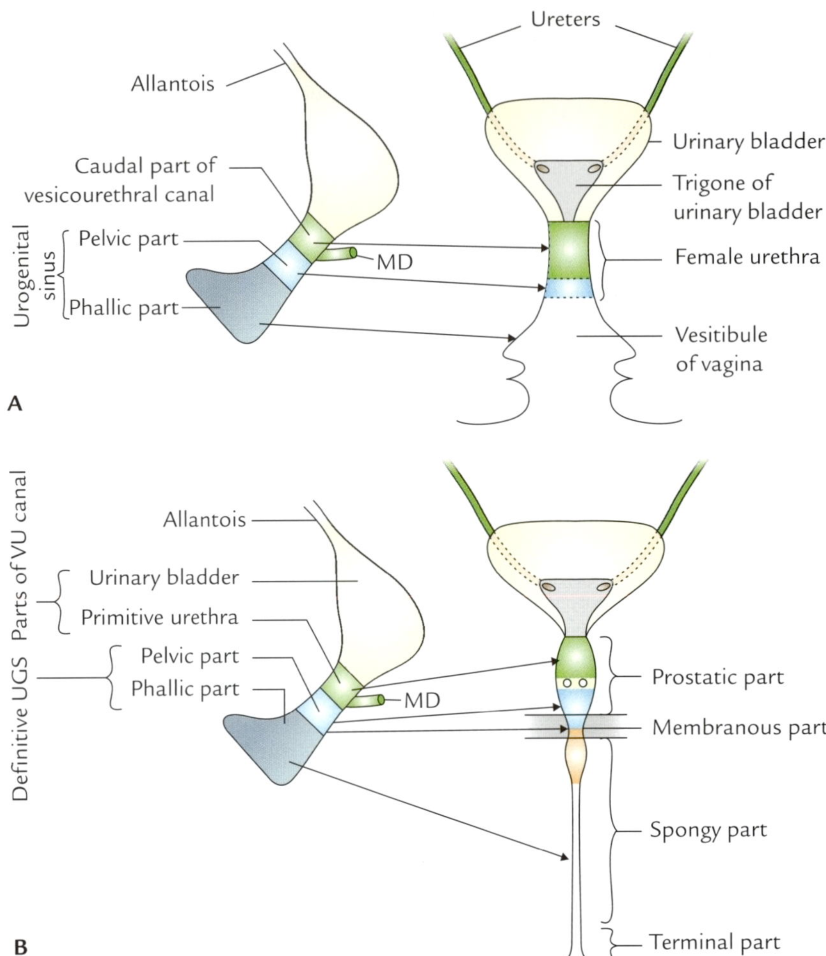

Fig. 24.19 Development of urethra. (A) Female urethra. (B) Male urethra. MD, mesonephric duct.

terminal part, which develops from the **pelvic part** of the **definitive urogenital sinus**. The **phallic part of the definitive urogenital sinus** forms vestibule of vagina into which the urethra opens.

N.B.
- The female urethra corresponds to the prostatic part of the male urethra above the colliculus seminalis.
- The whole of the female urethra is endodermal in origin (derived from urogenital sinus) except its dorsal wall that is mesodermal in origin, derived from absorption of mesonephric ducts.

Male Urethra (Fig. 24.19B)

The male urethra is divided into three parts: (a) prostatic part, (b) membranous part, and (c) spongy part.

1. **Prostatic part:** The part of prostatic urethra above the openings of ejaculatory ducts develops from the *caudal part of vesicourethral canal*. The posterior wall of this part is derived from **absorbed mesonephric ducts** (mesoderm). The part of the prostatic urethra below the openings of ejaculatory ducts develops from *upper pelvic part of definitive urogenital sinus*.
2. **Membranous urethra:** This small part of the urethra lies in deep perineal pouch. It develops from *lower pelvic part of definitive urogenital sinus*.
3. **Spongy part:** It is a part of the urethra that lies in the bulb (*bulbar part*) and shaft of the penis (*penile part*). Both these parts are derived from the *phallic part of definitive urogenital sinus*, except the terminal part of the urethra, which lies in glans penis (*glandular part*) that is derived from the *surface ectoderm*. Development of spongy part of the urethra is intimately related to development of male external genitalia; hence, it is described in detail in Chapter 25.

N.B. Only the lining epithelium of the urethra is derived from endoderm of urogenital sinus. Connective tissues and smooth muscles of urethra are derived from surrounding splanchnopleuric layer of intraembryonic mesoderm.

The development of male and female urethrae is summarized in Table 24.4 (for easy understanding, see also Fig. 24.19A and B).

Table 24.4 Development of male and female urethrae

Urethra	Embryonic Source of Development
Female urethra	• Caudal part of vesicourethral canal • Pelvic part of definitive urogenital sinus
Male urethra	
1. Prostatic part	
(a) Above the level of opening of ejaculatory ducts (colliculus seminalis)	• Caudal part of vesicourethral canal
(b) Below the level of openings of ejaculatory ducts	• Upper pelvic part of definitive urogenital sinus
2. Membranous part	• Lower pelvic part of definitive urogenital sinus
3. Penile part	• Phallic part of definitive urogenital sinus
4. Terminal part (which occupies the glans penis)	• Surface ectoderm

GESTATIONAL AGE OF KEY DEVELOPMENTAL EVENTS

Developmental Event	Time of Occurrence
➢ Development of kidney begins in the beginning of	4th week
➢ Pronephros forms at the beginning of	4th week
➢ Mesonephros forms at the end of	4th week
➢ Metanephros begins to form primordia of permanent kidneys in	5th week
➢ Newly formed permanent kidneys become functional at the beginning of	3rd month (12th week)
➢ Permanent kidneys ascend to their definitive position within abdomen in	9th week
➢ Cloaca divides into urogenital sinus and primitive rectum by urorectal septum during	4th to 7th weeks

GOLDEN FACTS TO REMEMBER

➢ **Precursor of nephron**	Renal vesicle
➢ **Commonest congenital anomaly of kidney**	Polycystic kidney
➢ **Commonest cause of failure of ascent of kidney**	Presence of sickle-shaped fold of peritoneum containing umbilical arteries
➢ **Accessory/supernumerary renal arteries**	Persisting fetal renal arteries
➢ **Epithelial lining of entire urinary bladder is derived from endodermal urogenital sinus *except***	In the region of trigone of urinary bladder, which is derived from absorbed mesodermal mesonephric ducts
➢ **Commonest urethral anomaly associated with exstrophy of urinary bladder**	Epispadias
➢ **Most common primary renal tumor of childhood**	Wilms tumor

CLINICAL PROBLEM SOLVING

PROBLEMS

1. Give the embryological basis of **accessory or supernumerary renal arteries** and discuss their clinical significance.
2. If the **ectopic ureteric orifice** opens inferior to the urinary bladder, it **results in urinary incontinence**. Give the anatomical basis.
3. **What is Wilms tumor**? Give its embryological/genetic basis.
4. **Give the embryological basis of congenital polycystic kidney (CPK).** Give its types and discuss the prognosis of each type.
5. Agenesis of the kidney is not fatal for fetus but is fatal for newborn baby (i.e., after the birth). Why?

SOLUTIONS

1. **Persistence of fetal arteries** form accessory or supernumerary renal arteries. For details, see *Clinical Correlation on p. 281.*
   - These are more common on the left side.
   - These are twice as common as supernumerary renal veins.
   - These usually arise at the level of the kidney and enter the lower pole of the kidney.

   Clinical significance: The supernumerary renal arteries may cross the pelviureteric junction and hinder the urine outflow. This causes dilatation of renal pelvis and calyces (*hydronephrosis*). The hydronephrotic kidney frequently becomes infected (*pyelonephritis*), which may lead to the destruction of the kidney.
2. Normally, the ureter takes a sinuous course through the bladder wall musculature (**detrusor muscle**) before it opens into its cavity. The oblique passage of the ureter through the bladder wall allows the contraction of detrusor muscle to act as a sphincter for the ureter and controls the flow of urine from it. If ectopic ureteric orifice opens below the urinary bladder, there is no such control; hence, the urinary incontinence results.
3. The **Wilms tumor is a malignant tumor of the kidney that usually affects children up to 5 years of age.** It occurs due to mutation in *WT1* gene on 11p13 chromosome.

   Clinically, the Wilms tumor presents as large, soft, solitary, and well-circumscribed mass, which on section appears homogenous and grayish in color.
4. In congenital polycystic kidney, numerous **cysts filled with urine appear in the substance of the kidney.** These are formed due to dilatation of parts of the nephrons, particularly the loops of Henle. Also, see *Clinical Correlation on p. 280.*

   The polycystic kidney disease is of two types: (a) childhood type of polycystic kidney disease (CPKD) and (b) adult type of polycystic kidney disease (APKD). The differences between the two types are given as follows:

Childhood Type of Polycystic Kidney Disease (CPKD)	Adult Type of Polycystic Kidney Disease (APKD)
Autosomal recessive	Autosomal dominant
Less common (occurs in 1:5000 births)	More common (occurs in 1:500 to 1:1000 births)
Disease manifests in childhood	Disease manifests above the age of 20 years
More progressive	Less progressive
Renal failure occurs in infancy or childhood	Renal failure usually does not occur until adulthood
Death occurs at an early age	Death occurs at a late age (longevity of life may extend up to 60 years of age)

5. The kidney becomes functional at the end of the first trimester of pregnancy. Urine is excreted into the amniotic cavity. It is swallowed by the fetus, absorbed into the blood from the gut, and circulated into the placenta. From placenta, it is excreted into the maternal blood. Thus, **placenta functions as true kidney in fetal life**; hence, agenesis of the kidney is not fatal for the fetus but is fatal after *birth.*

25 Genital System: Gonads and Genital Ducts

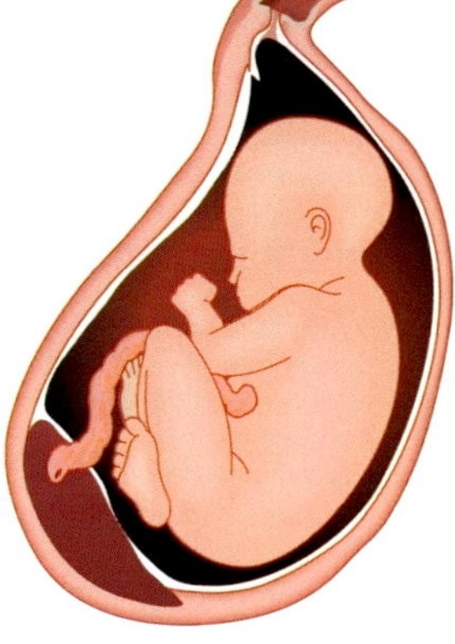

LEARNING OBJECTIVES

After studying this chapter, the student should be able to:

- Describe the development of male and female reproductive systems. AN 52.8
- Describe the development of gonads in brief. Give the differences in the development of testis and ovary in the tabular form.
- Enumerate derivatives of (a) mesonephric duct, (b) paramesonephric duct, and (c) urogenital sinus.
- Describe the development of uterus in brief and discuss associated common congenital anomalies.
- Write short notes on (a) hypospadias, (b) descent of testis, (c) ectopic testis, and (d) congenital hydrocele.

OVERVIEW

The **genital system** consists of (a) a pair of **gonads** (testes or ovaries), (b) **duct system** of gonads that carries the germ cells, and (c) **external genital organs**. It develops from the following three sources:

- Intermediate mesoderm
- Part of cloaca
- Coelomic epithelium covering the intermediate mesoderm

The development of genital system begins during the 4th week of intrauterine life (IUL). The genetic sex (genotype XY or XX) of embryo is established at the time of fertilization, but gonads do not acquire male or female morphological characteristics till 7th week of the development. Initially (weeks 1–6 of development), the gonads are structurally similar and hence this is called **indifferent stage of gonad**. From 7th week onward, the development proceeds in different directions in males and females, and gonadal sex can then be determined morphologically. By 12th week, some male and female characteristics of the external genitalia can also be recognized. By the end of 20th week, phenotypical differentiation is complete. This difference of development between male and female is because of chromosomal and hormonal factors.

The phenotypical differentiation is determined by ***SRY* gene** located on the short arm of Y chromosome (Yp11).

The ***SRY* gene** encodes for a protein called **testis-determining factor (TDF)**. The presence of TDF leads to development of male genital organs. As the indifferent gonad develops into the testis, the Leydig and Sertoli cells differentiate to produce **testosterone** and **Müllerian-inhibiting factor (MIF)**. This results in phenotypically male embryo.

In the absence of the **TDF, testosterone, and MIF**, the indifferent gonad will develop into ovary and embryo will be phenotypically female. The genetic basis of phenotypical differentiation of sex is summarized in Flowchart 25.1.

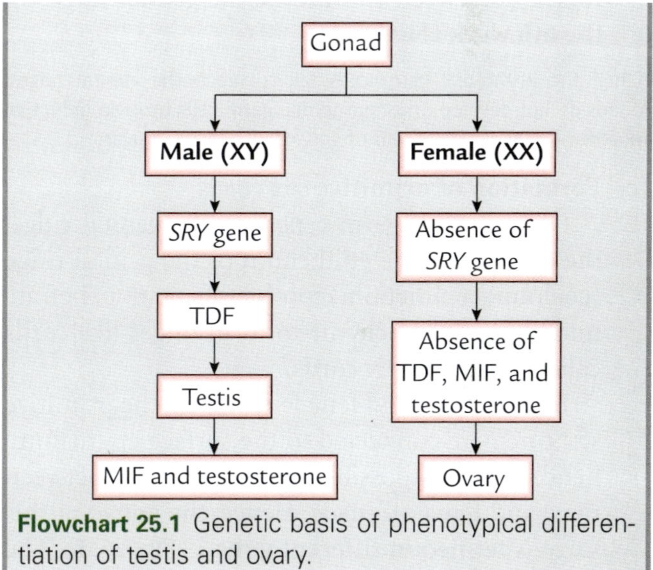

Flowchart 25.1 Genetic basis of phenotypical differentiation of testis and ovary.

DEVELOPMENT OF GONADS AN 52.8

The gonads develop from the following three sources:

1. **Intermediate mesoderm**
2. **Coelomic epithelium covering the intermediate mesoderm**
3. **Primordial germ cells**

Initially, the development of testis or ovary is similar (**indifferent stage**) and only after this stage the development proceeds in either male or female direction (**definitive stage**).

Indifferent Stage

(a) **Formation of genital ridge**

The gonads develop in the **intermediate mesoderm – medial** to middle part of mesonephros.

The first indication of development of **primitive gonad** is seen at about 4th week. An elongated elevation called **genital ridge** appears on medial side of **mesonephric ridge**. The genital ridge is formed by condensation of intermediate mesoderm and proliferation of overlying coelomic epithelium (Fig. 25.1).

(b) **Formation and migration of primordial germ cells (PGCs)**

The **primordial germ cells** arise from epiblast of bilaminar germ disc in **2nd week of IUL** and soon migrate into the wall of yolk sac close to allantois and become recognizable. During the **4th week**, the primordial germ cells migrate along dorsal mesentery of hindgut by active amoeboid movement and reach the genital ridges at beginning of 5th week and invade the genital ridges in the **6th week** (Fig. 25.2).

N.B. If the primordial germ cells fail to reach the genital ridges, gonads do not develop. Thus, primordial germ cells have an inductive influence on the development of gonads into testis or ovary.

(c) **Formation of primitive sex cords**

On arrival of germ cells into the genital ridge, the cells of surface epithelium of the genital ridge (coelomic epithelium) proliferate and penetrate underlying mesenchyme to form finger-like cords called **primitive sex cords**.

In both male and female embryos, the primitive sex cords are connected to the surface epithelium; hence, it is impossible to differentiate between male and female gonads. Hence, the gonad at this stage is termed **indifferent gonad** (Fig. 25.3). The outer part of the indifferent gonad is called **cortex** and its central part is called **medulla**.

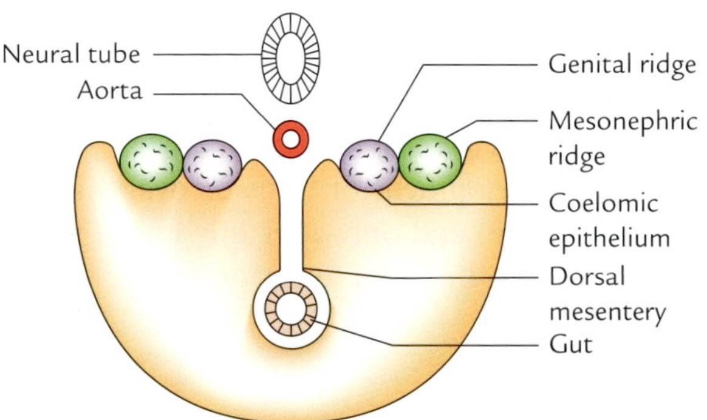

Fig. 25.1 Site of development of gonadal ridges.

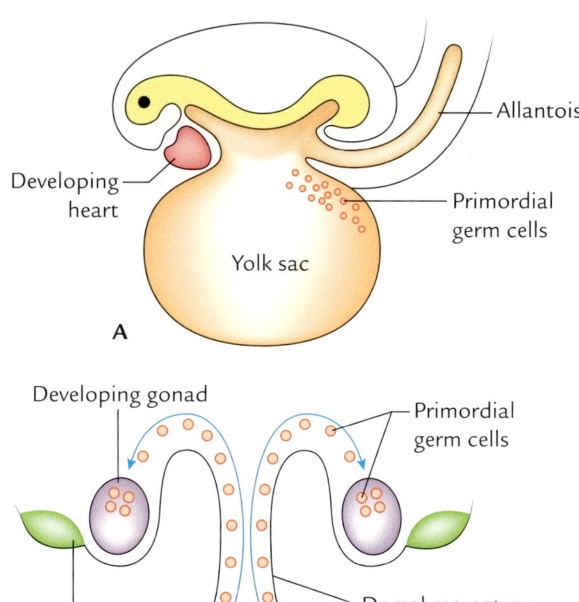

Fig. 25.2 Primordial germ cells. (A) Primordial germ cells developing in the wall of yolk sac close to the attachment of allantois. (B) Migration of primordial germ cells along the wall of hindgut and its dorsal mesentery into the developing gonad.

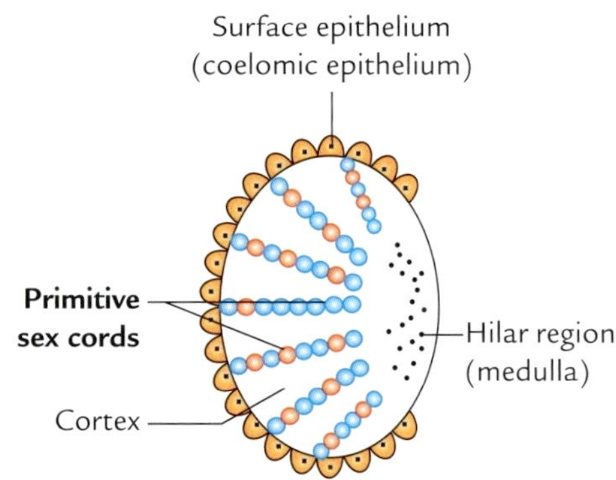

Fig. 25.3 Indifferent gonad.

Till this stage, the development of testis and ovary is similar. From here onward, the development of testis and ovary follow a different path, i.e., the development of testis and ovary proceeds into a **definitive stage**.

Definitive Stage

The indifferent gonad enters the *definitive stage*, i.e., it develops into testis or ovary depending on the chromosome complement of the primordial germ cells. If the primordial germ cells carry XY sex chromosome complement, the indifferent gonad will develop into **testis**;

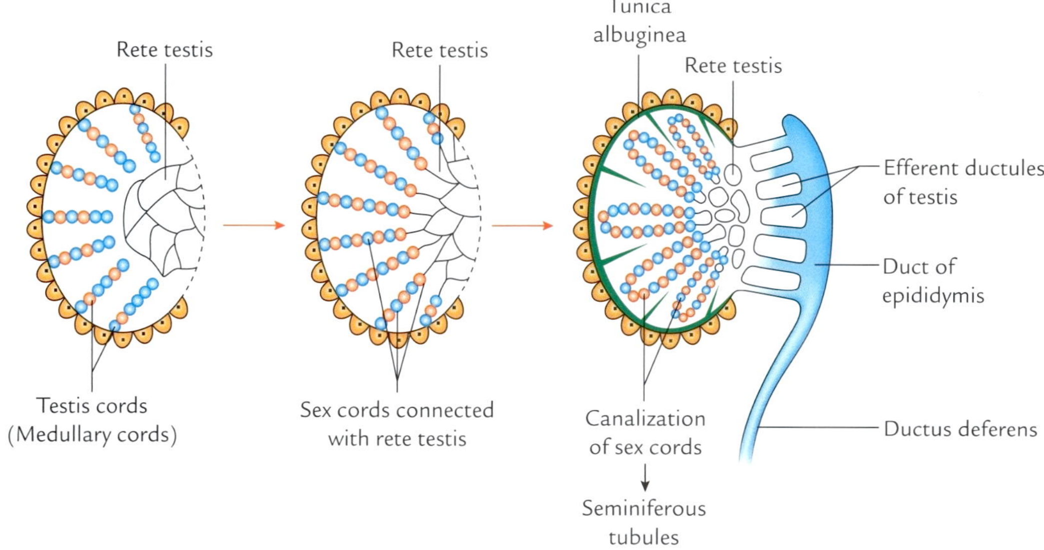

Fig. 25.4 Development of testis.

and if the primordial germ cells carry XX chromosome complement, the indifferent gonad will develop into an ovary. The development of testis and ovary is described in the following text.

Development of Testis (Fig. 25.4)

If the embryo is genetically male (i.e., the primordial germ cells carry XY chromosome complement; Flowchart 25.1) under the influence of *SRY* gene on the short arm of Y chromosome (Yp11), which encodes for the TDF, the primitive sex cords increase in length and extend deep into central part – *medulla* of the indifferent gonad. These are called **testis or medullary cords**. Toward the hilum of gonad, the medullary cords regress and break up into tiny cell strands that anastomose with each other. The sex cords then become horseshoe shaped and subsequently get canalized to form **seminiferous tubules**. The anastomosing tiny cell strands in medulla also get canalized to form "**rete testis.**" In the 4th month, communication is established between the seminiferous tubules and the rete testis.

The **seminiferous tubules** are lined by two types of cells: (a) sex cord cells (cells derived from surface coelomic epithelium) and (b) primordial germ cells (derived from wall of the yolk sac). The primordial germ cells form spermatogonia and the sex cord cells form **sustentacular cells of Sertoli**.

Now the mesenchyme migrates beneath the coelomic epithelium, forms a tough fibrous layer around the developing testis, and separates (cuts off) the sex cords from the coelomic epithelium (germinal epithelium), thus blocking its contribution to the formation of sex cords permanently. This tough fibrous layer covering the testis is called **tunica albuginea**. Mesoderm also forms mediastinum testis. The fibrous septa arise from mediastinum, extend toward periphery, and divide the testis into various lobules. Mesoderm around the seminiferous tubules forms **interstitial cells of Leydig**. By 8th week, the Leydig cells start secreting testosterone – the male hormone that influences sexual differentiation of genital ducts (from mesonephric duct) and external genitalia.

The tubules of rete testis extend into the mesonephric tissue, where they join the mesonephric tubules. The mesonephric tubules become **efferent ductules of the testis**. **Duct of epididymis**, **vas deferens**, **seminal vesicle**, and **ejaculatory duct** are formed from the mesonephric duct.

As the testes develop, they project in the coelomic cavity and are suspended from posterior abdominal wall by a mesentery called "**mesorchium.**"

CLINICAL CORRELATION

Seminoma

The medullary cords/sex cords of testes (primordia of seminiferous tubules) remain solid until puberty. Spermatogonia develop and form sperms only after puberty when the seminiferous tubules are formed by canalization of the sex cords. For this reason, testicular tumor called **seminoma** is unknown before puberty as the seminoma arises from the seminiferous tubules, which do not develop before puberty.

Development of Ovary (Fig. 25.5)

If the embryo is genetically female (i.e., primordial germ cells carry XX chromosome complement. Further

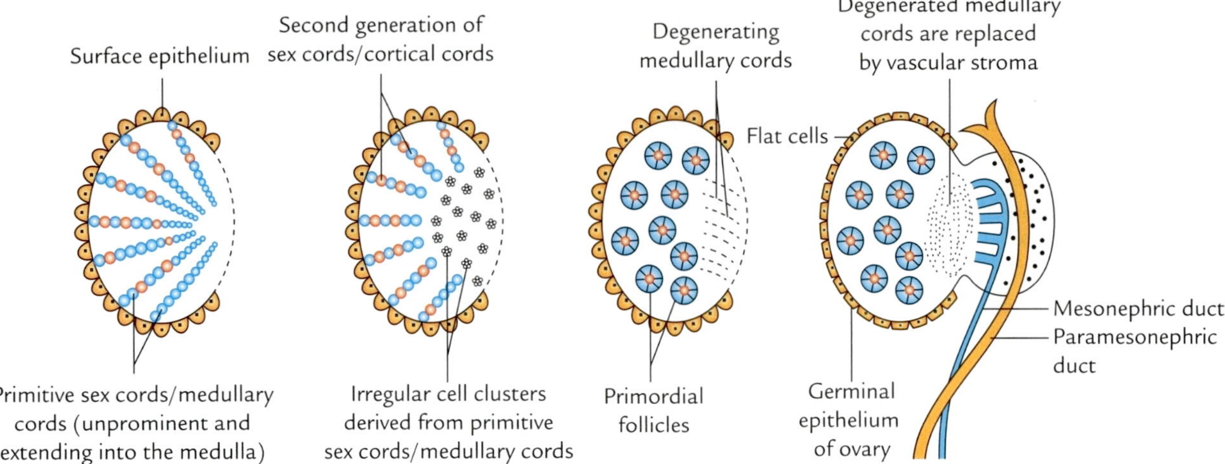

Fig. 25.5 Development of the ovary.

the Y chromosome with *SRY* gene, TDS, MIF and testosterone are absent (Flowchart 25.1). Therefore, the indifferent gonad develops into an ovary. The **primitive sex cords** containing the primordial germ cells do not become prominent but extend into the medulla. These cords dissociate into irregular cell clusters called **rete ovarii**, which occupy the medullary part of the ovary close to the mesonephric tubules. Later they disappear and are replaced by vascular stroma, which forms **ovarian medulla.**

N.B. The X chromosomes bear genes for ovarian development.

The surface epithelium (germinal epithelium) of female gonad, unlike that of male gonad, continues to proliferate and in the 7th week forms **second generation of sex cords. The second generation of sex cords containing the primordial germ cells does not extend into medulla.** Hence, they are also called **cortical cords.** In the 3rd month, the cortical cords get fragmented and form isolated cell clusters. Each cell cluster consists of a primordial germ cell in the center surrounded by a layer of coelomic epithelial cells. The primordial germ cells form **oogonia** and coelomic epithelial cells form **follicular cells.** The resulting structure is called "**primordial follicle.**" All the primordial follicles remain confined in cortex of the ovary.

N.B. A large number of primordial follicles are formed during fetal life. *No new primordial follicles are formed after birth. Further development of the primordial follicles takes place after puberty.*

The mesoderm does not form thick fibrous layer (tunica albuginea) around ovary as in case of testis. Therefore, the ovarian follicles are not separated from surface epithelium of the ovary. The surface epithelium of ovary flattens to form a single layer of cells that is continuous with the peritoneum at hilum of the ovary.

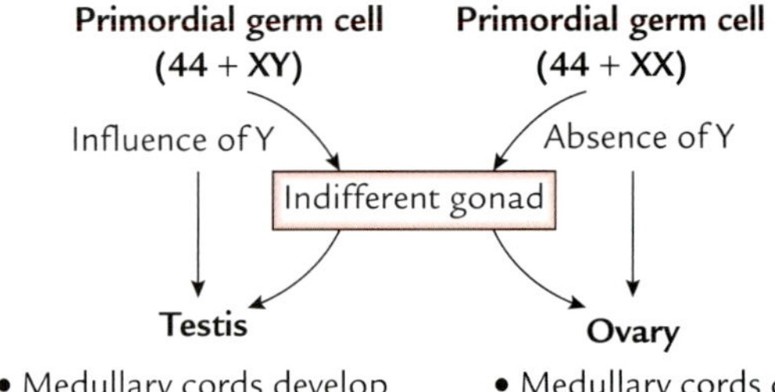

Flowchart 25.2 Influence of chromosome complement of primordial germ cells on indifferent gonad.

The layer of these cells is called **germinal epithelium,** although it does not form germ cells anymore. The mesoderm forms a thin connective tissue covering for the ovary and connective tissue stroma of the ovary.

The ovary is suspended from posterior abdominal wall by a mesentery called "**mesovarium.**"

The influence of genetic constitution of primordial germ cells on the indifferent gonad is shown in Flowchart 25.2.

The differences in the development of testis and ovary are summarized in Table 25.1.

N.B. The testis and ovary are not identifiable histologically until 10th week.

DEVELOPMENT OF GENITAL DUCTS

The genital ducts of male include *vasa efferentia, duct of epididymis, vas deferens,* and *ejaculatory duct*; the genital ducts of female include *fallopian tube, uterus,* and *vagina.*

Table 25.1 Differences in development of testis and ovary

Testis	Ovary
Formation of only one generation of sex cords (medullary cords) that produce seminiferous tubules and rete testis	Formation of two generations of sex cords: (a) First generation of sex cords (medullary cords) forms stroma of ovarian medulla (b) Second generation of sex cords (cortical cords) forms primordial follicles (ovarian follicles)
Formation of tunica albuginea separating seminiferous tubules from surface epithelium	No formation of tunica albuginea; hence, ovarian follicles are not separated from surface epithelium

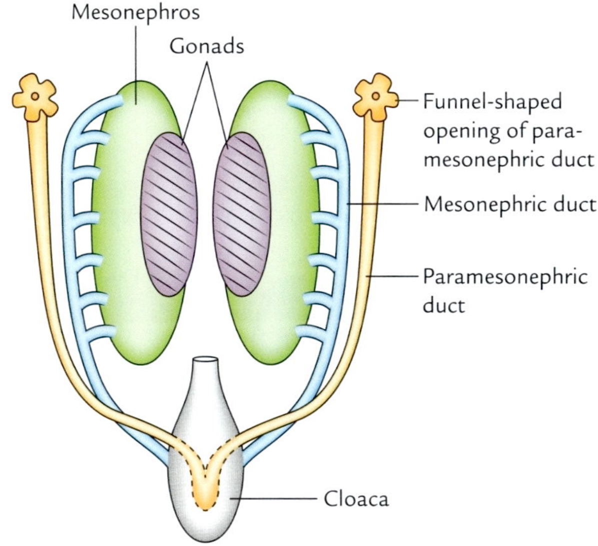

Fig. 25.6 Two pairs of genital ducts during the indifferent stage of development of gonads.

Initially two pairs of genital ducts develop in both the sexes (Fig. 25.6): (a) **mesonephric ducts (Wolffian ducts)** and (b) **paramesonephric ducts (Müllerian ducts)**.

In male, the mesonephric ducts form the definitive genital ducts while paramesonephric ducts mostly disappear, whereas in female paramesonephric ducts form the female genital ducts while the mesonephric ducts mostly disappear.

The differentiation of genital ducts and external genitalia into male and female directions is influenced by the gonads.

Influence of Gonads on Sex Differentiation

The influence of gonads on further sex differentiation (i.e., development of genital ducts and external genitalia) is as follows:

- The secretion of **Müllerian-inhibiting substance** by **Sertoli cells** of testis inhibits the development of paramesonephric ducts – the primordia of female genital ducts.
- The production of **testosterone** by interstitial cells (**Leydig cells**) stimulates the mesonephric ducts to form genital ducts, i.e., **efferent ductules, epididymis, vas deferens, seminal vesicles, and ejaculatory ducts**. The secretion of **dihydrotestosterone** by Leydig cells stimulates the development of male external genitalia, i.e., penis, scrotum, and prostate.
- The secretion of **estrogens** by the ovaries stimulates the paramesonephric ducts to form **uterine tube, uterus, and upper part of the vagina**. It also stimulates the development of female external genitalia, i.e., **labia majora, labia minora, clitoris, and lower portion of vagina**.

The influence of gonads on further differentiation of genital ducts and external genitalia is shown in Flowchart 25.3.

Development of Genital Ducts in Male (Fig. 25.7)

The **genital ducts in male** develop from **mesonephric duct**. Mesonephric duct develops in relation to mesonephros and opens into the cloaca (urogenital sinus). When the mesonephros is functional, the **mesonephric tubules** open into the mesonephric duct (Fig. 25.6).

When mesonephros degenerates, most of the **mesonephric tubules** disappear. Only few mesonephric tubules in the vicinity of testis persist and establish connection with **rete testis** to form the **vasa efferentia** or **efferent ductules of testis.**

The upper part of mesonephric duct, which receives the efferent ductules, becomes elongated and highly coiled to form **duct of epididymis**. This highly coiled duct of epididymis becomes wrapped in connective tissue to form a comma-shaped structure called **epididymis**. The epididymis is attached to the posterior border of testis. Next part of the mesonephric duct develops a thick muscular coat and forms the **vas deferens**. Just before the mesonephric duct opens into the definitive urogenital sinus (future prostatic urethra), it gives a diverticulum that develops into **seminal vesicle**. The part of mesonephric duct distal to seminal vesicle forms the **ejaculatory duct** that opens into prostatic urethra.

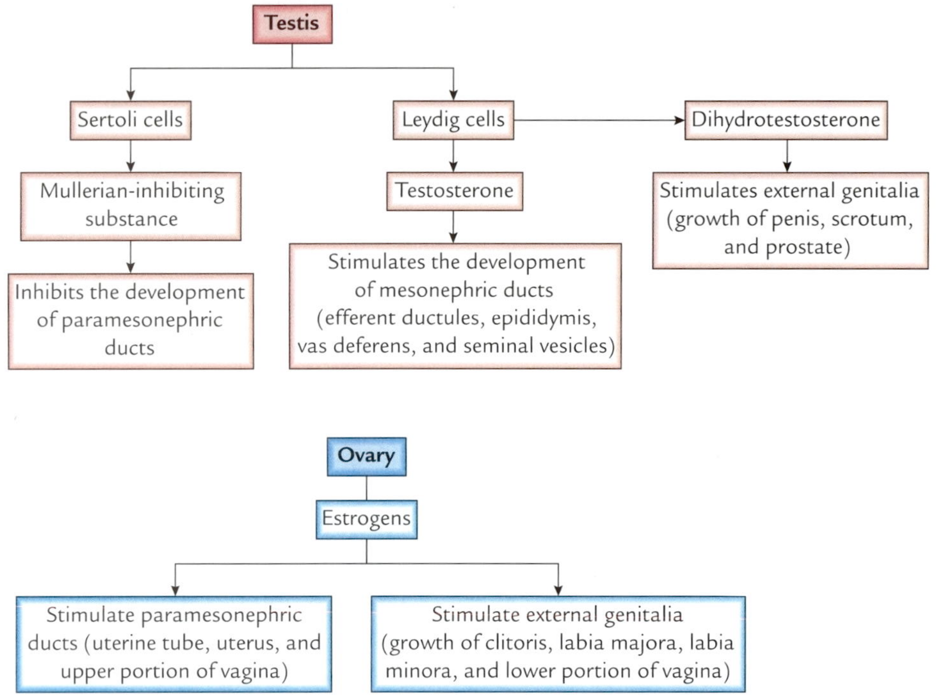

Flowchart 25.3 Influence of gonads on further sex differentiation.

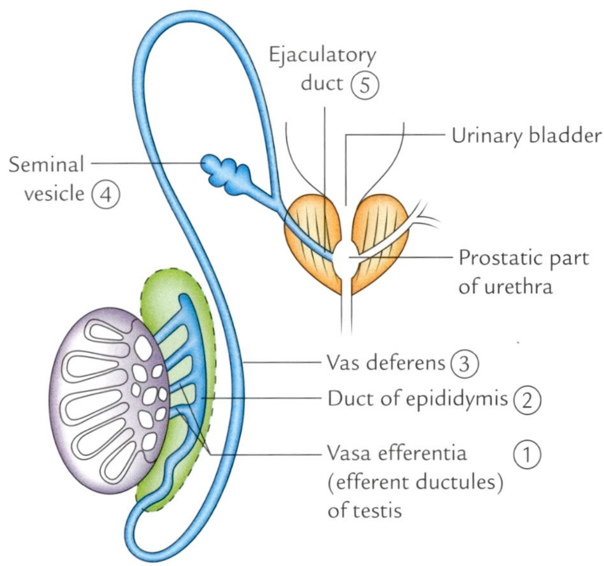

Fig. 25.7 Derivatives of mesonephric duct.

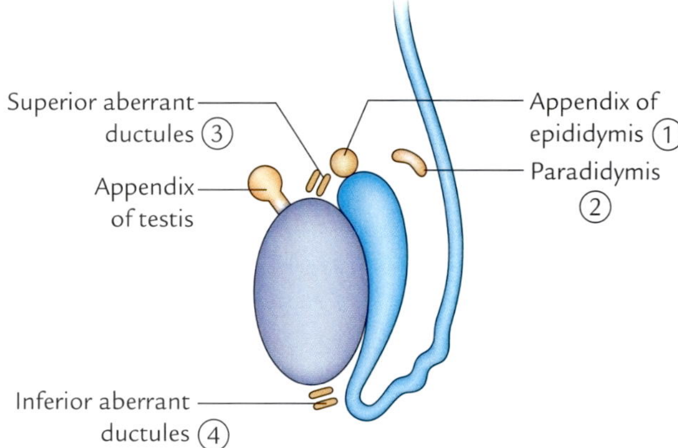

Fig. 25.8 Vestigial remnants of mesonephric duct.

N.B.

1. **Vestigeal remnants of mesonephric duct and mesonephric tubules in male** (Fig. 25.8)
   (a) *Appendix of epididymis:* The cranial end of the mesonephric duct may persist as a small body called *appendix of the epididymis,* which is usually attached to head of the epididymis.
   (b) *Paradidymis:* The mesonephric tubules that fail to connect with the rete testis may persist and form a small body called *paradidymis,* which lies close to the upper part of the epididymis.
   (c) *Superior aberrant ductules:* These are remnants of mesonephric tubules cranial to efferent ductules (vasa efferentia) of the testis.
   (d) *Inferior aberrant ductules:* These are remnants of mesonephric tubules caudal to efferent ductules (vasa efferentia) of testis.
2. **Vestigeal remnants of paramesonephric (Müllerian duct) in male**
   (a) *Appendix of testis:* The cranial end of paramesonephric duct may persist as a small vesicular body called *appendix of the testis.* It is found attached to the upper pole of the testis.
   (b) *Prostatic utricle:* It is a small blind sac that opens into the posterior wall of the prostatic urethra. The prostatic utricle is homologous to *uterus and vagina in females.*

N.B. **Appendix of epididymis** is a remnant of mesonephric duct, whereas **appendix of testis** is a remnant of paramesonephric duct.

Development of Prostate and Bulbourethral Glands

Although these two structures do not form part of the male genital duct, but due to their close anatomical and functional relationship with the male genital duct, they are described here.

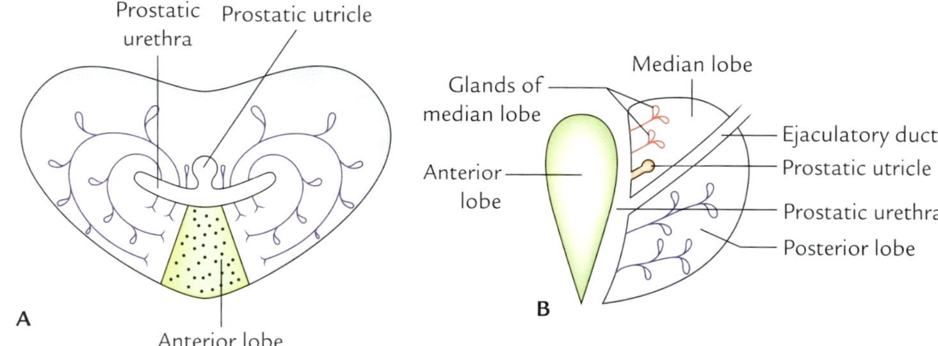

Fig. 25.9 Development of the prostate gland. (A) Transverse section of the prostate gland above the level of openings of ejaculatory ducts. (B) A sagittal section of the prostate gland. Note that the glands of median lobe which open into the posterior wall of the prostatic urethra above the openings of ejaculatory ducts are mesodermal in origin.

Development of Prostate Gland (Fig. 25.9)

The prostatic gland develops from epithelial buds that arise from the epithelial lining of the embryonic urogenital sinus (prostatic urethra) during 2nd week of IUL under the influence of androgen and fetal testosterone, and grow in the surrounding mesoderm as follows:

(a) The buds arising from mesodermal posterior wall of the urethra above the openings of ejaculatory ducts form **inner glandular zone of the gland.**

(b) The buds arising from rest of the prostatic urethra (endodermal in origin) form **outer glandular zone of the prostate.**

(c) The surrounding mesoderm forms dense fibrous stroma and smooth muscle of the prostate gland. It also forms **prostatic capsule.**

Stages of prostatic development The prostatic development is divided into five stages:

1. Formation of solid prostatic epithelial buds
2. Elongation and branching of buds
3. Canalization of solid buds
4. Differentiation of luminal and basal epithelial cells
5. Secretory cytodifferentiation

N.B. The reproductive function of prostate begins at puberty.

CLINICAL CORRELATION

The **outer glandular zone** of the prostate gland differentiates earlier than the **inner glandular zone.** In later life (older than 50 years), the outer (endodermal) zone is prone to develop **prostate cancer,** whereas the inner (mesodermal) zone is prone to undergo **benign hypertrophy of prostate.**

The reproductive function of prostate becomes active at puberty.

Development of Bulbourethral Glands

These are small pea-sized paired glands that develop during 10th–12th weeks of gestational age (IUL) from paired outgrowths from the spongy part of urethra. The secretion of bulbourethral glands lubricates the urethral lumen.

Development of Genital Ducts in Female

The genital ducts in female consist of **fallopian tubes, uterus,** and **vagina.** They develop from **paramesonephric ducts.**

The paramesonephric duct develops in 6th week of IUL, lateral to mesonephric ducts by a vertical invagination of coelomic epithelium (mesothelium) (Fig. 25.10); when traced caudally, they cross in front of the mesonephric ducts from lateral to medial side and come close to each other in the midline (Fig. 25.10). Here, two paramesonephric ducts fuse together in midline to form a vertical duct called **uterovaginal canal.** Upper ends of the paramesonephric ducts remain open into the coelomic cavity (future peritoneal cavity). The caudal end of uterovaginal canal grows down and comes in contact with the dorsal wall of the phallic part of the definitive urogenital sinus (Fig. 25.11). At first, fusion between the two paramesonephric ducts is incomplete, being separated by a fenestrated septum.

The paramesonephric duct is divided into three parts: (a) cranial vertical part, (b) middle horizontal part, and (c) caudal vertical part.

The various components of female genital duct develop as follows:

Fate of paramesonephric ducts in female (Fig. 25.12)

In females, the paramesonephric ducts form the following:

1. Uterine tubes
2. Uterus
3. Upper part of vagina

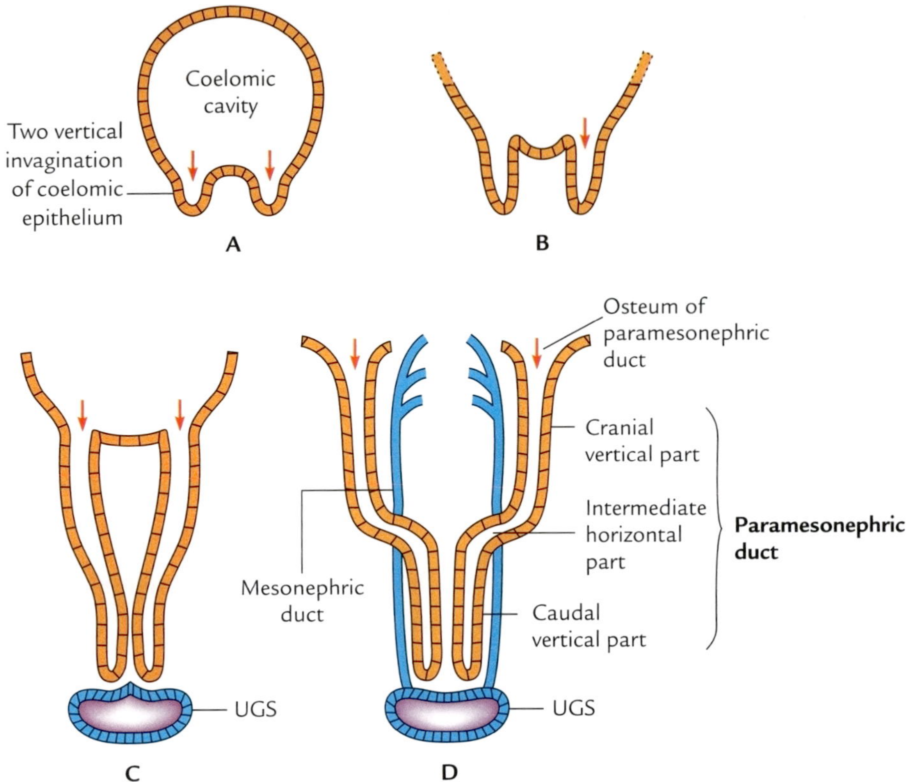

Fig. 25.10 Stages of development of paramesonephric ducts. UGS, urogenital sinus.

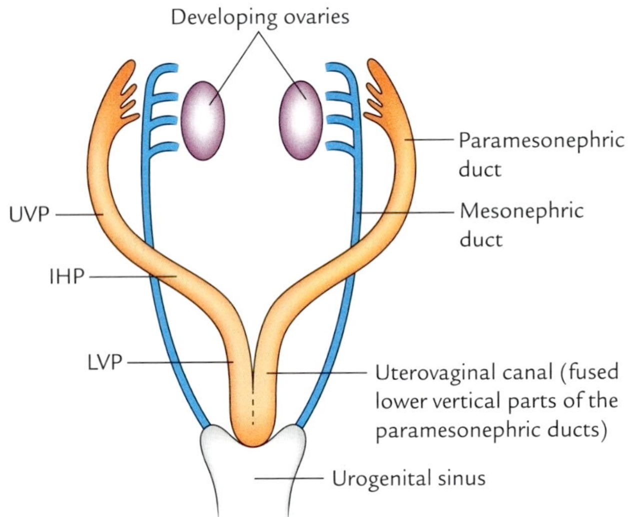

Fig. 25.11 Formation of uterovaginal canal. IHP, intermediate horizontal part; LVP, lower vertical part; UVP, upper vertical part.

Development of Uterine Tubes

The uterine tube, on each side, is formed by unfused part (the cranial vertical and middle horizontal parts) of the paramesonephric duct. The fallopian tube elongates and becomes tortuous.

The original site of evagination of the paramesonephric duct from coelomic cavity forms **abdominal ostium** of uterine tube. The fimbria develops later around the margin of the ostium.

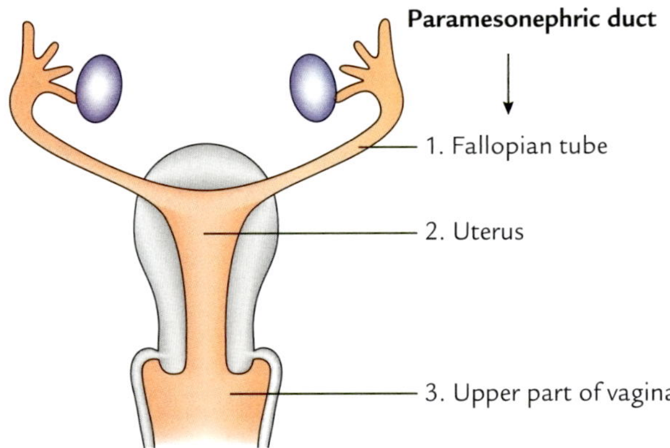

Fig. 25.12 Fate of paramesonephric ducts in females.

Development of the Uterus (Fig. 25.13)

The uterus is formed from the uterovaginal canal (fused, caudal vertical parts of the paramesonephric ducts). The primitive uterus soon differentiates into two parts: (a) **body** and (b) **cervix. In fetus, cervix is larger than the body of uterus** but later (particularly after puberty) the body of uterus elongates and becomes longer than cervix. The initial angular junction between the two paramesonephric ducts becomes a convex dome and forms fundus of uterus.

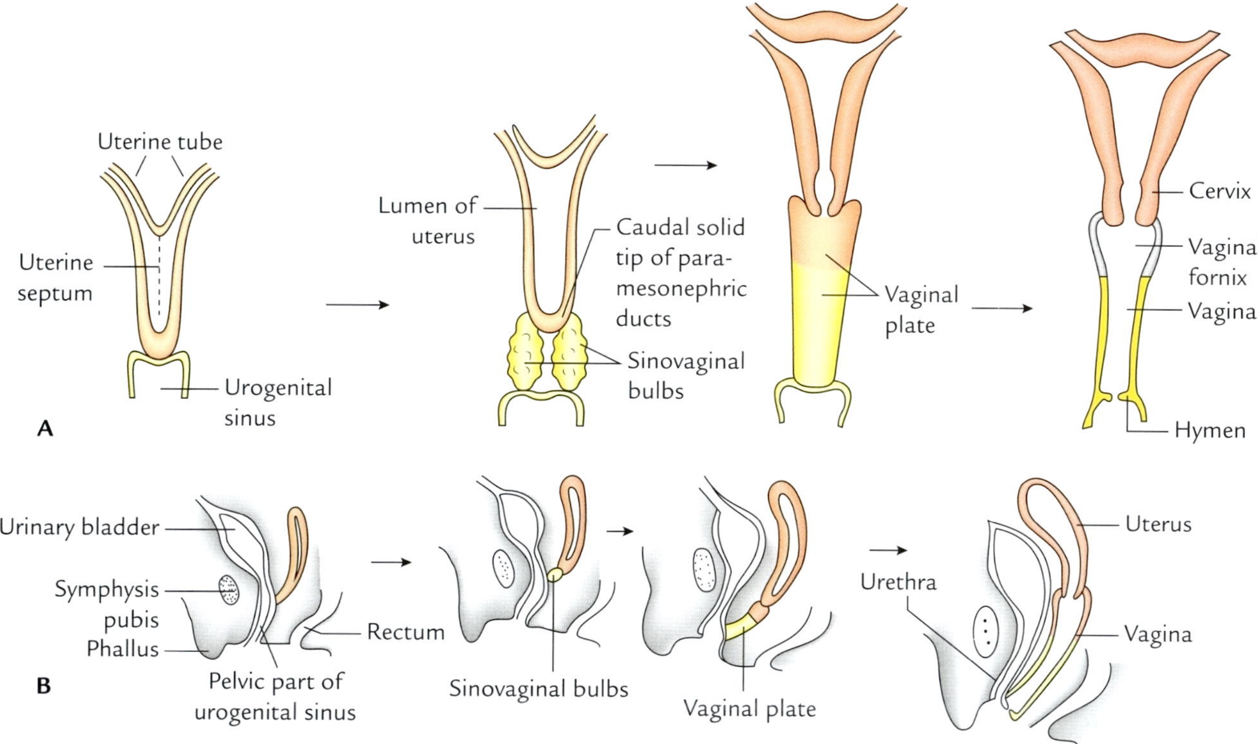

Fig. 25.13 Development of the uterus and vagina. (A) Frontal view. (B) Side view.

Myometrium of the uterus is derived from surrounding mesoderm.

Development of the Vagina (Fig. 25.13)

A little recapitulation of various parts of primitive urogenital sinus (see p. 282, and Fig. 24.14) helps students to understand the development of vagina.

The vagina develops as follows:

As solid caudal tip of the **uterovaginal canal** comes in contact with dorsal wall of pelvic part of the definitive urogenital sinus, it induces formation of two outgrowths (evaginations) from the dorsal wall of the pelvic part of the definitive urogenital sinus called **sinovaginal bulbs**. The endodermal cells of the sinovaginal bulbs proliferate rapidly and form solid plate of cells called **vaginal plate**. The cells from tip of the uterovaginal canal (mesodermal) also proliferate and add to the *vaginal plate*. Now the vaginal plate is interposed between the uterovaginal canal and the urogenital sinus. The vaginal plate is therefore of composite origin – the upper part of vaginal plate is derived from the mesodermal cells of uterovaginal canal, whereas the lower part of vaginal plate is derived from the endodermal cells of sinovaginal bulbs.

The upper end of vaginal plate expands and surrounds the caudal end of uterovaginal canal.

N.B. There is a controversy regarding the formation of *vaginal plate*. Some authorities consider that whole vaginal plate is derived from endodermal sinovaginal bulbs, whereas others believe that upper part of vaginal plate is derived from mesodermal uterovaginal canal and lower part is derived from endodermal sinovaginal bulbs.

The central cells of vaginal plate break down and by the 5th month the plate is completely canalized to form lumen of the vagina. The wing-like expansion of vagina around the cervix forms **fornices of vagina**. The vagina remains separated from the phallic part of definitive urogenital sinus by a thin plate of tissue called **hymen**, which consists of a thin layer of vaginal cells superiorly and epithelial lining of sinus inferiorly. Thus, both the surfaces of the hymen are lined by endoderm. The hymen usually develops a small opening in its center during perinatal life.

N.B. At first, the phallic part of the definitive urogenital sinus is closed/separated from the surface by the **urogenital membrane**. But this membrane breaks and the phallic part opens to the exterior. The phallic part of definitive urogenital sinus forms the vestibule of vagina, into which vagina and urethra open (derived from pelvic part of definitive urogenital sinus).

The development of vagina and associated structures, i.e., hymen and vestibule of vagina, is summarized in Table 25.2.

Table 25.2 Development of vagina and its associated structures

Adult Derivatives	Embryonic Structures
Upper part of vagina including fornices of vagina	From mesodermal upper part of vaginal plate (derived from uterovaginal canal)
Lower part of vagina	From endodermal lower part of vaginal plate (derived from sinovaginal bulbs)
Hymen	From thin plate of tissue separating vagina and phallic part of urogenital sinus
Vestibule of vagina	From phallic part of definitive urogenital sinus

CLINICAL CORRELATION

Congenital anomalies of the uterus (Fig. 25.14)

1. ***Double uterus with double vagina (Fig. 25.14A):*** In this condition, there are two uteruses (uterus didelphys) and two vaginas. It occurs due to *complete lack of fusion of the paramesonephric ducts and the sinovaginal bulbs.*
2. ***Double uterus with single vagina (Fig. 25.14B):*** It occurs when paramesonephric ducts fail to fuse but lie close to each other. As a result, there are two uteruses (**uterus didelphys**). The *vaginal plate* formed in relation to each duct fuses with each other to form a single vagina.

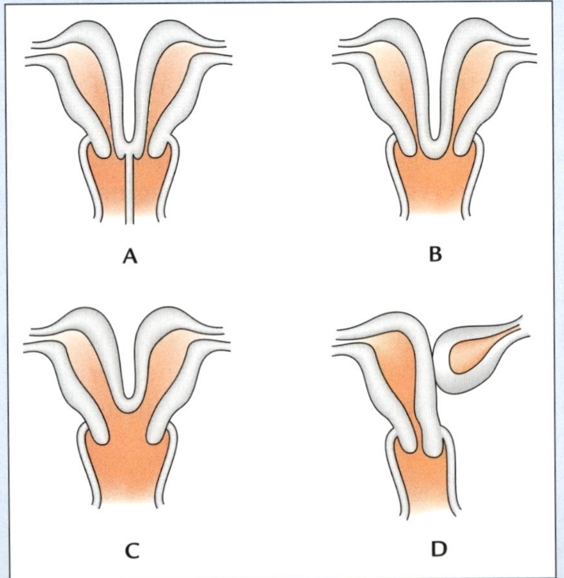

Fig. 25.14 Main congenital anomalies of the uterus. (A) Double uterus (uterus didelphys) with double vagina. (B) Double uterus with single vagina. (C) Bicornuate uterus. (D) Unicornuate uterus.

3. ***Bicornuate uterus (Fig. 25.14C):*** In this condition, there is one vagina and one cervix but the body of uterus is duplicated. Each half of the body is called horn or cornu of the uterus. One fallopian tube opens in each horn of the uterus.

   It occurs when the paramesonephric ducts fuse with each other only in their lower parts while they remain separate in upper part, thus giving rise to two horns of the uterus.
4. ***Unicornuate uterus (Fig. 25.14D):*** In this condition, half of the uterus is missing. It occurs when one paramesonephric duct degenerates so that only one horn of the uterus with one fallopian tube persists.
5. ***Septate uterus:*** In this condition, the two paramesonephric ducts fuse with each other but the septum separating them does not disintegrate. As a result, a vertical septum separates cavity of the uterus into two halves.
6. ***Agenesis of uterus:*** It is a rare condition in which uterus is completely absent. It occurs due to failure of the paramesonephric ducts to develop.
7. **Infantile uterus:** It is a clinical condition in which an adult female possesses a much smaller uterus than normal. The infantile uterus resembles to that present before puberty. The vagina and ovaries are normal. Clinically, it presents as *amenorrhea*.

Congenital anomalies of vagina

1. ***Agenesis of vagina:*** In this condition, the vagina is absent. It occurs when the urogenital sinus fails to form the sinovaginal bulbs and hence the vaginal plate. Absence of the vagina is usually associated with absence of the uterus and uterine tubes.
2. ***Atresia of vagina (imperforate vagina):*** This occurs when the vaginal plate fails to get canalized. Sometimes only middle part of the vaginal plate fails to disintegrate, giving rise to horizontal septum in the lumen of vagina.
3. ***Imperforate hymen:*** It occurs when the endodermal cells of the vaginal plate adjacent to the urogenital sinus fail to disintegrate. This condition causes retention of menstrual flow – a clinical condition called **hematocolpos**.
4. ***Duplication of vagina:*** This condition is generally associated with double uterus.
5. ***Rectovaginal and vesicovaginal fistulae:*** In these conditions, the vagina communicates with rectum and urinary bladder, respectively (Fig. 25.15).

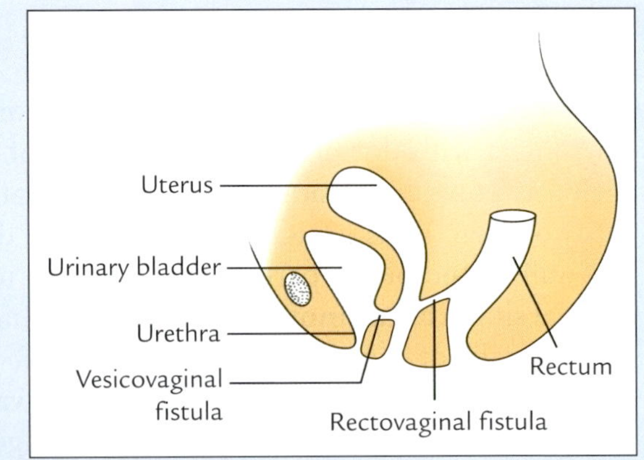

Fig. 25.15 Rectovaginal and vesicovaginal fistulae.

Vestigial remnants of mesonephric duct in females

These are the following (Fig. 25.16):

(a) ***Epoophoron:*** It consists of a longitudinal duct running parallel to the uterine tube (persistent cranial part of the mesonephric duct), and a

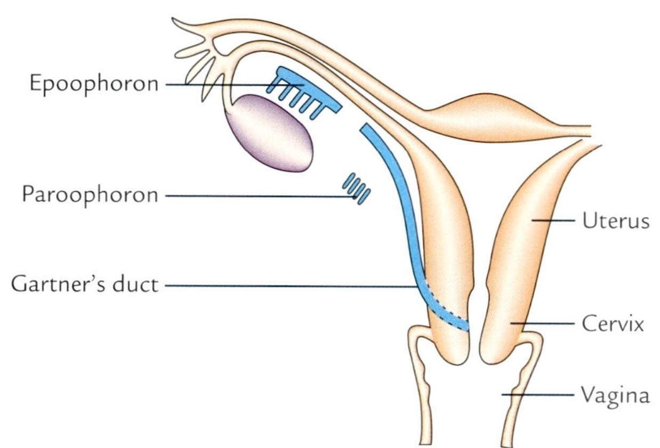

Fig. 25.16 Vestigial remnants of mesonephric duct in females.

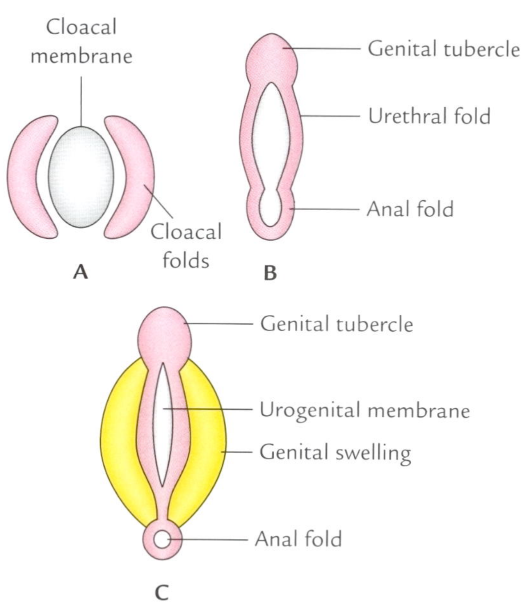

Fig. 25.17 Indifferent stages of external genitalia. Till the end of 6th week, external genitalia of two sexes cannot be differentiated.

number of transverse ductules that open into this duct (persistent mesonephric tubules) are present vertically above the ovary in the mesovarium. The *epoophoron* corresponds to efferent ductules of testes and epididymis of males (epi, above; oo, egg; and phoron, basket).

(b) ***Paroophoron:*** A few mesonephric tubules are detached from the mesonephric duct and persist as small blind tubules between the ovary and the uterus. These are called *paroophoron* (para, near; oo, egg; and phoron, basket).

(c) ***Gartner's duct:*** A part of the mesonephric duct persists and lies between the two layers of broad ligament by the side of the body of uterus. It may open into the cervix or vagina. This corresponds to the vas deferens in males. This duct may undergo abnormal cystic dilatations to form *Gartner's cysts.*

DEVELOPMENT OF EXTERNAL GENITALIA

OVERVIEW

The development of external genitalia is similar in both males and females till the 6th week of IUL (**during indifferent stage**). After this stage, the development proceeds in either male or female direction under the influence of hormones.

Indifferent Stage (Fig. 25.17)

The **external genitalia** develop in the region of **cloacal membrane.**

Early in the 4th week, the embryonic mesoderm from primitive streak migrates around the cloacal membrane to form a pair of swellings called **cloacal folds**. Cranial to the cloacal membrane, these folds unite to form **genital tubercle**. Caudally each fold is subdivided into two parts: (a) a large anterior part called **urethral fold** and (b) a small posterior part called **anal fold.**

Simultaneously the cloacal membrane is divided in two parts by **urorectal septum:** (a) the anterior part called **urogenital membrane** and (b) the posterior part called **anal membrane.** The genital tubercle and urethral folds are now related to the urogenital membrane. In the meantime, another pair of elevations called **genital swellings** appears – one on each side of the urethral folds. At this stage, the urogenital membrane in each sex is related on each side to the **urethral fold** medially, **genital swelling** laterally, and **genital tubercle** anteriorly. The morphological sex cannot be differentiated at this stage, hence the name **indifferent stage.** From this stage onward, development proceeds in different directions in male and female.

Definitive Stage

Development of Male External Genitalia (Figs 25.18 and 25.19)

Under the influence of androgens (*testosterone* and *dihydrotestosterone*) secreted by Leydig cells of fetal testes, the development of external genitalia proceeds in the male direction.

At *9th week of gestational age*, genital tubercle enlarges rapidly and becomes cylindrical to form **phallus**

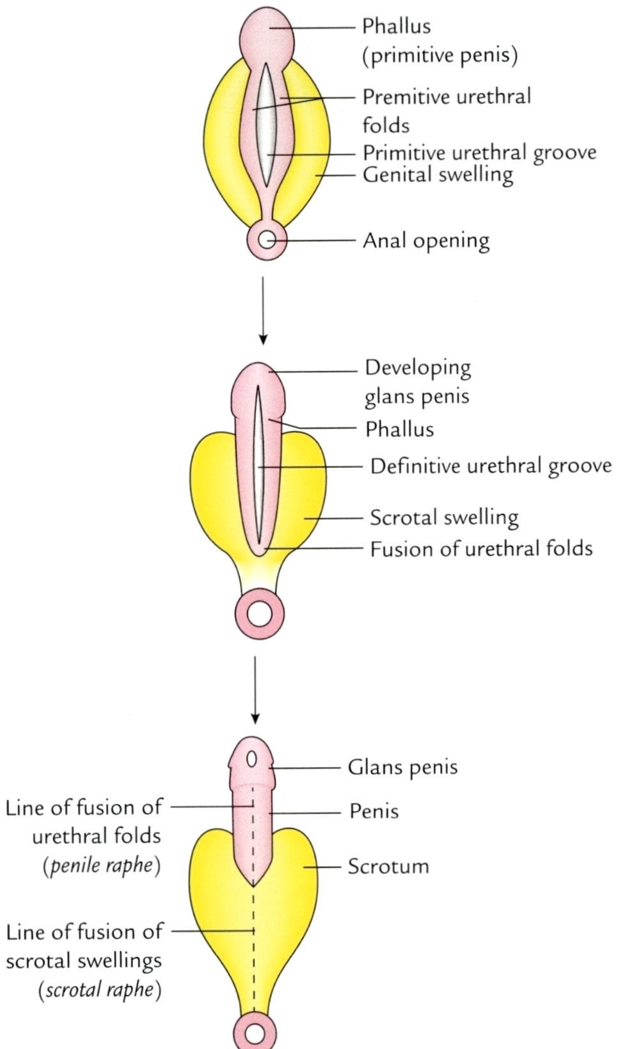

Fig. 25.18 Development of male external genitalia.

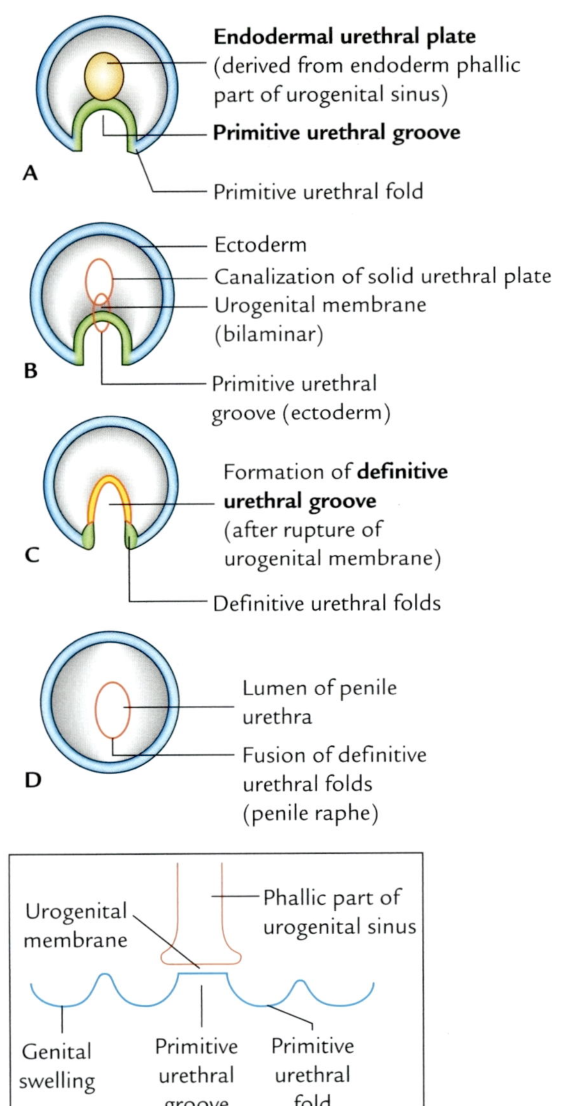

Fig. 25.19 Stages in the development of penile urethra in the body of penis (as seen in cross-sections of the body of phallus). The inset shows relationship of phallic part of urogenital sinus and primitive urethral groove.

(**primitive penis**). The enlargement of phallus forms the **penis**.

1. **Development of penile urethra:** As the phallus elongates, it pulls the primitive urethral folds forward under it. With extension of primitive urethral folds on the undersurface of phallus, the **primitive urethral groove** also extends on the undersurface of phallus, up to the tip of phallus (primordia of the glans penis). Concurrently, the phallic part of the urogenital sinus also extends up to base of the developing glans penis.

   The endodermal epithelial lining of the phallic part of the urogenital sinus proliferates to form **urethral plate** (Fig. 25.19A).

   The solid urethral plate gets canalized to form hollow tube. The bilaminar urogenital membrane separates the newly formed endodermal tube from the **primitive urethral groove**. Now the urogenital membrane breaks to form the **definitive urethral groove** flanked by the **definitive urethral folds**. At the end of 3rd month, the two definitive urethral folds fuse in craniocaudal direction to form **penile urethra** up to the base of the glans. The surface ectoderm fuses in the median plane of penis to form the **penile raphe**.

   The **spongy part of penile urethra** thus formed extends only up to the base of the glans.

   During the 4th month, the ectodermal cells from the tip of glans penis **penetrate inward** and form a short solid ectodermal epithelial cord. The cord canalizes and forms **terminal part of the urethra** and **external urethral meatus** (Fig. 25.20).

2. **Development of prepuce of the penis** (Fig. 25.21): Close to the tip of the phallus (primitive penis), a circular sulcus (**coronary sulcus**) appears, which separates

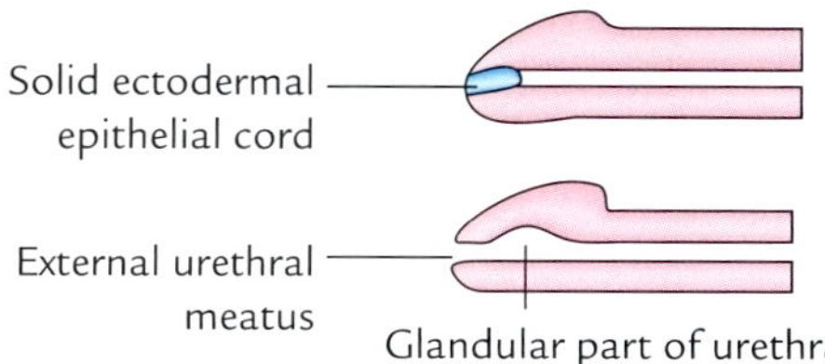

Fig. 25.20 Development of penile urethra in the glans penis.

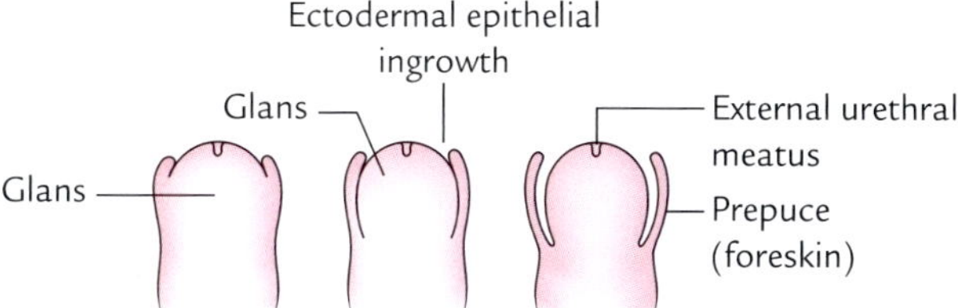

Fig. 25.21 Development of the prepuce of the penis.

the glans penis from rest of the penis. The surface ectoderm covering the glans proliferates and grows inward forming double-layered fold of ectoderm. Later, these two layers of ectoderm separate from each other to form the *prepuce*. The prepuce is retractable fold of skin that can slide over the surface of the glans penis.

3. **Development of scrotum:** After fusion of the definitive urethral folds, the two genital swellings enlarge to form **scrotal swellings**. They move medially and fuse with each other to form the scrotum. The scrotum thus lies below root of the penis. Each scrotal swelling forms half of the scrotum. The two halves of scrotum are separated from each other by **scrotal septum**. The line of fusion of these folds in the midline forms **scrotal raphe**.

CLINICAL CORRELATION

1. *Congenital anomalies of urethra*
   (a) **Hypospadias:** It is the **most common congenital anomaly of the urethra** (occurring in 3–5/100 births). In this condition, external urethral orifice (EUO) is located on ventral aspect of penis, instead of at the tip of the penis. It occurs due to failure of canalization of the ectodermal cord in the glans and/or failure of fusion of the urethral folds. Usually the penis is underdeveloped and curved ventrally, producing a clinical condition called **chordae**.

   Types of hypospadias (Fig. 25.22): Depending on the location of EUO, the hypospadias is classified into the following five types.
   (i) *Glandular:* When the EUO is located on the ventral aspect of the glans (it is the least severe form)
   (ii) *Coronal/balanic:* When urethra opens at the base of glans penis (in this case, the glans is often grooved on its ventral aspect)

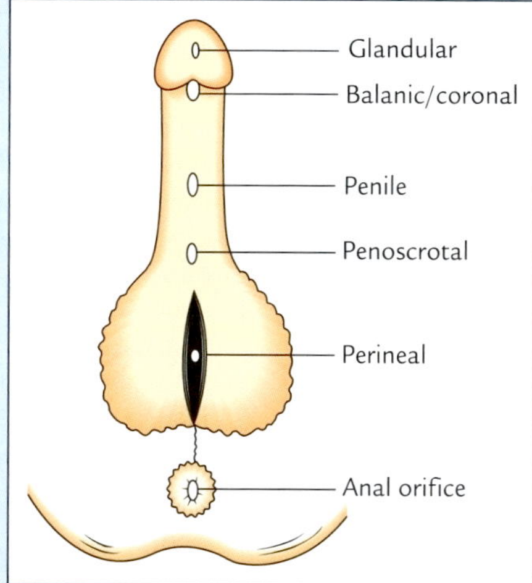

Fig. 25.22 Hypospadias. Note its various types according to the location of urethral orifice.

   (iii) *Penile:* When urethra opens anywhere between the base of the glans and in front of the scrotum
   (iv) *Penoscrotal:* When urethra opens at junction of the penis and scrotum
   (v) *Perineal:* When a wide sagittal slit is found along entire length of the penis and scrotum (the two scrotal swellings closely resemble labia majora; it is the **most severe form**)

N.B.

The chordae (downward curved/bent penis) is often seen in hypospadias.

The hypospadias occurs due to inadequate production of androgens by fetal testes.

The incidence of hypospadias has doubled in the last 15–20 years probably due to rise in environmental estrogens.

   (b) **Epispadias:** In this condition, the urethral orifice is located on the dorsal aspect of the penis. It is a rare anomaly and occurs in 1/30,000 births. Although epispadias may occur as an isolated defect, it is mostly associated with exstrophy of the urinary bladder (ectopia vesicae). The exact embryological basis for this condition is not clear. Probably it occurs when genital tubercle, instead of being formed cranial to the cloacal membrane, is formed more dorsally in the region of urorectal septum, and thus part of the urogenital membrane is seen cranial to the genital tubercle. When this membrane ruptures, the urogenital sinus opens on the dorsal aspect of the penis and then the urethral groove extends on the dorsal aspect of the penis.

2. *Congenital anomalies of penis*
   (a) **Agenesis of penis (absence of penis):** It occurs when the genital tubercle fails to develop.
   (b) **Micropenis (very small penis):** It occurs due to underdevelopment of the genital tubercle.
   (c) **Bifid penis and double penis:** The bifid penis occurs when the genital tubercle splits. The double penis is formed when the two genital tubercles develop.

3. *Congenital anomalies of prepuce (foreskin)*
   (a) **Phimosis:** The prepuce is a fold of skin covering the glans of penis. It develops during 12th week of IUL. It remains adherent to the glans up to 3 years of age and is not easy to retract. Thereafter, it separates progressively from glans and is nonadherent by 6 years of age. The phimosis is a condition in which prepuce is so tight that it cannot be retracted fully from glans. It is usually congenital and is often associated with *pinhole meatus*.

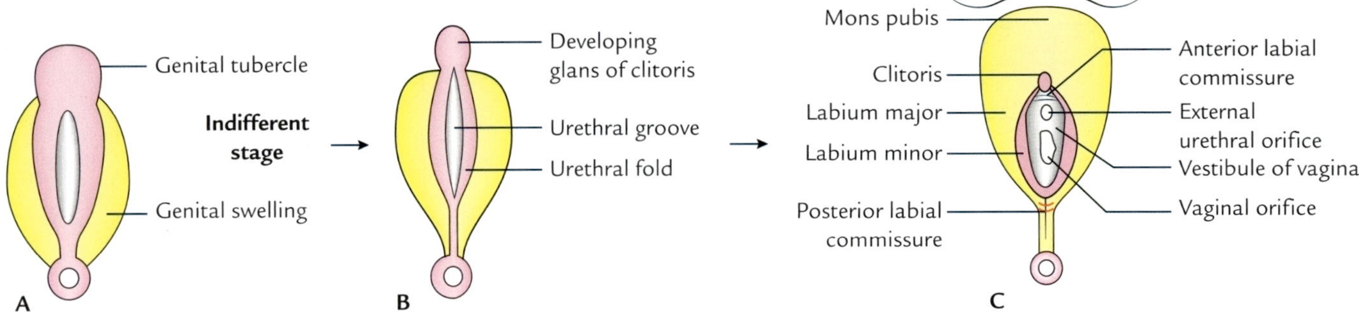

Fig. 25.23 Development of female external genitalia.

Development of Female External Genitalia (Fig. 25.23)

The female external genital organs develop from the indifferent stage of external genitalia due to influence of estrogens (derived from maternal and paternal sources). The estrogen stimulates the development of external genitalia of female. The changes are less extensive in the indifferent external genitalia than those in the males. The female external genital organs develop as follows:

1. The genital tubercle elongates only slightly to form small phallus, which bends to from **clitoris. The clitoris does not contain urethra.**
2. The **primitive urethral folds** do not fuse and form the **labia minora.**
3. The **genital swellings** now enlarge to form the **labia majora.** The labia majora fuses with each other posterior to the urogenital membrane but anterior to the anal membrane to form **posterior labial commissure.** It also fuses anteriorly to form **mons pubis** and **anterior labial commissure.** The labia majora overlaps the labia minora.
4. The urogenital membrane ruptures so that the phallic part of urogenital sinus forms the **vestibule of vagina,** which has openings of the urethra and vagina and communicates to the exterior (Fig. 25.24).

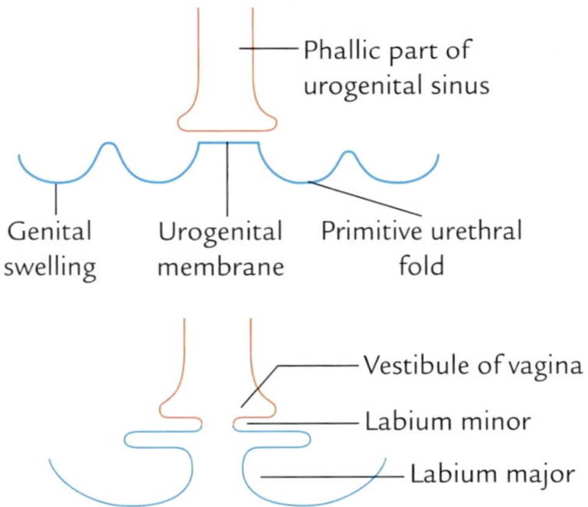

Fig. 25.24 Development of the vestibule of vagina, and labia minora and majora. Note that endoderm is shown in red color and ectoderm in blue color.

N.B. Although genital tubercle does not elongate extensively in female, it is larger than that in male during early stages of the development.

The labia minora has outer ectodermal and inner endodermal lining.

CLINICAL CORRELATION

1. ***Klinefelter syndrome*** (Fig. 25.25): It is the most common major abnormality of sexual differentiation occurring in 1/500 births. It is a trisomic condition found only in males with a karyotype of 47XXY. The most common cause is nondisjunction of XX homologues. The characteristic clinical features are as follows:
   - Hypogonadism associated with testicular atrophy
   - Infertility
   - Gynecomastia
   - Eunuchoid habitus
   - Elevated gonadotropin levels
   - Poorly developed secondary sexual characters

   For details, see Chapter 29.
2. ***Hermaphrodites:*** The sexual development of males and females begins in an identical fashion. Hence, it is not surprising that abnormalities in sex differentiation and sex determination may occur.
   (a) **True hermaphrodites:** The *true hermaphroditism* is an extremely rare condition in which both testes and ovaries are present (usually combined as ovotestes) and the external genitalia are ambiguous (neither completely male nor completely female).

   The testes and ovaries are usually nonfunctional. The chromosomal sex is usually female (80%) with 46XX karyotype.

   The uterus is present but the external genitalia are ambiguous or predominantly female. Most of these individuals are brought up as females.

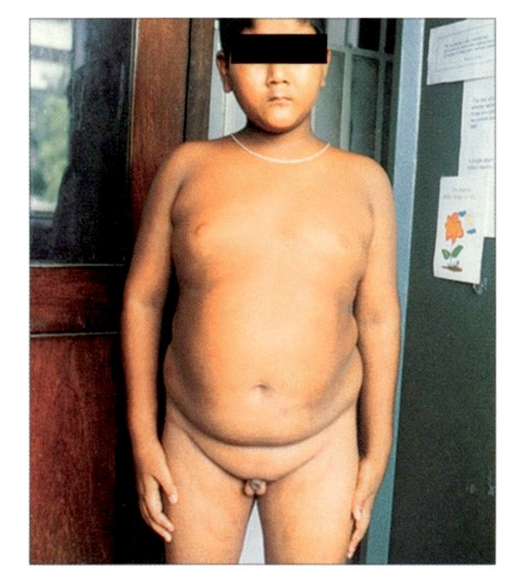

Fig. 25.25 Klinefelter syndrome.

(b) **Pseudohermaphrodites:** These are individuals in whom *genotypic sex* is masked by *phenotypic appearance*, which closely resembles the other sex.

If a pseudohermaphrodite has a testis, the individual is called *male pseudohermaphrodite* and if a pseudohermaphrodite has an ovary, the individual is called *female pseudohermaphrodite*. The differences between male and female pseudohermaphrodites are given in Table 25.3.

3. ***Androgen insensitivity syndrome (AIS):*** It is a clinical condition in which affected individual is phenotypically female (i.e., normal-appearing female) despite the presence of testes and 46XY chromosome complement. It is also called **testicular feminization syndrome**. It occurs in 1/20,000 births due to a defect in androgen receptor mechanism.

   Characteristic clinical features are as follows:
   - Normal-appearing female
   - Normal female external genitalia
   - Normal development of breasts at puberty
   - Vagina short and usually ending in a blind pouch
   - Uterus and uterine tubes absent or rudimentary
   - Absence of menstruation
   - Psychosexual orientation of women
   - Testes in inguinal canal

N.B.
- Socially, mentally, and psychologically, the women with AIS are entirely female.
- Embryologically, these females represent an extreme form of male pseudohermaphroditism.

Table 25.3 Differences between male and female pseudohermaphrodites

	Male Pseudohermaphrodite	Female Pseudohermaphrodite
Gonads	Testes	Ovaries
Chromosome complement	46XY	46XX
External genitalia	Resemble those of female • Phallus remains rudimentary and looks like clitoris • Scrotal swellings fail to fuse, giving an appearance of labia majora	Resemble those of male • Excessive enlargement of clitoris resembling penis • Partial fusion of labia majora, giving an appearance of a scrotum
Most common cause	Lack of androgen receptors (hence, androgens produced by fetal testes are ineffective in inducing differentiation of male genitalia)	Congenital adrenal hyperplasia with excessive production of androgens; masculinizes external genitals

DESCENT OF TESTES AND OVARIES

Descent of Testis (Fig. 25.26)

The testis develops within abdomen on its posterior wall in upper lumbar region. From here, it descends to lie outside the abdomen into the scrotum at or just after birth. The various stages of the descent of testis are given in Table 25.4.

Factors Responsible for Descent of Testis

These are the following:

1. Differential growth of the posterior abdominal wall.
2. **Formation of inguinal bursa:** The various layers of anterior abdominal wall form an outpouching toward the scrotum called **inguinal bursa**. The cavity of inguinal bursa forms the *inguinal canal*. Note that inguinal bursa is formed before the testis enters into it.

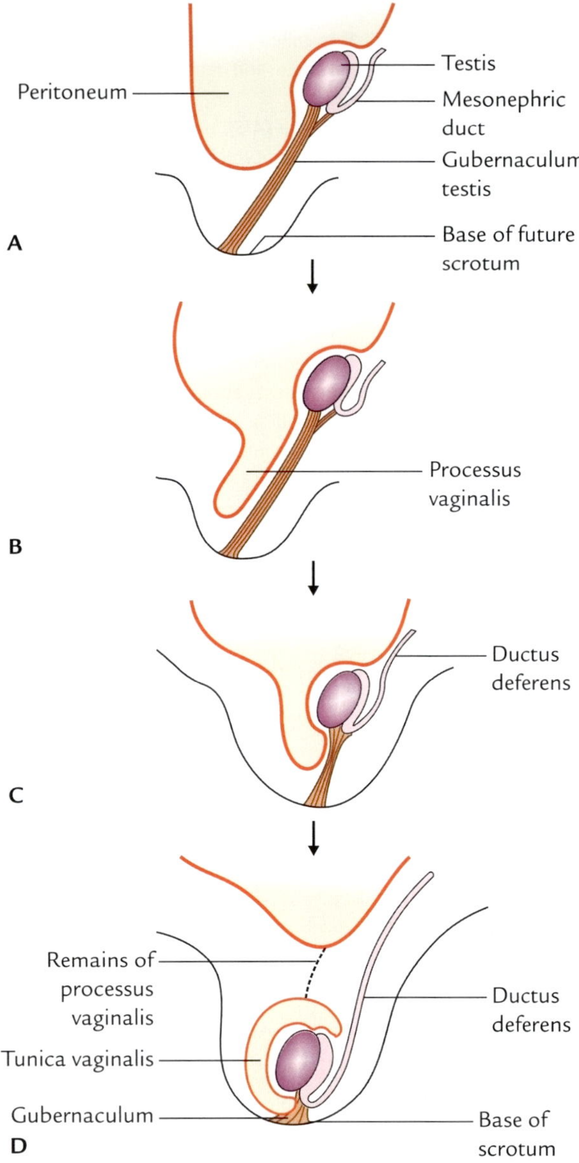

Fig. 25.26 Descent of testis.

Table 25.4 Stages of descent of testis (Fig. 25.26)

Extent of Descent	Time
Testis reaches iliac fossa	During 3rd month
Reaches deep inguinal ring	At the end of 6th month
Travels through inguinal canal	During 7th month
Reaches superficial inguinal ring	At 8th month
Reaches scrotum	By end of 9th month

3. **Gubernaculum testis:** It is a mesenchymal band extending from lower pole of the testis to bottom of the scrotum. It helps to dilate inguinal bursa and lays down the path for the descent of testis.

   During growth of the posterior abdominal wall, there is no corresponding increase in length of gubernaculum. Due to relative shortening of gubernaculum, the testis progressively assumes a lower position.
4. **Processus vaginalis:** It is a diverticulum of peritoneal cavity that grows into the inguinal canal and scrotum. As the testis descends into the scrotum, it invaginates processus vaginalis from behind. Once the descent of testis is completed, the part of processus vaginalis between the testis and the deep inguinal ring is obliterated. The part of processus vaginalis that covers the testis is now known as **tunica vaginalis of testis.**
5. **Increased intra-abdominal pressure** helps to push the testis out of abdomen.
6. **Male sex hormones** greatly influence the descent of testis.
7. A specific neurotransmitter called calcitonin gene–related peptide is secreted by genitofemoral nerve supplying muscle fiber of the gubernaculum testis.

N.B. When testis descends into scrotum from the posterior abdominal wall, it carries vas deferens and blood vessels along with it. This provides an embryological basis of "*crossing of vas deferens anterior to ureter near the urinary bladder.*"

CLINICAL CORRELATION

1. ***Cryptorchidism (undescended testis):*** It is a clinical condition in which one or both the testes may fail to descend from the abdomen into the scrotum.
   - In about 97% of newborns, the testes are present in the scrotum before birth; in remaining cases, the descent occurs postnatally during the first 3 months.
   - In less than 1% of infants, one or both testes fail to descend.
   - The cryptorchidism may occur due to decreased androgen (testosterone) production.
   - The testes may become arrested at any point during their journey from the upper lumbar region of abdominal cavity to the scrotum.

   Depending on their location, the cryptorchidism is classified into five types (Fig. 25.27; Table 25.5).

N.B. The term cryptorchidism means hidden testis.

Clinical significance of cryptorchidism

- The undescended testes fail to produce mature spermatozoa due to higher abdominal temperature. In bilateral cryptorchidism, the individual is sterile.
- The undescended testes are susceptible to injury.
- The undescended testes are likely to develop malignancy.
- The undescended testes are likely to atrophy.

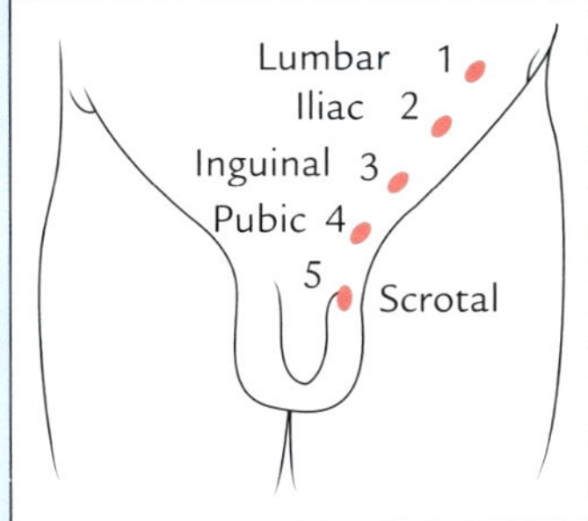

Fig. 25.27 Location of testis in cryptorchidism.

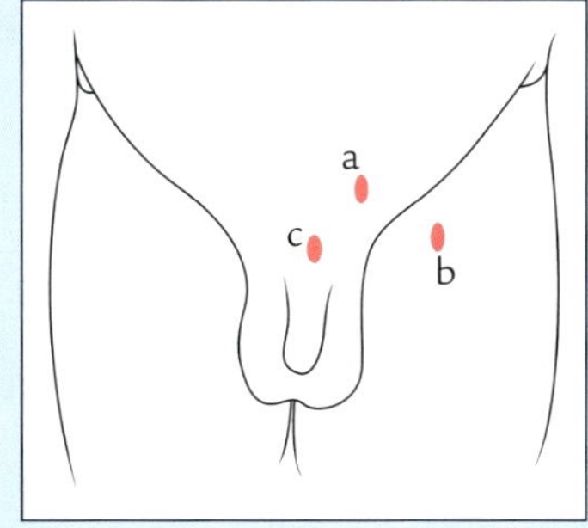

Fig. 25.28 Ectopic testis. a = superficial fascia; b = thigh; c = root of penis.

Table 25.5 Types of cryptorchidism according to location

Type	Location
1. Lumbar	Lumbar region of abdomen
2. Iliac	At deep inguinal ring
3. Inguinal	Within inguinal canal
4. Pubic	At superficial inguinal ring
5. Scrotal	High up in the scrotum

Table 25.6 Type of congenital hydroceles

Types of Hydrocele	Feature
Vaginal	Confined to scrotum
Congenital	Extends upward into the peritoneal cavity
Infantile/infundibular	Extends upward up to the deep inguinal ring
Hydrocele of cord	Confined only in the spermatic cord

N.B. In case of cryptorchidism, testicular hormones are used to promote the descent. If it fails, the testes are surgically mobilized and fixed to the scrotal floor (**orchidopexy**).

2. ***Ectopic testis*** (Fig. 25.28): It is a clinical condition in which the testis is located in an aberrant position off the normal path of its descent, i.e., present elsewhere away from expected path of descent. The sites of ectopic testis are as follows:
   (a) **In superficial fascia of the anterior abdominal wall (interstitial type**; it is the most common site of ectopic testis)
   (b) **Anteromedial aspect of thigh (in the region of femoral triangle)**
   (c) **At the root of penis**
   (d) **In the perineum, i.e. behind scrotum** (not shown in figure)

N.B. The ectopic testis occurs due to **hypothetic bands of Lockwood** (fibrous bands extending from the lower pole of testis to the ectopic sites).

3. ***Congenital indirect inguinal hernia:*** The processus vaginalis (diverticulum of peritoneal cavity) forms a communicating channel between the peritoneal cavity within the abdomen and the tunica vaginalis within the scrotum. Normally, it obliterates by the 1st year of life.

   If the processus vaginalis fails to obliterate and remains open, the loops of intestine may descend through it into the scrotum causing **congenital indirect inguinal hernia**. Clinically it presents as sac-like bulge in inguinoscrotal region in boys or in inguinolabial region in girls.

4. ***Congenital hydrocele (intermittent hydrocele):*** Hydrocele is accumulation of fluid in the peritoneal sac within the scrotum and/or inguinal canal. It occurs due to **incomplete obliteration of the processes vaginalis** providing a tiny communication between the peritoneal cavity and the tunica vaginalis, which permits the escape of fluid but not entry of intestine into the sac.

   Clinically it presents as swollen scrotum.

   The **various types of hydroceles** (Fig. 25.29) are given in Table 25.6.

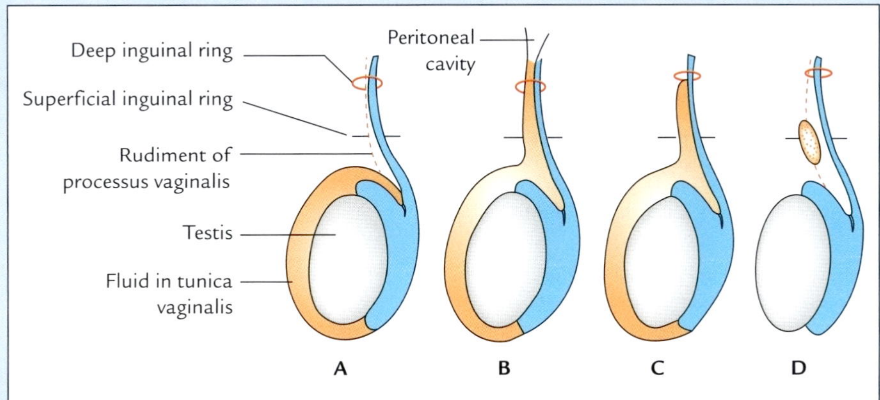

Fig. 25.29 Types of hydroceles. (A) Vaginal. (B) Congenital. (C) Infundibular. (D) Hydrocele of cord.

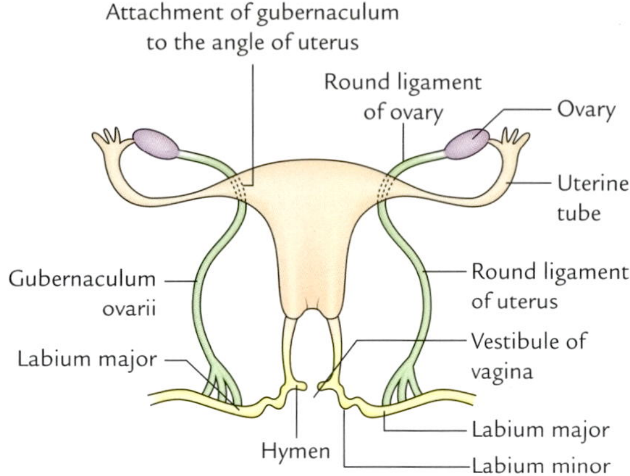

Fig. 25.30 Descent of ovary.

Descent of Ovary (Fig. 25.30)

The ovary develops on the posterior abdominal wall in the upper lumbar region. From here, it descends into the true pelvis, where it lies on its lateral wall in a fossa called **ovarian fossa**.

The caudal end of ovary is attached to the genital swelling (primordium of labium majus) by a fibromuscular band called **gubernaculum ovarii**. It is believed that the descent of ovary occurs due to pull of the gubernaculum. Its descent is arrested at the pelvis due to development of the uterus and broad ligament. This is because the gubernaculum gets attached to angle of the developing uterus. As a result, it gets divided into two parts: proximal and distal. The proximal part of gubernaculum drags the ovary into the pelvic cavity and becomes the **ligament of ovary**. The distal part of the gubernaculum becomes **round ligament of the uterus**. The round ligaments of uterus pass through the inguinal canal and terminate in the labium major.

During the descent of the ovary, a tubular prolongation of peritoneum, the **processus vaginalis** (also called **canal of Nuck**), extends into the inguinal canal along the gubernaculum. The processus vaginalis (canal of Nuck) usually obliterates and disappears much before birth.

N.B. The **ovaries mostly do not descend through inguinal canal** but if the gubernaculum of ovary fails to attach to angle of the uterus, the ovary may be present in the inguinal canal or in the labium, although it is very rare.

CLINICAL CORRELATION

- If the processus vaginalis (**canal of Nuck**) persists after birth, it may **cause congenital inguinal hernia in female.**

The embryonic structures, their adult derivatives, and homologies in male and female are given in Table 25.7.

Table 25.7 Embryonic structures and their homologous adult derivatives in males and females

Embryonic Structure	Adult Derivatives	
	In Males	**In Females**
1. Indifferent gonad (a) Primordial germ cells (b) Surface epithelium of gonad (c) Mesenchyme	• Testis • Spermatogonia • Sertoli cells/supporting cells • Leydig cells (interstitial cells)	• Ovary • Oogonia • Follicular cells • Theca cells (forming theca interna and externa)
2. Gubernaculum	Gubernaculum testis	• Round ligament of ovary • Round ligament of uterus
3. Mesonephric tubules (a) Cranial tubules (b) Caudal tubules	 • Efferent ductules • Paradidymis	 • Epoophoron • Paroophoron
4. Mesonephric duct	• Duct of epididymis • Vas deferens • Seminal vesicle • Ejaculatory duct	Gartner's duct
5. Paramesonephric duct	• Appendix of testis • Prostatic utricle	• Uterine tubes • Uterus • Cervix • Upper part of vagina

Table 25.7 Embryonic structures and their homologous adult derivatives in males and females—cont'd

Embryonic Structure	Adult Derivatives	
	In Males	**In Females**
6. Urogenital sinus	• Urinary bladder • Urethra (prostatic membranous and penile) • Prostate gland • Bulbourethral glands	• Urinary bladder • Urethra (membranous) and vestibule of vagina • Paraurethral glands (of Skene) • Greater vestibular glands
7. Müllerian tubercle	Seminal colliculus (verumon-tanum)	Hymen
8. Genital tubercle	Penis	Clitoris
9. Urethral folds	Penile urethra	Labia minora
10. Genital swellings	Scrotum	Labia majora

GESTATIONAL AGE OF KEY DEVELOPMENTAL EVENTS

Developmental Event	Time of Occurrence
➢ Genital system begins to develop during	4th week
➢ Gonads differentiate morphologically into male and female type by	7th week
➢ Morphological differentiation of male and female external genitalia is possible by the end of	12th week
➢ Testis begins its migration from abdominal cavity to scrotum around	2nd month
➢ Least common location of testis in cryptorchidism	Abdomen

GOLDEN FACTS TO REMEMBER

➢ **Master gene for development of testes**	*SRY* gene on short arm of chromosome "Y"
➢ **Commonest congenital anomaly of the urethra**	Hypospadias
➢ **Most common type of hypospadias**	Glandular type (urethra opens on the undersurface of the glans)
➢ **True hermaphrodite**	Individual with both testes and ovaries or ovotestes
➢ **Extreme form of male pseudohermaphroditism**	Complete androgen insensitivity syndrome
➢ **Pseudohermaphrodite**	Individual with gonads of one sex and external genitalia of other sex
➢ **Commonest site of ectopic testis**	Superficial fascia of anterior abdominal wall (interstitial type)
➢ **Canal of Nuck**	Persistence of processus vaginalis in female
➢ **Organ of Rosenmüller**	Remnant of mesonephric tubules
➢ **Gartner's duct**	Mesonephric duct in female

CLINICAL PROBLEM SOLVING

PROBLEMS

1. **There is enormous variation in sperm counts between individual men, whether fertile or infertile. Give the embryological basis.**
2. The **antenatal sex determination during 3rd and 4th months of gestation by ultrasonography is often misleading** (i.e., gives false results). **Give the embryological basis.**
3. During physical examination of a male infant, the pediatrician noted **presence of urethral orifice on the ventral aspect of shaft of the penis**. He also noted that the glans was curved ventrally. What is the most likely diagnosis? Give its embryological basis.
4. A mother brought her 1.5-year-old boy to OPD and complained to the doctor on duty that few days ago she noticed a lump in groin of her child. After a thorough physical examination, the boy was diagnosed as a case of **congenital indirect inguinal hernia**.

   Give the embryological basis of congenital indirect inguinal hernia and mention whether or not congenital indirect inguinal hernia can occur in females.
5. A 19-year-old girl was disqualified to take part in the Olympic Games because her buccal smear test was sex chromatin negative. On the basis of your embryological knowledge, tell whether she is male or female and provide the genetic basis for her failing to pass the sex chromatin test.

SOLUTIONS

1. The supporting **Sertoli cells** of testis develop from the surface epithelium of early gonad. They proliferate throughout antenatal development and may do so up to childhood. Then they stop proliferating. Once they stop proliferating, they cannot be activated. Each Sertoli cell can support only a fixed number of germ cells during their development into spermatozoa, i.e., the number of Sertoli cells determines the maximum limit of sperm output.

   Therefore, the **variation in the Sertoli cell number is probably the most important factor in accounting for the enormous variation in sperm counts between individual men.**
2. The genital tubercle elongates extensively in males to form penis, whereas it does not elongate much in females and forms clitoris.

   During early stages of development (3–4 months of gestation), the rate of growth of genital tubercle is same in both males and females, and often larger in females than that in males. Therefore, using length of the genital tubercle as a criterion (as monitored by an ultrasound) for sex determination is often misleading.
3. The most likely diagnosis is **hypospadias**. The hypospadias is a clinical condition in which the urethral orifice is located on the ventral aspect of the penis instead of the tip of the glans penis. For details, see Clinical Correlation on p. 301.
4. The **indirect inguinal hernia** is herniation of a loop of intestine into the inguinal canal through deep inguinal ring.

   The embryological basis of indirect inguinal hernia is persistence of the processus vaginalis (for details, see p. 305).

   Since the **processus vaginalis** also forms in females, the persistent processus vaginalis in female is called the **canal of Nuck**, into which abdominal contents may herniate. Hence, congenital inguinal hernia can also occur in females, although it is rare as compared with males.
5. Phenotypically this girl is entirely female but genetically she is male. Such an individual is an example of extreme form of **male pseudohermaphroditism**. This girl had 46XY chromosome complement; hence, cells of her buccal smear are sex chromatin negative. For this reason, she could not pass her **sex chromatin** test.

26 Development of Nervous System: Spinal Cord and Brain

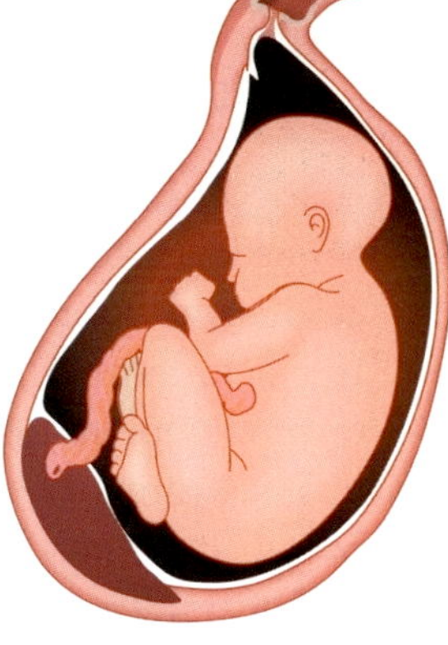

LEARNING OBJECTIVES

After studying this chapter, the student should be able to:

- Describe the development of neural tube and spinal cord. AN 64.2
- Describe the process of **neurulation** and give the embryological basis of **neural tube defects** with emphasis on **open neural tube defects.** AN 79.3, AN 64.3, AN 79.5
- Describe the development of brain, viz., medulla oblongata, pons, cerebellum, midbrain, and cerebral hemispheres. AN 64.2
- Describe the development of neural crest cells in brief. Give structures derived from them.
- Discuss the formation of brain vesicles from neural tube and enumerate the various parts of brain derived from these vesicles.
- Write short notes on (a) ventricular system of brain, (b) positional changes of spinal cord, and (c) hydrocephalus.

OVERVIEW

Study of development of the nervous system helps to understand its complex organization and occurrence of various congenital anomalies.

The nervous system develops from ectoderm following induction from notochord.

The specific cell population of early ectoderm, which gives rise to entire nervous system and special sense organs, is termed **neural ectoderm**. The neural ectoderm later differentiates into two structures: **neural tube** and **neural crest cells. The neural tube gives rise to the central nervous system (CNS)** while **neural crest cells** form nearly entire **peripheral nervous system.**

NEURULATION (FORMATION OF NEURAL TUBE) (FIG. 26.1) AN 64.2

It involves the formation of **neural plate** from ectoderm above notochord and folding of neural plate to form **neural tube.**

In early embryonic disc, at about 16th day of embryonic life, the ectoderm overlying the newly formed notochord thickens in midline forming **neural plate**. Initially the neural plate is flat and slipper shaped with narrow end toward the primitive node. The somatic mesoderm develops on either side of the notochord. The margins of neural plate are elevated as **neural folds**. As a result, center of the plate sinks, creating **neural groove**. The neural folds gradually move together

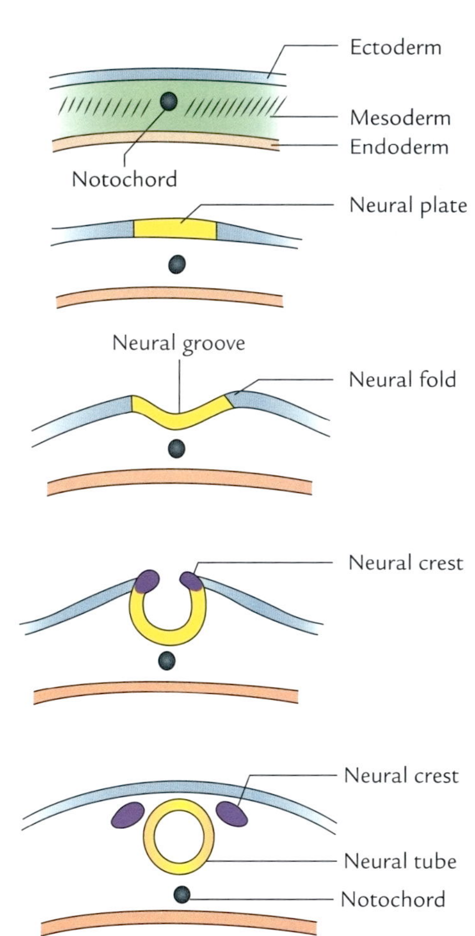

Fig. 26.1 Formation of neural tube and neural crest.

toward the midline and finally fuse to form a cylindrical **neural tube** that loses its connection with the surface ectoderm. The process of neural tube formation is termed **neurulation.**

The fusion of neural folds begins in the middle (region of fourth somite on 20th day of embryonic development) and it simultaneously proceeds in the cephalic and caudal directions. The fusion at the cranial and caudal ends of neural tube is somewhat delayed, forming small openings called **anterior** and **posterior neuropores**. The neural tube and overlying amniotic cavity, therefore, remain temporarily in open communication with each other through these pores. The anterior neuropore closes earlier, in the middle of the 4th week at 18- to 20-somite stage (i.e., on 25th day), and the posterior neuropore closes later at the end of 4th week at about 25-somite stage (i.e., on 27th day). By the time the neural tube is completely closed, it is divided into an enlarged cranial part and an elongated caudal part, which later on give rise to the **brain** and **spinal cord**, respectively.

Secondary Neurulation

The secondary neurulation forms the caudal part of spinal cord distal to S2 spinal segment and the filum terminale.

The **secondary neurulation begins on day 27**, in tissue located within caudal cell mass (representing **Hensen's node**) present caudal to the posterior neuropores at the caudal end of embryo.

First, small tubules form within this tissue (caudal cell mass) which coalesce to form **secondary neural tube.** The secondary neural tube eventually fuse with the neural tube (vide supra).

FORMATION OF NEURAL CREST CELLS

As the neural folds come together and fuse, cells at the tips of neural folds break away from the neuroectoderm to form the neural crest cells. The surface ectoderm of one side becomes continuous with the surface ectoderm of opposite side over the neural tube.

Thus, cells at the tips of neural folds (**neural crest cells**) do not participate in the neural tube formation. The neural crest cells at first remain in the midline between the dorsal surface of the neural tube and the surface ectoderm, and then form two-cell clusters dorsolaterally, one on either side of the neural tube.

The neural crest cells differentiate to form cells of dorsal root ganglia, sensory ganglia of cranial nerves, autonomic ganglia, adrenal medulla, chromaffin tissue, melanocytes, and Schwann cells (Fig. 26.2).

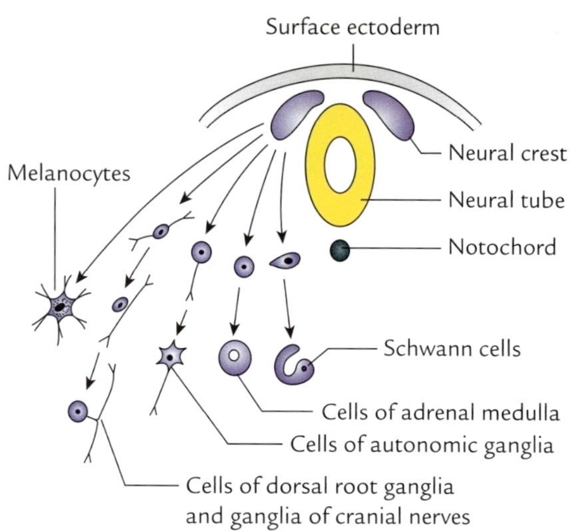

Fig. 26.2 Structures derived from neural crest cells (differentiation of neural crest cells).

CLINICAL CORRELATION AN 64.3

Neural tube defects (NTDs)

These are defects of CNS which occur in 1st month of pregnancy when neural tube fails to close.

The causes of NTDs are multifactorial. The vitamin B_6 (folic acid) can reduce the occurrence of NTDs by more than 70% if given during pregnancy.

Two most common neural tube defects are **anencephaly** (defect of brain) and **spina bifida** (defects of spinal cord).

1. ***Anencephaly (craniorachischisis):*** Failure of the cephalic part of the neural tube to close and associated defective development of the vault of the skull produces a congenital anomaly called **anencephaly** (Fig. 26.3).

   Characteristic features
   - Vault of skull is absent.
   - Brain is represented by a mass of degenerated tissue exposed to the surface.
   - Cord is open in the cervical region.
   - Appearance of child is characteristic, with prominent eyes bulging forward and chin continuous with chest due to absence of neck.
2. ***Spina bifida*** (Fig. 26.4)
   - It occurs due to nonfusion of vertebral arches posteriorly usually in the lumbosacral region.
   - Their presence is suspected by the presence of (a) abnormal tuft of hair, (b) a birth mark, or (c) protruding spinal cord tissue.

   Types: Depending on the severity, it is classified into the following four types:

   (a) **Spina bifida occulta**
   - It is the mild type of spina bifida and does not cause any disability.
   - It usually goes unnoticed.
   - Skin over the defect presents port-wine stain or tuft of hair.

   (b) **Meningocele**
   - In this, sack of leptomeninges (pia and arachnoid) → filled with Cerebrospinal fluid (CSF) protrudes through the defect.
   - Clinically it presents as a cystic swelling on baby's back.

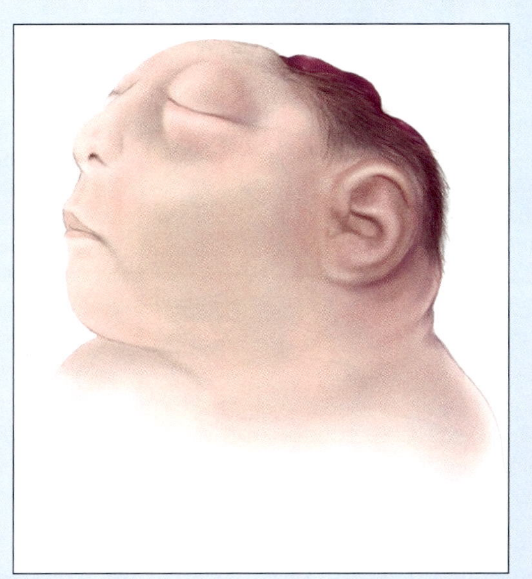

Fig. 26.3 Anencephaly. (*Source:* Functional and Clinical Neuroanatomy: A Guide for Health Care Professionals, Jahangir Moini, Pirouz Piran, Fig. 2.6, Elsevier Inc., 2020.)

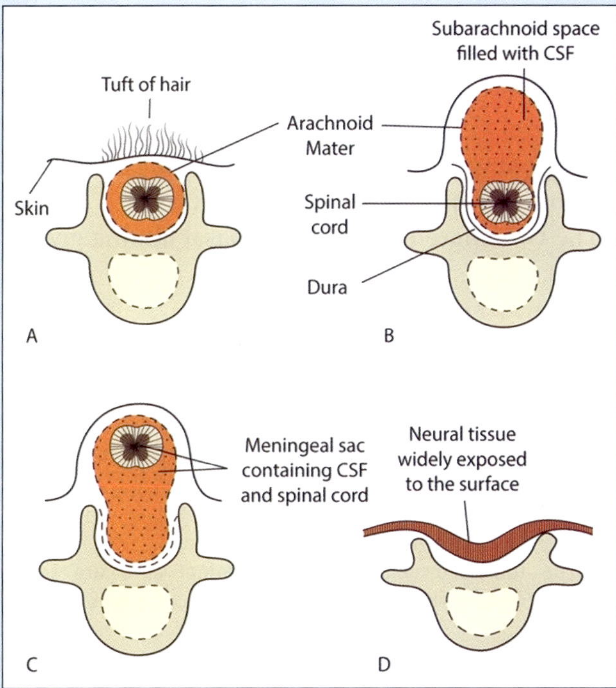

Fig. 26.4 Schematic diagrams to show types of spina bifida. (A) Spina bifida occulta. (B) Meningocele. (C) Meningomyelocele. (D) Rachischisis.

(c) **Meningomyelocele**
- In this, a large meningeal sac containing spinal cord protrudes through the gap on the lower part of baby's back which may or may not be covered by the skin.
- Clinically it presents as follows:
  - Weak or paralyzed leg muscles
  - Involvement of bowel and bladder

(d) **Myelocele (rachischisis)**
- It is the most severe form of spina bifida and often associated with anencephaly.
- Neural tissue or spinal cord is directly exposed to the surface on baby's back.
- It is incompatible with life.
- Defect involves a number of vertebrae or entire vertebral column.

N.B. **Anencephaly** and **rachischisis** are common and severe forms of congenital anomalies of CNS due to defective development of the neural tube.

DEVELOPMENT OF SPINAL CORD AN 64.2

The spinal cord develops from caudal elongated part of the neural tube. The transverse section of this tube is in the form of a dorsoventral cleft with thick lateral wall and thin roof (dorsal) and floor (ventral).

Histogenesis of Neural Tube

The neural tube increases in thickness due to repeated mitosis of its epithelial lining.

Classical Theory

According to classical theory, by the middle of 5th week of embryonic development, the transverse section of recently closed neural tube reveals **three distinct layers or zones**. From within outward, these are (a) **matrix (ependymal) zone**, (b) **mantle zone**, and (c) **marginal zone** (Fig. 26.5).

Matrix (ependymal) zone is thick and lines the enclosed cavity (neurocele). Its numerous cells undergoing mitosis produce **neuroblasts** and **spongioblasts**; the former develops into **neurons** and the latter into **neuroglial cells.**

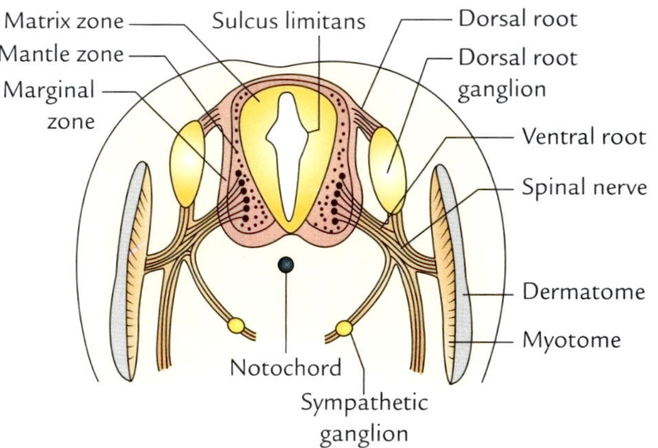

Fig. 26.5 Differentiation of the neural tube into three distinct layers/zones, and associated structures.

The neuroblasts migrate to the adjacent **mantle zone**, the future spinal gray matter; and their axons enter the external **marginal zone**, the future white matter.

Some central processes of dorsal root ganglia ascend in the marginal zone, whereas others synapse with neurons in the mantle zone.

Once histogenesis is complete, the remaining matrix cells differentiate into ependymal cells lining the central canal.

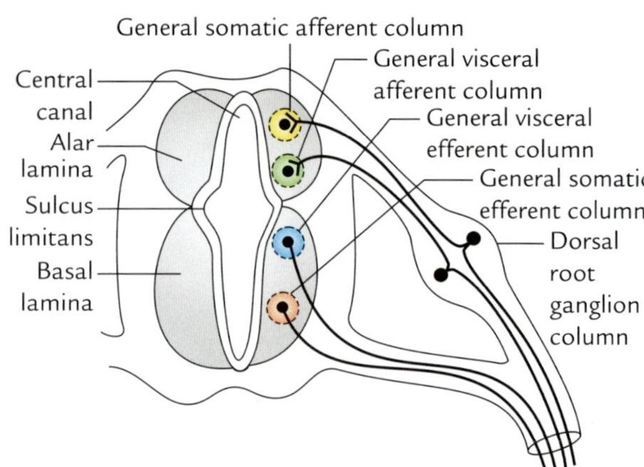

Fig. 26.6 Transverse section of the developing spinal cord showing four longitudinal cell columns.

Current Theory

Recently, on the basis of **microspectrophotometric**, **radioautographic**, and **electron microscopic observation**, the concept of classical theory is changed.

Now according to current theory, wall of recently closed neural tube consists of only one cell type – the *pluripotent neuroepithelial cells*. These cells extend over the entire thickness of the wall and form a thick pseudostratified neuroepithelium. This zonal appearance merely reflects different phases of their proliferative cycle – the sequence being termed *interkinetic migration*.

As development proceeds, these neuroepithelial cells give rise to another cell type having round nuclei *with dark-staining nucleoli called nerve cells or neuroblasts*. The neuroblasts form a zone that surrounds the neuroepithelial layer. It is known as **mantle zone.** Mantle zone later forms the gray matter of the spinal cord. The outermost layer of the spinal cord contains fibers emerging from neuroblasts in the mantle layer and is known as the *marginal layer*. Myelination of nerve fiber gives this layer a white appearance and is referred as the white matter of the spinal cord.

Development of Functional Columns

On cross-section, the cavity of neural tube appears like a vertical slit. Due to formation of vertical slit, the dorsal and ventral walls of neural tube remain thin and are called roof and floor plates, respectively. The lateral walls of neural tube get thickened. On each side, the lateral wall of neural tube is demarcated into dorsal and ventral regions by an inner longitudinal sulcus called **sulcus limitans.**

The cells of dorsal region or **alar lamina** are functionally afferent/sensory, whereas those of **basal lamina** are efferent/motor. The axons of cells of basal lamina leave the cord as ventral roots and join with peripheral processes of dorsal root ganglia to form **spinal nerves** (Fig. 26.6).

The cells of alar and basal laminae are arranged into longitudinal columns. Each lamina reveals two columns.

The **two afferent columns of alar lamina** receive axons from dorsal root ganglia:

1. **General somatic afferent column:** It extends throughout the spinal cord and receives impulses from superficial (cutaneous) and deep (proprioceptive) receptors.
2. **General visceral afferent column:** It is confined to thoracolumbar and sacral regions only and receives impulses from viscera and blood vessels.

The **two efferent columns of basal lamina** give rise to motor fibers:

1. **General visceral efferent column:** It is confined only to the thoracolumbar and sacral regions and provides preganglionic fibers (synapsing in ganglia) to viscera, glands, and blood vessels.
2. **General somatic efferent column:** It extends throughout the spinal cord and provides fibers that innervate skeletal muscles.

N.B. The four cell columns in the spinal cord are termed "general" because three additional "special" columns exist in the brainstem.

Positional Changes of the Spinal Cord (Fig. 26.7)

- **At week 8** (Fig. 26.7A), lengths of spinal cord and vertebral column are equal. The spinal cord extends along entire length of vertebral canal and the spinal nerves exit intervertebral foramina at the level of their origin.

  Due to differential growth of the cord and vertebral column, the intervertebral foramina do not remain at the level of the spinal nerves. In order to exit from corresponding intervertebral foramina due to

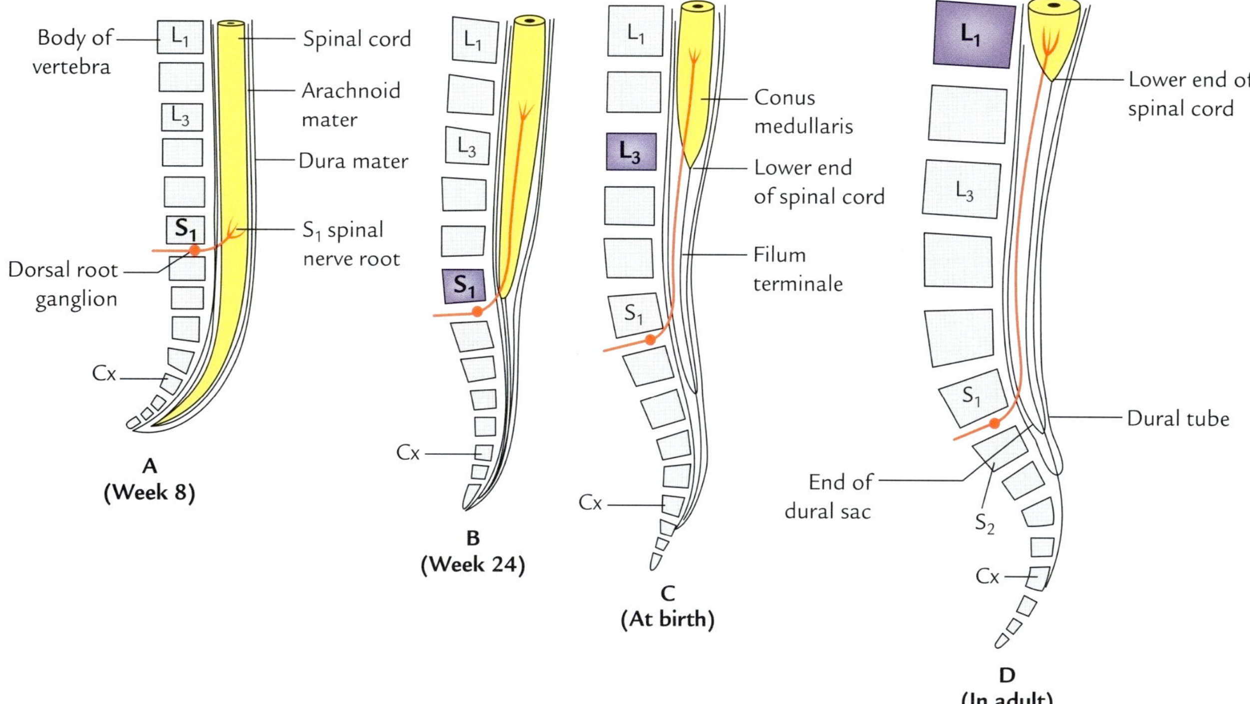

Fig. 26.7 Positional changes of spinal cord. Note the termination of spinal cord in relation to vertebral canal at various stages of development: (A) at week 8, (B) at week 24, (C) at birth, and (D) in adult. Note that lower end of spinal cord moves cranially, relative to the vertebral column.

recession of the spinal cord, the spinal nerves are forced to go down in oblique direction.

- **At week 24** (Fig. 26.7B), the lower end of spinal cord ends at S1 vertebrae.
- **At birth** (Fig. 26.7C), the lower end of spinal cord ends at the level of L3 vertebra.
- **In adults** (Fig. 26.7D), due to further recession of the cord, the lower end of spinal cord ends at the lower border of **L1 vertebra**.
- The nerve roots (i.e., lumbar, sacral, and coccygeal) that descend below the lower end of spinal cord (the **conus medullaris**) surround thin thread-like prolongation of pia mater from tip of conus medullaris (the **filum terminale**) and form **cauda equina**.

N.B. The obliquity of spinal nerves is minimum in cervical region and maximum in sacral and coccygeal regions.

DEVELOPMENT OF BRAIN AN 64.2

The brain develops from enlarged cranial part of the neural tube. At about end of 4th week, enlarged cephalic part of neural tube shows three distinct dilatations called **primary brain vesicles** (Fig. 26.8). Craniocaudally, these are (a) prosencephalon (forebrain), (b) mesencephalon (midbrain), and (c) rhombencephalon (hindbrain). Their cavities form ventricular system of adult brain. During 5th week, both prosencephalon and rhombencephalon subdivide into two vesicles, thus producing five **secondary brain vesicles.**

The **prosencephalon** gives a rostral telencephalon and caudal diencephalon (interbrain). The *telencephalon* develops lateral diverticula by evagination, which enlarge, overgrow and cover the caudal diencephalon to form cerebral hemispheres. The *diencephalon* thus becomes hidden in the lower parts of the cerebral hemispheres and forms thalamus, hypothalamus, epithalamus, etc.

The **mesencephalon** gives rise to midbrain. It does not show much changes in early part of development, except that its cavity gets progressively narrowed to form *cerebral aqueduct.*

The **rhombencephalon** divides into rostral *metencephalon*, which eventually develops into pons and cerebellum, and caudal *myelencephalon*, which gives rise to medulla oblongata.

The adult derivatives of brain vesicles are summarized in Table 26.1.

Flexures of the Brain

Primitive brain presents three flexures:

1. *Pontine flexure* at the middle of rhombencephalon
2. *Cervical flexure* at the junction of rhombencephalon and spinal cord

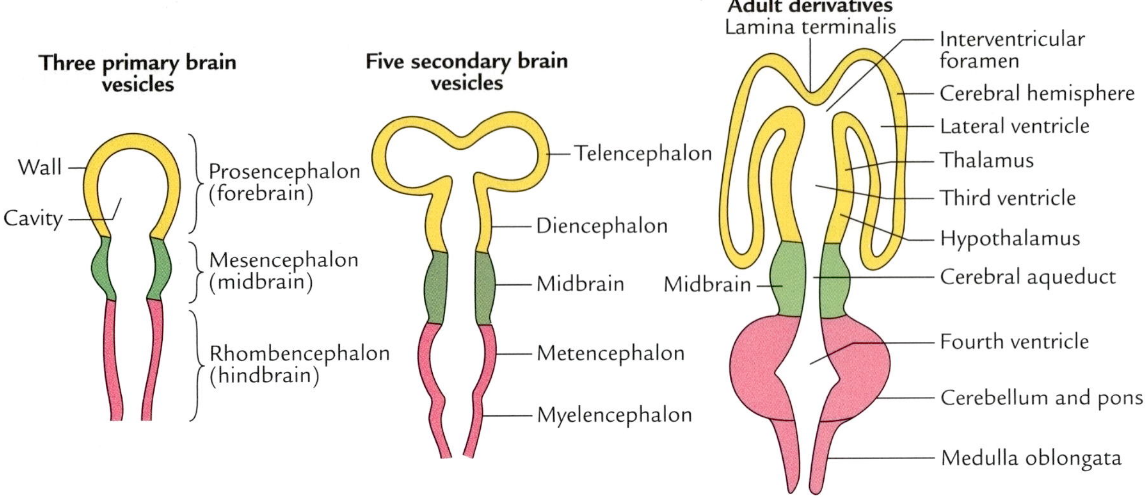

Fig. 26.8 Stages in differentiation of brain vesicles and ventricular system.

Table 26.1 Adult derivatives of brain vesicles

Primary Brain Vesicles (Three in Number)	Secondary Brain Vesicles (Five in Number)	Parts of Adult Brain	Parts of Ventricular System
Prosencephalon (forebrain)	• Telencephalon • Diencephalon	Cerebral hemispheres • Thalamus • Metathalamus • Hypothalamus • Subthalamus • Epithalamus	• Lateral ventricles • Third ventricle
Mesencephalon (midbrain)	Mesencephalon	Midbrain	Cerebral aqueduct
Rhombencephalon (hindbrain)	• Metencephalon • Myelencephalon	• Pons • Cerebellum • Medulla oblongata	Fourth ventricle

3. *Cephalic (mesencephalic) flexure* in the region of midbrain

The cephalic and cervical flexures are concave ventrally, whereas the pontine flexure exhibits a ventral convexity (Fig. 26.9).

The cervical flexure makes a 90° bend between hindbrain and spinal cord, causing the brain to be oriented almost at 90° to the spinal cord.

The brain assumes its configuration as a result of differential growth of its vesicles and flexures.

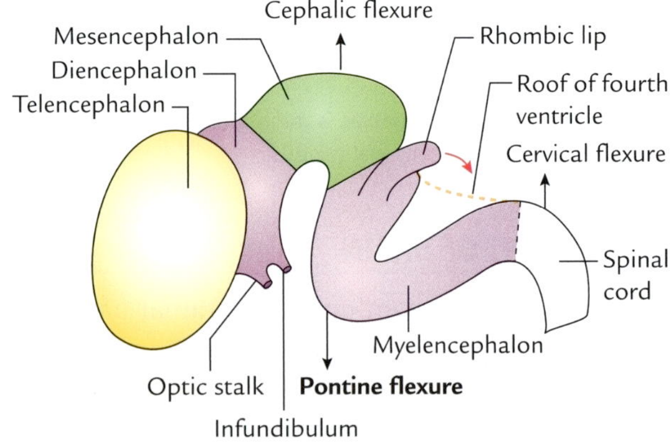

Fig. 26.9 Three flexures of the developing brain. The arrow from the rhombic lip indicates the direction of growth of the cerebellum.

Pontine Flexure

Hindbrain is folded at its middle so that it forms an acute angle ventrally. This changes shape of the tube dramatically. The cavity becomes a diamond-shaped

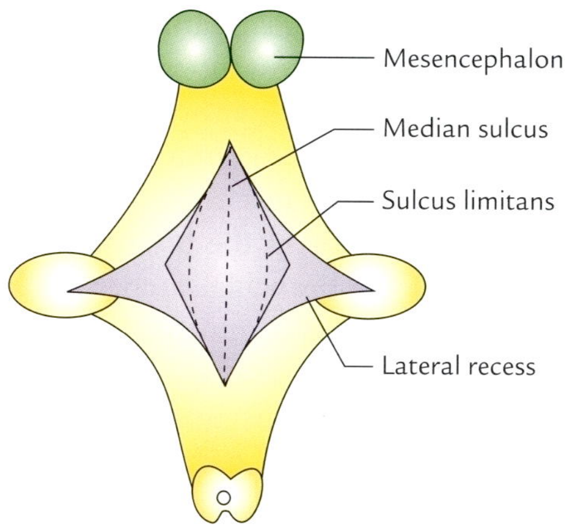

Fig. 26.10 Posterior view of developing rhombencephalon showing role of pontine flexure in the formation of fourth ventricle. Note that, opposite to the line of pontine flexure, the neural tube is flattened out. As a result, slit-like cavity of rhombencephalon becomes diamond shaped.

space called **fourth ventricle**, which is widest at line of folding (junction of two parts of the hindbrain – pons and medulla oblongata) and tapers superiorly to narrow canal of the midbrain, the aqueduct of Sylvius and inferiorly to the central canal in the lower part of medulla oblongata (Fig. 26.10). The thin roof is pulled out to cover the space posteriorly, and the line of folding extends far laterally as roof of the lateral recesses of the fourth ventricle. At tips of these recesses and inferior angle of the ventricle, the thin roof breaks down, forming apertures (lateral foramina of Luschka and median foramen of Magendie) through which the cavity of neural tube communicates with the surrounding subarachnoid space.

N.B. To understand the formation of rhomboid-shaped cavity of fourth ventricle due to pontine flexure, take a 4-inch-long piece of a rubber tube, make a vertical slit, and then bend it. This converts linear slit into a rhomboid-shaped aperture.

I have a pleasant memory of my teacher Prof. A. Halim, the most popular teacher of anatomy of his time, of bringing a rubber tube in the pocket of his white apron to demonstrate it to students.

The flattening of the hindbrain, which results from folding, displaces alar laminae so that they lie lateral to basal laminae (buckling effect). Thus, sensory nuclei, which arise from the alar laminae, are lateral to motor nuclei, which arise from the basal laminae. *For this reason, sensory cranial nerves are attached laterally and motor cranial nerves medially to the brainstem.*

The part of hindbrain caudal to the pontine flexure is called *myelencephalon* (the future medulla oblongata) and rostral part from which pons and cerebellum develop is called *metencephalon*.

Cervical Flexure

Cervical flexure is convex dorsally and appears at the junction of hindbrain and spinal cord, making a right-angled bend between them.

Cephalic Flexure

Cephalic flexure is convex dorsally and appears at the midbrain level.

N.B. The closed rostral end of the neural tube persists as a thin *lamina terminalis*.

Development of Ventricular System (Fig. 26.11)

The cavities of brain vesicles form the ventricular system of adult brain:

- The hindbrain cavity becomes the fourth ventricle.
- The narrowed mesencephalic cavity becomes the cerebral aqueduct (aqueduct of Sylvius).
- The diencephalic cavity becomes the third ventricle.
- The twin telencephalic cavities become lateral ventricles.

Thus, the brain contains four ventricles: **two lateral ventricles**, a **third ventricle**, and a **fourth ventricle**. The **two lateral ventricles** communicate with the third ventricle via interventricular **foramina (of Monro)**. The third ventricle communicates with the fourth ventricle through the cerebral aqueduct. The fourth ventricle is continuous below with central canal of the spinal cord, which presents a small dilatation at inferior end called **terminal ventricle**.

CSF is formed in the ventricles, mainly in lateral ventricles by choroid plexuses. It leaves the ventricular system through apertures in the roof of ventricle (i.e., foramen of Magendie and foramina of Luschka) into subarachnoid spaces around the brain and spinal cord.

N.B. The enlargement of brain in Dandy–Walker syndrome is limited to the posterior cranial fossa.

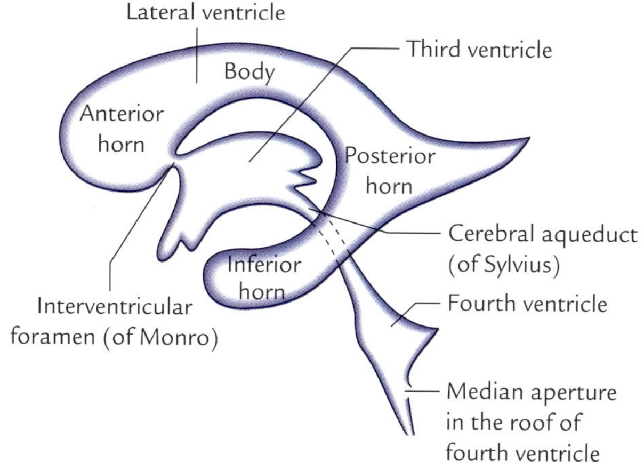

Fig. 26.11 Ventricular system of the brain.

Further development of hindbrain, midbrain, and forebrain is discussed next in brief.

CLINICAL CORRELATION

1. ***Hydrocephalus*** *(*Fig. 26.12*)***:** It is a clinical condition characterized by dilatation of ventricles due to excess accumulation of CSF within them. It occurs due to either overproduction of CSF or obstruction to its circulation. (For details, see *Textbook of Clinical Neuroanatomy* by Dr Vishram Singh.)
2. ***Dandy–Walker syndrome:*** It occurs due to atresia and blockage of apertures in the roof of fourth ventricle (e.g., foramen of Magendie and foramina of Luschka). This syndrome consists of dilatation of fourth ventricle, agenesis of cerebellar vermis, occipital meningocele, and often agenesis of splenium of corpus callosum.

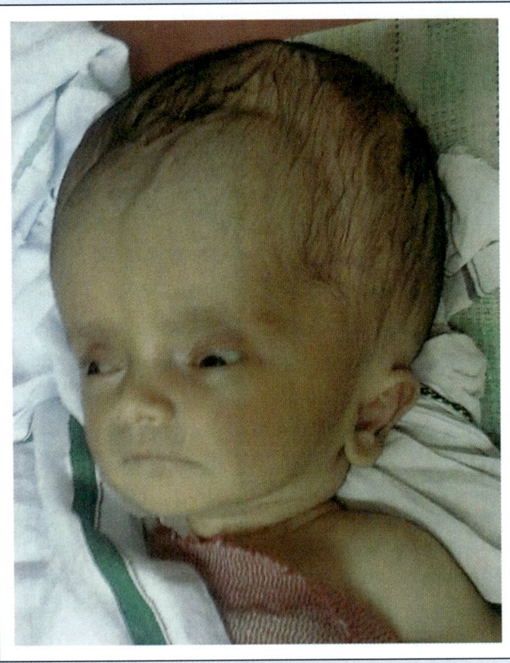

Fig. 26.12 Hydrocephalus. Note the disproportionately large size of head and typical setting-sun appearance of the eyes. (*Courtesy* of Dr Basant Kumar, Assistant Professor, Department of Pediatric Surgery, SGPGIMS, Lucknow.)

Hindbrain (Rhombencephalon)

The hindbrain consists of **medulla, pons**, and **cerebellum**. The caudal part of myelencephalon has a central canal and forms the **closed part of medulla oblongata**. Rostrally the central canal expands as the cavity of the fourth ventricle, and thus the rostral part of myelencephalon forms the open part of the medulla oblongata.

The floor of fourth ventricle is derived from myelencephalon (medulla) and metencephalon (pons). On either side of midline, the floor consists of the basal and alar laminae, which are separated from each other by a longitudinal sulcus called **sulcus limitans**. The basal and alar laminae, similar to those of spinal cord, contain motor and sensory nuclei, respectively. These nuclei are arranged into longitudinal columns. In spinal cord, as discussed earlier, each lamina contains two columns, somatic and visceral, but **in the brainstem to supply the derivatives of the branchial arches that develop around this region, a special branchial column appears between somatic and visceral columns of each lamina**. In addition, a special somatic column appears in the most lateral part of the alar lamina to receive impulses of special sensations of hearing and balance. Thus, in brainstem, the basal lamina contains three columns and alar lamina contains four columns as follows:

1. Functional column with basal lamina of brainstem
   (a) General somatic efferent
   (b) Special visceral efferent
   (c) General visceral efferent
2. Functional columns in the alar lamina of brainstem
   (a) General visceral afferent
   (b) Special visceral afferent
   (c) General somatic afferent
   (d) Special somatic afferent

Note: All motor nuclei of the brainstem are derived from functional columns of its basal plate, and all the sensory nuclei from the functional columns of the alar plate (Fig. 26.13).

The stretched roof plate of rhombencephalic vesicle forms the roof of fourth ventricle. The roof consists of a single layer of ependymal cells covered by a vascular mesenchyme – the pia mater. Pia mater along with covering layer of ependymal cells forms **tela choroidea**. Due to active proliferation of vascular mesenchyme, the tuft of capillaries of blood vessels invaginates into the ventricular cavity. These sac-like invaginations consisting of tela choroidea and tuft of capillaries form **choroid plexus** (Fig. 26.14).

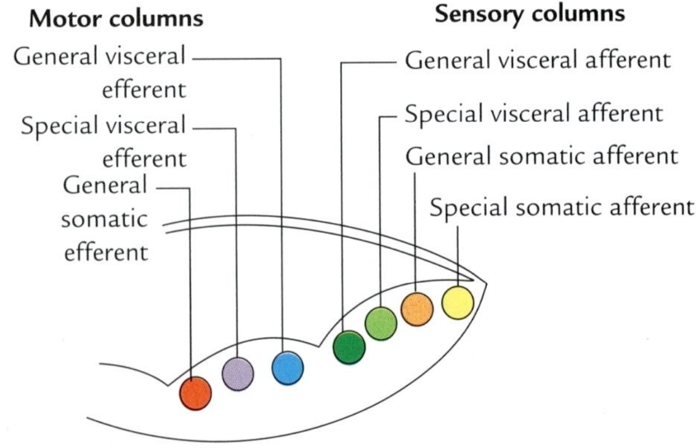

Fig. 26.13 Functional columns of gray matter in the brainstem.

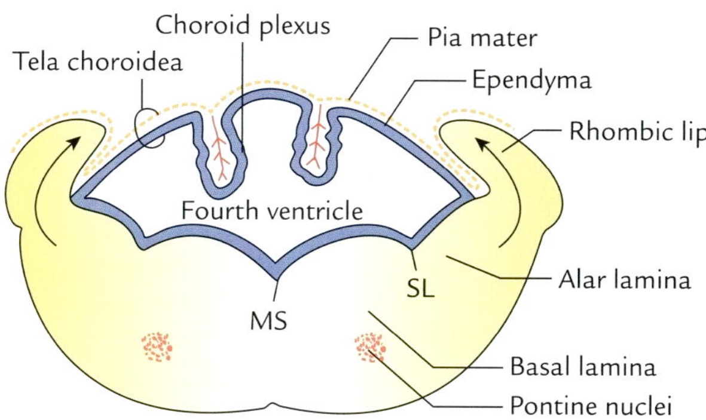

Fig. 26.14 Developing fourth ventricle and cerebellum. Note: (A) vascular pia mater invaginates ependyma to form choroid plexus, (B) alar lamina lies lateral to basal lamina, and (C) rhombic lips derived from alar laminae grow together to form cerebellum dorsal to the roof of fourth ventricle. MS, median sulcus; SL, sulcus limitans.

Dorsolateral parts of the alar laminae of metencephalon extend medially and dorsally to form **rhombic lips.** These meet and fuse in the midline over the roof of the fourth ventricle and then grow dorsally to form **cerebellum.**

The marginal layer of basal plates of metencephalon expands considerably to serve as a bridge for nerve fibers connecting cerebral cortex and cerebellar cortex (corticopontocerebellar pathways). Since this portion of metencephalon serves as a bridge, it is known as **pons** (pons, bridge).

1. Medulla Oblongata

The medulla oblongata develops from myelencephalon. For descriptive purposes, it is divided into two parts: **caudal closed part** and **cranial open part.**

- **Lower closed part** is more or less similar to upper part of spinal cord and presents the following:
  - A vertical central canal
  - Narrow thin roof and foot plates
  - Sulcus limitans in the center of lateral wall
  - Thick alar and basal laminae in the lateral wall (Fig. 26.6)
- **Upper open part** forms due to expansion (widening) of central canal of spinal cord and presents the following:
  - Thin, highly elongated roof plate
  - Narrow base plate
  - Alar laminae lying dorsolaterally
  - Basal laminae lying ventromedially

  Note: Due to dorsal widening of central canal of spinal cord, both alar and basal laminae lie in the floor of developing 4th ventricle.

N.B. Both the alar and basal laminae contain functional columns of cranial nerve nuclei (Fig. 26.13).

2. Pons

- The pons develops from two sources:
  (a) Ventromedial part of metencephalon
  (b) Alar laminae of myelencephalon
- The *roof plate* of metencephalon becomes thin and broad, similar to myelencephalon, to form roof of the 4th ventricle.
- The alar laminae become dorsolateral to the basal laminae.
- The cells of alar laminae of myelencephalon migrate ventrally to form **bulbopontine extensions.**
- The bulbopontine extension forms the following:
  (a) Olivary group of nuclei
  (b) Pontine nuclei
- The basal and alar laminae differentiate into motor and sensory columns of cranial nerve nuclei.

3. Cerebellum (Fig. 26.15)

The cerebellum develops from two rhombic lips which arise on either side from alar lamina of metencephalon on day 45 of gestational age.

- The rhombic lips enlarge and move toward midline where they fuse to form **cerebellar plate.**

The cerebellar plate differentiates to form a median vermis and two lateral cerebellar hemispheres.

Histogenesis of cerebellar hemisphere (Fig. 26.15A)

Initially, the cerebellar primordium consists of three layers from superficial to deep; these are the following:

- Superficial marginal layer
- Middle mantle layer, and
- Inner layer of neuroepithelial cells

Later some cells of mantle layer migrate into marginal layer to form **external granular** layer along its **superficial surface.**

Formation of cerebellar cortex

- The cells of superficial granular layer proliferate and migrate inwards into the mantle layer to form three layers of cerebellar cortex (Fig. 26.15B). From superficial to deep, these are as following:
  (i) **Molecular layer**, consisting of stellate and basket cells
  (ii) **Purkinje cell layer**, consisting of a single row of large flask-shaped Purkinje cells
  (iii) **Granular layer**, consisting of granule cells and Golgi cells

N.B. Remaining cells of **mantle layer** form intracerebellar nuclei (viz., nucleus dentatus, nucleus globosus, nucleus emboliformis, and nucleus fastigial).

Formation of cerebellar peduncles

- **Superior cerebellar peduncle** is formed by outgoing (efferent) fibers and dentate nucleus.

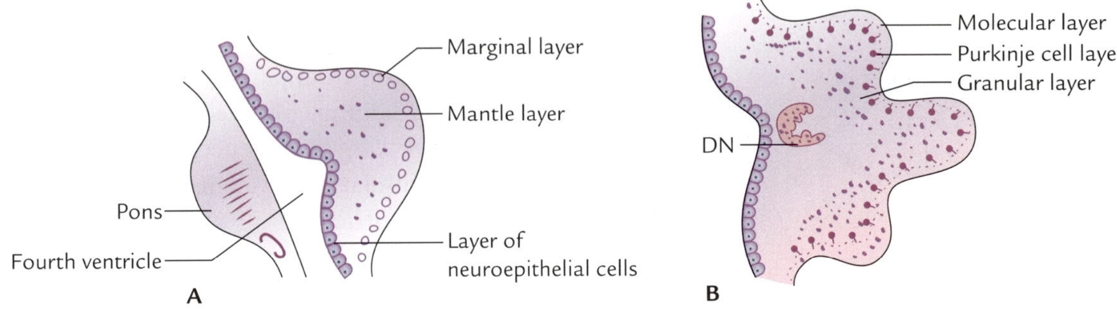

Fig. 26.15 Development of cerebellum. (A) Layer of neuroepithelial cells. (B) Histogenesis of cerebellum. DN, dentate nucleus.

- **Middle cerebellar peduncle** is formed by axons of pontine nuclei growing into cerebellum.
- **Inferior cerebellar peduncle** is mainly formed by fibers from medulla (inferior olivary nucleus) growing into cerebellum.

Formation of fissures and folia

These are formed by intricate folding of cerebellar cortex.

Midbrain (Mesencephalon)

Morphologically, the midbrain is the most primitive of the brain vesicles. It generally retains a cylindrical form and its narrowed cavity forms the cerebral aqueduct, which is continuous below with the fourth ventricle and above with the third ventricle.

- Anterior to the cerebral aqueduct, the basal laminae give rise to **tegmentum** and **substantia nigra**. The marginal layer of each basal lamina enlarges and forms **crus cerebri**. These crura serve as pathways for nerve fibers descending from the cerebral cortex to the lower centers in pons, medulla, and spinal cord.
- The cells of alar laminae invade the roof plate to form bilateral longitudinal elevations separated by a shallow midline groove. With further development, each elevation is subdivided by a transverse groove into upper and lower parts called **superior and inferior colliculi**, respectively. Thus, four colliculi (also called corpora quadrigemina) develop in the roof plate dorsal to the aqueduct of Sylvius and form **tectum**.

Forebrain (Prosencephalon)

The forebrain gives rise to diencephalon and two cerebral hemispheres.

1. Development of Diencephalon

The diencephalon develops from the median portion of the prosencephalon. Its cavity is called the **third ventricle.** The primitive diencephalon consists of two thick lateral walls, a thin roof, and floor plates.

Each lateral wall presents a sulcus, the **hypothalamic sulcus**, which appears to be rostral continuation of **sulcus limitans.** The hypothalamic sulcus divides lateral wall into dorsal and ventral regions. The dorsal region develops into **thalamus.** The ventral region encroaches on the floor plate and forms **hypothalamus.**

A downgrowth from the floor of anterior hypothalamus, the *neurohypophysis*, joins an upgrowth from the stomodeum, the *adenohypophysis*, to form **hypophysis cerebri (pituitary gland).**

The **epithalamus** comprising *pineal gland* and *habenular nuclei* develops posteriorly in the roof plate. The **pineal gland** grows posteriorly from the roof plate at its junction with the midbrain, and lies on the dorsal surface of midbrain between the two superior colliculi.

2. Development of Cerebral Hemisphere

The cerebral hemispheres are the derivatives of telencephalon.

The telencephalon consists of a median part and two lateral diverticula or cerebral vesicles. The median part forms a small anterior part of the third ventricle and the **lamina terminalis**, which limits the ventricle rostrally.

The lamina terminalis represents the cephalic end of the primitive neural tube and corresponds with the site of closure of anterior neuropore.

The lateral diverticula or cerebral vesicles represent **rudiments of cerebral hemispheres.** The cavities of hemispheres, the **lateral ventricles**, communicate with the cavity of diencephalon, the third ventricle, through the interventricular foramina.

The developing cerebral hemisphere enlarges forward, upward, and backward in that order. As the vesicle grows backward, it overlaps successively diencephalon, mesencephalon, and cerebellar rudiments. The lowest parts of medial walls of hemispheres in the region where they are attached to the roof of diencephalon remain very thin due to disproportionate growth of various parts of the hemispheres.

Through this thin wall, the choroid plexus of third ventricle protrudes laterally into lateral ventricle along a line known as **choroid fissure**.

Immediately above the choroid fissure, the medial wall of the hemisphere thickens to form **hippocampus**. With subsequent massive expansion of the cerebral hemispheres (neocortex), the hippocampus is displaced posteroinferiorly into the lateral ventricle; the **fornix** is drawn out as an efferent tract on its medial aspect. The choroid fissure also becomes curved, interposed between the fornix and the diencephalon.

Corpus striatum develops bilaterally in the floor of telencephalon adjacent to thalami. Primitively these areas of gray matter (corpus striatum) are **sensory–motor control centers**. Subsequent to massive development of neocortex, a major pathway must develop for descending fibers from the cerebral cortex and ascending fibers from the thalamus to the cerebral cortex; the only possible route is through this region. Hence, these fibers that form **internal capsule** on each side divide the corpus striatum into two parts: (a) a dorsomedial portion, the **caudate nucleus**; and (b) a ventrolateral portion, the **lentiform nucleus** (Fig. 26.16A and B).

N.B. The *cerebral hemisphere* starts growing/expanding in the region of interventricular foramen. It grows rapidly forward (forming frontal lobe), dorsally (forming parietal lobe), posteriorly (forming occipital lobe), and then anteroinferiorly (forming temporal lobe). This curved pattern of expansion of cerebral hemisphere from interventricular foramen around the diencephalon causes structures related to it (i.e., lateral ventricle, corpus callosum, fornix, choroid fissure, and caudate nucleus) to acquire C-shaped forms.

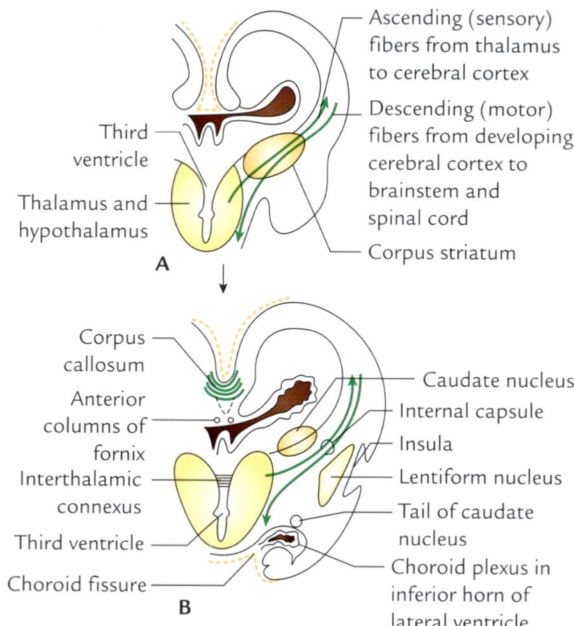

Fig. 26.16 Coronal sections through the developing forebrain showing development of internal capsule and establishment of corpus striatum. Note the ascending and descending fibers traversing through corpus striatum (A), and the division of corpus striatum into caudate and lentiform nuclei, and formation of internal capsule (B).

Meninges of Brain and Spinal Cord

The **three meninges/membranes** (i.e., *pia mater, arachnoid mater,* and *dura mater*) surrounding the brain and spinal cord are derived from mesenchyme surrounding the neural tube. However, according to some workers, the pia mater and the arachnoid mater *(leptomeninges)* are derived from the neural crest and not form mesenchyme.

CLINICAL CORRELATION

The mitotic activity within the neural tissue is completed during prenatal development. Thus, **a person is born with all neurons he or she was destined to have**. However, the nervous tissue continues to grow and specializes even after birth, particularly in initial several years of postnatal life.

GESTATIONAL AGE OF KEY DEVELOPMENTAL EVENTS

Developmental Event	Time of Occurrence
➢ Nervous system begins to develop during	3rd week
➢ Anterior (rostral) neuropore closes approximately on	25th day
➢ Posterior neuropore closes approximately on	27th day
➢ Primary brain vesicles develop at the end of	4th week
➢ Secondary brain vesicles develop during	5th week
➢ Flexures of brain develop during	5th week

GOLDEN FACTS TO REMEMBER

➢ **First indication of development of nervous system**	Formation of neural plate and neural groove
➢ **Most common serious birth defect seen in stillborn infants**	Anencephaly
➢ **Most common congenital anomaly of brain involving cerebellum**	Arnold–Chiari malformation
➢ **Most severe congenital anomaly of brain in fetal alcohol syndrome**	Holoprosencephaly (telencephalon with single ventricular cavity)
➢ **Most common cause of congenital hydrocephalus**	Congenital stenosis of aqueduct of Sylvius (cerebral aqueduct)
➢ **Hortega cells**	Microglia
➢ **Site of secondary neurulation**	**Caudal cell mass (a remnant of Hensen's node)**
➢ **Structures formed by secondary neurulation**	(a) Spinal cord distal to S2 (b) Filum terminale
➢ **First fissure to appear in cerebellum**	Posterolateral fissure
➢ **Growth of cerebellar cortex after birth**	Up to 1.5 years
➢ **Arnold–Chiari malformation**	Herniation of medulla oblongata and cerebellar vermis into spinal canal through foramen magnum

CLINICAL PROBLEM SOLVING

PROBLEMS

1. **A newborn has no cranial vault, and its brain substance is exposed to the surface as an irregular, degenerated mass. Name the congenital anomaly and mention whether a physician can detect it prenatally (i.e., before birth).**
2. **Why is anencephalic fetus associated with polyhydramnios?**
3. What do you understand by **meningocele**, **meningoencephalocele**, and **meningohydroencephalocele**? Give their embryological basis.
4. What do you understand by a clinical condition called **spina bifida** and its several forms? Give their embryological basis.
5. **What is Arnold–Chiari malformation? Discuss its clinical features.**

SOLUTIONS

1. This is a typical case of **anencephaly**, in which the brain tissue and associated vault of skull fail to develop due to failure of closure of anterior neuropore. A physician can detect this anomaly by (a) **ultrasonography in later part of pregnancy** or (b) **detecting the α-fetoprotein level** of amniotic fluid after transabdominal amniocentesis.

   N.B. The level of α-fetoprotein is increased in anencephaly.

2. The amniotic cavity is normally filled with clear, watery fluid derived mainly from maternal blood and partly from amniotic cells, and amounts to about 300–1000 mL at 37th week of gestation.

   From beginning of the 5th month, the fetus swallows about 400 mL of fluid every day. The swallowed fluid is absorbed through gut and passes into maternal blood. In anencephalic baby, the **swallowing reflex does not develop due to defective development of the brain**, leading to excessive accumulation of amniotic fluid (1500–2000 mL). It is termed **polyhydramnios**.

3. These are congenital malformations of the nervous system, which occur due to defective ossification of skull bones, particularly squamous part of the occipital bone.

   A gap in the skull caused by defective ossification makes meninges surrounding the brain to bulge out of the cranial cavity producing meningocele. If the defect is large, a part of brain tissue may also herniate producing **meningoencephalocele**. If herniated part of the brain contains a part of ventricular cavity, it is termed **meningohydroencephalocele**.

4. The **spina bifida** is a congenital malformation produced due to failure of fusion of vertebral arches. Consequently, vertebral canal (also called spinal canal) remains defective posteriorly. Depending on herniation of structures present within the spinal canal through the defect, it is classified into the following forms:
   (a) **Spina bifida occulta:** There is no herniation of structures of spinal canal through the gap. A tuft of hair is often present over the skin at the site of defect.
   (b) **Meningocele:** Meninges surrounding the spinal cord bulge out through the defect in the vertebral arches, forming a cystic swelling beneath the skin containing CSF.
   (c) **Meningomyelocele:** Spinal cord and spinal nerve roots also herniate along with the meninges if the defect is large.
   (d) **Rachischisis:** The neural tissue is exposed to surface. It is, in fact, due to failure of fusion of caudal neuropore. For details, see Page 310.

5. The **Arnold–Chiari malformation** occurs when **medulla oblongata**, inferior vermis, and tonsils of cerebellum herniate through foramen magnum. Clinically, it presents as (a) hydrocephalus due to obstruction of CSF circulation, (b) spastic dyspnea, (c) difficulty in swallowing, (d) laryngeal stridor, (e) diminished gag reflex, etc., due to compression of medulla oblongata and stretching of X, XI, and XII cranial nerves.

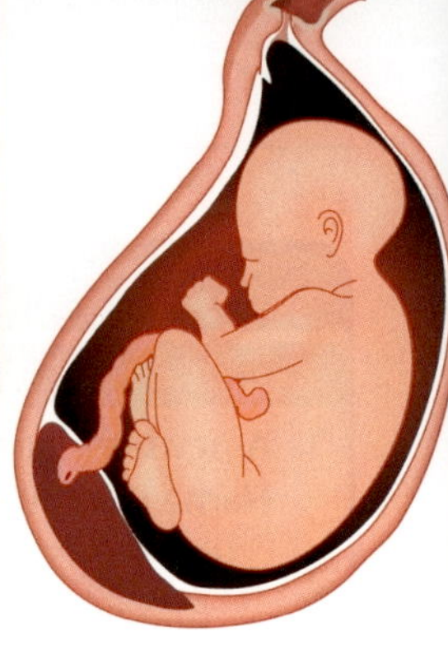

27 Endocrine System: Pituitary, Pineal, and Adrenal Glands

LEARNING OBJECTIVES

After studying this chapter, the student should be able to:

- Describe the development of pituitary gland and give the embryological basis of its congenital anomalies, viz., craniopharyngioma and pharyngeal hypophysis. AN 43.4
- Write short notes on (a) development of pineal and adrenal glands and (b) pheochromocytoma.
- Describe the development of suprarenal gland and associated common congenital anomalies.

OVERVIEW

- The **pituitary gland/hypophysis cerebri** develops from two entirely different sources: (a) *ectoderm*, lining the roof of stomodeum; and (b) *neuroectoderm* of hypothalamus.
- The **pineal gland** develops as a diverticulum from the roof of the third ventricle.
- The **adrenal gland** develops from two entirely different sources: (a) coelomic epithelium and (b) neural crest.

PITUITARY GLAND (HYPOPHYSIS CEREBRI)

The pituitary gland is an endocrine gland, about the size of a pea and weighing about 0.5 g. It consists of two distinct parts: (a) **adenohypophysis** (**anterior pituitary**) and (b) **neurohypophysis** (**posterior pituitary**). These two parts develop from two different sources as follows:

1. **Adenohypophysis** develops from an evagination of ectoderm lining the roof of primitive oral cavity called **Rathke's pouch** (Fig. 27.1). The Rathke's pouch develops in the 3rd week of intrauterine life (IUL). Later the Rathke's pouch is cut off from the primitive mouth or stomodeum.
   (a) **Anterior wall of Rathke's pouch** proliferates extensively to form **pars anterior** (**anterior lobe**) of the hypophysis cerebri.
   (b) **Posterior wall of Rathke's pouch** remains thin and forms **pars intermedia**.
   (c) **Cleft of Rathke's pouch** persists as hypophyseal cleft, which separates the two parts of adenohypophysis (anterior pituitary).

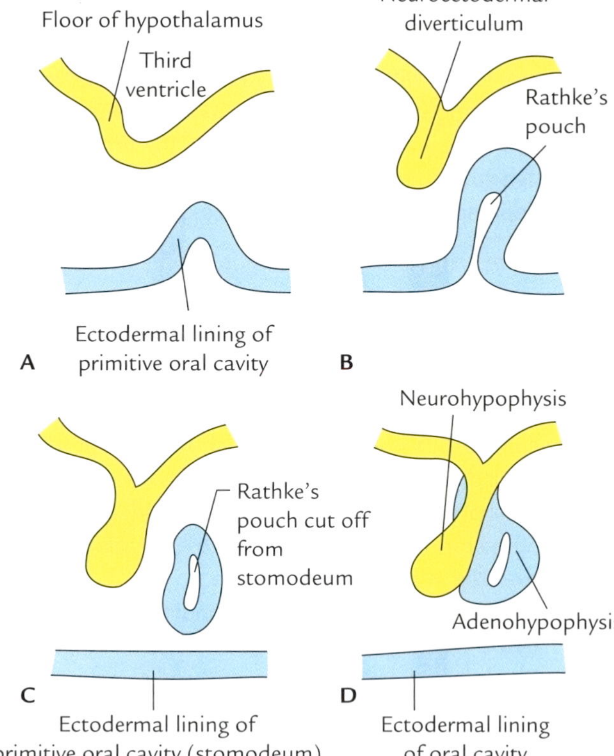

Fig. 27.1 Stages of development of the pituitary gland.

   (d) A small extension of pars anterior grows upward along the infundibular stalk and eventually surrounds it to form **pars tuberalis.**
2. **Neurohypophysis** develops from an evagination of neuroectoderm of hypothalamus/floor of the third ventricle. It differentiates into two parts: pars posterior

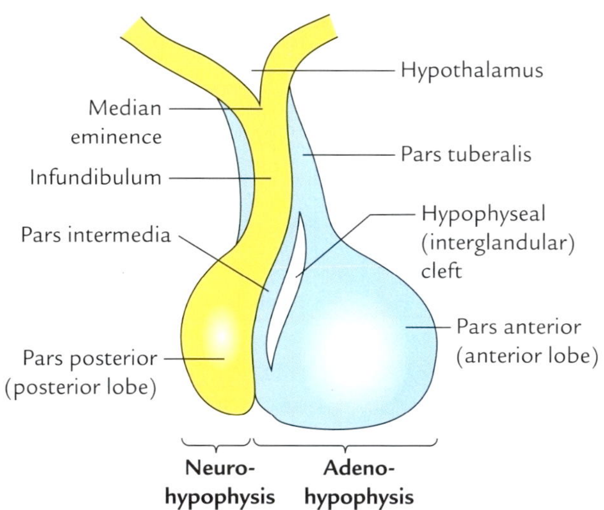

Fig. 27.2 Subdivisions of hypophysis cerebri.

(posterior lobe/pars nervosa) and **stalk of the hypophysis** (infundibulum).

The neuroectodermal diverticulum from the floor of the third ventricle and the ectodermal pouch from the roof of stomodeum (two primordia of hypophysis cerebri) fuse with each other to form hypophysis cerebri.

The various components of definitive pituitary gland are shown in Fig. 27.2 and Flowchart 27.1.

CLINICAL CORRELATION

Congenital anomalies of pituitary

The common ones are described as follows:

(a) ***Craniopharyngiomas:*** It is a rare noncancerous tumor arising from remnant of Rathke's pouch. The **Rathke's** pouch is detached from the primitive oral cavity to form **adenohypophysis**. With the formation of definitive oral cavity and pharynx, the original site of attachment of this pouch to the roof of primitive oral cavity (stomodeum) comes to lie in roof of nasopharynx. The *tract of Rathke's pouch* forms *craniopharyngeal canal.* Remnant of the craniopharyngeal canal sometimes gives rise to peculiar tumors called **craniopharyngiomas** that are seen in relation to sphenoid bone forming the roof of nasopharynx.
Clinically it presents as follows:
- Headache, nausea and vomiting
- Excessive thirst and increased urination
- Blurring of vision/gradual changes in vision
- Obesity and excessive weight gain

N.B. The *craniopharyngeal canal* runs between the roof of nasopharynx and the floor of hypophyseal fossa. In the event of agenesis (nondevelopment) of the hypophysis, the **accessory hypophyseal tissue** may develop in the posterior wall of the pharynx.

(b) ***Pharyngeal hypophysis:*** It is a remnant of the stalk of the Rathke's pouch in the roof of oropharynx.

THYROID GLAND

The development of thyroid gland is described in detail in Chapter 15, page no. 164.

PINEAL GLAND (EPIPHYSIS CEREBRI) (FIG. 27.3)

The pineal gland is very small endocrine gland (about 7 mm long) shaped like a **pine cone.** It is situated in the center of brain and a source of **melatonin.**

The **pineal gland** develops as a small median diverticulum from caudal part of the roof of the third ventricle. The cells of diverticulum proliferate to fill its lumen. As a result, the diverticulum becomes a solid structure – the **pineal gland.** The pineal gland is made up of modified neuroglial cells called **pinealocytes.** The pinealocytes secrete a hormone called **melatonin.**

The melatonin inhibits the secretion of gonadotropin (GnRH) from the hypothalamus and thus has an inhibitory effect on the reproductive system. The pineal gland probably holds back the development of reproductive system until a suitable age. For details, see *Textbook of Clinical Neuroanatomy*, 4th ed., by Dr Vishram Singh.

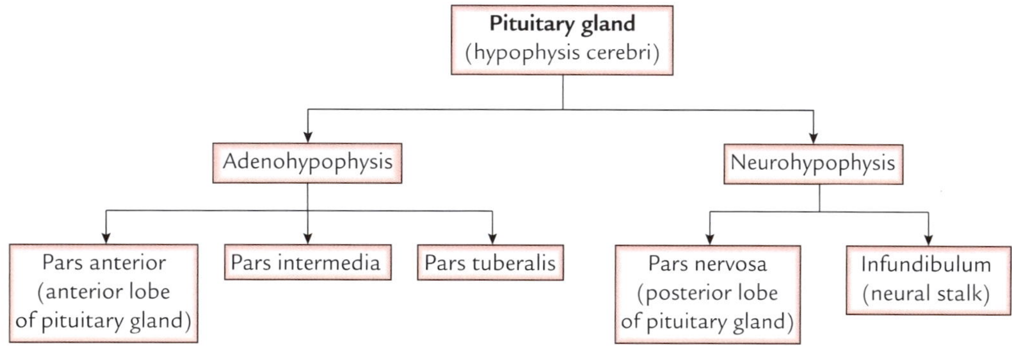

Flowchart 27.1 Subdivisions of the pituitary gland.

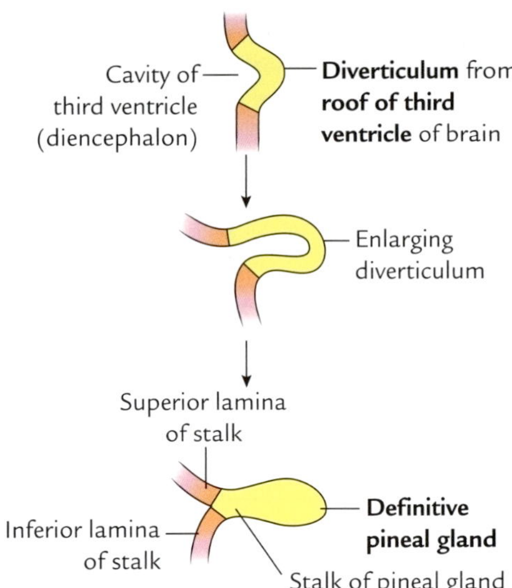

Fig. 27.3 Development of the pineal gland.

ADRENAL GLAND/SUPRARENAL GLAND

The suprarenal glands are paired triangular glands weighing about 4 g and situated on the upper pole of each kidney. They secrete **steroid hormones** and **catecholamines.**

The adrenal gland, weighing about 4 g, consists of two parts: (a) a large outer part called **cortex** and (b) a small inner part called **medulla.**

The adrenal gland develops from two entirely different sources:

1. The **adrenal cortex** is mesodermal in origin and develops from *coelomic epithelium.*
2. The **adrenal medulla** is neuroectodermal in origin and develops from *neural crest.*

The adrenal gland begins to develop in the 5th week of IUL.

The details of development are shown in Fig. 27.4.

Development of Adrenal Cortex

The cells from dorsal wall of coelomic epithelium (in the region of angle between developing gonad and root of dorsal mesentery) proliferate to form a ridge called **suprarenal ridge.**

The **adrenal cortex develops from two episodes of mesodermal proliferation of suprarenal ridge. First batch of cells of suprarenal ridge** consists of large acidophilic cells; they reach the site of development and surround the cells of the adrenal medulla to form **fetal cortex** of the adrenal gland.

Subsequently, **second batch of cells of suprarenal ridge** consists of small cells that reach the site of development and surround the fetal cortex from outside to form **definitive cortex** of the adrenal gland.

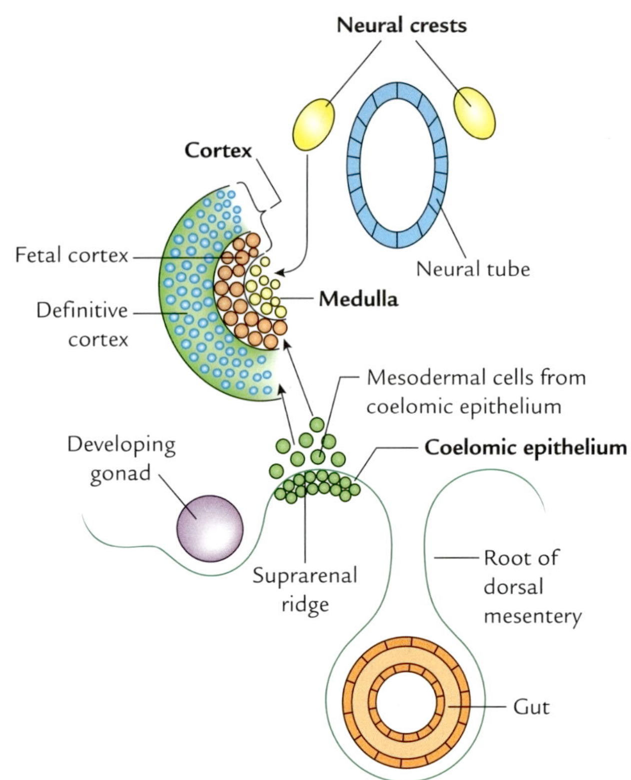

Fig. 27.4 Development of the adrenal gland.

At birth, the fetal cortex retrogresses and its involution is mostly completed in the first few weeks of life.

Formation of Zones in Adrenal Cortex (Fig. 27.5)

The adrenal cortex consists of three layers. From superficial to deep, these are as follows:

1. **Zona glomerulosa**
2. **Zona fasciculata**
3. **Zona reticularis**
   - The **zona glomerulosa** and **zona fasciculata** are formed at birth due to differentiation of the cells of the definitive cortex.
   - The **zona reticularis,** however, is identifiable only during the 3rd year of life.

Development of Adrenal Medulla

The adrenal medulla is formed by **sympathochromaffin cells** derived from **neural crests.** The cells of the adrenal medulla are similar to postganglionic neurons of sympathetic ganglia. Preganglionic sympathetic neurons terminate by synapsing with these cells.

The cells forming the medulla of the adrenal gland migrate from neural crest and enter the fetal cortex from the medial side.

N.B. The fetal adrenal gland is 10–20 times larger than adult adrenal gland.

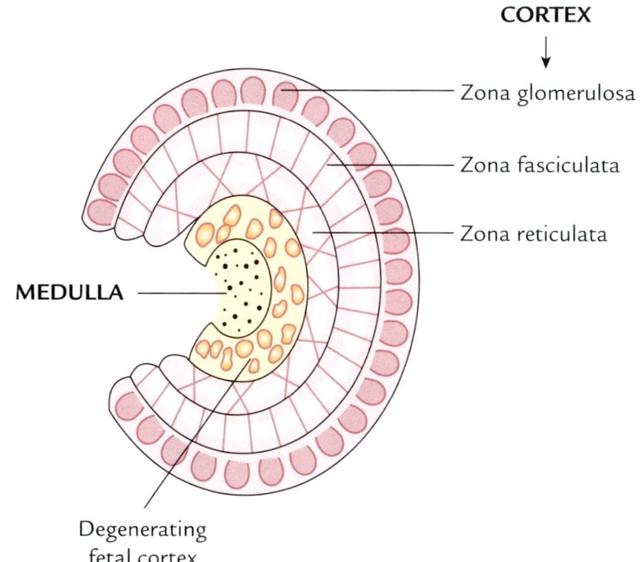

Fig. 27.5 Differentiation of various zones of definitive cortex.

CLINICAL CORRELATION

1. ***Ectopic adrenal tissue/adrenal gland:*** The adrenal tissue or complete adrenal gland may be found fused to kidney, deep to its capsule or in the right lobe of the liver.
2. ***Congenital adrenal hyperplasia:*** It is most commonly caused by mutation of genes for enzymes involved in adrenocortical steroid biosynthesis (e.g., 21-hydroxylase deficiency), which may cause elevation of androgen levels that may culminate in pseudointersexuality.
3. ***Adrenogenital syndrome:*** It occurs due to congenital hyperplasia of the cells of the adrenal cortex, which secrete androgen. The clinical manifestations differ in males and females as follows:
   (a) **In males:** It leads to a very early development of secondary sexual characters. This condition is termed **adrenogenital syndrome**.
   (b) **In females:** It leads to an enormous enlargement of the clitoris, and the child may be mistaken as a male. This condition is termed **pseudohermaphroditism**.

Chromaffin Tissue

The chromaffin tissue is made up of cells similar to those of the adrenal medulla. Like the cells of the adrenal medulla, the cells of chromaffin tissue are derived from neural crests.

Sites of Chromaffin Tissue

The chromaffin tissue is found at the following sites:
1. In relation to the abdominal aorta, where it forms **para-aortic bodies (organ of Zuckerkandl)**
2. Along sympathetic chain near sympathetic ganglia
3. Along sympathetic plexuses
4. Near splanchnic nerves

CLINICAL CORRELATION

Pheochromocytoma: It is a tumor arising from chromaffin cells. It usually arises from extra-adrenal chromaffin tissue. There is an excessive secretion of both adrenaline and noradrenaline. Clinically, pheochromocytoma presents as hypertension and features of sympathetic overdrive such as palpitation, sweating, apprehension, and fear of death.

GESTATIONAL AGE OF KEY DEVELOPMENTAL EVENTS

Developmental Event	Time of Occurrence
➢ Pituitary gland begins to develop during	3rd week
➢ Rathke's pouch forms from roof of stomodeum	4th week
➢ Adrenal cortex begins to develop during	6th week
➢ Adrenal medulla begins to develop during	7th week

GOLDEN FACTS TO REMEMBER

➢ **Most complex endocrine gland in the body**	Pituitary gland
➢ **Master endocrine gland**	Pituitary gland
➢ **Third eye**	Pineal gland
➢ **Principal seat of soul**	Pineal gland
➢ **Fetal adrenal gland is**	10–20 times larger than adult adrenal gland
➢ **Organs of Zuckerkandl**	Para-aortic bodies made up of chromaffin tissue
➢ **Thickest zone of adrenal cortex**	Zona fasciculata (forms 65% of cortical volume)

CLINICAL PROBLEM SOLVING

PROBLEMS

1. **Fetal adrenal gland is 10–20 times larger than the adult adrenal gland.** Give its embryological basis.
2. A mother told her family physician that her 10-year-old son is getting tall very fast. The physician after thorough physical examination and investigation made the diagnosis of **gigantism**. On the basis of your knowledge of embryology, answer the following questions:
   (a) What is gigantism?
   (b) In what way does gigantism differ from acromegaly?
3. Give the source of development of following endocrine glands:
   - Pituitary gland
   - Adrenal gland
   - Thyroid gland
   - Parathyroid glands
   - Pineal gland

SOLUTIONS

1. The large size of fetal adrenal gland is attributed to **large size of fetal cortex.**
   The regression of fetal cortex begins at birth and completes by the end of 1st year of life.

N.B. One-third weight of the adrenal gland is lost during first 3 months after birth.

2.
   (a) **Gigantism** is a clinical condition characterized by excessive growth of body. It occurs due to excessive production of growth hormone by the pituitary gland when it is affected by pituitary adenoma.
   (b) The main **difference between gigantism and acromegaly** is that acromegaly occurs when the limb bones have stopped growing, and gigantism occurs when they are still growing.
3. The source of development of these endocrine glands is given in the box below:

Endocrine gland	Source of development
• Pituitary gland (a) Adenohypophysis (b) Neurohypophysis	 From Rathke's pouch Downgrowth from floor of diencephalon
• Suprarenal gland (a) Cortex (b) Medulla	 From coelomic epithelium From neural crest cells
• Pineal gland	From roof of diencephalon

N.B. The thyroid gland is described on page 164 while parathyroid glands are described on page 155.

28 Development of Eye and Ear

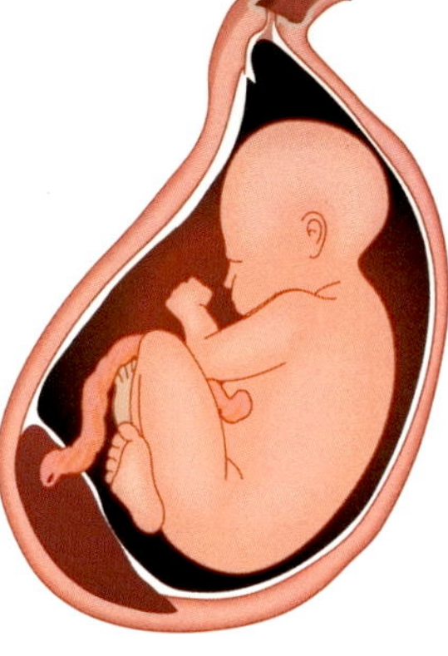

LEARNING OBJECTIVES

After studying this chapter, the student should be able to:

- Give a brief account of development of eyeball and accessory structures associated with it.
- Describe the developmental basis of congenital anomalies of eye. AN 43.4
- Write short notes on (a) development of lens, (b) development of iris, and (c) embryological basis of coloboma iris.
- Describe the development of external and middle ears in brief and discuss the congenital anomalies associated with external ear.
- Describe the development of (a) external ear, (b) tympanic membrane, and (c) ear ossicles.

DEVELOPMENT OF EYE

The eye is the organ of vision. It is divided into two components: (a) eyeball and (b) accessory structures of the eyeball. The development of eye begins on day 22.

Development of Eyeball

OVERVIEW

The eyeball develops from four sources:

1. Neuroectoderm of forebrain
2. Surface ectoderm of head
3. Mesoderm between neuroectoderm of forebrain and surface ectoderm of head
4. Neural crest cells

The **neuroectoderm** of forebrain forms retina, posterior layers of iris, and optic nerve.

The **surface ectoderm** of the head forms lens of the eye and corneal epithelium (epithelium covering the superficial surface of the cornea).

The **mesoderm** between the neuroectoderm of forebrain and the surface ectoderm of the head forms fibrous and vascular coats of the eye.

The **neural crest cells** migrate into mesenchyme from the neural crests and form choroid, sclera, and corneal epithelium.

The development of eyeball is described under the following heads:

(a) Optic cup and lens vesicle
(b) Various parts of eyeball

Optic Cup and Lens Vesicle (Figs 28.1–28.3)

At first, a pair of shallow groove or sulcus appears on either side in the forebrain. It is called **optic groove/ sulcus**. The optic sulcus invaginates the surrounding mesenchyme to form **optic vesicle**.

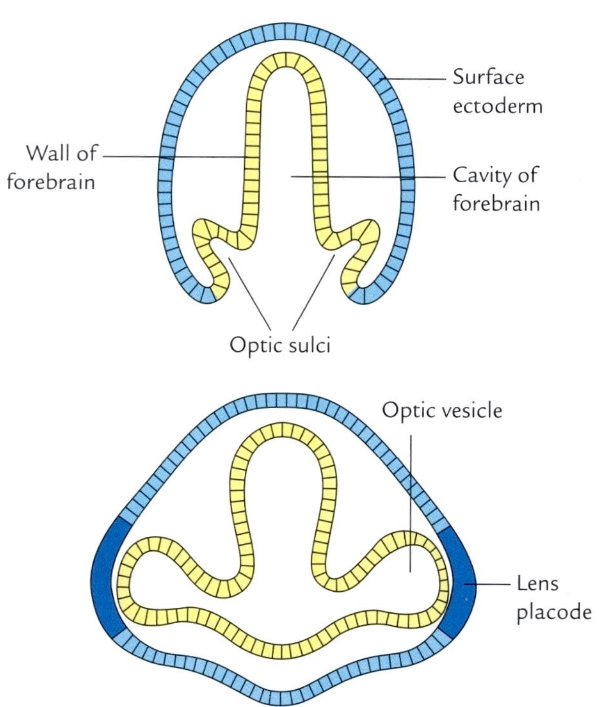

Fig. 28.1 Development of the optic vesicle and lens placode.

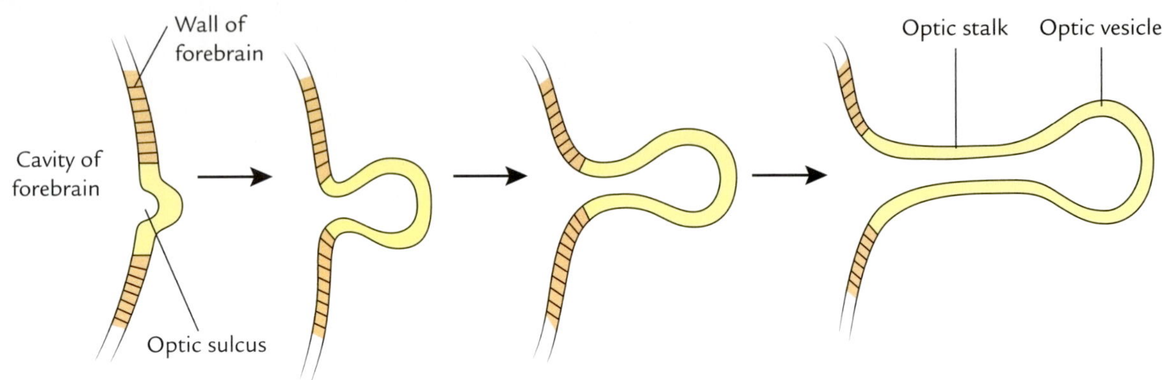

Fig. 28.2 Formation and development of the optic vesicle.

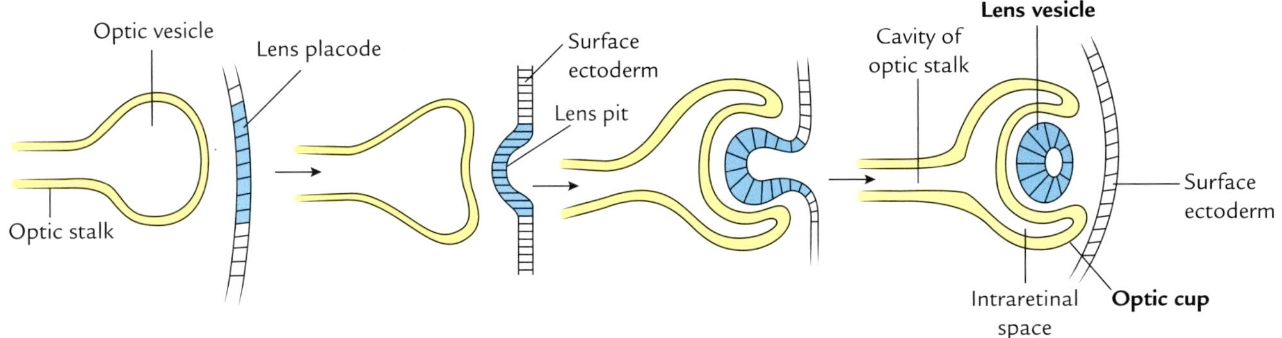

Fig. 28.3 Development of the lens vesicle and optic cup. Note the invagination of lens vesicle into the optic cup.

Each optic vesicle grows laterally. Its distal part expands and invaginates to form **optic cup**; its proximal part connected to the forebrain constricts to form **optic stalk**. As the optic vesicle comes in contact with the surface ectoderm, it induces it to thicken and forms **lens placode** – the **primordium of lens.**

The lens placode gets depressed below the surface to form **lens pit.** As the lens pit deepens, its edges approach each other and fuse to form spherical **lens vesicle**, which is soon cut off from the surface ectoderm.

As the lens vesicle is being formed, optic vesicle begins to invaginate to form double-layered **optic cup.** The margins of the optic cup grow and enclose the lens vesicle, i.e., lens vesicle enters the optic cup.

The optic cup forms *retina*, whereas optic stalk forms *optic nerve.*

Subsequently, a fissure called **retinal/choroidal fissure** develops on the inferior aspect of the optic cup and the optic stalk. The vascular mesoderm enters the choroidal fissure and gets trapped in the optic vesicle and optic stalk. The choroid fissure is closed. This vascular mesoderm within it forms hyaloid vessels (**hyaloid artery and hyaloid vein**), which supply to the layers of the optic cup, mesoderm in the optic cup, and lens vesicle (Fig. 28.4).

The distal parts of hyaloid vessels eventually degenerate, whereas their proximal parts persist as **central artery and vein of retina.**

Development of Various Parts of Eyeball

Retina (Fig. 28.5)

The retina develops from walls of the optic cup. Outer thin layer of the optic cup forms **pigment layer of the retina.** Inner thick layer of the optic cup forms **neural layer of the retina**. The cells of the neural layer proliferate to form various cells of retina, i.e., **photoreceptor cells** (**rods and cones**), **bipolar cells**, and **ganglionic cells.** The rods and cones are modified neurons. The axons of ganglionic cells form nerve fiber layer, which passes through the optic stalk and forms **optic nerve.** During embryonic and early fetal periods, the pigment and neural layers of the retina are separated from each other by an **intraretinal space** representing the original cavity of the optic cup. Before birth, the space between

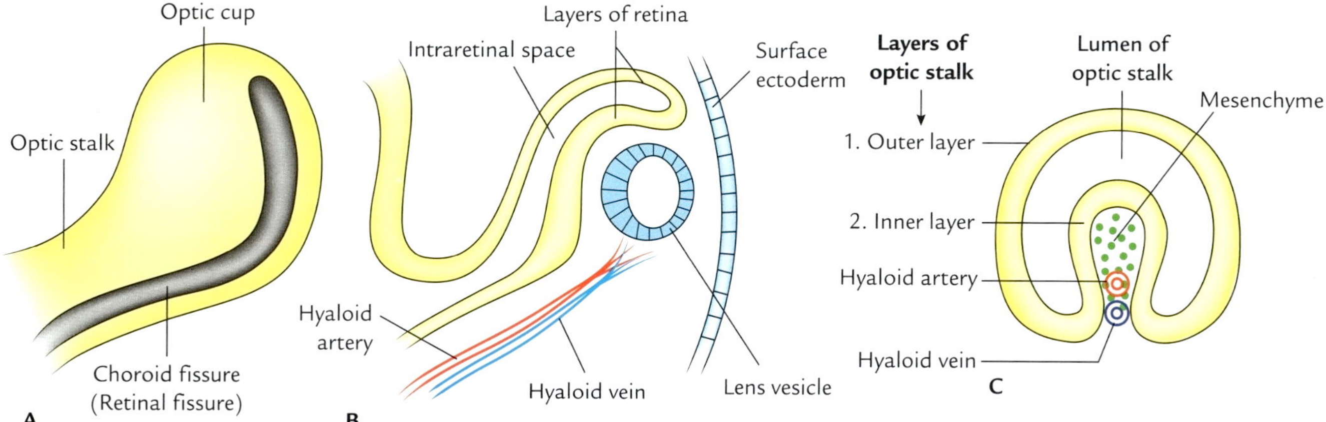

Fig. 28.4 Development of choroid fissure and hyaloid vessels. (A) Ventrolateral view of optic cup and optic stalk with choroid fissure on their undersurfaces. (B) Section through lens vesicle, optic cup, and optic stalk at the planes of choroid fissure. (C) Transverse section through optic stalk showing choroid fissure and its contents.

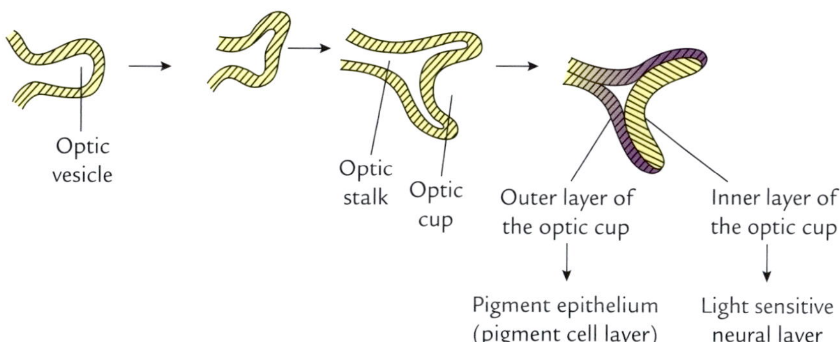

Fig. 28.5 Stages in the development of retina.

the inner and outer layers of the optic cup is obliterated with the proliferation of cells of the inner layer. As a result, the rod and cone cells come in contact with pigment layer of the retina.

Optic Nerve

As discussed earlier, the optic stalk contains choroid fissure, which contains hyaloid vessels. The hyaloid vessels later become **central artery and vein of retina**. The optic stalk contains nerve fibers derived from ganglionic cells of the retina. The choroid fissure closes in week 7. As a result, the optic stalk along with axons of ganglionic cells forms the optic nerve.

N.B. The **optic nerve is a tract of diencephalon** and not a peripheral nerve because:

1. It is myelinated by oligodendrocytes in the 3rd month.
2. It is not capable of regeneration after transaction.
3. It is surrounded by meninges and subarachnoid space filled with cerebrospinal fluid (CSF).

CLINICAL CORRELATION

1. ***Retinal detachment:*** There is a separation of pigment epithelium from the neural layer of the retina in retinal detachment. The retinal detachment may be congenital or can occur because of a blow to the eye.

   This can be easily explained embryologically, because during development the two layers of the retina are separated by a space called the **intraretinal space**, which later gets obliterated.

   The integrity of the retina depends on the pressure of the vitreous humor in adults, which keeps the two layers of the retina adhered to each other. When a hole or tear occurs in retina, the fluid may accumulate between the pigment and neural layers of the retina and may separate these layers.
2. ***Papilledema:*** The optic nerve is surrounded by three meninges that were invaginated by developing optic vesicle and stalk. Consequently, it is surrounded by subarachnoid space (filled with CSF), which is continuous with the subarachnoid space around the brain.

   Therefore, an increase in CSF pressure due to increased intracranial pressure hampers the venous return from retina. As a result, fluid accumulates in the optic disc leading to its swelling (**papilledema**).

   This occurs because the retinal vessels are covered by pia mater and lie in the subarachnoid space that surrounds the optic nerve.

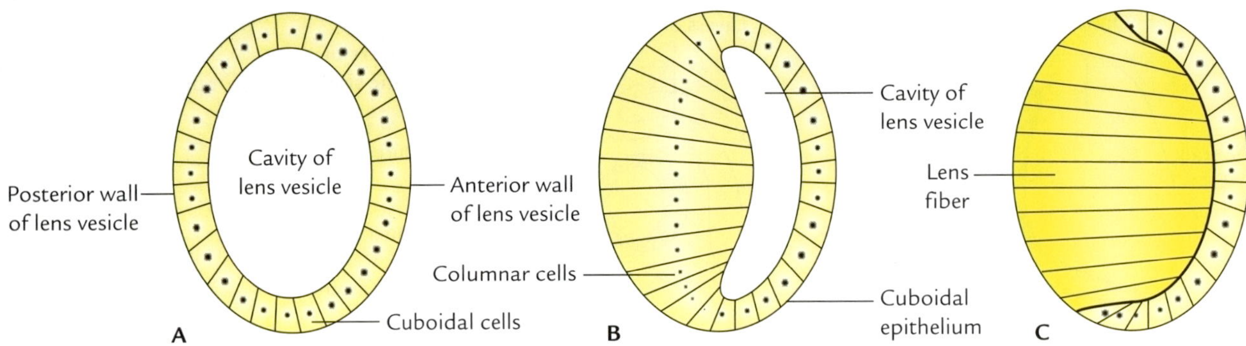

Fig. 28.6 Developmental stages in the formation of the lens. (A) Lens vesicle lined by cuboidal cells. (B) Cells of anterior wall remain cuboidal; the cells of posterior wall elongate and become columnar. (C) Columnar cells of posterior wall elongate to form lens fibers.

Lens (Fig. 28.6)

The lens develops from the **lens vesicle** – a derivative of surface ectoderm (see p. 328). Initially, the lens vesicle is lined by a single layer of cuboidal cells. The cells of anterior wall of the vesicle remain cuboidal, whereas the cells of posterior wall of the lens vesicle elongate, become columnar, and extend into the cavity of lens vesicle. As a result, the cavity of lens vesicle is obliterated. The elongated cells of posterior wall of the lens vesicle further elongate considerably and lose their nuclei to form highly transparent **primary lens fibers.** The lens grows because new lens fibers (**secondary lens fibers**) are added to it by cells in the **equatorial zone of lens.** The cells of anterior layer persist as **epithelium.**

Although the secondary lens fibers continue to form during childhood and lens increases in its diameter, the primary lens fibers become old and harder.

N.B. Lens is formed during 7th week.

N.B. At first, the lens is supplied by hyaloid artery – a branch of the ophthalmic artery. Later on, the distal part of hyaloid artery disappears, and blood supply to the lens is stopped. Consequently, the lens becomes an avascular structure.

CLINICAL CORRELATION

Cataracts

The **cataract** is opacity **of the lens.** It may be congenital or acquired.

1. ***Congenital cataracts:*** The congenital cataracts are opacities of the lens since birth. They are usually bilateral. They are caused by rubella virus, toxoplasmosis, Down syndrome (trisomy 21), or galactosemia (an inborn error of metabolism due to enzymatic deficiency).

   Note: The lenses are vulnerable to rubella virus between 4th and 7th weeks, when the primary lens fibers are formed.
2. ***Acquired cataract:*** They occur due to ageing. In old age, central part of the lens becomes harder than peripheral part. Old primary lens fibers complete their lifetime and degenerate. As a result, there is accumulation of a special set of proteins called *crystalline* within the lens, which causes opacity of the lens.

Sclera and Choroid (Fig. 28.7)

The mesoderm around the optic cup differentiates into two layers: (a) an inner vascular layer that forms choroid and (b) an outer fibrous layer that forms sclera. Anteriorly the sclera is continuous with substantia propria of the cornea, whereas posteriorly it is continuous with the dura mater surrounding the optic nerve. The choroid is continuous anteriorly on each side with ciliary body, whereas posteriorly it is continuous with pia arachnoid around the optic nerve.

Ciliary Body (Fig. 28.7)

The ciliary body is a wedge-shaped extension of the choroid anteriorly. It is formed by the mesoderm around the anterior part of the optic cup. The ciliary muscle and connective tissue of the ciliary body are derived from mesoderm. The pigment epithelium lining inner aspect of the ciliary body, including the ciliary processes, is derived from the outer layer of the optic cup. It is continuous with the retinal pigment epithelium.

The nonpigmented epithelial layer of the ciliary body is derived from the inner layer of the optic cup. Thus, there are two layers of the ciliary epithelium. The ciliary epithelium over the ciliary processes becomes secretory and secretes the **aqueous humor.**

The nonpigmented ciliary epithelium represents anterior prolongation of the neural layer of the retina.

Iris

The iris develops from the rim of optic cup (i.e., anterior extension of two layers of the optic cup), which grows inward and partially covers the lens. Thus, the epithelium of iris is derived from both layers of the optic cup. It is continuous posteriorly with the double-layered

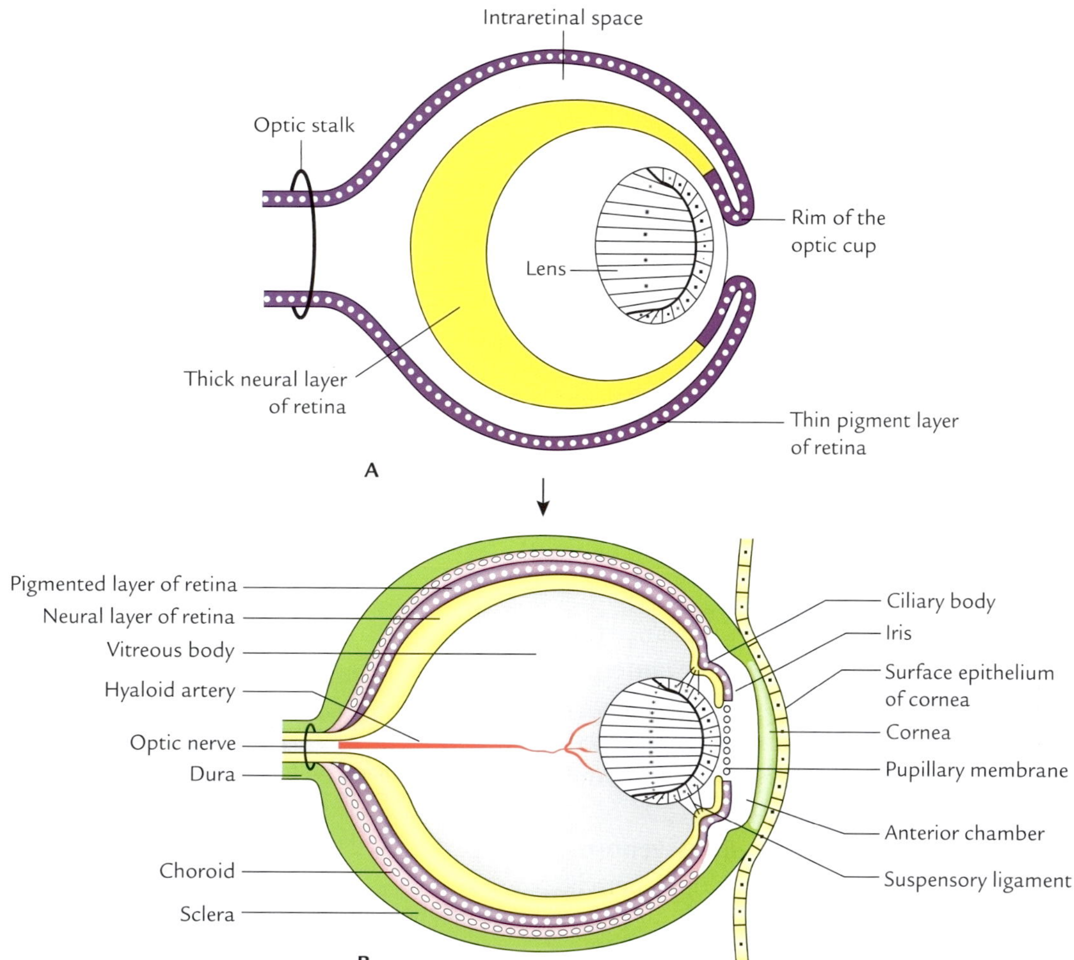

Fig. 28.7 Development of the coats of the eye. (A) Development of retinal layers. (B) Development of sclera, choroid, ciliary body, and iris.

epithelium of the ciliary body. The neuroectodermal cells of the optic cup give rise to muscles of the iris (**sphincter and dilator pupillae**). The two layers of epithelium of the iris constitute iridial part of the retina. The vascular connective tissue of the iris is derived from mesoderm located anterior to the optic cup.

The anterior extension from the rim of the optic cup, which forms iris, does not extend up to the center. As a result, almost circular gap remains in the center of the iris – the **pupil**.

N.B. The smooth muscle of the sphincter and dilator pupillae results from the transformation of epithelial cells into smooth muscle fibers.

CLINICAL CORRELATION

Color of the iris: The color of the iris depends on concentration and distribution of pigment-containing cells (**chromatophores**) in the iris. When melanin pigment is confined to the pigment epithelium on the posterior surface of the iris, the iris appears blue and when the melanin is also distributed in the stroma of the iris, the eye appears brown.

Cornea

The development of cornea is induced by the lens vesicle.

The cornea is derived from the following:

1. *Outer stratified squamous epithelium* is derived from the **surface ectoderm**.
2. *Lamina propria of the cornea* is derived from the **mesoderm**. It is continuous with sclera.
3. *Inner corneal epithelium* is derived from the **neural crest cells**.

Anterior and Posterior Chambers of the Eye (Fig. 28.8)

The mesoderm located between developing iris and cornea splits to form a space called the **anterior chamber**. The mesoderm anterior to this space forms substantia propria of the cornea and mesothelium of the anterior chamber.

The mesoderm located between the developing iris and the lens splits to form a space called the **posterior chamber**.

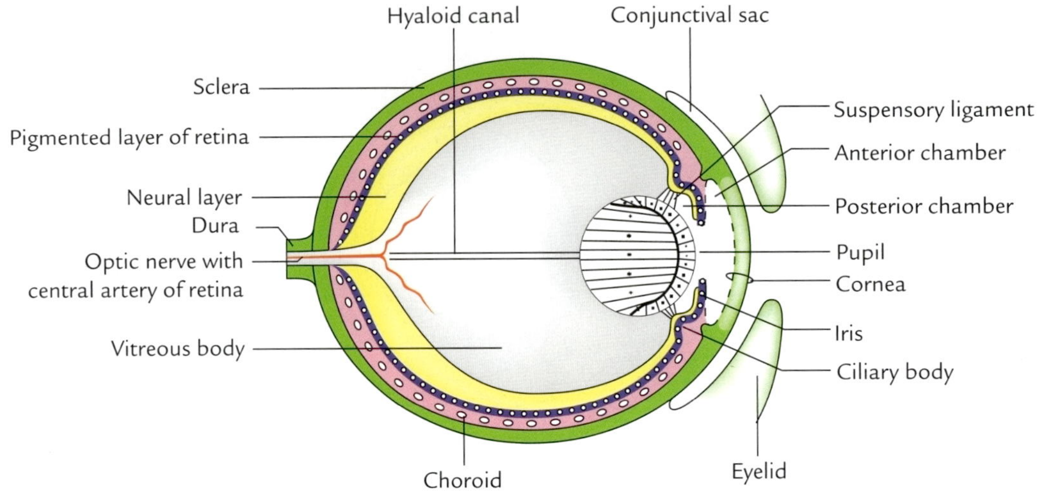

Fig. 28.8 Formation of anterior and posterior chambers.

When the pupillary membrane disappears, the pupil forms a communication between the anterior and posterior chambers of the eye.

The anterior and posterior chambers are filled by aqueous humor secreted by ciliary processes of the ciliary body.

The aqueous humor is drained by **sinus venosus sclerae** (a circumferential scleral venous sinus encircling the anterior chamber).

Vitreous Body (Vitreous Humor)

At first, the vitreous humor is formed by neural crest mesoderm present in the optic cup. It is called **primary vitreous humor**. Later on, it is replaced by gelatinous **secondary vitreous humor** derived mainly from the inner layer of the optic cup and a little bit from the lens vesicle. Vitreous body is made up of a vascular mass of transparent gel-like intracellular substance. It contains hyaloid artery that later obliterates to form a **hyaloid canal** of adult eye.

The adult components of eyeball derived from various embryonic structures are given in Table 28.1.

Table 28.1 Adult components of eye derived from various embryonic structures

Embryonic Structure	Adult Derivatives
Neuroectoderm (of forebrain)	
(a) Optic cup	• Retina • Dilator pupillae • Sphincter pupillae • Epithelium of iris and ciliary body
(b) Optic stalk	• Optic nerve
Surface ectoderm	• Lens • Anterior epithelium of cornea
Mesoderm	• Sclera • Substantia propria and posterior epithelium of cornea • Choroid, ciliary body, and stroma of iris • Vitreous body • Central artery and vein of retina • Extraocular muscles

CLINICAL CORRELATION

Congenital anomalies of the eye (Fig. 28.9)

1. ***Anophthalmia (absence of an eye):*** It occurs when the optic vesicle fails to form.
2. ***Microphthalmia (a small eye):*** It occurs when the optic vesicle is small or there is underdevelopment of eye. The lens is usually not formed. The microphthalmia is usually associated with intrauterine infections from *Toxoplasma*, rubella virus, cytomegalovirus, and herpes simplex virus group of organisms.
3. ***Cyclopia (single eye)*** (Fig. 28.9A): The cyclopia is a severely uncommon anomaly of the face. There develops a single median eye. The nose is usually absent at the normal site but may be represented by a tubular appendage called proboscis above the median eye. The cyclopia is transmitted by recessive inheritance. The two eyes may fuse (synophthalmia) to form a single eye.
4. ***Persistent pupillary membrane*** (Fig. 28.9B): The pupillary membrane may persist as a whole or it may persist in the form of few strands of connective tissue. It may obstruct the vision completely or partially.
5. ***Coloboma of the iris*** (Fig. 28.9C) (Gr. *Coloboma*, a part that is cut off or missing): It is a congenital notch or cleft on the inferior aspect of the iris. It occurs due to failure of choroid fissure to close.

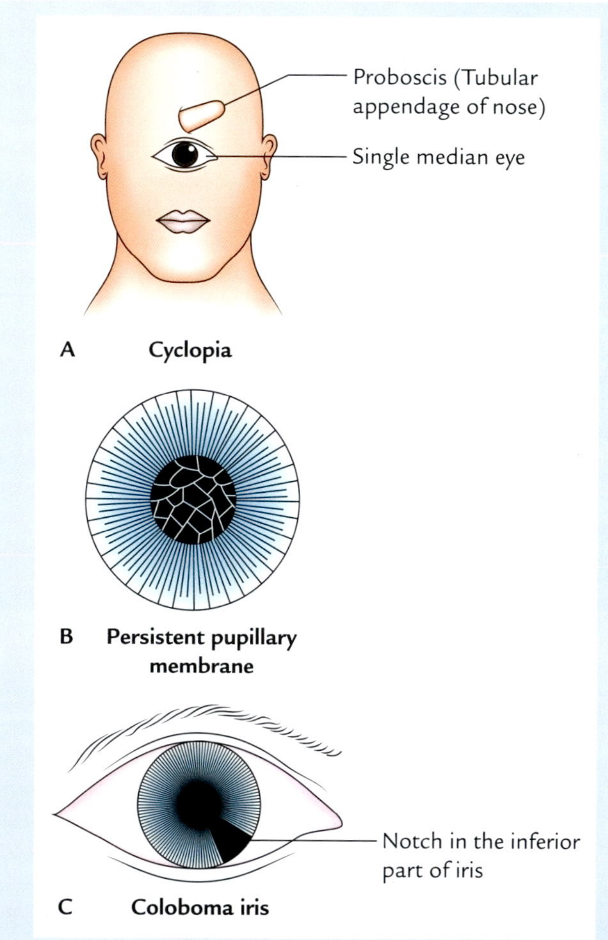

Fig. 28.9 Some congenital anomalies of the eye.

6. ***Congenital aniridia (complete absence of the iris):*** It occurs from an arrest of development at the rim of the optic cup.
7. ***Congenital glaucoma (buphthalmos):*** It is an increased intraocular pressure that results due to impaired drainage of the aqueous humor, following abnormal development of *canal of the Schlemm* or *iridocorneal filtration angle.*
8. ***Congenital aphakia (aphakia, absence of the lens of the eye):*** It occurs if lens placode fails to develop following failure of lens induction by the optic vesicle.

Accessory Structures of the Eyeball

OVERVIEW

The accessory structures of the eyeball include eyelids, conjunctival sac, lacrimal gland, lacrimal sac, and nasolacrimal duct.

Eyelids (Fig. 28.10)

The upper and lower eyelids develop from reduplication of surface ectoderm above and below the cornea, respectively. These ectodermal folds contain a core of mesoderm. As the upper and lower folds grow, they approach and fuse with each other, thus enclosing a space between them and cornea called **conjunctival sac.** Therefore, the conjunctival sac is of ectodermal origin and lined by ectoderm.

The eyelids remain fused with each other till the beginning of 10th week and remain adhered to each other until 28th week (7th month) of intrauterine life (IUL). Thereafter, the eyelids get separated from each other to form the upper and lower eyelids, respectively. (cf. *In many lower mammals, e.g., cats, the offsprings are born with closed eyelids.*)

The central core of the mesoderm in the ectodermal folds (developing eyelids) forms **tarsal plate** and connective tissue of the eyelids.

The **eyelashes** and **glands in the eyelids** develop from surface ectoderm covering the eyelids in a similar manner as in the skin (see Chapter 11).

Lacrimal Glands (Fig. 28.10)

Each lacrimal gland develops from 15 to 20 buds that grow from the superolateral angle of the conjunctival sac. These buds elongate and get canalized to form the ducts. The secretory acini develop at the ends of these ducts. The ducts of lacrimal gland, therefore, open in the conjunctival sac.

Lacrimal Sac and Nasolacrimal Duct

They develop from the ectoderm of **nasolacrimal/naso-optic groove** present along the line of fusion of maxillary and lateral nasal processes. It is described in detail on p. 170.

The **lacrimal canaliculi** develop from canalization of the ectodermal buds that grow from the margin of each eyelid near their medial ends to the lacrimal sacs.

CLINICAL CORRELATION

1. **Anomalies of the eyelids**
   (a) ***Coloboma of eyelid:*** It is an uncommon congenital condition in which part of the eyelid is missing. Coloboma of eyelid usually occurs as a small notch in the upper eyelid. The coloboma of inferior eyelid is rare. It is caused by failure of fusion of lid folds.
   (b) ***Entropion and ectropion:*** When the lid margins are turned inward, the condition is called *entropion*, and when the lid margins are turned outward, the condition is called *ectropion*.
   (c) ***Congenital ptosis (drooping of the upper eyelid):*** It occurs if the levator palpebrae superioris muscle fails to develop; it may be transmitted as an autosomal dominant trait.
   (d) ***Epicanthus:*** It is the development of crescentic fold of skin that extends from upper eyelid to canthus. It is a normal feature in Mongolian races.

Continued

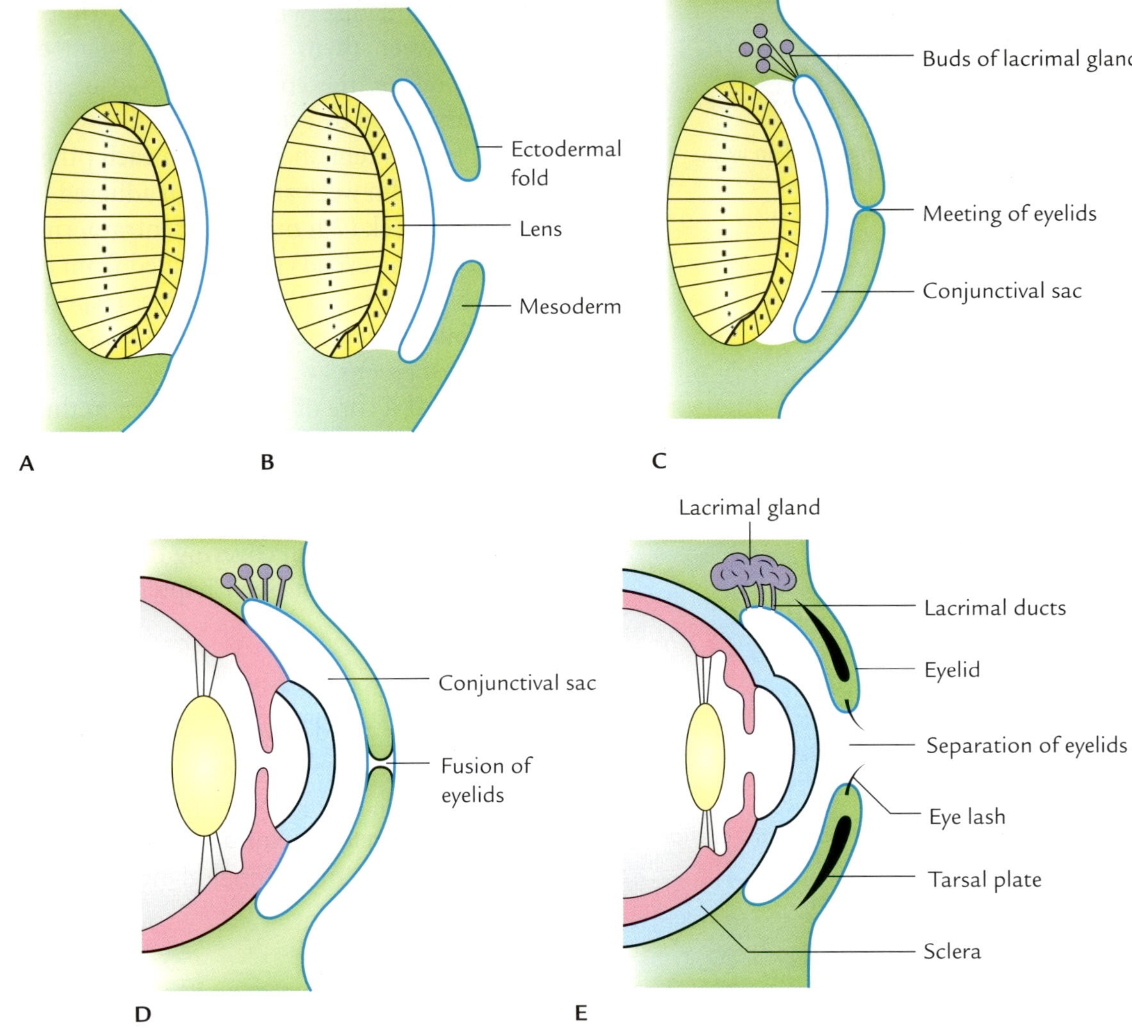

Fig. 28.10 Development of eyelids, conjunctival sac, and lacrimal gland.

(e) ***Cryptophthalmos (L. kryptos, hidden):*** It occurs due to congenital absence of the eyelids. The eyeball is small and defective. It is covered by the skin (i.e., absence of palpebral fissure between the eyelids).

2. **Anomalies of the lacrimal apparatus**
   (a) Lacrimal gland may be absent or nonfunctional.
   (b) There occurs **complete absence of lacrimal passages** in whole, in part, or atresia of some part.
   (c) Supernumerary puncta or canaliculi are present.
   (d) Cysts are present in any part of the lacrimal apparatus, mostly close to the lacrimal puncta.

DEVELOPMENT OF EAR

OVERVIEW

The ear is an **organ of hearing and balance**. It consists of three anatomical parts. From the lateral to the medial side, they are arranged as follows:

1. **External ear** consisting of the pinna and external auditory meatus
2. **Middle ear** consisting of a slit-like cavity containing three small ear ossicles
3. **Internal ear** consisting of bony and membranous labyrinths

The external, middle, and internal ears develop from three distinctly different sources. However, in adults, they form a single anatomical unit to serve the function of hearing as well as balance.

1. **The external ear collects the sound waves.**
2. **The middle ear transfers the sound waves from the external to the internal ear.**
3. **The internal ear performs dual functions.**
   (a) It converts sound waves into nerve impulses that lead to **hearing.**
   (b) It registers changes in **equilibrium and balance,** and subsequently maintains them.

N.B.

- Developmentally internal ear appears first.
- Internal ear, tympanic cavity (middle ear), mastoid antrum, and ear ossicles assume adult size at the time of birth.

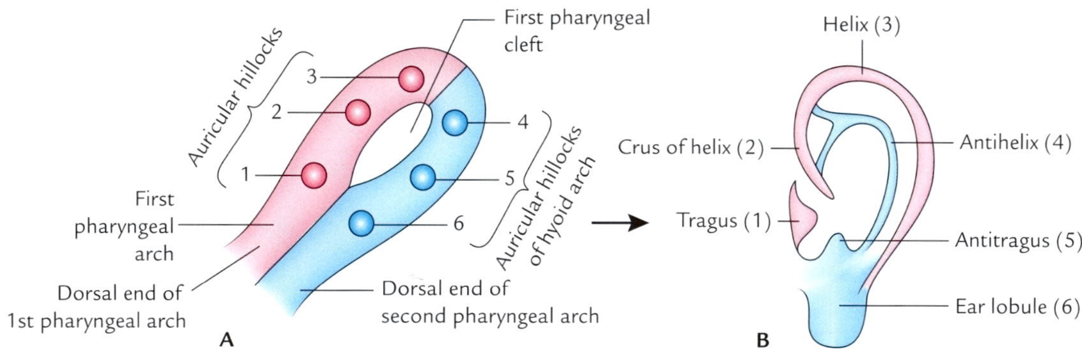

Fig. 28.11 Development of auricle or pinna.

External Ear

The external ear consists of two parts: (a) auricle/pinna and (b) external auditory meatus.

1. **Auricle or pinna** (Fig. 28.11): **It develops from six mesodermal thickenings** (called **auricular hillocks/tubercles**) around the first pharyngeal cleft during 5th week of IUL, three along caudal border of the dorsal end of first pharyngeal/mandibular arch, and three along cephalic border of the dorsal end of second pharyngeal (hyoid) arch.

   These hillocks fuse with one another to contribute in the formation of auricle of the ear. It is believed that the tragus, crus of helix, and helix are derived from auricular hillocks of the mandibular arch, whereas antihelix, antitragus, and ear lobule are derived from auricular hillocks of the hyoid arch.
2. **External auditory meatus** (Fig. 28.12): It develops from **ectodermal first pharyngeal cleft**.

   At first, it gets filled with the ectodermal cells forming a temporary solid **meatal plug**. These ectodermal cells are derived from ectodermal lining epithelium of the first pharyngeal cleft. The meatal plug gets canalized during 7th month of IUL to form external auditory meatus.

Tympanic Membrane (Figs 28.12 and 28.13)

It develops by the apposition of the tubotympanic recess and first pharyngeal cleft, i.e., from the **first pharyngeal membrane**.

1. The *outer cuticular layer* of the tympanic membrane is derived from the ectodermal lining of the first pharyngeal cleft.
2. The *inner endodermal layer* of the tympanic membrane is derived from the endodermal lining of the first pharyngeal pouch.
3. The *intermediate fibrous layer* of the tympanic membrane is derived from the mesoderm intervening between the first pharyngeal cleft and the first pharyngeal pouch.

N.B. The **handle of malleus** and **chorda tympani nerve** extends into the tympanic membrane between its intermediate fibrous layer and inner endodermal (mucous) layer.

CLINICAL CORRELATION

Congenital anomalies of external ear

1. ***Anotia (absence of the auricle):*** It occurs due to failure of mesenchymal proliferation to form auricular hillocks. It is rare but commonly associated with *first arch syndrome*.
2. ***Preauricular appendages and pits:*** These are skin tags and shallow depressions that are usually seen anterior to the ear. The *preauricular appendages* occur due to development of accessory hillocks, whereas the *preauricular pits* occur due to abnormal development of auricular hillocks. Most of the anomalies of the external ear are associated with various chromosomal syndromes such as Down syndrome (trisomy 21), Patau syndrome (trisomy 13), and Edward syndrome (trisomy 18).
3. ***Atresia of the external auditory meatus:*** It occurs due to failure of the meatal plug to canalize. Clinically, it presents as *conduction deafness* and is often associated with first arch syndrome.

N.B. The ear is most sensitive to teratogens during 4th to 9th weeks of gestation.

Middle Ear (Figs 28.12, 28.13, and 28.14)

1. The **middle ear** (**tympanic cavity**) develops from the distal part of tubotympanic recess, which develops mainly from the dorsal part of the first pharyngeal pouch with a little contribution from the second pharyngeal pouch. The mastoid antrum and mastoid air cells are formed by extensions of the tympanic cavity.
2. The **ear ossicles** (**malleus**, **incus**, and **stapes**) develop as follows:
   (a) The **malleus** and **incus** develop from the cartilage of the first pharyngeal arch – the *Meckel's cartilage*.

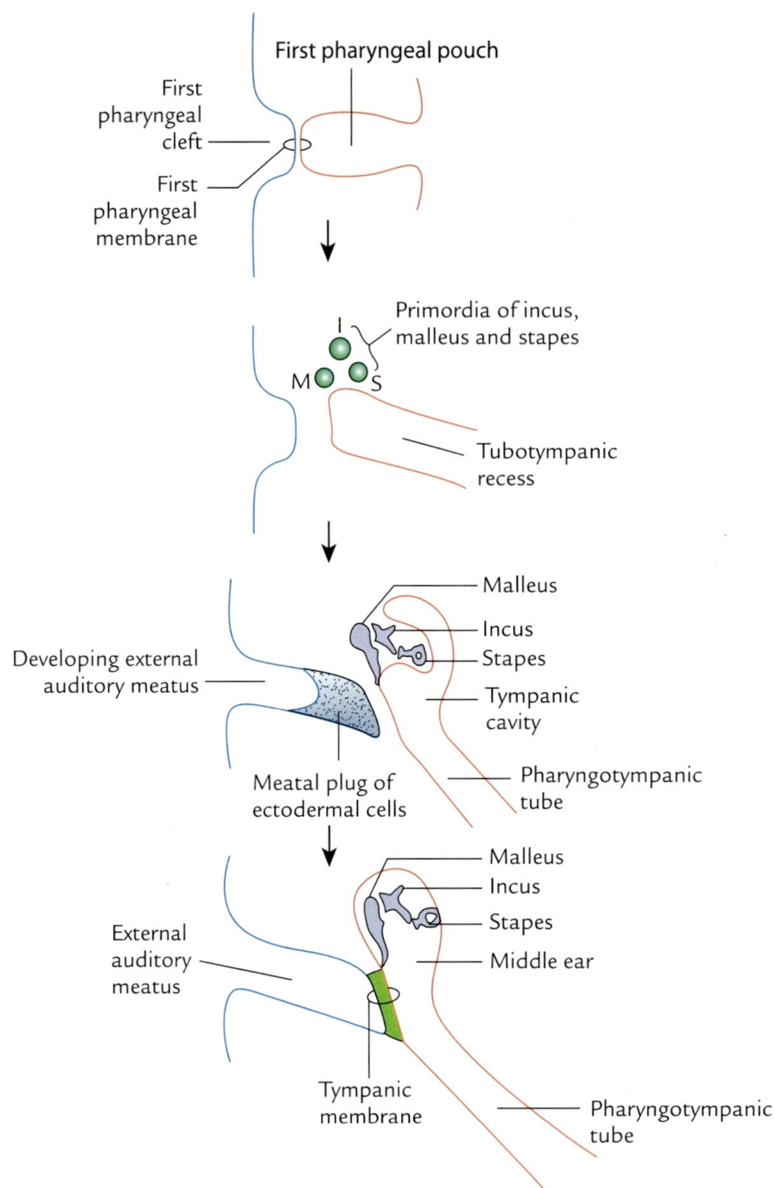

Fig. 28.12 Development of external auditory meatus, middle ear, and tympanic membrane. M, malleus; I, incus; S, stapes.

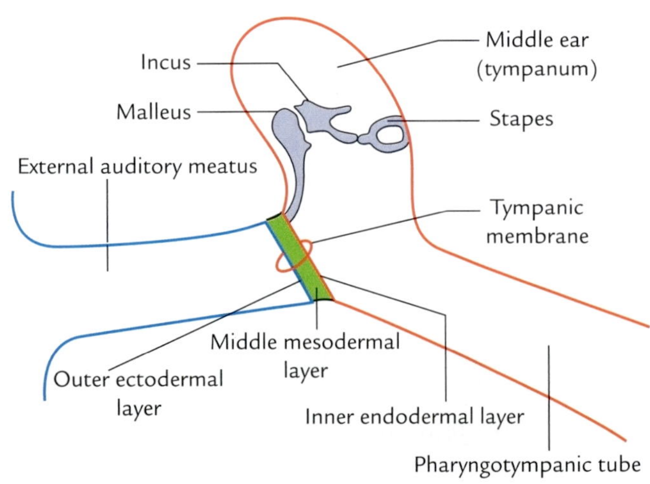

Fig. 28.13 Tympanic membrane.

(b) The **stapes** develops from the cartilage of the second pharyngeal arch – the *Reichert's cartilage.*

The ear ossicles are initially embedded in mesenchyme. When the mesenchyme surrounding the ossicles dissolves, the endodermal epithelial lining of primitive tympanic cavity extends along the newly developing space and connects the ossicles with the wall of tympanic cavity in a mesentery-like fashion. The supporting ligaments of the ossicles develop later within the mesenteries.

Mastoid Antrum

The dorsal expansion of tympanic cavity gives rise to the **mastoid antrum.** The mastoid antrum is almost of

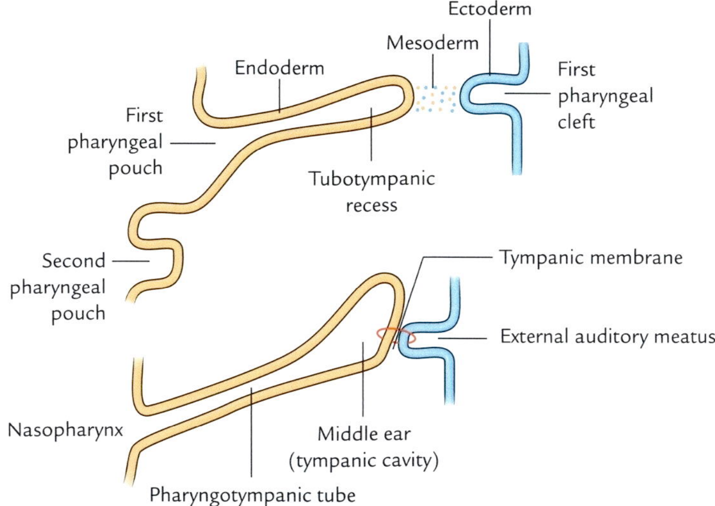

Fig. 28.14 Development of middle ear (tympanum) and pharyngotympanic tube.

adult size at birth; however, mastoid air cells are not present in the newborn infants. The mastoid air cells develop at the age of 2 years.

Muscles of Middle Ear

1. **Tensor tympani muscle:** It is attached to the upper part of handle of malleus and also develops from the first pharyngeal arch like malleus. It is supplied by **mandibular branch of trigeminal** nerve – the nerve of the first arch.
2. **Stapedius muscle:** It is attached to the stapes and also develops from the second pharyngeal arch like stapes. It is supplied by **facial nerve** – the nerve of the second pharyngeal arch.

Pharyngotympanic Tube

(Auditory Tube/Eustachian Tube) (Fig. 28.14)

It is derived from narrow proximal part of the tubotympanic recess. It connects the tympanic cavity with nasopharynx.

Internal Ear

The **internal ear is first of the three parts of the ear to develop**. Early in the 4th week, the surface ectoderm on either side of rhombencephalon shows a localized thickening called **otic placode**. The otic placode soon invaginates the underlying mesoderm to form **otic pit**. Margins of the otic pit approach each other and fuse together to form **otic vesicle** or otocyst (Fig. 28.15). The otic vesicle gets separated from the surface. The **otic vesicle is primordium of the membranous labyrinth.**

Otic vesicle then grows and forms various parts of the membranous labyrinth of the internal ear as follows:

The otic vesicle divides into two components: **ventral saccular portion** and **dorsal utricular portion.**

1. The **saccular portion of otic vesicle** gives rise to **saccule, cochlear duct** (organ of Corti), and **spiral ganglion** of **vestibulocochlear nerve.**
2. The **utricular portion of otic vesicle** gives rise to **utricle, semicircular ducts, endolymphatic duct and sac**, and **vestibular ganglion of vestibulocochlear nerve.**

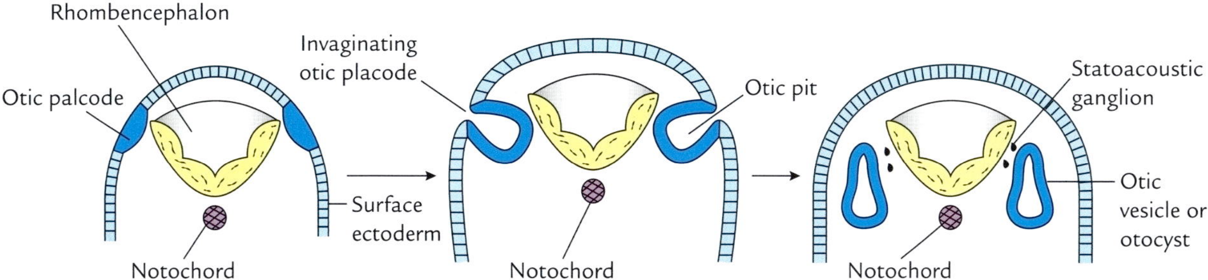

Fig. 28.15 Formation of the otic vesicle. Note the appearance of statoacoustic ganglion.

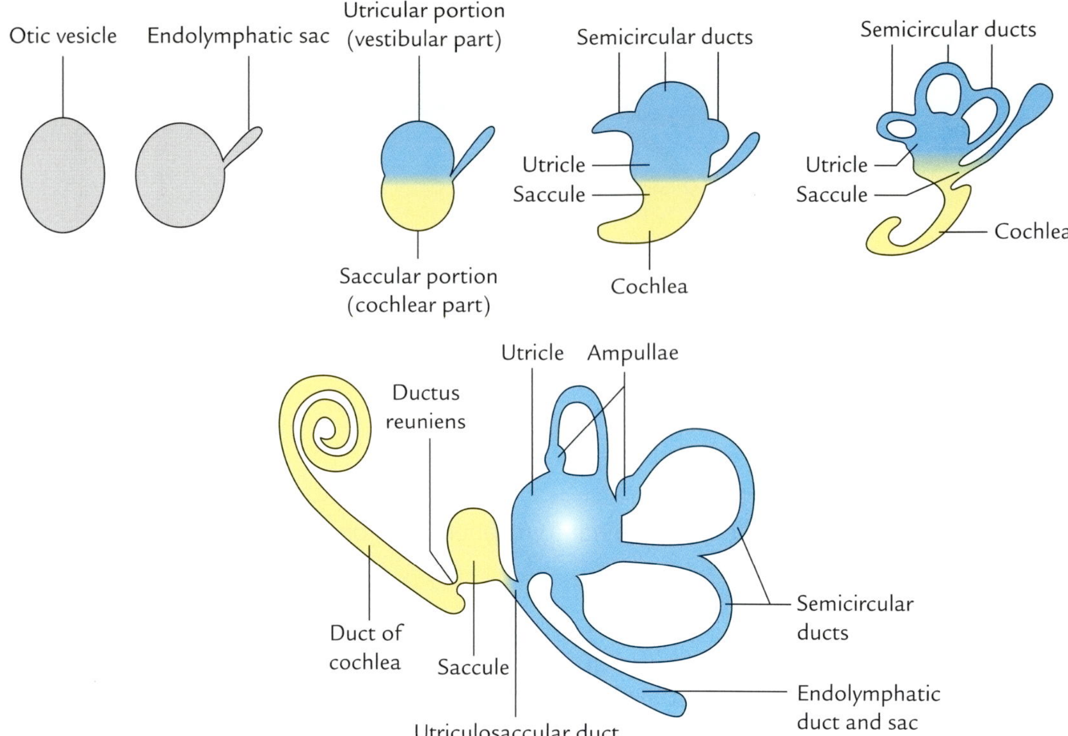

Fig. 28.16 Development of the membranous labyrinth.

All these components, i.e., cochlear duct, saccule, utricle, and endolymphatic duct and sac, together constitute the membranous labyrinth.

Saccule, Cochlear Duct, and Organ of Corti (Fig. 28.16)

During the 6th week, the saccule forms a tubular diverticulum – the **cochlear duct** that grows in a spiral fashion till it completes two and half turns. Later its connection with the saccule becomes narrow, forming **ductus reuniens**.

The mesenchyme condenses around the membranous labyrinth. This condensation is converted into cartilage to form **otic capsule**. The space between the otic capsule and the membranous labyrinth is called **perilymphatic space**. Cartilage of the otic capsule is converted into bone to form bony labyrinth. The perilymphatic space between the bony labyrinth and the membranous labyrinth is filled with a fluid called **perilymph**. The membranous labyrinth is filled with a fluid called **endolymph**. Special sense organs for hearing and equilibrium develop in the wall of membranous labyrinth. They are innervated by vestibulocochlear nerve that is attached to the brainstem at the junction of pons and medulla.

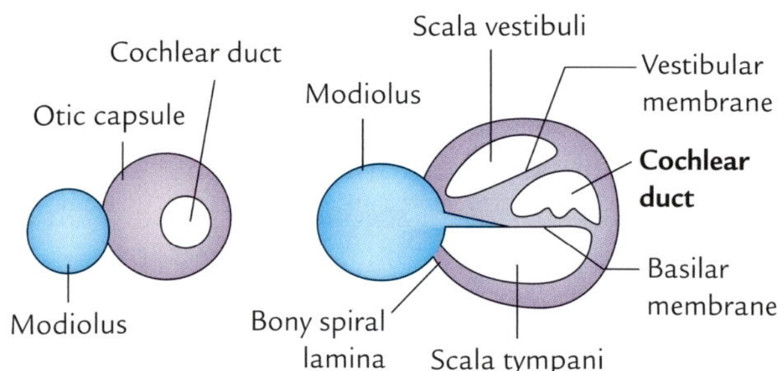

Fig. 28.17 Development of perilymphatic spaces around the cochlear duct.

The mesenchyme of the bony labyrinth forms two perilymphatic spaces around the cochlear duct (Fig. 28.17):

- *Scala vestibuli* above the duct
- *Scala tympani* below the duct

The scala vestibuli is separated from the duct by **vestibular membrane (Reissner's membrane)** and scala tympani is separated from the duct by **basilar membrane.**

The lateral end of the cochlear duct is attached to the surrounding cartilage by **spiral ligament**, whereas its medial end is connected to a long cartilaginous process, the **modiolus** – the future axis of bony cochlea.

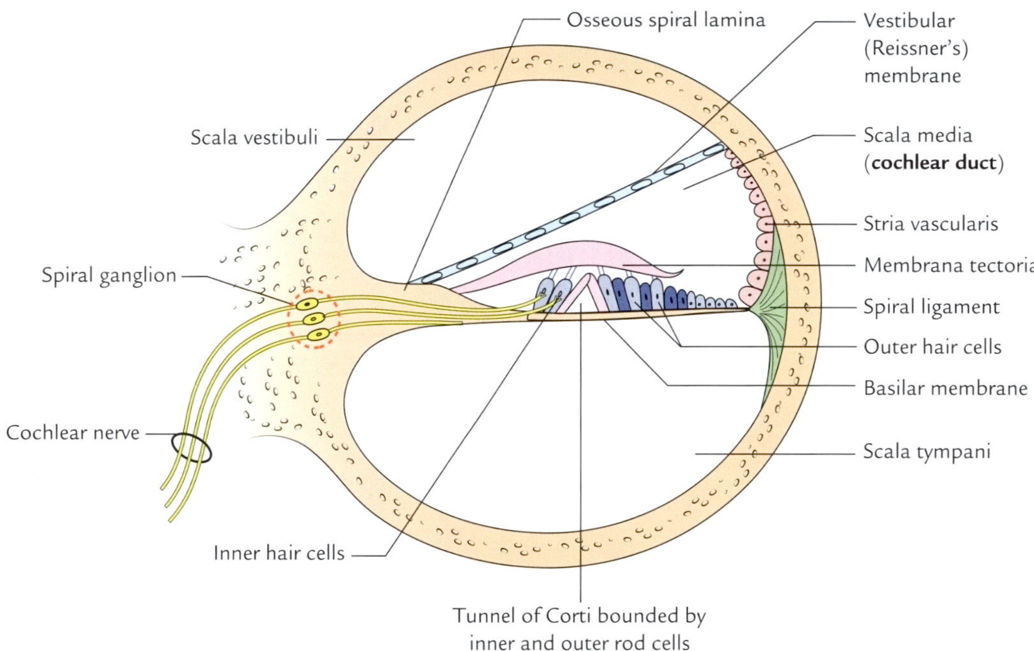

Fig. 28.18 Cross-section of cochlear canal showing boundaries of the cochlear duct and organ of Corti within it.

Two ridges develop on the basilar membrane. These are called **inner** and **outer ridges**.

1. Cells of the inner ridge form **spiral limbus**, which gives attachment to ***membrana tectoria***.
2. Cells of the outer ridge form two rows of **inner hair cells** and three or four rows of **outer hair cells**. The hair cells are sensory cells of the auditory system.
   (a) These sensory cells and tectorial membrane together form **organ of Corti**.
   (b) When the membrana tectoria touches the hair cells, it produces sound waves in the form of vibrations that are carried to the brain through **auditory nerve** (Fig. 28.18).

Utricle and Semicircular Canals

During the 6th week of IUL, three **semicircular canals** develop as outpouchings of the utricle. One end of each duct dilates to form the **ampulla**, whereas its other end remains narrow to form **crus nonampullare**. The crus ampullare of anterior and posterior semicircular canals fuse. As a result, the **three semicircular canals communicate with utricle by five openings**.

The cells in the crus ampullare form a crest called ***crista ampullaris*** – the sensory receptors of equilibrium. The cristae ampullare are sensory receptors for kinetic balance.

In the same manner, **maculae** (the **sensory receptors for *static balance/gravity***) develop in the medial walls of utricle and saccule.

The impulses generated in sensory cells of **maculae** and **cristae ampullaris** due to change in position of the body are carried to the brain by ***vestibular nerve***.

For details, see *Anatomy of Head, Neck, and Brain* by Vishram Singh.

The adult components of ear derived from various embryonic structures are given in Table 28.2.

Table 28.2 Derivatives of various components of the ear

Embryonic Structure	Adult Derivatives
Internal ear	
• Saccular portion	• Saccule and cochlear duct
• Utricular portion	• Utricle, semicircular ducts, endolymphatic duct, and sac
Middle ear	
• First pharyngeal arch	• Malleus, incus, and tensor tympani muscle
• Second pharyngeal arch	• Stapes and stapedius muscle
• First pharyngeal pouch	• Pharyngotympanic tube and middle ear (tympanum)
• First pharyngeal membrane[a]	• Tympanic membrane
External ear	
• First pharyngeal cleft	• External auditory meatus
• Auricular hillocks in mandibular and hyoid arches	• Pinna/auricle

[a]First pharyngeal membrane is trilaminar. From outside to inside, it consists of ectoderm, mesoderm, and endoderm.

GESTATIONAL AGE OF KEY DEVELOPMENTAL EVENTS

Developmental Event	Time of Occurrence
➢ Development of the eye begins on	22nd day
➢ Lens is formed during	7th week
➢ Auricle/pinna starts forming at the end of	5th week
➢ External auditory meatus gets canalized by	7th week
➢ Internal ear starts developing during	4th week
➢ Mastoid air cells develop at the age of	2 years

GOLDEN FACTS TO REMEMBER

➢ **First indication of the development of eye**	Formation of optic sulcus (optic groove)
➢ **Most important refractive medium of the eye**	Cornea
➢ **First of the three parts of the ear (external, middle, and internal) to develop**	Internal ear
➢ **Most common cause of congenital deafness**	Failure of canalization of the meatal plate
➢ **Ear is most sensitive to teratogens during**	Weeks 4–9 of the development
➢ **Parts of ear which assume adult size at birth**	**Middle ear, ear ossicles, mastoid antrum, and internal ear**
➢ **Eye is most susceptible to teratogens during**	Weeks 4–8 of the development

CLINICAL PROBLEM SOLVING

PROBLEMS

1. A male baby was born with partial **detachment of retina** in both eyes. Give the embryological basis.
2. An infant was born with the absence of lens (**aphakia**) in both the eyes (**bilateral aphakia**). Give the embryological basis of bilateral aphakia.
3. A pregnant woman during the 6th week of gestation contracted **rubella virus**. On the basis of your knowledge of embryology, what types of **congenital defects** might occur in her offsprings.
4. While taking the round of ward, Professor and HOD of ENT asked the final-year MBBS student to tell the role played by the **otic placode** in the development of internal ear. Discuss the differentiation of **otic vesicle** into **different components of internal ear.**
5. An infant was born with **bilateral microtia**. Give its embryological basis and tell whether the presence of microtia makes the ENT surgeon to think of other associated anomalies.

SOLUTIONS

1. The retinal detachment occurs due to **separation of two layers of the retina** pigment layer and neural layer. For details, see p. 329.
2. The lens develops from thickening of surface ectoderm (**lens placode**) adjacent to the optic cup of forebrain. In addition to molecular and cellular signals essential for lens development, the contact of optic cup with lens placode is utmost essential for its differentiation into the lens.

   Therefore, when molecular and cellular signals essential for lens development are disrupted or when the optic cup fails to contact the lens placode, the lens fails to develop, causing aphakia.
3. The rubella virus is a well-known teratogenic agent to cause **congenital cataracts, deafness**, and other congenital malformations, especially if the mother contracts this virus during 4th to 8th weeks of gestation (pregnancy).
4. The **otic placode** forms as a result of thickening of surface ectoderm and appears on each side of rhombencephalon, as they can be seen in an approximately 22-day-old embryo. They rapidly invaginate to form **otic vesicles** (otocysts). The tubular outpouchings from otocyst differentiate into various components of the internal ear, i.e., **saccule, utricle, semicircular canals, and endolymphatic and cochlear ducts.**
5. **The term microtia stands for a small or rudimentary auricle.** The auricle develops from six mesenchymal proliferations at the dorsal ends of first and second pharyngeal arches. The microtia results from suppressed mesenchymal proliferation. The presence of microtia serves as an indicator of associated congenital anomalies such as an atresia of external auditory meatus and hemifacial microsomia.

N.B. The neural crest cell population plays a key role in most of ear malformations.

29 Medical Genetics

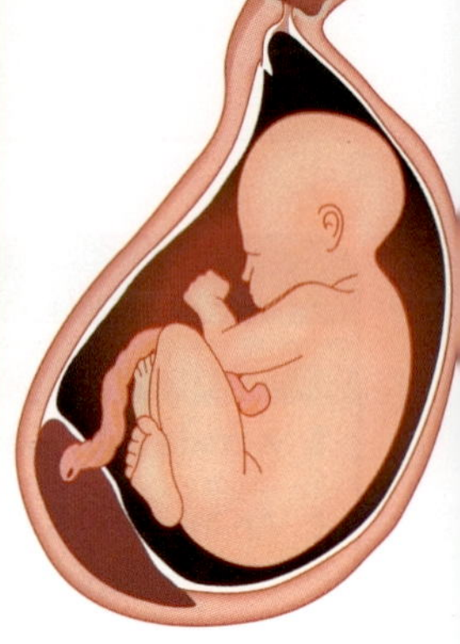

LEARNING OBJECTIVES

After studying this chapter, the student should be able to:

- Give brief description of (a) DNA and (b) sex chromatin.
- Describe the structure of chromosomes with their classification. AN 73.1
- Describe the technique of karyotyping with its applications. AN 73.2
- Describe the Lyon's hypothesis. AN 73.3
- Describe the various modes of inheritance with one example of an associated disease. AN 74.1
- Describe the genetic basis and clinical features of (a) achondroplasia, (b) cystic fibrosis, (c) vitamin D–resistant rickets, (d) hemophilia, (e) Duchene muscular dystrophy, and (f) sickle cell anemia. AN 74.4
- Describe the structural and numerical chromosomal aberrations. AN 75.1
- Write short notes on (a) Down syndrome, (b) Klinefelter syndrome, (c) Turner syndrome, and (d) Marfan syndrome.
- Describe the genetic basis and clinical features of (a) Prader–Willi syndrome, (b) Edward syndrome, and (c) Patau syndrome. AN 75.3
- Explain the term mosaics and chimeras with examples AN 75.2
- Draw pedigree charts for the various type of inheritance and give examples of diseases of each mode of inheritance. AN 74.2
- Describe the multifactorial inheritance with examples. AN 74.3
- Describe the genetic basis of variation: (a) polymorphism and (b) mutation. AN 75.4
- Describe the principles of genetic counseling. AN 75.5

OVERVIEW

Genetics is the study of heredity – a process by which children inherit certain characteristics (traits) from their parents.

These are called **inherited traits** that include physical, mental, normal, and abnormal characteristics in an individual.

The characteristics (traits) pass from parents to children through the inheritable material **(genetic code)** present in the nucleus of the cell. The genetic code is carried by the deoxyribonucleic acid (DNA) molecules. The functional unit of DNA is called **gene**.

The DNA molecules are arranged in linear sequences in chromosomes inside the nucleus of the cell. The total genetic information present in a cell is called **genome**. The human genome comprises about 50,000–100,000 genes.

The gene expression occurs by formation of different types of proteins. The protein is synthesized by transcription of genetic code into the ribonucleic acid (RNA), perpetuated by DNA replication. The RNA forms protein by translation using genetic code. Thus, RNA is an intermediary molecule to execute gene expression.

INTRODUCTION TO GENETICS

The genetics is the study of heredity and inherited variations. The foundation of genetics was laid down by Gregor Mendel in 19th century. He is known as the **father of genetics**.

Basic Fundamentals of Genetics

1. Inheritance of each trait/character is determined by DNA units called **genes**.
2. An individual inherits two genes, one from each parent for one trait (character).
3. Genes are transmitted from one generation to other through gametes.
4. Genes for each trait (character) come in pair.
5. Trait may not show up in an individual but can be passed on to the next generation.
6. At the time of formation of gametes (gametogenesis), members of a pair of gene are separated from each other.
7. When individuals of contrasting traits mate, only one trait is expressed in the first generation. However, both the traits are expressed in the next generation.

HUMAN GENETICS

The human genetics is the study of inheritance in human beings. The term medical genetics refers to application of knowledge of genetics to medical practice.

Branches of Genetics

1. **Cytogenetics:** It deals with the study of chromosomes and genes.
2. **Molecular genetics:** It deals with the study of chemical structure of genes at molecular level.
3. **Developmental genetics:** It is the study of genetic control of embryonic development.
4. **Immunogenetics:** It deals with the genetics of production of various types of antibodies.
5. **Behavioral genetics:** It deals with influence of genes on the behavior of individual.
6. **Population genetics:** It deals with the laws of genetics applicable on human population.
7. **Biochemical genetics:** It deals with the inborn errors of metabolism.

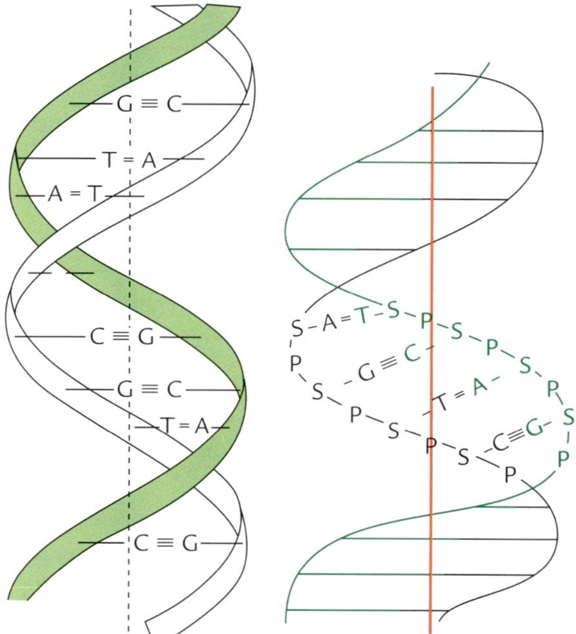

Fig. 29.1 Double helical model of DNA.

Applications of Genetics in Medicine

- To study various diseases that have a genetic background.
- To study factors that control embryonic development.
- To study immunological status of an individual.
- To study the inborn errors of metabolism.
- To make prenatal diagnosis and treatment.
- To do genetic counseling for helping in planning pregnancies.
- To do gene therapy in patients who have a genomic defect.

DEOXYRIBONUCLEIC ACID

DNA is a double-stranded molecule, made up of two chains of nucleotides, coiled around each other, forming what is commonly described as a **double helix.** The double helix model of DNA was first introduced by **James Watson and Francis Crick in 1953** (Fig. 29.1).

The nucleotides are the basic structural units of the DNA.

Each **nucleotide** consists of three subunits:

1. A sugar
2. A phosphate group
3. A nitrogenous base

Each strand of the double helix consists of alternate units of sugar and phosphate. The sugar is **deoxyribose.** The two strands are held together by **hydrogen bonds** between the nitrogenous bases, which are attached to the sugars as side groups and point toward center of the helix. Thus, structure of a DNA molecule is like a twisted ladder. The nitrogenous bases are **adenine** (A), **guanine** (G), **thymine** (T), and **cytosine** (C). The nitrogenous base of two strands in normal conditions pair by hydrogen bonds in a specific manner. For example:

- **Adenine binds with thymine** by two hydrogen bonds (A=T).
- **Guanine binds with cytosine** by three hydrogen bonds (G≡C).

However, under abnormal conditions, when the bases are in **enol form**, adenine may pair with cytosine and guanine with thymine. This is the basis of **mutation of genes.**

The two strands of a DNA molecule are complementary to each other, i.e., if the base sequence of one strand is known, the base sequence of the other strand can be formulated.

The functions of DNA molecule are as follows:

1. **Self-replication:** During nuclear division, the two strands of DNA separate and each strand acts as a template to form a new complementary strand.
2. **Synthesis of RNA and proteins:** Certain regions of DNA serve as a template for the synthesis of RNA, which in turn synthesizes proteins.
3. **Recombination:** During crossing-over in meiosis, there is an exchange of genetic material between homologous chromosomes, which leads to shuffling of genes, and the process is called **recombination.**

4. **Mutation:** It is the major source of genetic variation. Change of base sequence in a gene or gene sequence in the DNA molecule is called **gene mutation.** The mutation may be spontaneous or induced. The inducing agents include chemicals, radiation, etc.

GENE

The gene is a part of single DNA strand made up of distinct **sequence of nucleotides** which can code for a sequence of amino acids to form protein. There are about **1,000 nucleotide pairs** of coding sequence per gene. The genes are described in detail on page 351.

RNA

RNA is structurally similar to single strand of DNA with following two differences:

(a) Sugar molecule in RNA is **ribose sugar,** i.e., **deoxyribose sugar** of DNA is replaced by **ribose** sugar.
(b) Nitrogen base **thymine** is replaced by **uracil.**

Further **uracil** can bind to **adenine** only by hydrogen bond.

Synthesis of RNA and Proteins

DNA molecule acts as a template for synthesis of RNA (Fig. 29.2), which conveys genetic message to synthesize a protein. Therefore, **central dogma of molecular genetics is that genetic information flows from DNA to proteins during gene expression.** It involves two steps as follows:

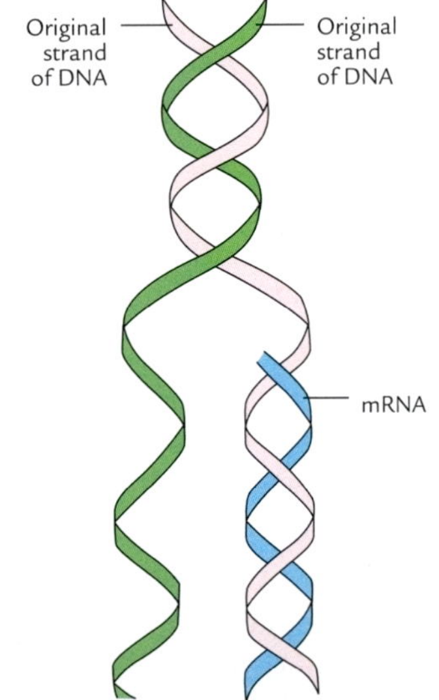

Fig. 29.2 Transcription of mRNA.

*All the cells of body are somatic cells *except* the germ cells.

- DNA $\xrightarrow{\text{transcription}}$ RNA
- RNA $\xrightarrow{\text{translation}}$ Protein

CHROMOSOMES

AN 73.1

The chromosomes (Gr. *Chromosome* = a readily staining body) are deeply stained minute rod-like structures in the nucleus of the cell formed by condensation of chromatin during cell division. These contain DNA encoding genetic information inherited from parents. The individual chromosomes are best defined (visible) under microscope only during metaphase stage of cell division.

Morphological Structure of Chromosomes

Each chromosome presents a primary constriction called **centromere** or **kinetochore.** During cell division (prophase), each chromosome splits longitudinally into two **chromatids**, except at centromere. The centromere divides each chromatid into two arms and is associated with movement of chromosomes during cell division. The free ends of chromatids are known as **telomeres.** The chromatids of some chromosomes present a secondary constriction near one end. The segment of chromatid distal to secondary constriction is called a **satellite body** (Fig. 29.3). Such chromosomes are sometimes called **SAT chromosomes.**

Morphological Types

Depending on the location of centromere, the chromosomes are classified into four types (Fig. 29.4):

1. **Metacentric:** Centromere is located in the middle.
2. **Submetacentric:** Centromere is located close to the middle.
3. **Acrocentric:** Centromere is located close to the end of chromosome.
4. **Telocentric:** Centromere is located at the end of the chromosome.

Number of Chromosomes

The number of chromosomes is constant in a species. In humans, this number is 46 in somatic cells* and 23 in germ

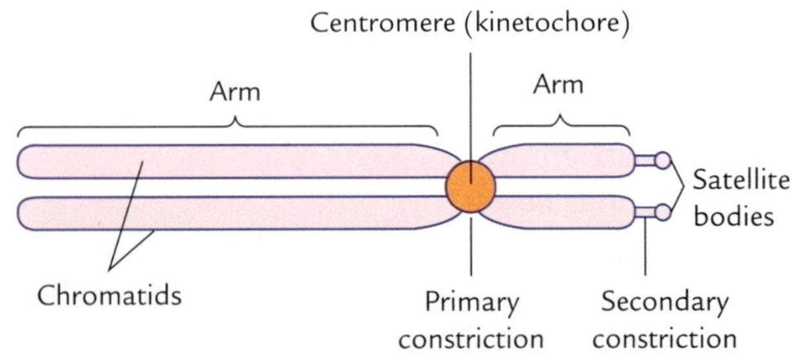

Fig. 29.3 Morphological structure of a chromosome.

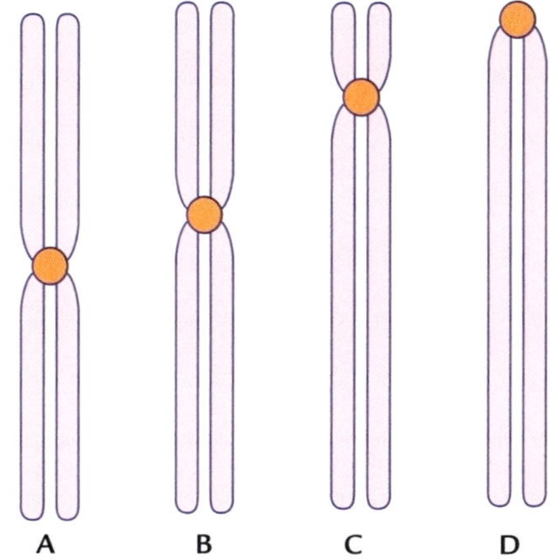

Fig. 29.4 Morphological types of chromosomes: (A) Metacentric, (B) submetacentric, (C) acrocentric, and (D) telocentric.

cells. In somatic cells, these are arranged into 23 pairs, whereas in germ cells, these are not arranged in pairs. A cell with 23 pairs of chromosomes is called **diploid cell** and a cell with 23 chromosomes is called **haploid cell.**

In each pair of chromosomes, one is inherited from mother and one from father. The chromosomes belonging to the same pair are called **homologous chromosomes.** The complete set of chromosomes from a cell is called its **karyotype.**

Two of the 46 chromosomes are called **sex chromosomes** and remaining 44 chromosomes are called **autosomes.**

A normal female has two **X** chromosomes (XX) in each somatic cell, whereas a normal male has one **X** and one **Y** chromosome (XY) in each somatic cell. For convenience, the autosomes are numbered in pairs from 1 to 22. Some genetic disorders occur due to abnormal chromosomal number, e.g., Turner syndrome occurs due to absence of one X chromosome (XO).

KARYOTYPING

AN 73.2

It is a process of sorting and arranging the metaphase chromosomes of a cell **to study the complete chromosomal complement of an individual.**

According to Denver System of Classification (1960), the chromosomes, including sex chromosomes, are arranged into seven groups depending on their (a) size, (b) position of centromere, (c) length ratio between their arms, and (d) presence of satellite bodies on their arms. These groups are referred to by capital letters A–G. This arrangement of chromosomes is called a **karyotype** (Fig. 29.5). The karyotype provides the chromosomal constitution of a cell of an individual.

The features of chromosomes in different groups are presented in Table 29.1.

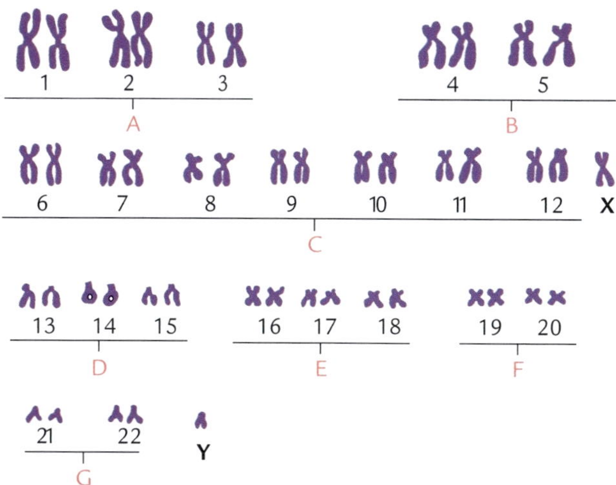

Fig. 29.5 Karyotype of a normal male.

Table 29.1 The characteristic features of pairs of chromosomes in karyotype

Group	Pairs of Chromosomes	Features
A	1, 2, and 3	Long and metacentric
B	4 and 5	Fairly long and submetacentric
C	6–12 + X chromosome	Medium sized and submetacentric
D	13–15	Medium sized and acrocentric; a *satellite body* is attached to the free end of short arm of each chromosome
E	16–18	Fairly short and submetacentric
F	19 and 20	Short and metacentric
G	21 and 22 + Y chromosome	Very short and acrocentric with *satellite bodies* on their short arms

N.B.

- Group A consists of longest metacentric chromosomes.
- Group G consists of shortest acrocentric chromosomes.

The precise identification of individual chromosome is now made possible by noting the patterns of bands on chromosomes by special staining techniques such as G-banding (Fig. 29.6).

CLINICAL CORRELATION

Applications of **karyotyping are in** identifying the structural and numerical variations in chromosomes. Further with chromosomal banding pattern, one can even note certain abnormalities of chromosome structure such as *deletion* and *translocation* of specific regions of chromosomes.

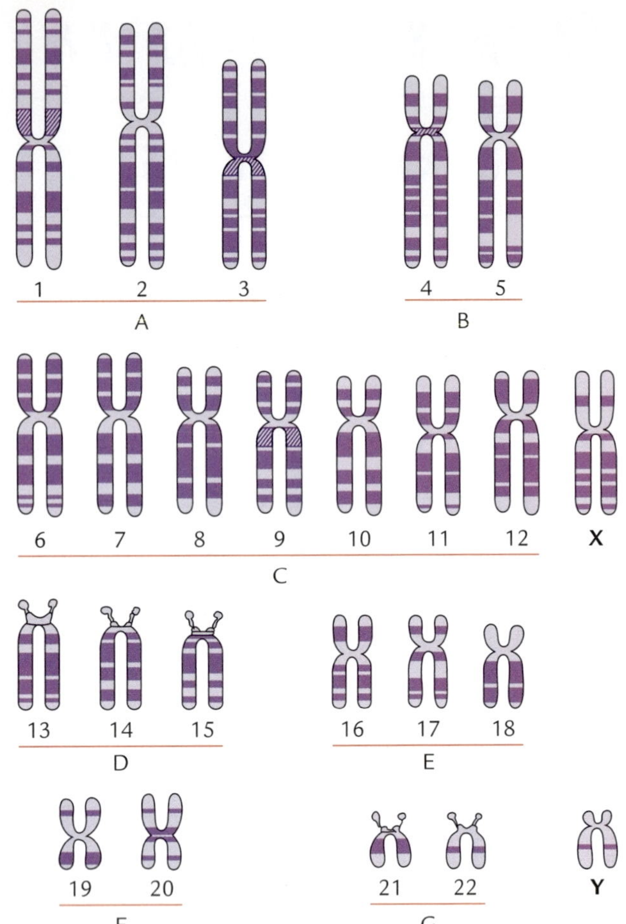

Fig. 29.6 G-banding pattern of chromosomes.

SEX CHROMATIN (BARR BODY; FIG. 29.7)

It is a darkly stained condensed clump of chromatin located subjacent to the nuclear membrane of somatic cells of normal (XX) females. It represents inactivated X chromosome.† During interphase (resting phase) of cell cycle, the chromosomes become uncoiled and thinned-out; consequently, these cannot be identified. The nucleus thus contains a network of **chromatin threads**. However, at some places the chromosome still remains coiled and these are visualized as **chromatin granules**. The uncoiled segments of chromosomes, the **euchromatin**, are genetically active. The coiled segments of chromosomes, the **heterochromatin**, are genetically inactive, i.e., inert. During cell division, each chromosome becomes thicker, shorter, and tightly coiled along its entire length. As a result, the individual chromosomes are visualized and identified.

†In female embryo, at a particular stage of embryogenesis (usually at the blastocyst stage), one of the two X chromosomes is inactivated on a random basis.

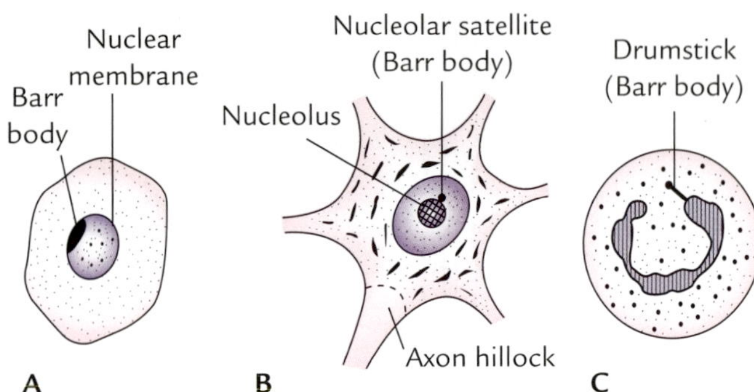

Fig. 29.7 Location of Barr body in (A) buccal smear, (B) neuron, and (C) neutrophil.

During interphase in females, out of two X chromosomes, one becomes highly coiled (genetically inactive) and other remains uncoiled (genetically active). The coiled (genetically inactive) X chromosome is seen as heterochromatic body called **sex chromatin.** It is also called **Barr body** after the name of a Canadian geneticist Murray Barr. It was first noticed by Barr and Bertram (in 1949) in the nucleus of nerve cell of a female cat.

The Barr body is generally located on the inner surface of nuclear membrane as a dark basophilic body of chromatin in most of the cells of the body. It is generally ovoid or plano-convex (Fig. 29.7A). However, in neurons it appears as a small, dark body opposite to the nucleolus (Fig. 29.7B), and in neutrophils, it appears as a knob of 1.5 μmin diameter, known as drumstick (Fig. 29.7C).

N.B. Structurally, the **sex chromatin** is an extra X chromosome which is heterochromatic and genetically inactive.

Y chromosome: During interphase, the Y chromosome in male exhibits within the nucleus of a cell an intensely fluorescent mass called "***F body***" when stained with fluorochrome dye and examined under fluorescent microscope.

Lyon's Hypothesis

According to this hypothesis (formulated by Lyon), the number of Barr bodies in a cell is equal to the total number of X chromosomes minus one. It is also known as "***n*** **– 1 rule,**" where ***n*** represents the number of X chromosomes in the cell. The number of Barr bodies per cell in different conditions in given in Table 29.2.

CHROMOSOMAL ABNORMALITIES

The study of chromosomal abnormalities is of great clinical importance because these produce number of genetic disorders causing various clinical conditions.

Table 29.2 Individual's sex chromosomal constitution and number of Barr bodies per cell

Individual	Sex Chromosomal Constitution	Number of Barr Bodies
Normal male	XY	Nil
Turner syndrome	XO	Nil
Normal female	XX	One
Klinefelter syndrome	XXY	One
Triple X syndrome (superfemale)	XXX	Two

Classification

The chromosomal abnormalities may be classified in a number of ways.

1. **On the basis of type of abnormality:**
   (a) ***Numerical:*** Involving changes in the number of chromosomes, e.g., polyploidy and aneuploidy.
   (b) ***Structural:*** Involving changes in the structure of chromosomes, e.g., deletion and translocation.
2. **On the basis of types of chromosomes involved:**
   (a) ***Involving autosomes***, e.g., Down syndrome.
   (b) ***Involving sex chromosomes***, e.g., Turner syndrome and Klinefelter syndrome.

Numerical Abnormalities

AN 75.1

The numerical abnormalities of chromosomes occur due to failure of meiotic division to occur or due to abnormal meiotic division during the formation of gametes. In normal meiotic division during gametogenesis, both primary spermatocytes and primary oocytes produce four daughter cells, each with 23 chromosomes; and when haploid sperm fertilizes haploid ovum, the diploid zygote (46 chromosomes) is produced (Fig. 29.8).

Sometimes separation of two chromosomes does not occur (**nondisjunction;** Fig. 29.9), either during first meiotic division (Fig. 29.9A) or during second meiotic division (Fig. 29.9B), and then both the members of a pair move into one cell.

As a result of the nondisjunction of the chromosome (Fig. 29.10), one gamete receives 24 chromosomes and the other 22. Consequently, at fertilization, when a gamete (e.g., sperm) having 23 chromosomes fuses with a gamete (e.g., ovum) having 24 or 22 chromosomes, the result will be an individual with either 47 chromosomes (**trisomy**) or 45 chromosomes (**monosomy**), respectively.

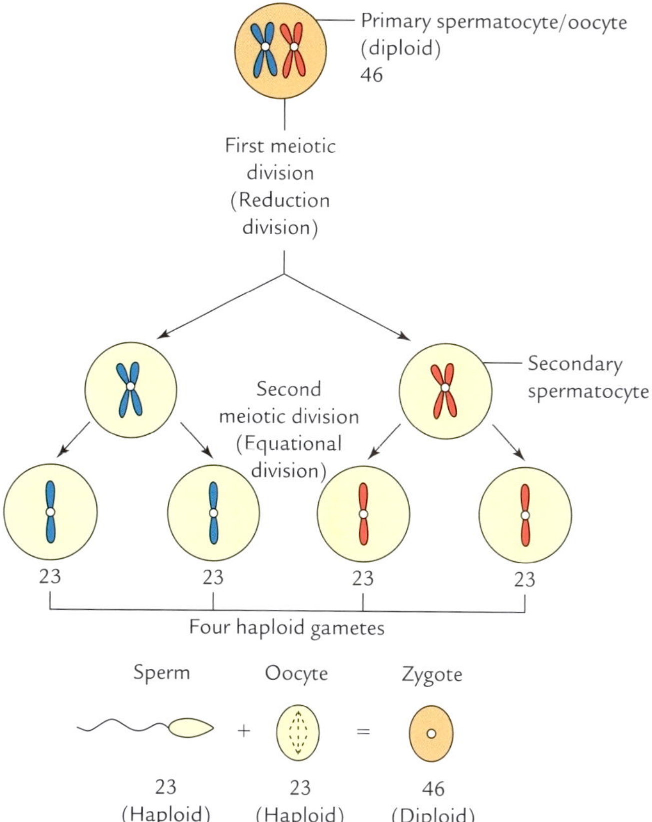

Fig. 29.8 Normal meiotic division producing gametes with 23 chromosomes.

The numerical abnormalities include following conditions:

1. **Polyploidy:** It is a condition in which chromosome number is increased in a multiple of haploid (23) set of chromosomes, of course, in addition to the diploid number. In other words, polyploidy is the condition of extra haploid set/sets of chromosomes (i.e., 23) to normal diploid set of chromosomes (i.e., 46). The examples are given as follows:
   (a) ***Triploidy:*** In this condition, the cells contain 69 chromosomes (23 × 3). It occurs either due to failure of meiosis in germ cell, e.g., fertilization of diploid ovum by a haploid sperm or fertilization of haploid ovum by two haploid sperms (dispermy).

N.B. Triploidy results in spontaneous abortion of the conceptus or brief survival of live-born infant after birth.

   (b) ***Tetraploidy:*** In this condition, the cells contain 92 chromosomes (23 × 4). It occurs due to failure of first cleavage division.

N.B. Tetraploidy results in spontaneous abortion of the conceptus.

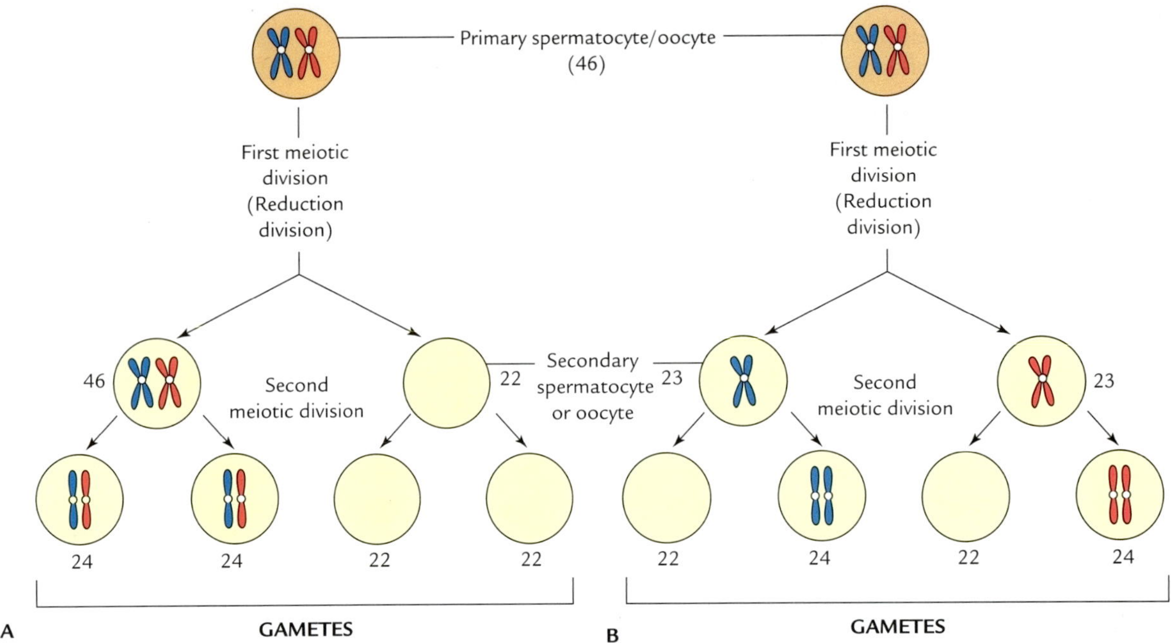

Fig. 29.9 Nondisjunction occurring during meiosis. (A) Nondisjunction in meiosis I producing gametes with 24 and 22 chromosomes. (B) Nondisjunction in meiosis II producing gametes with 24 and 22 chromosomes.

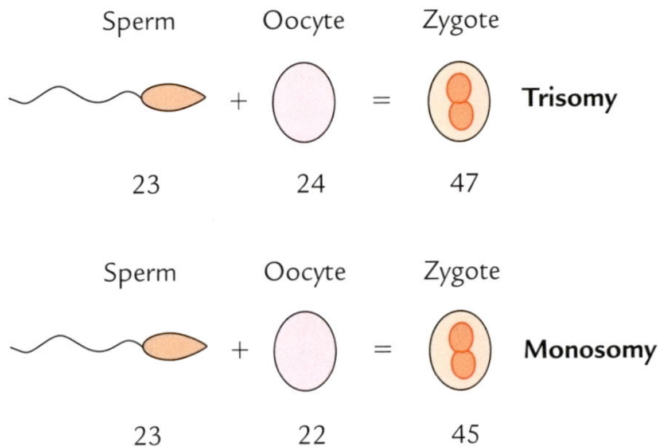

Fig. 29.10 Nondisjunction during oogenesis. Note that if an abnormal oocyte with 24 chromosomes is fertilized by a normal sperm with 23 chromosomes, a zygote with 47 chromosomes is produced (i.e., trisomy). If an abnormal oocyte with 22 chromosomes is fertilized by a normal sperm with 23 chromosomes, a zygote with 45 chromosomes is produced (i.e., monosomy).

2. **Aneuploidy:** It is a condition in which chromosome number is altered by one, i.e., there is an addition of one chromosome (**trisomy**) or loss of one chromosome (**monosomy**). It occurs due to nondisjunction during meiosis (Figs 29.9 and 29.10).

N.B. *Trisomy* usually results in spontaneous abortion of the conceptus; however, *trisomy 13* (Patau syndrome), *trisomy 18* (Edward syndrome), *trisomy 21* (Down syndrome), and Klinefelter syndrome are found in live-born population.

Monosomy also usually results in spontaneous abortion of the conceptus; however, monosomy of X chromosome (45XO), i.e., Turner syndrome is found in live-born population.

Structural Abnormalities

These abnormalities involve change in the structure of chromosome. The types of structural abnormalities include ***deletions, microdeletions, translocation, fragile sites, isochromosomes, inversions,*** and ***breakage.***

The abnormalities in structure cause the following conditions:

1. **Deletions:** It is a condition in which there is a loss of segment of a chromosome, i.e., cri-du-chat syndrome or cat's cry syndrome.

N.B. Sometimes, chromosome is deleted at both the ends, and then the two broken ends adhere/unite in the form of ring called *ring chromosome*, commonly seen due to break points of chromosome 14.

2. **Microdeletions:** In this condition, there is a loss of a segment of chromosome, which can be detected only by a high-resolution banding. The clinical conditions caused by microdeletions include *Prader–Willi syndrome, Angelman syndrome or happy puppet syndrome*, etc.
3. **Translocation:** In this condition, there is breakage and exchange of segments between chromosomes. The examples include the following:
   (a) ***Robertsonian translocation:*** It is a special type of translocation in which breaks occur at the centromeres, e.g., translocation between long

arms of chromosomes 13 and 14 (**most common translocation found in humans**), and chromosomes 21 and 22. The short arms of these chromosomes involved in Robertsonian translocations are generally lost.

(b) ***Reciprocal translocation between chromosome 15 and chromosome 17***: It leads to *acute promyelocytic leukemia*.

(c) ***Reciprocal translocation between chromosome 9 and chromosome 22 (Philadelphia chromosome)***: It leads to *chronic myeloid leukemia*.

4. **Fragile sites:** In this condition, there are gaps or breaks in chromosomes. The clinical examples caused by this condition include **fragile X syndrome** (*Martin–Bell syndrome*).
5. **Isochromosomes:** In this condition, the centromere divides transversely instead of longitudinally. As a result, two arms of a chromosome are separated forming two isochromosomes.
6. **Inversions:** In this condition, a part of chromosome is detached and later unites with the same chromosome in inverted position. As a result, there is a reversal of order of DNA between two breaks in the chromosome. It can be **pericentric** if inversions occur on sides of the centromere, or **paracentric** if inversions occur on the same side of the centromere.
7. **Breakage:** In this condition, there occurs a break in chromosome due to ultraviolet radiation and ionizing radiation.

CLINICAL CORRELATION

DISORDERS DUE TO CHROMOSOMAL ABNORMALITIES AN 75.3

Disorders due to chromosomal abnormalities can be due to numerical or structural abnormalities of chromosomes.

A. **Numerical abnormalities**

1. ***Numerical chromosomal abnormalities affecting autosomes***

(a) **Down syndrome (mongolism) or trisomy 21:** In this disorder, there are three copies of chromosome 21 (**trisomy 21**), i.e., there is an extra chromosome 21. The karyotype of patient is 47XY + 21.

The trisomy 21 is of two types:

(i) **Triplo-21 (nonfamilial mongolism):** It is common and the affected babies possess 47 chromosomes, including two X chromosomes. It occurs during meiosis due to nondisjunction of 21st pair of chromosomes.

(ii) **Translocation mongolism (familial mongolism):** In this, an individual possesses 46 chromosomes. In this condition, the extra chromosome becomes attached to one of the other autosomes.

The Down syndrome occurs 1 in every 700 births (1/700).

Majority of the mongoloid babies have 47 chromosomes with trisomy 21, but about 3% have normal 46 chromosomes with translocation of two 21 chromosomes.

Characteristic clinical features (Fig. 29.11):

The affected individual presents the following features:

- Round face with oblique palpebral fissures and inner epicanthic folds, i.e., mongoloid facies, hence the name mongolism.
- Small nose with shallow bridge and low-set square ears.
- Short and broad hands with single transverse crease in the palm (*Simian crease*) across the bases of four fingers.
- Open mouth with long protruding tongue.
- Mental retardation (IQ 29–50).
- Short stature with hyperflexibility of joints (hypotonia).

N.B.

- **Down syndrome is the best known and one of the most common chromosomal abnormalities in humans.** It was first described in 1886 by L. Down.
- Down syndrome is the most common numerical chromosomal abnormality.

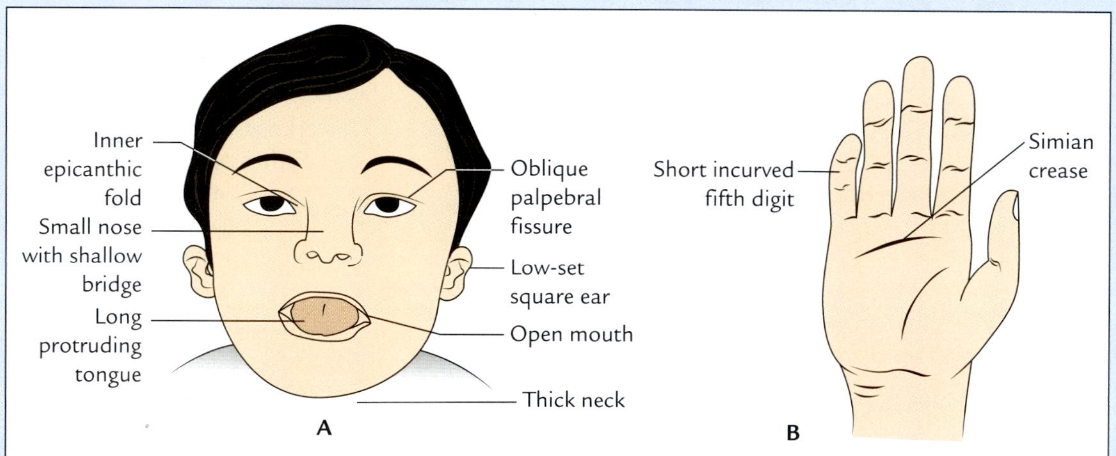

Fig. 29.11 Down syndrome (47XY + 21). (A) Facial features of an infant with Down syndrome. (B) Simian crease.

Continued

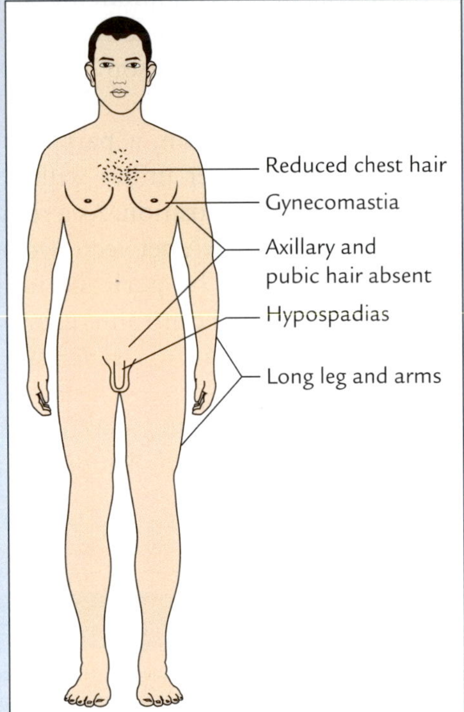

Fig. 29.12 An individual with Klinefelter syndrome (47XXY karyotype; individual is tall, thin, shy, and nervous).

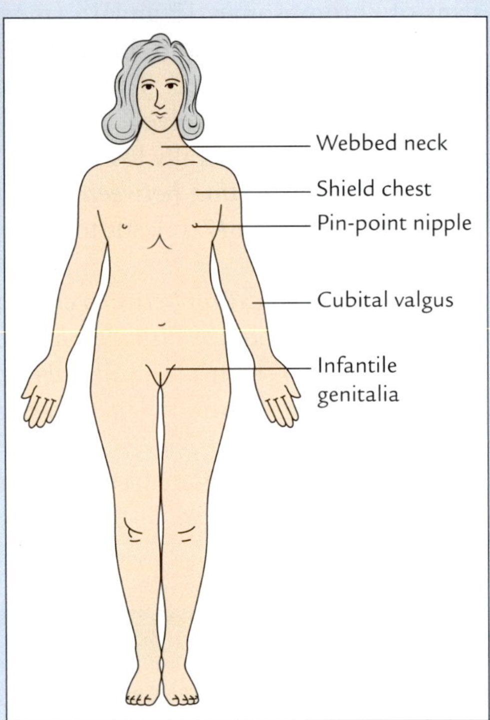

Fig. 29.13 An individual with Turner syndrome (45XO karyotype).

(b) **Patau syndrome:** In this disorder, there are three copies of chromosome 13 (***trisomy 13***). For details see p. 87.

(c) **Edward syndrome:** In this disorder, there are three copies of chromosome 18 (***trisomy 18***). For details see p. 87.

N.B. The Patau and Edward syndromes are very rare conditions and infants with these syndromes usually die within few weeks after birth.

2. ***Numerical abnormalities affecting sex chromosomes***

(a) **Klinefelter syndrome:** It is a trisomic condition found only in males. It is caused by nondisjunction of XX chromosomes during gametogenesis. As a result, the chromosomal complement in somatic cells is XXY. The individual is phenotypically a male but is sex chromatin (Barr body)—positive due to presence of an extra X chromosome. **The karyotype of the individual is 47XXY.**

Characteristic clinical features (Fig. 29.12)

- Affected individual is phenotypically a male with eunuchoid habitus
- Hypogonadism and associated azoospermia and sterility
- Gynecomastia
- Axillary and pubic hair absent, chest hair reduced
- Mental retardation
- Length of legs and arms are usually longer than normal
- Increased gonadotropin levels

N.B. The incidence of Klinefelter syndrome is about 1:500 male births and it increases with advancing maternal age.

(b) **Turner syndrome:** It is a monosomic condition found only in females. It occurs due to loss of one X chromosome following nondisjunction of X chromosome during meiosis. As a result, the chromosomal complement in somatic cells is 45XO. The karyotype of an individual is 45XO.

Characteristic clinical features (Fig. 29.13)

- Affected individual is phenotypically a female
- Short stature and webbing of neck (due to delayed maturation of lymphatics)
- Shield chest with pin-point nipples
- Bilateral cubital valgus
- Low-set ears
- Infantile external genitalia
- Gonadal dysgenesis associated with amenorrhea
- Coarctation of aorta

N.B. The incidence of Turner syndrome is 2:3000 female births. This syndrome is the common cause of *primary amenorrhea.* In 75% of Turner patients, the X chromosome is maternal in origin. Turner syndrome is the only viable monosomy in human beings.

The key differences between Klinefelter and Turner syndromes are presented in Table 29.3.

Table 29.3 Differences between Klinefelter and Turner syndromes

Klinefelter Syndrome	Turner Syndrome
Trisomic condition found only in males	Monosomic condition found only in females
Chromosomal complement in somatic cells is 47XXY	Chromosomal complement in somatic cells is 45XO
Affected individuals are phenotypically males	Affected individuals are phenotypically females
Long stature	Short stature

(c) **Superfemale or triple X syndrome:** It occurs due to fertilization of XX-containing oocyte by an X-containing sperm (gynosperm). The karyotype shows 47 chromosomes. The individual is phenotypically a female with two Barr bodies, hence referred to as "**superfemale.**" The chromosome complement in somatic cell is 47XXX.

Characteristic clinical features

- Female phenotype
- Some degree of mental retardation
- Scanty menses
- Infantile personality

B. *Structural chromosomal abnormalities affecting autosomes*

1. **Cri-du-chat syndrome (cat's cry syndrome):** This condition is caused by a deletion in the short arm of chromosome 5 so that part of chromosome 5 is missing.

   Characteristic clinical features
   - Round face
   - Characteristic cat-like cry (i.e., meowing cry) of a child
   - Hypertelorism
   - Congenital heart defects
   - Microcephaly
   - Mental retardation

2. **Prader–Willi syndrome:** This condition occurs due to microdeletion in the long arm of chromosome 15 derived from father (i.e., *paternal imprinting*).

   Characteristic clinical features

   The affected children present the following features:
   - Hyperphagia (insatiable appetite) and obesity
   - Short stature with small hands and feet
   - Hypotonia
   - Hypogonadism
   - Mild-to-moderate mental retardation
   - Behavioral problems such as rage and violence

3. **Angelman syndrome (happy puppet syndrome):** It occurs due to microdeletion in the long arm of chromosome 15 derived from mother (i.e., *maternal imprinting*). Angelman syndrome is the counterpart of Prader–Willi syndrome.

   Characteristic clinical features
   - Happy disposition with inappropriate laughter
   - Severe mental retardation (IQ: 5–10)
   - Ataxic gait (stiff, jerky, unsteady)
   - Seizures

GENES

Gene, a *functional unit of DNA,* is the unit of inheritance. The term "**gene**" was coined by Johannsen (1909). *The properties of gene include*:

1. To determine traits, e.g., color of skin, intelligence, and height
2. To undergo replication
3. To undergo mutation

About 50,000–100,000 genes are present in the **human genome**; out of these, about 450 genes are linked to human diseases.

Functions of Genes

1. Maintain the genetic specificity of an individual.
2. Play key role in transmission of traits from the parents to the offspring.
3. Synthesize various proteins and enzymes of cell.

Types of Genes

The genes are classified into various types. It is beyond the scope of this book to describe all the types. The present account deals with only two (major) types of genes. These are as follows:

1. **Structural genes:** These are those DNA segments that code for specific amino acid sequences in a protein.
2. **Regulatory genes:** These are those DNA segments that control structural genes being transcribed for synthesis of a protein.

Location of Genes

Each gene occupies a specific **locus** on a chromosome. Both chromosomes of a given pair contain similar genes. The two homologous chromosomes of a pair contain alleles of same genes occupying the same locus. If two allelic genes are identical, the person is **homozygous** for the trait specified by that gene locus. For example, ability to roll one's tongue is coded on a single gene. Since one chromosome of each pair is inherited from father and one from mother, an individual has two genes controlling the ability to roll the tongue. Such paired genes are **alleles.**

If the two alleles are different, the person is **heterozygous** for that trait. For example, one copy of tongue rolling gene may code for the ability to roll the tongue, whereas the corresponding gene on the other chromosome may code for inability to roll the tongue. Note that this example involves only two forms of the same gene. Some traits like eye color are controlled by more than one gene.

During reproduction, each male and female contribute 23 chromosomes to the zygote. Therefore, for any given pair of alleles controlling a given trait, the female contributes one allele and male contributes one allele.

An exception occurs with X and Y chromosomes as there are no alleles on the Y chromosome for most of the loci on the X chromosome.

The paired chromosomes are called homologous chromosomes (Fig. 29.14). In females, the two sex chromosomes (XX) are identical in length; hence, these are homologous. In males, the two sex chromosomes (XY)

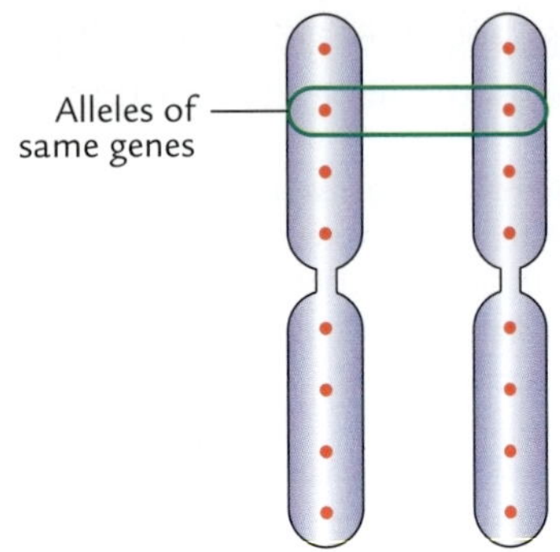

Fig. 29.14 Homologous chromosomes with genes located on same loci.

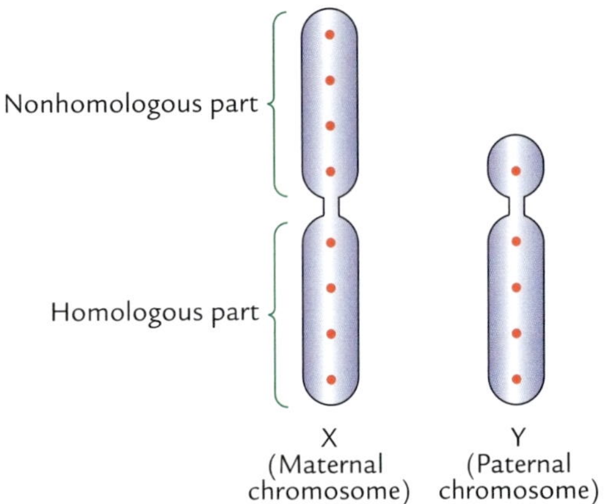

Fig. 29.15 Nonhomologous male sex chromosomes (XY) with homologous and nonhomologous parts.

Table 29.4 Differences between homologous and nonhomologous pairs	
Homologous Chromosomes	**Nonhomologous Chromosomes**
Chromosomes belong to same homologous pairs, one from father and one from mother	Chromosomes belong to different homologous pairs
Consists of alleles of same genes located on the same loci	Consists of alleles of different genes located on different loci
Pair during meiosis I for exchange of genetic recombination	Do not pair during meiosis I for genetic recombination (however, parts can be exchanged during translocation)
Examples: • 22 pairs of autosomal chromosomes • XX pair of sex chromosomes in female	Examples: • 23rd pair of XY sex chromosomes in male

are unequal in length – X chromosome is longer than Y chromosome; hence, these have homologous and nonhomologous parts. Therefore, a pair of XY chromosome is called nonhomologous pair (Fig. 29.15).

The differences between homologous and nonhomologous pairs of chromosomes are given in Table 29.4.

Dominant and Recessive Genes

If gene produces its effect, whether it is present on one or both chromosomes of a pair, it is called **dominant gene.** If it produces its effect only when it is present on both chromosomes, it is called **recessive gene.** In other words, the **dominant traits** are always expressed even if they have only one copy of dominant allele. The recessive traits are expressed only if they have two copies of recessive alleles. Thus, diseases are inherited through both dominant and recessive genes called dominant inheritance and recessive inheritance, respectively.

N.B. Individuals receive two versions of each gene, one from mother and one from father, called **alleles.** If two alleles are different, only one allele will be expressed.

POLYMORPHISM AND MUTATION

The polymorphism is a variation or change in a DNA sequence which is common in a particular population, whereas mutation is a change in DNA sequence away from normal.

Polymorphism

It is normal genetic variation within a population due to presence of more than one form of a trait or gene, i.e., if more than one allele occupies a specific locus of a gene, then that gene is termed as **polymorphic gene.** In other words, it is inheritance of different forms (alleles) of a gene.

Clinical Significance

- The polymorphic genes can cause abnormal formation of proteins/enzymes which may be associated with many diseases such as **hypertension, ischemic heart disease,** and **angina pectoris.**
- Polymorphism plays an important role in **major histocompatibility complex** (MHC).
- Polymorphism plays an important role in production of drugs.

N.B.
- The polymorphism can be detected in genetic labs by performing a polymerase chain reaction (PCR).
- The genetic polymorphism is generally considered as a normal variant in population, when specific alleles occur at least in 1% population.

Mosaicism

In this condition, an individual contains cells of two genetically different types. It affects any type of cell, i.e., somatic cells and germ cells. It occurs when mutation occurs early in life.

The examples of mosaicism are as follows:
Mosaic Down syndrome
Mosaic Klinefelter syndrome
Mosaic Turner syndrome

Chimerism

In this condition, an individual contains two or more population of cells with different genotypes, similar to mosaicism but two or more genotypes arise from the fusion of two or more zygotes in the early stages of embryonic development.

The differences between mosaicism and chimerism are given in Table 29.5.

Mutation

The mutation is a permanent change in genomic sequence.

It can be caused by the alteration of a single base units in DNA, or the deletion, insertion, or rearrangement of larger sections of genes or chromosomes. These changes are irreversible and heritable.

Mutagens

Substances causing mutation are called mutagens.

For examples:

1. Radiation by UV light or X-rays
2. Chemicals
3. Viruses
4. Jumping genes (transposons) in a DNA sequence

The mutation can occur at the level of gene (**gene mutation**) or at the level of chromosome (**chromosomal mutation**).

About 70% mutations are harmful. The rest have either no effects or may even have some beneficial effects.

Types of Mutation

The eukaryotes have two primary cells types:
(a) Somatic cells
(b) Germ cells

The mutation can occur in the somatic cells or in the germ cells.

(a) **Somatic mutations**

As the name indicates, these occur in somatic cells, hence not passed into the subsequent generation. Furthermore, majority of these mutations are phenotypically silent but some are expressed in the individual containing the mutation.

(b) **Germline mutations**

- As the name indicates, these occur in germ cells.
- Only some gametes arising from germ cells will carry mutant gene. Then it can be passed into the subsequent generation by sexual means.

Usually, the germ cell mutations are not expressed in the individual carrying the mutation.

The differences between somatic and germline mutations are given in Table 29.6.

N.B. Mutation of gene or genes leads to genetic disorders.

INHERITANCE AN 74.1

Inheritance is the process of transmission of characters/traits from generation to generation. The reproduction is an essential requisite for the inheritance to take place. The inheritance of traits from parents to offspring takes

Table 29.5 Differences between mosaicism and chimerism

Mosaicism	Chimerism
• Presence of two or more population of cells with different genotypes	• Presence of two or more population of cells with different genotypes
• Two or more population of cells arise from single zygote	• Two or more population of cells arise due to fusion of two zygotes
• Occurs due to somatic cells and germ cells	• Occurs due to fusion of two or more zygotes

Table 29.6 Differences between the somatic and germline mutations

Somatic Mutation	Germline Mutation
Occurs in somatic cells, hence not transmitted to the children	Occurs in germ cells, hence transmitted to children
Can cause cancer	Can cause certain types of cancer, e.g.: – Retinoblastoma (eye tumor) – Wilms tumor (malignancy of kidney)
People are mosaics	People are not mosaics

place through genes which carry all information about all types of traits. The genes are located in both autosomes and sex chromosomes. The inheritance occurring through genes of autosomes is called **autosomal inheritance**, whereas inheritance occurring through genes of sex chromosomes is called **sex-linked inheritance**.

The inheritance which occurs due to interaction of gene and environmental factors, i.e., infectious agents, drugs, or ionizing radiation is called **multifactorial inheritance**.

Types of Inheritance

There are three types of inheritance (vide supra) as follows:

1. Autosomal inheritance
2. Sex-linked inheritance
3. Multifactorial inheritance

Principles of Inheritance

- A disease exhibits **autosomal dominant inheritance** when an abnormal allele in an autosomal locus is sufficient to cause disease in both homozygous and heterozygous states (e.g., TT or Tt; T = tall and t = short).
- A disease exhibits autosomal recessive inheritance when one abnormal allele in an autosomal locus is able to express only in a homozygous state (e.g., tt; t = short).

Sex-linked genes are abnormal genes located on X or Y chromosome.

Each chromosome of a homologous pair contains genes for the same traits.

PUNNETT SQUARE

The Punnett square is a chart which is used in genetics to predict all possible outcomes of a particular breeding or cross, i.e., to determine the probability of offspring having a particular genotype.

Thus, **Punnett square is a tabulated visual representation of Mendelian inheritance**.

While constructing the Punnett square, the genotype of father (paternal alleles of genes) is kept in top squares of the horizontal row and genotype of mother (maternal alleles of genes) is kept in the squares of vertical row (i.e., side squares).

The genotype of offspring in all possible combinations is then entered into remaining large squares. For example, the Punnett square of tongue rolling parents is shown in Fig. 29.16.

		PATERNAL GENES	
		T	t
MATERNAL GENES	T	TT	Tt
	t	Tt	tt

Fig. 29.16 Punnett square showing sex-linked inheritance.
TT = Tongue-roller homozygous
Tt = Tongue-roller heterozygous
Tt = Tongue-roller heterozygous
tt = Nonroller homozygous

PEDIGREE CHART (FIG. 29.17)

AN 74.2

The preparation of a pedigree chart is a procedure through which gene mapping is done.

- It is dependent on the study of segregation of *marker genes* in families with genetic disorders.
- The pedigree chart is a useful document that helps in determining mode of inheritance of a

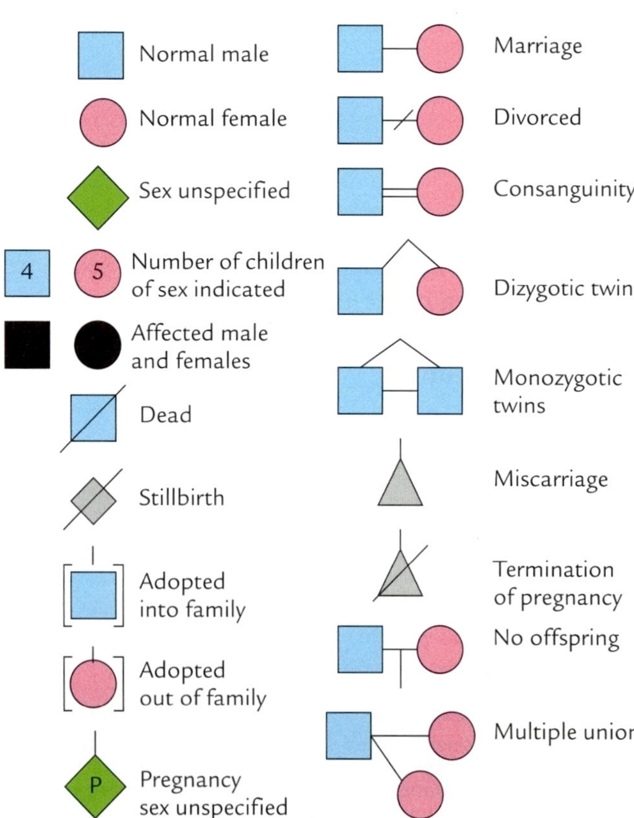

Fig. 29.17 Symbols used in pedigree chart.

particular genetic disorder, which is an essential requisite in *genetic counseling*. By preparing pedigree chart, one can explain the inheritance patterns and predict risks for various family members to have offspring with genetic diseases (recurrence risks).

Methodology of Preparing a Pedigree Chart

A graphic representation of a generation of a family is made by using various symbols. The symbols represent relationships, clinical findings, etc.

The steps of making pedigree chart are as follows:

- Extract information
- Use standard symbols with key for interpretation
- Identify information and use other family members for documentation of information
- Ask details about adoption, abortion, stillbirth, etc.
- Ask about history of consanguinity

The standard symbols used for making pedigree chart are given in Fig. 29.17.

Autosomal Inheritance

AN 74.4

Autosomal Dominant Inheritance (Fig. 29.18)

When one parent is affected (i.e., have an abnormal dominant allele), then 50% children are affected. The pedigrees involving autosomal dominant disease exhibit vertical pattern of inheritance from one generation to the other. The examples of disorders caused by autosomal inheritance are as follows:

- **Marfan syndrome**
- **Achondroplasia**
- **Brachydactyly**
- **Neurofibromatosis**
- **Osteogenesis imperfecta**
- **Huntington's disease**

N.B. The unaffected members of family do not transmit the trait further.

Affected parent (Aa)

Normal parent (aa)		A	a
	a	Aa	aa
	a	Aa	aa

Aa = An affected heterozygous (50%)
aa = Normal homozygous (50%)

Affected parent (Aa)

Affected parent (Aa)	Parent	A	a
	A	AA	Aa
	a	Aa	aa

AA = An affected homozygous (25%) (severely affected)
Aa = An affected heterozygous (50%)
aa = Normal homozygous (25%)

A. Percentage of genetic risk in an autosomal dominant disorder.

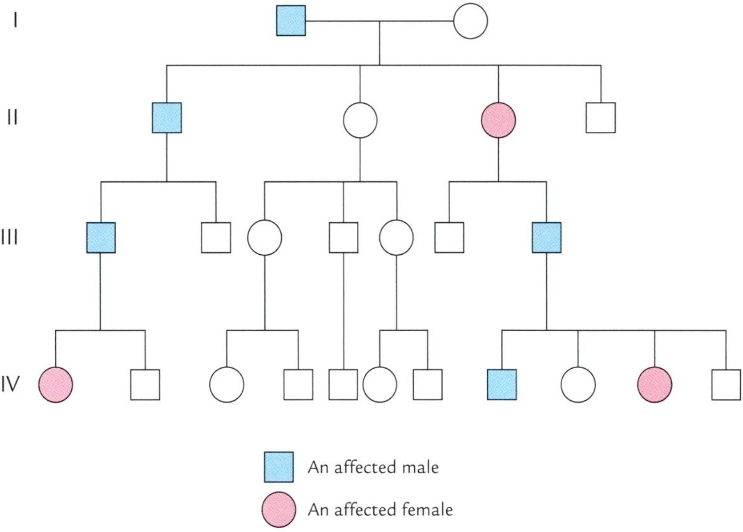

B. Pedigree of an autosomal dominant disorder.

Fig. 29.18 Autosomal dominant disorder.

Autosomal Recessive Inheritance (Fig. 29.19)

In this, the disease is transmitted by a couple, both of whom are carriers of an abnormal gene, but they themselves are not affected, i.e., only siblings are affected but parents are normal. This inheritance shows horizontal pattern where many individuals in a single generation are affected. The risk of children affected is 25% in carrier couple. The parents are usually close relatives (cousins). The examples of autosomal recessive disorders are as follows:

- Cystic fibrosis
- Inborn errors of metabolism
- Hemoglobinopathies, e.g., sickle cell anemia and thalassemia

N.B. The presence of consanguinity alerts parents to the possibility of an autosomal recessive disorder in children.

Sex-Linked Inheritance

The **Y** chromosome is shorter than **X** chromosome. Therefore, traits coded on the nonhomologous part of X chromosome have no corresponding traits on the Y chromosome. These genes on sex chromosomes are called **sex linked,** those on X chromosome are X linked, and those on Y chromosome are Y linked.

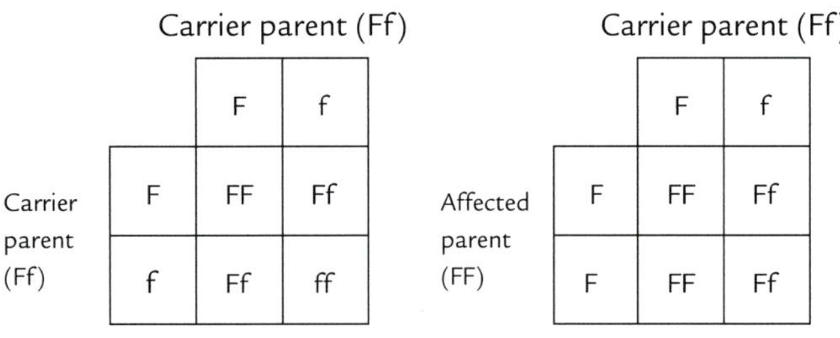

ff = Normal homozyous (25%)
Ff = Heterozygous carrier (50%)
FF = Affected heterozygous (25%)

FF = Affected heterozygous (50%)
Ff = Heterozygous carrier

A. Percentage of genetic risk in autosomal recessive disorder.

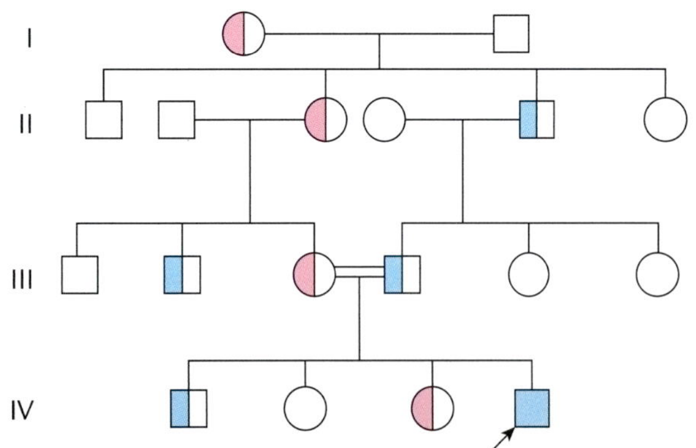

B. Pedigree of autosomal recessive trait.

Fig. 29.19 Autosomal recessive disorder.

The genes that are carried by sex chromosomes are called **sex-linked genes.**

Since men inherit only one **"Y"** chromosome, they inherit only Y-linked inheritance. The question of dominant and recessive inheritance does not arise.

On the contrary, women inherit two XX chromosomes; hence, they have both X-linked dominant inheritance as well as X-linked recessive inheritance.

X-Linked Inheritance

X-linked genes are exclusive to X chromosome. For example, the gene that codes for normal **color vision** is carried only on the X chromosome. It is the dominant form of gene. There is a **rare, faulty, recessive form of this gene** that codes **for red–green blindness.** If female inherits a faulty gene, she is likely to have a normal gene on her other chromosome that provides normal color vision. A female carrying the faulty gene (color blindness gene), even though she is not a color blind, may pass the faulty gene onto her children and thus she is called a **carrier**. If the gene is faulty in male, he will be color blind because he has only one X chromosome and so will have only one copy of the gene.

N.B. The ability to discern red–green color depends entirely on X chromosome.

X-linked dominant inheritance (Fig. 29.20)

- ***It is less common than sex-linked recessive disorder.***
- It occurs more frequently in females than males (2:1).
- The affected male transmits the trait to all his daughters and none to his sons.
- The affected females if homozygous, they will transmit the trait to all of her children.

The affected females, if heterozygous, they will transmit the trait to half of her children.

For examples:

- **Vitamin D—resistant rickets**
- **Hypophosphatemia**
- **Xg blood group**

X-linked recessive inheritance (Fig. 29.21)

The females are carriers. Their one X chromosome contains abnormal gene. The gene on other X chromosome is normal.

- The trait is transmitted by male through daughters to half of their sons.
- No male-to-male transmission occurs because father contributes only Y chromosome to his sons.

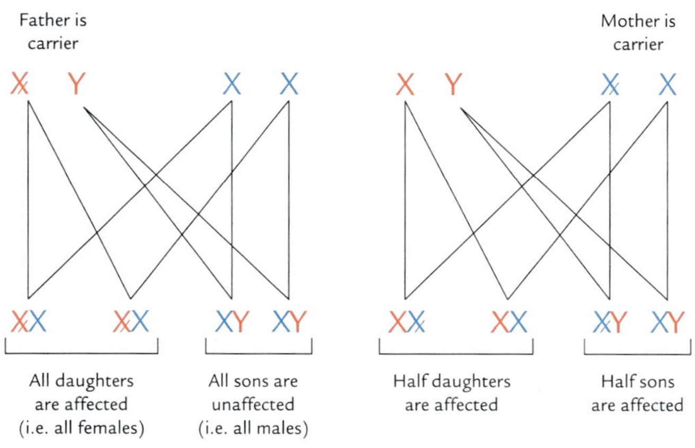

A. Percentage of risk affecting sons and daughters.

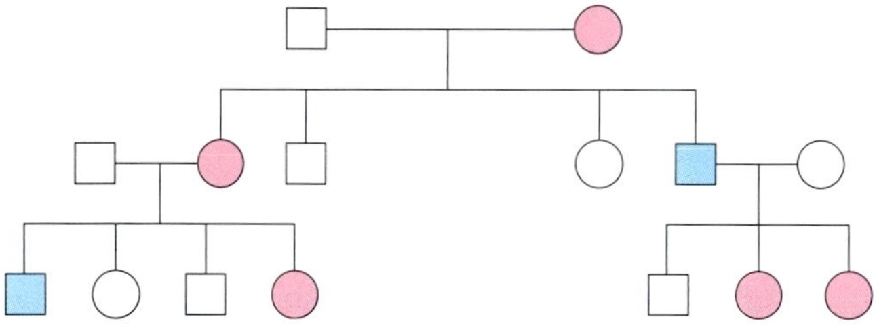

B. Pedigree of X-linked dominant disorder.

Fig. 29.20 X-linked dominant inheritance.

For examples:

- **Hemophilia**
- **Color blindness (red-green color blindness)**
- **Diabetes mellitus**
- **Duchenne muscular dystrophy (DMD)**

N.B.

- The trait usually affects males.
- For a female to be color blind for red and green color, she has to have a recessive allele (color blind gene) on both of her X chromosomes (XcXc). This is possible only if her mother is a carrier (XCXc) and her father is a color blind (XcY).
- Capital 'C' = Normal gene
- Small 'c' = Faulty gene

Y-Linked Inheritance (Holandric Inheritance)

Since males have only one Y chromosome, the gene is necessarily unpaired. Therefore, if present, it will be expressed and the question of dominance and recessiveness does not arise. Further the gene will be passed on from affected male to all his sons, e.g., characteristic growth of hair on the pinna of ear. This is the only Y-linked gene inheritance and hence **for all practical purposes, sex linked means X linked.**

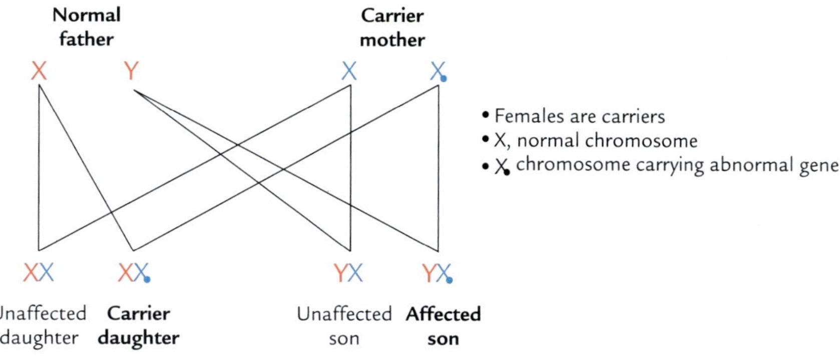

A. Percentage of risk affecting sons and carrier daughters.

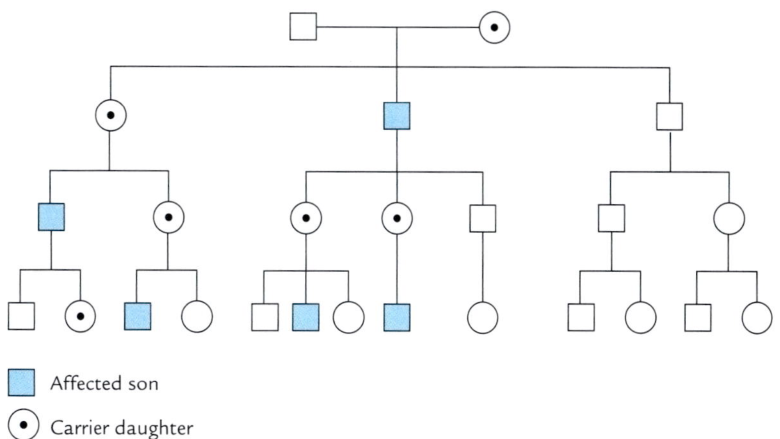

B. Pedigree of X-linked recessive disorder.

Fig. 29.21 X-linked recessive inheritance.

Multifactorial Inheritance AN 74.3

The multifactorial inheritance occurs as a result of interaction of genes and environmental factors. Some examples of congenital disorders caused by multifactorial inheritance are as follows:

- Neural tube defects
- Cleft lip
- Cleft palate
- Club foot
- Congenital dislocation of hip
- Congenital heart defects

N.B. Nongenetic factors that contribute to multifactorial inheritance include:

- *Drugs*, e.g., thalidomide and anticonvulsants.
- *Infections*, e.g., rubella virus.
- *Ionizing radiations*, e.g., X-rays and radioactive substances.

SINGLE-GENE INHERITED DISEASES AN 75.3

1. ***Autosomal dominant disorders:***
   (a) ***Marfan syndrome*** (Fig. 29.22): It is an inherited autosomal dominant connective tissue disorder.
   Characteristic clinical features
   - Long spidery fingers (arachnodactyly)
   - Arm span greater than height
   - Saucer or funnel-shaped chest (pectus excavatum)
   - Scoliosis
   - A high-arched palate
   - Ectopic lens
   - Aortic dilatation or dissection

   (b) ***Achondroplasia***
   - It is an inherited autosomal dominant disorder which occurs due to mutation in FGFR3 gene.
   - Parents of persons with achondroplasia mostly have normal stature.
   - Interferes with growth of long bones due to defective bone formation in the epiphyseal regions.
   - Individual remains dwarf.

2. ***Autosomal recessive disorders:***
   (a) ***Cystic fibrosis (CF):***
   It is caused by autosomal recessive disorder due to mutation of CF gene which is located on the long arm of chromosome 7.
   It causes production of abnormally thick secretion of mucus by epithelial cells lining the respiratory and gastrointestinal tracts, particularly in the first one.
   Characteristic clinical features
   The affected individual presents the following features:
   - Obstruction of respiratory airways
   - Recurrent respiratory infections

   (b) ***Sickle cell anemia:***
   - Synthesis of abnormal hemoglobin.
   - Red blood cells become sickle shaped.
   - Cells die early leaving shortage of healthy blood cells, leading to anemia.
   - The sickle cell anemia is a recessive trait.
   - It occurs due to mutation in hemoglobin beta gene found on chromosome 11.
   - Being a recessive trait of gene, it can occur only if you have two copies of recessive alleles, one from father and one from mother.

3. ***X-linked dominant disorder:***
   Vitamin D–resistant rickets/hypophosphatemic rickets:
   - It occurs due to renal phosphate washing resulting in adequate mineralization of bones.
   - Bones become painfully soft and bend easily due to low level of phosphate in the blood.
   - Symptoms typically begin in early childhood, leading to characteristic bowing and deformity of lower limbs.

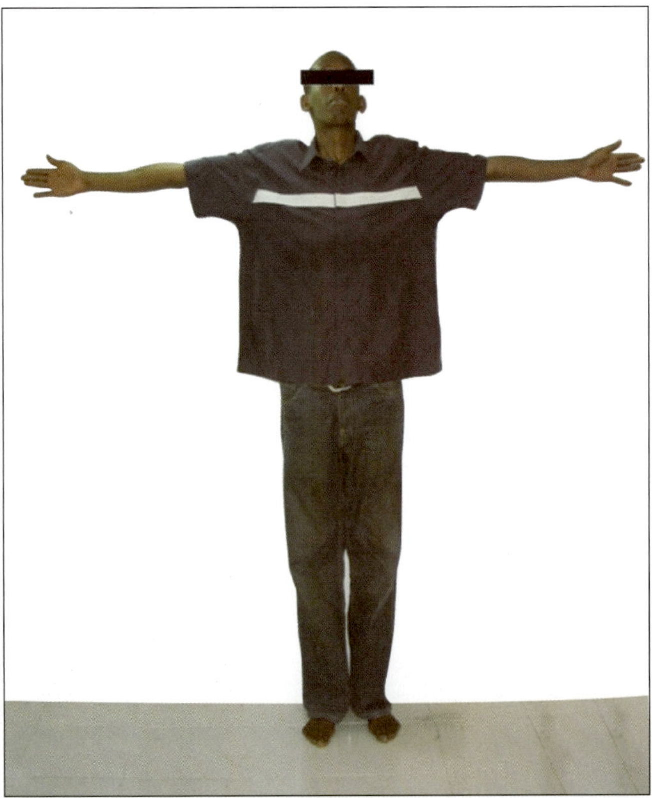

Fig. 29.22 Marfan syndrome.

4. ***X-linked recessive disorders:***
   (a) ***Duchenne muscular dystrophy (DMD):*** It is a hereditary disease of skeletal muscle which usually affects males. DMD is caused by an **X-linked recessive mutation**. The DMD gene is located on the short arm of chromosome X. The DMD gene encodes for a protein called **dystrophin**, on the inner surface of sarcolemma of muscle fibers which anchors the actin (cytoskeleton) of skeletal muscle cells to extracellular matrix. Thus, mutation of DMD gene destroys the ability of dystrophin to anchor actin to the extracellular matrix. Consequently, the skeletal muscles become progressively weak from early childhood, and by the time the patient reaches adolescence, he becomes completely immobile.

   Characteristic clinical features
   - Most common type of muscular dystrophy.
   - Affects 1 in 4000 males at birth.
   - Progressive muscle weakness and wasting.
   - Premature death due to cardiac and respiratory failure.

   (b) ***Hemophilia:*** The hemophilia results due to deficiency or dysfunction of clotting factor VIII. It occurs due to mutation of X-linked recessive gene located on one X chromosome, which is responsible for clotting factor VIII.

   Characteristic clinical features
   - Related episodes of excessive bleeding with little trauma particularly from gums, but virtually no tissue is exempted.
   - When bleeding follows trauma, it is characteristically prolonged.
   - Bleeding tendency may range from mild to severe.
   - Excessive bleeding is unusual until the baby is about 6 months old.

   N.B. In hemophilia, clotting factor VIII is abnormal.

   (c) ***Red and green color blindness:*** The gene that codes of normal color vision is a dominant gene and is located only on nonhomologous part of X-chromosomes.

   The red and green color blindness occurs due to presence of rare recessive form of gene that codes for color vision.

   This recessive gene codes for red and green color blindness.

   For example, if the mother is carrying color blindness gene on one of her X chromosomes, she is likely to have normal gene on her other X chromosome, which provides her normal color vision, but she may pass faulty gene on to her children. If the faulty gene passes to son, he will be color blind because he has only one copy of this faulty gene. The daughter will be normal but carrier (Fig. 29.23).

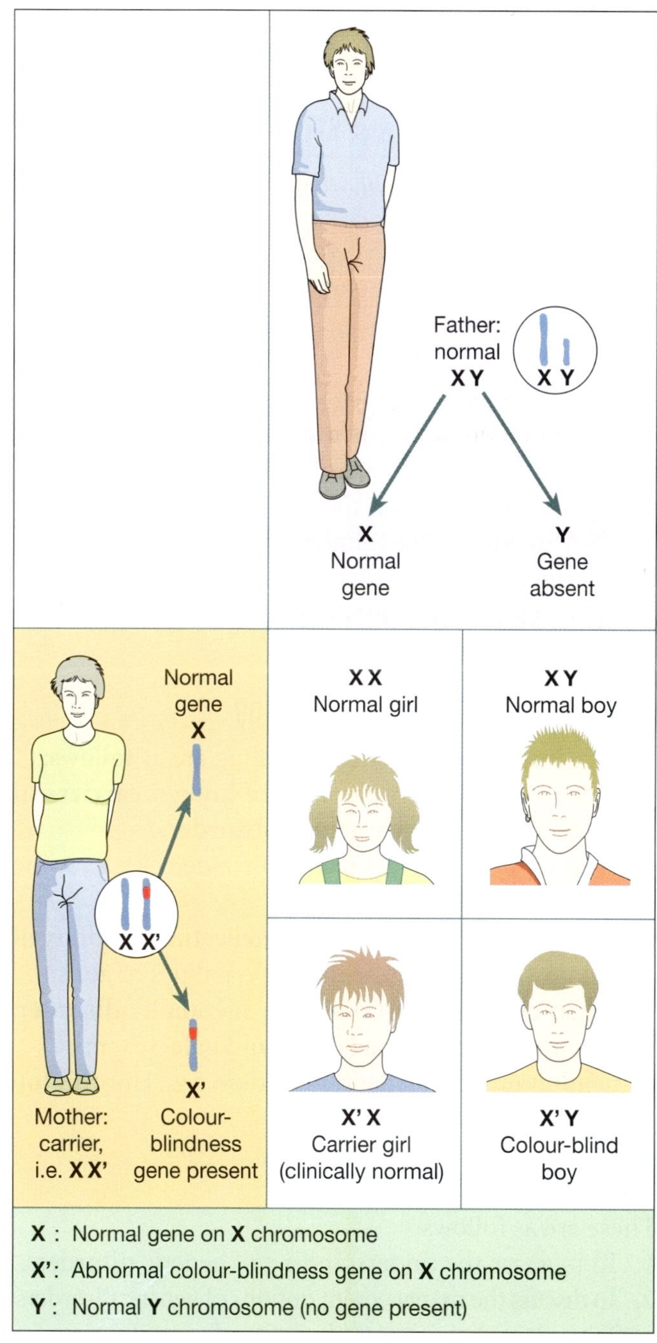

Fig. 29.23 Inheritance of the sex-linked red–green color blindness gene between generations. (*Source: Ross and Wilson Anatomy & Physiology in Health and Illness*: Anne Waugh and Allison Grant, Figure 17.11, page 445, 12th Edition, Churchill Livingstone, Elsevier, 2014.)

Clinical features

- Mostly affects males.
- Difficulty in distinguishing different shades of red, green, brown, and orange.
- Confusion in differentiating blue and purple hues.

The red and green color blindness is also described on p. 359.

GENETIC COUNSELING

SPECIFIC LEARNING OBJECTIVES

After studying this section, the student should be able to:

- Define genetic counseling.
- Tell the steps to follow in the process of genetic counseling.
- Calculate the recurrence risk of the genetic disorder.
- Enumerate the goals of genetic counseling.
- Enumerate the benefits of genetic counseling.

INTRODUCTION

The genetic counseling is a process by which parents and their relatives who are at the risk of inherited disorders are advised about the following three things:

(a) **Nature and consequences of genetic disorder.**
(b) **Chances of transmitting the genetic disorder.**
(c) **How to prevent, avoid, or improve the outcome of the disorder.**

Indications of Genetic Counseling

The indications of genetic counseling are as follows:

- When one or both parents are **known carriers of certain trait to cause genetic disorder.**
- When children are born with birth defect, e.g., **spina bifida** and **cleft lip/palate**
- When children are born with **intellectual disability of unknown cause,** e.g., learning disabilities or autism.
- When children are born with **metabolic disorder,** e.g., **phenylketonuria (PKU) and galactosemia.**
- In adult onset of genetic condition, e.g., **Huntington disease or hereditary cancers.**

Goals of Genetic Counseling

These are as follows:

1. To increase the understanding of genetic disorders.
2. To discuss the management options of genetic disorders.
3. To explain the risks and benefits of prenatal tests for genetic disorders.

Who Should Go for Genetic Counseling?

1. People having family history of genetic disorders.
2. Females older than 35 years planning to have a child.
3. When there is increased nuchal translucency measuring 3 mm or more detected by ultrasound scanning at 12 weeks and 5 days.

N.B. Nuchal translucency is produced due to fluid collecting behind the neck.

Benefits of prenatal counseling to parents

- Can calculate the likelihood of baby to be born with genetic disorder, e.g., **Down syndrome, cystic fibrosis,** and **sickle cell anemia**
- Can have better peace of mind.
- Can plan appropriate testing.
- Can plan early intervention.
- Can help in decision-making.

Steps followed in genetic counseling

1. Accurate diagnosis of disorder.
2. Survey of relatives with similar conditions.
3. Management – it includes early detection and interaction.
4. Follow-up to prevent occurrence in next generation.

GOLDEN FACTS TO REMEMBER

➤ **Father of genetics**	Gregor Johann Mendel (discovered fundamental laws of inheritance in 1865)
➤ **Correct structure of DNA was first deduced by**	James Watson and Francis Crick (1953)
➤ **Structural unit of DNA**	Gene
➤ **The term "gene" was first coined by**	Johannsen (1909)
➤ **Unit of inheritance**	Gene
➤ **Number of genes in human genome**	50,000–100,000
➤ **Most important intermediary molecule for gene expression**	RNA
➤ **Best known and most common chromosomal abnormality**	Down syndrome (trisomy 21)
➤ **Only viable monosomy in human beings**	Turner syndrome (45XO)
➤ **Most common translocation in chromosomes of human beings**	Robertsonian translocation
➤ **Most common hereditary bleeding disorder**	Hemophilia
➤ **Most common X-linked gene disorder**	Red and green color blindness
➤ **Most important process required for inheritance**	Reproduction
➤ **Most X-linked disorders are recessive conditions *except***	Vitamin D−resistant rickets that is X-linked dominant condition
➤ **Only known condition that is Y linked**	Hairy pinna in male
➤ **In all living organisms, the genetic information is stored in DNA *except***	In some viruses (RNA viruses) in which the genetic information is stored in RNA
➤ **All cells in the body contain 46 chromosomes *except***	Gametes (sex cells) that contain 23 chromosomes

CLINICAL PROBLEM SOLVING

AN 75.2

PROBLEMS

1. A mother took her 5-year-old son to the pediatrician and complained that her child always keeps his tongue protruded and appears dull as compared to other children of his age. His eyes also appear abnormal. On examination, the pediatrician made the following observations: (a) round face with epicanthic folds, (b) mental retardation, (c) hypotonia, and (d) single line in the palm. On the basis of these observations, the child was diagnosed as a case of Down syndrome. **Give the embryological and genetic basis of Down syndrome.**
2. **A 40-year-old woman went to a gynecologist for a checkup when she missed her period. On pelvic examination, the doctor told her that she is pregnant. The gynecologist was very much concerned as it was her first pregnancy. Answer the following questions on the basis of your knowledge of embryology and developmental genetics:**
   (a) Are women older than 35 years at risk of giving birth to abnormal children?
   (b) If a 40-year-old woman becomes pregnant, what tests would you like to advise?
   (c) What genetic abnormality is likely to occur?
3. **What is mosaicism**? Give its genetic basis.
4. **In consanguinity (marriage among cousins), which genetic disorders are likely to occur?**

SOLUTIONS

1. Down syndrome (trisomy 21) is the most common numerical abnormality that leads to various defects which are seen in this case.

   The most common cause of abnormal chromosome number is nondisjunction during meiosis. Nondisjunction during meiosis I or II results in half of the gametes having no copy and half having two copies of chromosomes.

   In this case, the fertilization had occurred between gamete with two copies and a normal one. As a result, the zygote has 47 chromosomes (**trisomy**). The trisomy 21 occurs during meiosis due to nondisjunction of 21st pair of chromosomes.
2. (a) Yes, because women older than 35 years are likely to have child with Down syndrome and other malformations.
   (b) She will be advised the following tests: (a) Ultrasonography to measure nuchal transluscency, (b) Chronic villus biopsy and/or amniocentesis to determine chromosomal disorders such as trisomy 21 and trisomy 13.
   (c) Down syndrome.
3. The mosaicism is a state of being mosaic: A person who has at least two cell lines with two or more different genetic constitutions. In this condition, either the autosomes or sex chromosomes are involved. The mosaicism usually occurs from nondisjunction during early cleavage of zygote.
4. Autosomal recessive disorders.

30 Application of Embryology in Clinical Practice

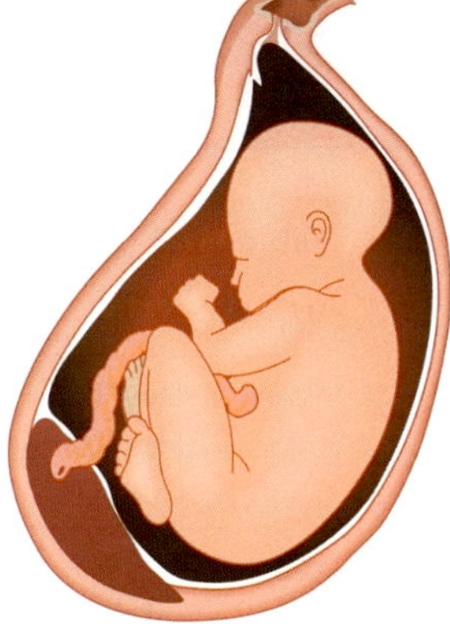

LEARNING OBJECTIVES

After studying this chapter, the student should be able to:

- Define pregnancy and divide it into three trimesters. AN 76.2 Discuss the important events occurring in each trimester.
- What is teratology? Define and classify teratogens.
- Enumerate the drugs that are absolutely contraindicated during pregnancy.

OVERVIEW

Gone are the days when embryology was learnt from models, charts, and museum specimens of aborted fetuses. Nowadays, with the advent of new imaging techniques, particularly ultrasonography, one can learn about developing embryo and fetus within the uterus along the entire period of pregnancy in a woman (**living embryology**), and apply this knowledge in one's clinical practice.

To learn living embryology, one should precisely know various developmental events that take place continuously from the date of fertilization to the birth of baby.

PREGNANCY (GESTATION PERIOD)

Pregnancy is a state of a woman carrying a baby (product of conception) starting from the time of conception until the delivery (L. *Pregnancy* = carrying products of conception), i.e., 266 days.

Length of pregnancy (gestation period) is **280 days** or **40 weeks** calculated from the **first day of last menstrual period (LMP)**.

Or

More accurately, the length of pregnancy (gestation period) is considered to be of **266 days** or **38 weeks** from the day of fertilization or 9 months ± 7 days.

Clinically, the pregnancy/gestation period responsible for prenatal development of an individual is divided into the following two parts:

1. **Embryonic period**
2. **Fetal period**

EMBRYONIC DEVELOPMENT IN DAYS

Gestation period from the fertilization to the end of 8th week is termed **embryonic period**. Development of embryo during this period in days is given in Table 30.1.

Some key developmental events that occur during the embryonic period are given in Table 30.2.

Criteria for Estimation of Age of Embryo in Days

The age of embryo in days can be accurately determined during early time period by counting somites because these appear with a specified periodicity (for details, see pages 71 and 365). Later, it can be determined by measuring the length of the embryo (Table 30.3).

FETAL DEVELOPMENT IN WEEKS

Gestation period from the beginning of 9th week to the birth is termed **fetal period**. The development of fetus during this period in weeks is given in Table 30.4.

Changes in external appearance of the fetus during the fetal period (from 9th to 38th week) are shown in Fig. 30.1. Size of head in relation to rest of the body at different periods of fetal development is shown in Fig. 30.2.

Criteria for Determination of Fertilization Age During Fetal Period AN 80.6

The criteria taken for the determination of age of the fetus are as follows:

1. Length of the fetus
2. Weight of the fetus

The length of a fetus is usually measured from top (vertex) of the skull to bottom of the buttock; it is termed **crown–rump length** (CRL)/**sitting height**. Otherwise, it is measured from top (vertex) of the skull to the heel; it is termed **crown–heel length** (CHL) (Fig. 30.3).

Table 30.1 Embryonic development in days

Weeks	Days					
Week 1	**Day 1** Fertilization	**Day 2** Embryo with two-cell stage	**Day 3** Formation of morula	**Day 4** Early stage of blastocyst	**Day 5** Late stage of blastocyst	**Days 6 and 7** Implantation	
Week 2	**Day 8** • Formation of bilaminar embryonic disk • Trophoblast differentiates into cytotrophoblast and syncytiotrophoblast	**Day 9** Formation of lacunae in syncytiotrophoblast	**Days 10 and 11** Embryo gets completely implanted in endometrium		**Day 12** Formation of extraembryonic mesoderm	**Day 13** Formation of primary villi	**Day 14** Formation of prechordal plate and connecting stalk
Week 3	**Day 15** Formation of primitive streak	**Day 16** • Migration of mesenchymal cells from epiblast • Formation of secondary and tertiary villi	**Day 17** Migration of cells from primitive streak	**Day 18** Formation of trilaminar embryonic disk	**Day 19** • Neurulation begins • Formation of neural plate	**Day 20** Formation of neural folds and neural groove	**Day 21** Formation of first pair of somites
Week 4	**Day 22** Closure of neural tube begins	**Day 23** • Closure of neural tube with cranial and caudal neuropore • Formation of lens and otic placodes	**Day 24** • Appearance of pericardial heart bulge • Rostral neuropore closes • Two pairs of pharyngeal arches appear	**Day 25** • Formation of optic pit • Three pairs of pharyngeal arches appear	**Day 26** Upper limb bud appears	**Day 27** Formation of otic pit	**Day 28** Neurulation completes
Week 5	**Day 29** Upper and lower limb buds become paddle shaped	**Day 30** Development of face begins	**Day 31** Formation of primitive gut tube	**Day 32** Embryo completely surrounded by amnion lies in chorionic cavity	**Day 33** Formation of: • Umbilical ring • Tertiary yolk sac • Umbilical cord	**Day 34** Formation of optic cup and lens placode	**Day 35** Formation of pharyngeal arches and cartilages
Week 6	**Day 36** Physiological umbilical hernia occurs	**Day 37** Developing face	**Day 38** Development of muscles	**Day 39** Endodermal derivatives of primitive gut	**Day 40** Formation of auricular hillocks	**Day 41** Atrial septum is formed	**Day 42** Formation of digital rays
Week 7	**Day 43** Formation of cartilages in developing limb	**Day 44** Developing face (an advanced stage)	**Day 45** Conotruncal and ventricular septa form	**Day 46** • Subdivision of decidua • Wellformed amniotic cavity and chorion	**Day 47** Indifferent stage of development of external genitalia	**Day 48** Fusion of facial prominences	**Day 49** • Formation of eyelid • Formation of external ear • Presence of digits
Week 8	**Day 50** • Upper limbs are longer and appear bent at elbow • Finger distinct but webbed	**Day 51** Eye, external ear, nose, finger, and toes are clearly visible	**Day 52** Large forehead	**Day 53** External genitalia begin to differentiate	**Day 54** Genital tubercle, urethral groove, and anus are clearly visible	**Day 55** Eye, ear, elbow, wrist, knee, and toes are clearly visible	**Day 56** Embryo acquires a miniature human form

Table 30.2 Key developmental events during the embryonic period

Developmental Events	Day/Days of Gestation
Fertilization	Day 1
Blastocyst	Day 4
Bilaminar embryonic disk	Day 8
Implantation	Day 10
Primitive streak appears	Day 15
Primitive heart tube	Day 17
Neurulation, first pair of somites	Day 21
Limb buds	Days 26–28
Primitive gut	Day 31
Physiological herniation	Day 36
Face appears	Day 37
External genitalia	Day 53
Miniature human form	Day 56

Table 30.3 Criteria for estimation of the age of embryo in days

Age (Days)	Number of Somites	Crown–Rump Length (mm)
20, 21	1–3	1.5–3
22, 23	4–12	2–3.5
24, 25	13–20	2.5–4.5
26, 27	21–29	3–5
28–30	30–35	4–6
31, 32	–	5–7
33–36	–	7–9
37–40	–	8–11
41–43	–	11–14
44–46	–	13–17
47, 48	–	16–18
49–51	–	18–22
52, 53	–	22–24
54, 55	–	23–28
56	–	27–31

Table 30.4 Development of fetus in weeks

Age (Weeks)	Developmental Events
9	Closed eyes or closing eyes, more rounded head, and herniation of intestines in umbilical cord
10	Intestines in abdomen and early development of fingernails
12	Differentiated external genitalia and well-defined neck
14	Erect head, well-developed lower limb, and early fingernail development
16	External ears standing out from the head
18	Vernix caseosa and early toenail development
20	Lanugo hair
22	Wrinkled and red skin
24	Fingernails and lean body
26	Partially open eyes and eyelashes
28	Open eyes, hair, and slightly wrinkled skin
30	Toenails and descending testes
32	Fingernails up to fingertips, and pink and smooth skin
36	Plump body, absence of lanugo hair, toenails up to toetips, flexed limbs, and a firm grasp
38	Prominent chest faintly protruding breasts, testes in the scrotum or inguinal canals, and fingernails beyond fingertips

During the fetal period, there is a rapid increase in weight due to maturation of tissues and organs. The weight is seen as 8 g at 9th week (beginning of fetal period) to 3400–3500 g at birth.

N.B. Most of the weight is gained during last 8 weeks (2 months) of the pregnancy.

Criteria for estimation (determination) of age of the fetus are given in Table 30.5.

PREGNANCY DATING

Estimated date of confinement is calculated on the basis of assumption that a woman has 28-day menstrual cycle, with ovulation on day 14. In general,

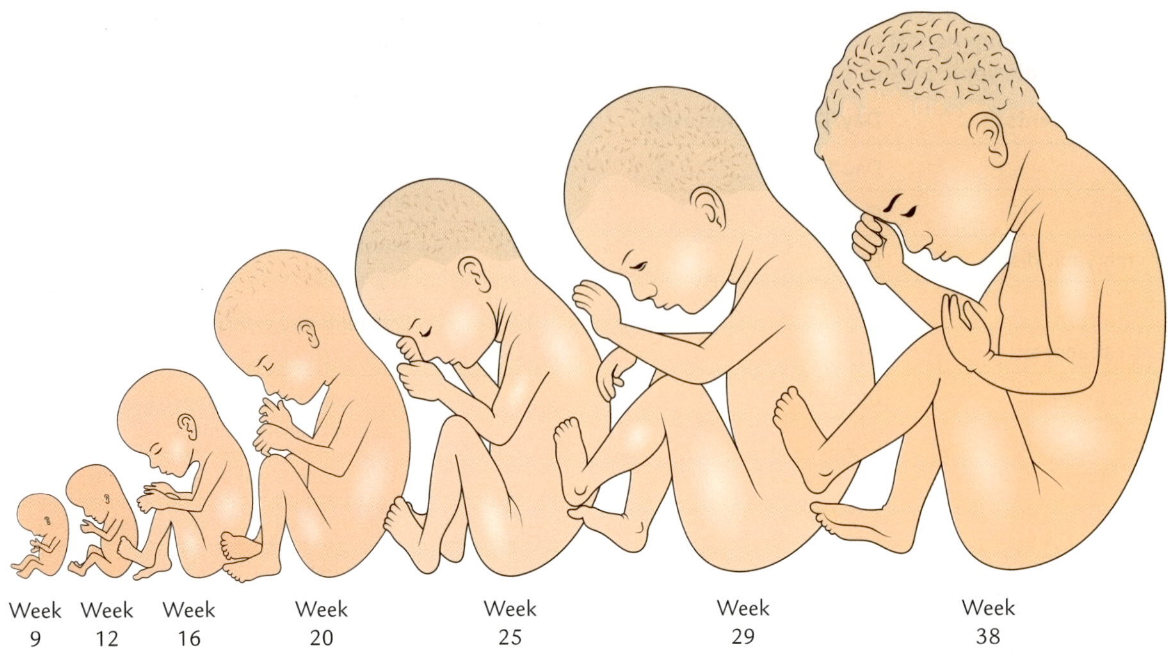

Fig. 30.1 Changes in the external appearance of fetus during fetal period (from weeks 9 to 38).

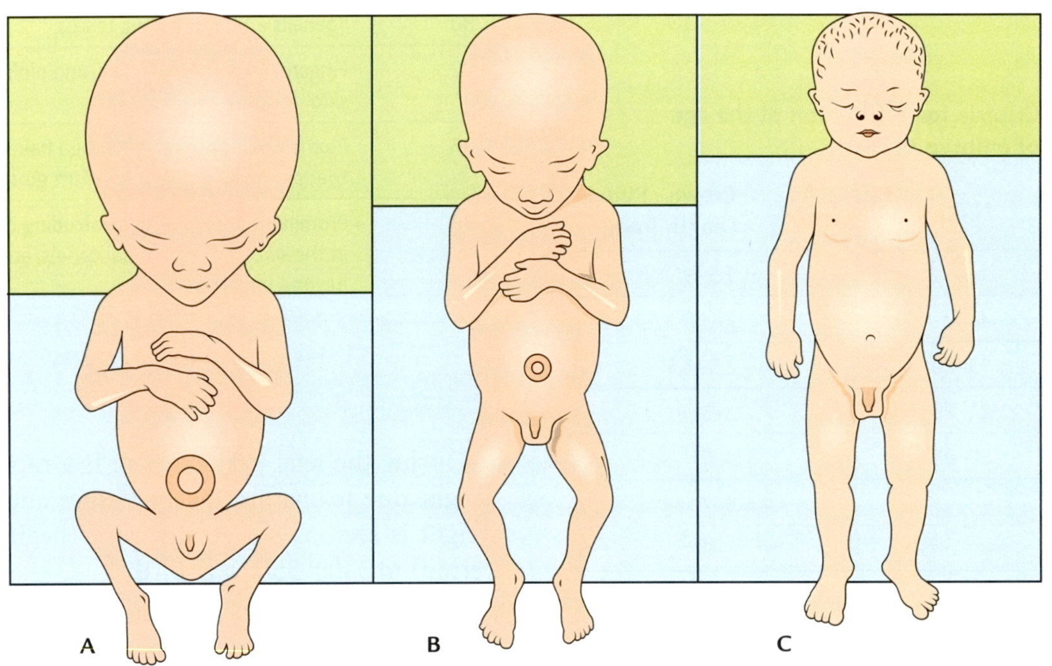

Fig. 30.2 Changing proportions of body during the fetal period. Note size of the head in relation to rest of the body at various gestation ages: (A) 3rd month, (B) 5th month, and (C) at birth.

duration of pregnancy is 280 days (40 weeks) from the first day of LMP.

N.B. **Naegele's rule for estimation of duration of pregnancy:** It is commonly used by gynecologists. According to this rule, first count back 3 months from the first day of LMP and then add 1 year 7 days. This method is reasonably accurate in women with regular menstrual cycles.

Trimesters of Pregnancy/Milestones of Pregnancy

AN 76.2

Clinically, pregnancy (gestation period) is divided into **three trimesters,** each lasting for about 3 months.

- **First trimester:** From week 1 to the end of week 12, i.e. it includes **preembryonic period, embryonic period,** and **early fetal period.**

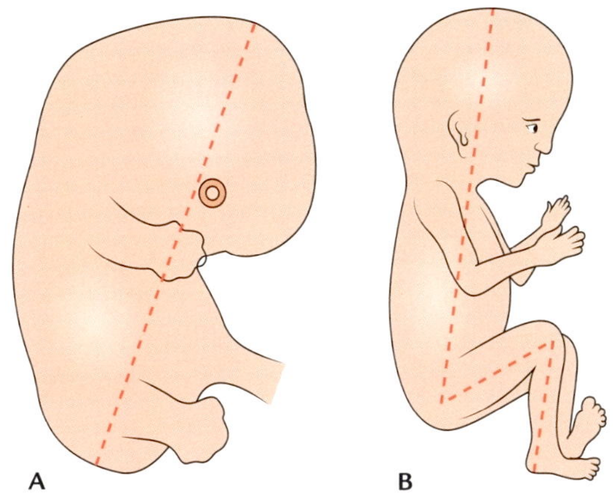

Fig. 30.3 Measurement of the length of the embryo. (A) Crown–rump length. (B) Crown–heel length.

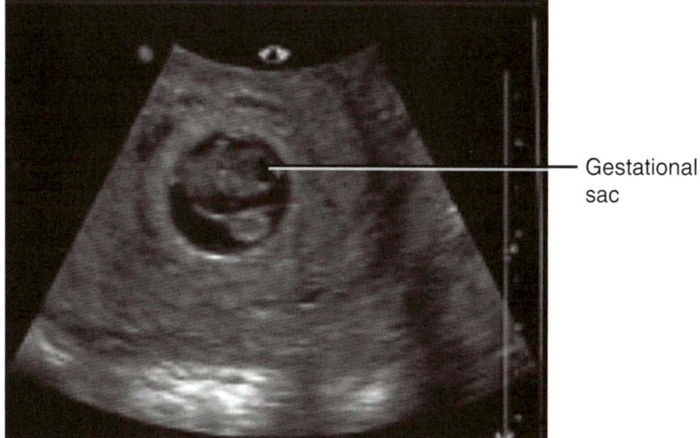

Fig. 30.4 Ultrasound showing gestation sac.

Table 30.5 Criteria for estimation of age of the fetus

Age (Weeks)	Crown–Rump Length (mm)	Foot Length (mm)	Weight (g)
9	50	7	8
10	61	9	14
12	87	14	45
14	120	20	110
16	140	27	200
18	160	33	320
20	190	39	460
22	210	45	630
24	230	50	820
26	250	55	1000
28	270	59	1300
30	280	63	1700
32	300	68	2100
36	340	79	2900
38	360	83	3400

During this trimester the crucial events of baby's development take place. For examples:
- Implantation
- Formation of 3-germ layer
- Organogenesis and functioning of heart

- **Second trimester**: From week 13 to the end of week 26, i.e., fetal period.
  This trimester is called golden period because most of unpleasant effects of pregnancy such as nausea, vomiting (morning sickness), increased frequency of passing urine, breast tenderness, etc. disappear.
- **Third trimester**: From week 27 to the end of week 40 or end of pregnancy, i.e., fetal period.
  This period is mainly concerned with functional growth of various organs and preparation of fetus for delivery.

The important events of each trimester are given as follows.

First Trimester (From the First Day of LMP to the End of Week 12)

1. From days 8–10, **pregnancy test** by human chorionic gonadotrophin (HCG) assay shows positive result, i.e., testing presence of hCG in maternal urine or serum.
2. At weeks 4.5–5, **gestational sac** is seen in the posterior wall of the uterus (Fig. 30.4) by ultrasound.
3. At weeks 5–6, embryonic heart rate is about 100 beats per minute; by weeks 8–9, it enhances to about 140 beats per minute.
4. At week 10, fetus starts swallowing amniotic fluid.
5. At week 12, fundus of the uterus is palpable above pubic symphysis.
6. Face becomes more human looking.
7. By week 12, **primary ossification centers** are present in long bones and skull.
8. By week 12, external genitalia develop to such an extent that **sex of the fetus can be determined by ultrasound.**

N.B. During the first trimester, pregnant woman experiences **morning sickness, increased urination, swollen breasts,** and **fatigue.**

Second Trimester (From the End of First Trimester, i.e., 13–27 Weeks)

1. At weeks 14–18, **amniocentesis** is performed to detect fetal chromosomal abnormalities.

2. At week 16, fundus of the **uterus is palpable** midway between pubic symphysis and umbilicus.
3. At weeks 14–16, respiratory movements begin.
4. At weeks 16–18, movements of the fetus (**quickening**) can be felt by women who have had one or more previous pregnancies.
5. At weeks 17–20, the **fetal heart sounds are audible** with fetoscope.
6. At week 18, female and male external genitalia can be distinguished by ultrasound (**antenatal sex determination**).
7. At weeks 18–20, movements of the fetus (**quickening**) can be felt by a woman in her first pregnancy.
8. At week 20, fundus of the uterus is palpable at the umbilicus.
9. At week 24, sucking movements begin.
10. At weeks 24–26, some sound can be heard.
11. At weeks 25–27, the fetal lungs become capable of respiration.
12. At week 28, eyes become sensitive to light.

N.B. There are 70%–80% chances of survival of an infant born at the end of second trimester.

Third Trimester (From the End of Second Trimester, i.e., 27 – 40 Weeks/Until Term)

1. **Pupillary light reflex** is present.
2. **Descent of the fetal head into pelvic inlet** occurs.
3. **Rupture of fetal membranes** (amniochorionic membranes) occurs with labor pains, which usually begins 24 h later.

Viability of fetus

The term **viability** means ability to survive successfully.

The term **viable fetus** means that fetus has reached such a stage of development that if born it can survive outside the uterus under normal conditions.

The general age of viability is 24 weeks of gestation. This means that a baby born after 24 weeks of gestation can survive.

ULTRASONOGRAPHY IN PREGNANCY

The **ultrasonography** is an extremely useful, safe, and noninvasive technique in hands of radiologists to confirm pregnancy and differentiate between normal and abnormal gestations.

Common ultrasonographic techniques used are (a) **transabdominal sonography (TAS)**, (b) **transvesical sonography (TVS)**, and (c) **endovaginal sonography (EVS)**.

Aims of Ultrasonography

The **ultrasonography during pregnancy** is performed for the following purposes:

1. Localization of gestational sac (if present)
2. Estimation of menstrual age of embryo or fetus
3. Early identification of embryonic death
4. Determination of the number of embryos
5. Determination of fetal abnormalities
6. Determination of growth, progress, or retardation of growth of embryo/fetus
7. Determination of ectopic pregnancy
8. Providing guidance to perform **chorionic villus biopsy** and/or **amniocentesis**

The ultrasonographic scanning is performed routinely for all pregnant women (Fig. 30.5).

N.B. Nowadays, the ultrasonography has become an inseparable and integral part of diagnostic care and management of pregnancies.

Ultrasonography During the First Trimester (i.e., 1 – 12 Weeks)

Indications

The ultrasounds during the first trimester are performed before 14 weeks of pregnancy to check:

- Presence of gestational sac to confirm pregnancy.
- Size of gestational sac to determine the gestational age.
- Location of gestational sac to detect ectopic pregnancy.
- Number of gestational sacs to detect multiple pregnancies.
- Gestational sac is seen at weeks 5–5.5 of gestation.
- Yolk sac and embryo within the gestational sac are visualized by weeks 5.5–6.

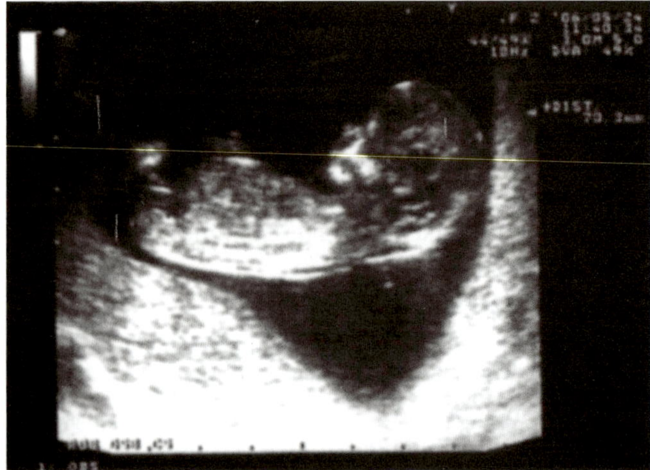

Fig. 30.5 Transabdominal ultrasound at week 12 showing measurement of the crown–rump length to calculate the gestational age.

- Embryonic heart beat is identifiable by weeks 6–6.5.
- Crown–rump length can be measured week 6 onwards.

Ultrasonography During the Second Trimester or Level II Ultrasound (i.e., 13–26 Weeks)

Indications. The ultrasounds during the second trimester or **"level II" ultrasounds** are performed between 18 and 20 weeks to examine the anatomy of fetus:

- Confirm whether the baby is developing normally or not
- Check position of placenta to rule out **placenta previa**
- Check amniotic fluid to rule out oligohydramnios etc.

N.B. Women with high-risk pregnancies may be advised multiple ultrasounds during the second trimester.

Ultrasonography During the Third Trimester or Level III Ultrasound (i.e., 28–32 Weeks)

Indications. The ultrasound during the third trimester may be advised to:

- Check growth of the baby
- Check amount of amniotic fluid, especially if the due date is crossed
- Check fetal abnormalities in high-risk pregnancies
- Evaluate status of placenta, and uterus

Determination of Gestation Age by Ultrasound

A. **During the first trimester**

It is determined by taking following measurements in millimeters:

1. **Diameter of gestational sac in the uterus:** The gestational sac is seen around 5th week and increases in size by 1 mm per day.
2. **Crown-rump length (CRL):** It is measured from the highest point of skull to the lowest point of buttock. It is the most accurate parameter for determination of gestational age during the first trimester.

B. **During second and third trimesters**

It is determined by taking the following parameters:

1. **Biparietal diameter (BPD):** It refers to the greatest transverse diameter of head which extends from one parietal eminence to the other in an axial plane. It is about 2.4 cm at 13th week to about 9.5 cm at term.
2. **Head circumference:** It is determined by measuring the greatest occipitofrontal circumference. The head circumference is obtained in the same plane as that of BPD.
3. **Abdominal circumference:** It is taken in axial plane at the level of fetal stomach or at the level of bifurcation of portal vein. It should be around skin surface and not deep to skin.
4. **Femur length:** It is measured from the tip of greater trochanter to the lateral epicondyle.

Table 30.6 Time of appearance of ossification centers

Bone	Time of Appearance of Ossification Centers
Clavicle	5th–6th weeks of IUL
Mandible and palate	9th week
Vertebral body and neural arch	9th week
Frontal bone	10 and 11 weeks
Femur, humerus, scapula, ileum, and phalanges	11th week
Skull base	12–14 weeks
Skull calvaria	16th week
Metatarsals and metacarpals	Early second trimester
Calcaneum	24–26 weeks

N.B.

- Ossification centers can be seen. The order in which ossification centers appear is given in Table 30.6.
- Abnormalities of digits are identifiable during early/middle second trimester.
- The fetal age and growth can be assessed by measuring the CRL during weeks 5–10 of gestation, and after that by measuring the length of femur and BPD and abdominal circumferences.
- The ultrasound measurements are taken to determine the size and probable age of the fetus to provide a prediction of the expected date of delivery (EDD).

GOLDEN FACTS TO REMEMBER

- **First sign of early pregnancy** — Presence of gestational sac on weeks 3–5
- **Gestational age (GA)** — Length of pregnancy after the first day of LMP
- **First fetal heart tones heard by Doppler** — ±2 weeks
- **First fetal heart tones heard by auscultation** — ±2–4 weeks
- **Most susceptive period of pregnancy for teratogenesis** — 3–8 weeks
- **Most common test for prenatal diagnosis** — Ultrasonography
- **Movements of the fetus can be felt by the mother during** — 5th month of pregnancy
- **Body part with the largest circumference at the end of 9th month of pregnancy** — Skull
- **Menstrual length of pregnancy** — 280 days or 40 weeks
- **Fertilization length of pregnancy/most accurate date of birth** — 266 days or 38 weeks after fertilization
- **Respiratory movements in fetus begin** — During weeks 14–16
- **Sucking movements in fetus begin** — At week 24
- **Fetus starts swallowing amniotic fluid** — At week 10
- **Three cardinal signs of preeclampsia** — Hypertension, proteinuria, and edema

CLINICAL PROBLEM SOLVING

PROBLEMS

1. **Are the multiple ultrasounds done during prenatal period, safe for the baby?**
2. **Can you determine the gender at 12 weeks of pregnancy?**
3. **What are the basic biometric parameters used in ultrasound to assess the fetal size?**
4. **What is implantation bleeding?**
5. **Can drugs taken during first 2 weeks of pregnancy cause birth defects?**
6. **What is gestational sac?**

SOLUTIONS

1. The multiple prenatal ultrasounds do not cause any harm to the fetus as regards to its growth and development.
2. May be, but sex of the baby is determined by ultrasound as early as 14 weeks.
3. These are (a) biparietal diameter, (b) head circumference, (c) abdominal circumference, and (d) femur length.
4. It refers to scanty (small amount of) bleeding per vaginum few days after the expected date of menstruation. It is not menstrual blood. It comes from intervillous space or chronic vessels. The blood comes out if implantation site is not closed by fibrinoid plugs.
5. Drugs taken during first 2 weeks of pregnancy do not cause birth defects, rather they kill few cells in which case embryo recovers and develops normally; or the drugs kill the embryo leading to abortion.
6. It is a fluid-filled structure surrounding an embryo during the first few weeks of pregnancy. It is the first structure seen in pregnancy by ultrasound as early as 4.5 to 5 weeks of gestational age. In 97.6% cases, it confirms pregnancy.

Appendix

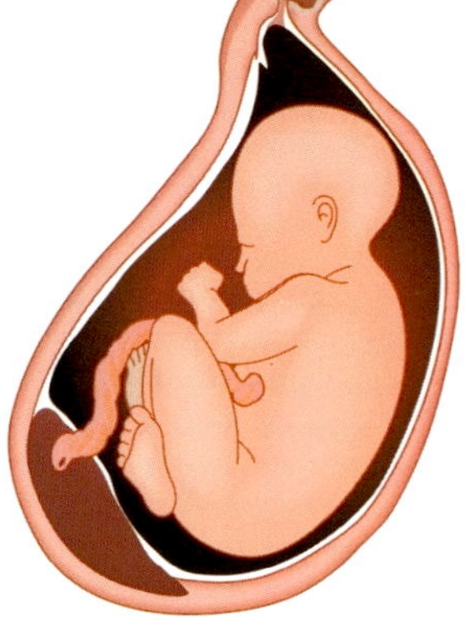

EMBRYONIC STRUCTURES AND THEIR DERIVATIVES

Embryonic Structure	Description	Derivatives/Functions
Primitive streak	It is a linear thickening of epidermal cells in the median plane caudally on the dorsal aspect of bilaminar embryonic disk. It is formed on day 15 of IUL.	• Formation of intraembryonic mesoderm • Cardiogenic mesoderm/septum transversum • Notochord
Notochord	It is the midline cord of cells (derived from primitive knot) extending between primitive knot and prechordal plate.	• Apical ligament of dens • Nucleus pulposus of intervertebral disks
Prechordal plate	It is a circular area near the cranial end of embryonic disk, where ectoderm and endoderm are in direct contact as mesoderm does not extend between above two layers here.	Buccopharyngeal membrane
Yolk sac	It is a membranous sac attached on the ventral aspect of the bilaminar embryonic disk. It is lined by Heuser's membrane derived from endoderm.	• Primitive gut • Formation of blood vessels • Houses primordial germ cells in this wall
Allantois (allantoenteric diverticulum)	• It is a small diverticulum from caudal wall of yolk sac which grows into connecting stalk. After formation of tail fold, it is absorbed into hindgut. • Blood vessels of allantois form umbilical blood vessels.	• Urachus (vestigial remnant) → median umbilical ligament
Decidua	It refers to modified uterine endometrium during pregnancy. It is divided into three parts: (a) Decidua basalis, (b) decidua capsularis, and (c) decidua parietalis.	• Facilitates embedding • Forms maternal part of placenta • Nourishes and protects embryo • Sheds off at birth
Amnion	It is a thin membrane that forms vesicle (amniotic cavity) dorsal to the embryonic disk. This cavity is filled with amniotic fluid. Later on, amniotic cavity enlarges and surrounds the entire embryo, and also wraps around the umbilical cord.	• Protects embryo from external injury • Helps form "**bag of waters**," which helps to dilate cervix during labor
Chorion	Chorion along with amnion forms the chorionic sac. (N.B. Inner wall of the sac is formed by amnion while outer wall is formed by chorion.) Within (chorionic sac), the embryo, amniotic sac, and yolk sac (umbilical vesicle) are suspended by connecting stalk. The chorion is formed by somatopleuric layer of extraembryonic mesoderm and trophoblast. It differentiates into two parts: (a) Chorion **frondosum** (b) Chorion laeve	• *Chorion frondosum* forms fetal part of placenta • *Chorion laeve* forms smooth chorion membrane

Continued

Embryonic Structure	Description	Derivatives/Functions
Bag of waters	It is a double-layered fluid-filled amniochorionic sac that encloses and protects the fetus in the womb. N.B. In fact, the amniotic fluid just before birth is enclosed in composite membrane called *membranes* formed by the fusion of amnion, chorion, and greatly thinned-out decidua capsularis.	At the time of birth, these membranes bulge into cervical canal due to increased pressure of amniotic fluid following contraction of uterine muscle. This bulging helps to dilate cervical canal. The bulging membranes can be felt per vaginum and are referred to as "**bag of waters**."
Intraembryonic mesoderm (secondary mesoderm)	• It is derived from primitive streak. • It lies between ectoderm and endoderm. • From medial to lateral, it is divided into three parts: (a) Paraxial mesoderm (b) Intermediate mesoderm (c) Lateral plate mesoderm	• **Paraxial mesoderm** forms (a) Axial skeleton (b) Axial and appendicular skeletal muscles (c) Skin related to above-mentioned structures • **Intermediate mesoderm forms** (a) Most of genitourinary system, i.e., kidneys, testes, and ovaries • **Lateral plate mesoderm** (a) Somatopleuric mesoderm which forms body wall (b) Splanchnopleuric mesoderm which forms walls of GIT and respiratory tracts
Intraembryonic coelom (coelomic cavity)	It is a horseshoe-shaped cavity within the intraembryonic mesoderm.	• **Derivatives of coelomic cavity** (a) Pericardial cavity (b) Pleural cavities (c) Peritoneal cavity **Functions** (a) Provides free and frictionless movements (b) Coelomic epithelium gives rise to: (i) Gonads (ii) Suprarenal cortex (iii) Mullerian ducts
Septum transversum	It is unsplit part of intraembryonic mesoderm near the cranial end of embryonic disk.	• Fibrous pericardium • Central tendon of diaphragm • Fibrous stroma of liver • Pleuroperitoneal membranes
Stomodeum	It is ectodermal pit at the cranial end of embryo, which is separated from foregut by **buccopharyngeal membrane**.	Anterior part of oral cavity
Cloacal membrane	• It is circular area at the caudal end of embryonic disk where intraembryonic mesoderm does not extend between ectoderm and endoderm. • It separates proctoderm from cloaca. • It is divided into ventral and dorsal parts by urorectal septum.	• Urogenital membrane (ventral part) • Anal membrane (dorsal part) • Part of cloacal membrane invaded by mesoderm forms (a) Perineal body (b) Anococcygeal body (c) Infraumbilical part of anterior abdominal wall
Proctodeum (ectodermal cloaca)	It is ectodermal pit at the caudal end of the embryo, which is separated from endodermal hindgut by **anal membrane**.	Lower part (ectodermal part) of anal canal
Cloaca	• It is a part of primitive hindgut caudal to allantois. • It is divided into two parts: (a) Primitive urogenital sinus (i) Vesicourethral canal (ii) Definitive urogenital sinus (b) Anorectal canal	 • Urinary bladder + primitive urethra (prostatic part above the opening of ejaculatory ducts) • Remaining urethra except terminal part • Rectum + upper part of anal canal

Embryonic Structure	Description	Derivatives/Functions
Tubotympanic recess	It refers to elongated recess of first pharyngeal pouch.	• Pharyngotympanic tube • Tympanic (middle ear) cavity • Tympanic (mastoid) antrum • Mastoid air cells
Primordial germ cells	• These are initially derived from epiblast of bilaminar embryonic disk and later get located in the wall of yolk sac. • In 4th week of IUL, they migrate into the genital ridge.	Male and female gametes
Somites	• These are paired blocks/segments of paraxial mesoderm. • These lie by the side of notochord and neural tube. • Parts: (a) Ventromedial part (*sclerotome*) (b) Dorsolateral part (*dermomyotome*)	Vertebral column Somatic muscles and overlying dermis of skin
Neural crest	It refers to segmentally arranged neuroectodermal cells on the dorsolateral aspects of neural tube.	• Ganglia of cranial nerves • Dorsal root ganglia of spinal nerves • Sympathetic and parasympathetic ganglia • Adrenal medulla • Paraganglia • Schwann cells • Melanoblasts • Leptomeninges • Pharyngeal arch mesoderm • Pharyngeal arch cartilages • Odontoblasts
Rathke's pouch	It refers to **ectodermal evagination (diverticulum) from roof of stomodeum** just in front of *buccopharyngeal membrane*.	Adenophysis of pituitary gland (i.e., pars distalis, pars tuberalis, and pars intermedia)
Thyroglossal duct	It refers to median endodermal thyroid diverticulum from floor of primitive pharynx.	• Thyroid gland • Levator glandulae thyroideae

Multiple Choice Questions

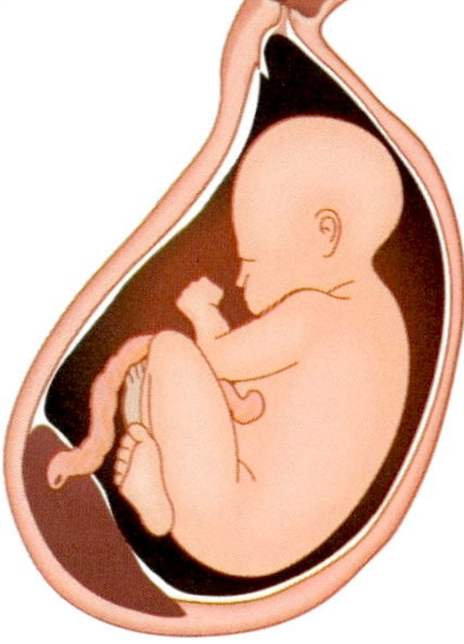

CHAPTER 1

1. Preembryonic period completes when
   (a) Blastocyst reaches the uterus
   (b) Blastocyst implants in the uterus
   (c) Placenta forms
   (d) Two primary germ layers form

2. All of the following are the features of preembryonic period, *except*
   (a) Cleaving of zygote
   (b) Formation of blastocyst
   (c) Implantation of blastocyst
   (d) Formation of extraembryonic membranes

3. All of the following are the features of embryonic period, *except*
   (a) Differentiation of germ layers into specific body organs (organogenesis)
   (b) Formation of extraembryonic membranes
   (c) Occurs from 3rd to 8th weeks
   (d) Body growth

4. Who is called the father of modern embryology?
   (a) Aristotle
   (b) Galen
   (c) Karl Ernst von Baer
   (d) Joham Ham van Arnheim

5. First mammal was cloned in the year
   (a) 1875
   (b) 1960
   (c) 1997
   (d) 2002

6. All of the following statements are correct regarding stem cells, *except*
   (a) These were first discovered by James Till
   (b) These were discovered in 1960
   (c) These can divide and develop into specialized cells
   (d) These are found only in embryonic tissue

7. Period of growth from birth to the end of 4th week is called
   (a) Neonatal
   (b) Infancy
   (c) Fetal
   (d) Childhood

8. Select the *incorrect statement.*
   (a) *Neonatal period* extends from birth to the end of 4th week
   (b) *Infancy period* extends from the birth until the end of the 1st year
   (c) *Childhood* extends from beginning of the 2nd year to the end of 12 years
   (d) *Adolescence* extends from 19 to 40 years

Answers

1, *d*; 2, *d*; 3, *d*; 4, *c*; 5, *c*; 6, *d*; 7, *a*; 8, *d*.

CHAPTER 2

1. Select the *correct statement* regarding basic processes of embryonic development.
   (a) Growth
   (b) Differentiation
   (c) Cell-to-cell interaction
   (d) All of the above

2. Select the *correct statement* regarding types of tissue growth.
   (a) Multiplicative growth
   (b) Auxetic growth
   (c) Accretionary growth
   (d) All of the above

3. Select the *incorrect statement.*
   (a) Primitive streak is secondary organizer
   (b) Notochord is secondary organizer
   (c) Neural tube is tertiary organizer
   (d) Primitive streak is primary organizer

4. Key signaling pathways involved during embryonic development include all, *except.*
   (a) Sonic hedgehog (SHH) pathway
   (b) Planer cell polarity (PCP) pathway
   (c) Notch pathways
   (d) Apoptosis signaling pathways

Answers

1, *d*; 2, *d*; 3, *a*; 4, *d*.

CHAPTER 3

1. All of the following statements are correct regarding testis, *except*
   (a) It is primary reproductive organ in males
   (b) It contains 50–100 seminiferous tubules
   (c) It forms sperms
   (d) It produces testosterone hormone

2. Select the *incorrect statement* about the epididymis.
   (a) It lies posteriorly and slightly lateral to the testis
   (b) It plays an important role in the maturation of sperms
   (c) Its duct is continuous with the vas deferens
   (d) Its duct begins in rete testis

3. Prostate gland
   (a) Is a pyramidal fibromuscular gland
   (b) Surrounds two ejaculatory ducts
   (c) Pours its secretion into the membranous urethra by 10–20 ducts
   (d) Secretes prostatic fluid, which forms the bulk of the semen

4. Bulk of semen is formed by
   (a) Seminal vesicles: 60%
   (b) Prostate: 30%
   (c) Testis: 5%
   (d) Bulbourethral gland: 5%

5. All of the following statements are correct regarding ovary, *except*
   (a) It is primary reproductive organ of female
   (b) It contains about 2 million primary oocytes (primordial follicles) at birth
   (c) It contains about 400,000 ovarian follicles at puberty
   (d) It is involved in the ovulation of only 40–50 ova during entire reproductive period of a woman

6. Select the *incorrect statement* about the ovarian cycle.
   (a) It usually consists of 28 days
   (b) It is regulated by estrogen and progesterone hormones
   (c) Unlike menstrual cycle, it is continuous during pregnancy
   (d) It is divided into follicular and luteal phases

7. All of the following statements are correct regarding menstrual cycle, *except*
   (a) It is characterized by monthly cyclic changes in the uterine endometrium
   (b) The changes in the endometrium occur due to hormones secreted by the ovaries
   (c) It is most obvious as monthly bleeding (menstruation) in females
   (d) It occurs throughout the life of a female

8. Ovulation usually occurs at
   (a) 7 days after menstruation
   (b) 14 days after menstruation
   (c) 7 days before menstruation
   (d) 14 days before the next menstruation

9. All of the following statements are correct regarding corpus luteum, *except*
   (a) It prepares the uterus for implantation of fertilized ovum
   (b) It lasts for 14 days if fertilization does not take place
   (c) It lasts for 3 months if the ovum is fertilized
   (d) It is formed whether ovulation takes place or not

10. Select the *incorrect statement.*
   (a) Proliferation of endometrium occurs due to estrogen secreted by the ovary
   (b) Ovulation occurs at 14th day before the start of next menstruation
   (c) Fertilization leads to persistent corpus luteum
   (d) LH hormone corresponds to the estrogenic phase of the ovary

Answers

1, *b*; 2, *d*; 3, *c*; 4, *a*; 5, *d*; 6, *c*; 7, *d*; 8, *d*; 9, *d*; 10, *d*.

CHAPTER 4

1. Number of sperms formed from single spermatogonium is
   (a) 2
   (b) 4
   (c) 6
   (d) 8

2. In which stage of spermatogenesis, the chromosome number is halved?
   (a) Spermatogonium to primary spermatocyte
   (b) Primary spermatocyte to secondary spermatocyte
   (c) Secondary spermatocyte to spermatid
   (d) Spermatid to sperm

3. An individual is likely to be sterile if the number of healthy sperms per milliliter of semen is below
   (a) 80 million
   (b) 60 million
   (c) 40 million
   (d) 10 million

4. The usual period of viability of an ovum in female genital tract is
   (a) 10–12 h
   (b) 24–48 h
   (c) 58–68 h
   (d) 72–82 h

5. At puberty, the number of ovarian follicles present in each ovary is about
   (a) 400,000
   (b) 40,000
   (c) 4000
   (d) 400

6. The number of ovarian follicles that undergo ovulation during the entire reproductive period of women is about
   (a) 40,000
   (b) 4000
   (c) 400
   (d) 100

7. Ovum completes its second meiotic division
   (a) Just before ovulation
   (b) Soon after ovulation
   (c) Just before fertilization
   (d) Soon after fertilization

8. Second meiotic division gives rise to
   (a) Primary spermatocytes
   (b) Secondary spermatocytes
   (c) Spermatids
   (d) Spermatozoa

9. Number of female gametes (ova) formed from a single oogonium is
   (a) 1
   (b) 2
   (c) 3
   (d) 4

10. Spermiogenesis is transformation of
    (a) Spermatogonium into primary oocyte
    (b) Primary spermatocyte into secondary spermatocyte
    (c) Secondary spermatocyte into spermatid
    (d) Spermatid into sperm

11. Number of chromosomes in the primary spermatocyte is
    (a) 22 + Y
    (b) 22 + XY
    (c) 44 + XY
    (d) 44 + X

12. Primary oocyte completes its first meiotic division at the time of
    (a) Ovulation
    (b) Fertilization
    (c) Puberty
    (d) None of the above

Answers

1, *b*; 2, *b*; 3, *d*; 4, *b*; 5, *a*; 6, *c*; 7, *d*; 8, *c*; 9, *a*; 10, *d*; 11, *c*; 12, *a*.

CHAPTER 5

1. Fertilization normally occurs
   (a) In the upper part of uterine cavity
   (b) In the lower part of uterine cavity
   (c) Inside the uterine tube
   (d) Inside the cervix

2. Oocyte usually remains viable after ovulation without fertilization up to
   (a) 8 h
   (b) 12 h
   (c) 24–48 h
   (d) 68 h

3. All of the following act as a barrier of oocyte, *except*
   (a) Corona radiata
   (b) Zona pellucida
   (c) Vitelline membrane
   (d) Perivitelline space

4. Process/processes which sperms must undergo to be able to fertilize an oocyte is/are
   (a) Capacitation
   (b) Acrosome reaction
   (c) Both capacitation and acrosome reaction
   (d) Zonal reaction

5. Conventional phases of fertilization include all of the following, *except*
   (a) Penetration of corona radiata
   (b) Penetration of zona pellucida
   (c) Fusion of oocyte and sperm cell membranes
   (d) Disintegration of sperm head

6. All of the following are primitive germ layers, *except*
   (a) Ectoderm
   (b) Neuroectoderm
   (c) Mesoderm
   (d) Endoderm

7. Process of gastrulation includes all of the following, *except*
   (a) Formation of primitive streak
   (b) Form of intraembryonic mesoderm
   (c) Formation of primitive gut
   (d) Formation of three germ layers

8. All of the following are results of fertilization, *except*
   (a) Restoration of diploid number of chromosomes
   (b) Determination of genetic sex of the embryo
   (c) Initiation of cleavage
   (d) Implantation of conceptus

Answers

1, *c*; 2, *c*; 3, *d*; 4, *c*; 5, *d*; 6, *b*; 7, *c*; 8, *d*.

CHAPTER 6

1. During 2nd week of development the blastocyst cavity becomes
   (a) Chorionic cavity
   (b) Extraembryonic coelom
   (c) Amniotic cavity
   (d) Primary yolk sac

2. Events occurring during 2nd week of development include all, *except*
   (a) Embryoblast differentiates into hypoblast and epiblast
   (b) Formation of amniotic cavity and primary yolk sac
   (c) Formation of intraembryonic mesoderm and intraembryonic coelom
   (d) Formation of amniogenic membrane and Heuser's membrane

3. Select *incorrect statement* about bilaminar germ disc.
   (a) Consists of epiblast and hypoblast
   (b) Is developed from embryoblast
   (c) Forms embryo proper
   (d) Forms trophoblast

4. During 2nd week of embryonic development, the blastocyst cavity is converted into:
   (a) Amniotic cavity
   (b) Primary yolk sac
   (c) Chorionic cavity
   (d) Extra embryonic cavity

Answers

1, *d*; 2, *c*; 3, *d*; 4, *b*.

CHAPTER 7

1. Which of the following structures represents remnant of notochord?
   (a) Centrum of body of vertebra
   (b) Nucleus pulposus
   (c) Membrana tectoria
   (d) Odontoid process of second cervical vertebra

2. All of the statements are true about notochord, *except*
   (a) It develops from Hensen's node
   (b) It induces formation of neural tube
   (c) It forms part of intervertebral disk
   (d) It extends headwards beyond prechordal plate

3. Somites differentiate to form all of the following, *except*
   (a) Notochord
   (b) Sclerotome
   (c) Myotome
   (d) Dermatome

4. Developing embryo has a distinct human appearance by the end of
   (a) 4th week
   (b) 5th week
   (c) 7th week
   (d) 8th week

5. Lateral plate mesoderm is divided into two distinct layers due to the formation of
   (a) Extraembryonic coelom
   (b) Amniotic cavity
   (c) Intraembryonic coelom
   (d) Yolk sac

6. Which of the following statements is *incorrect* regarding somites?
   (a) These are formed by the segmentation of paraxial mesoderm
   (b) Somite period extends from 20 to 30 days
   (c) First pair of somites appears in the occipital region
   (d) These form most of the appendicular skeleton

7. Chordoma arises from remnants of
   (a) Spinal cord
   (b) Nephrogenic cord
   (c) Notochord
   (d) Umbilical cord

8. All of the following are derivatives of intraembryonic mesoderm, *except*
   (a) Septum transversum
   (b) Somatopleuric mesoderm
   (c) Splanchnopleuric mesoderm
   (d) Connecting stalk

9. Select *incorrect statement* about notochord.
   (a) Lies between mesoderm and endoderm
   (b) Is connected to yolk sac via neurenteric canal
   (c) Extends from primitive knot to the *buccopharyngeal membrane*
   (d) Provides central axis for the development of axial skeleton

Answers

1, *b*; 2, *d*; 3, *a*; 4, *d*; 5, *c*; 6, *d*; 7, *c*; 8, *d*; 9, *a*.

CHAPTER 8

1. All of the following are derivatives of ectoderm *except*
   (a) Central nervous system
   (b) Mammary glands
   (c) Synovial membrane
   (d) Enamel of tooth

2. All are derivatives of mesoderm *except*
   (a) Skeletal muscles
   (b) Spleen
   (c) Sebaceous glands
   (d) Testes

3. Structures derived from endoderm include all *except*
   (a) Thyroid gland
   (b) Uterus
   (c) Thymus
   (d) Tonsils

4. Select the *incorrect statement.*
   (a) Pharyngeal arches appear on day 30
   (b) Buccopharyngeal membrane ruptures during 4th week
   (c) Cloacal membrane ruptures during 7th week
   (d) Upper limb buds appear before lower limb buds

5. Trilaminar embryonic disc acquires miniature human form at the end of
   (a) 7th week
   (b) 8th week
   (c) 9th week
   (d) 10th week

Answers

1, *c*; 2, *c*; 3, *b*; 4, *a*; 5, *b*.

CHAPTER 9

1. Select the *incorrect statement* regarding frequency of congenital anomalies involving various systems.
   (a) Integumentary system 20%
   (b) Central nervous system 14%
   (c) Musculoskeletal system 9%
   (d) Respiratory system 2%

2. Most susceptible period for teratogenesis is
   (a) 0 to 2 weeks
   (b) 3 to 8 weeks
   (c) 9 to 38 weeks
   (d) None of the above

3. All of the following drugs are absolutely contraindicated in pregnancy *except*
   (a) Thalidomide – an antinausea drug
   (b) Phenytoin – an antiepileptic drug
   (c) Triazolam – a hypnotic drug
   (d) Alprazolam – an antianxiety drug

4. Birth defects caused by multifactorial inheritance include all *except*
   (a) Neural tube defects
   (b) Cleft lip and cleft palate
   (c) Cri-du-chat syndrome (cat's cry syndrome)
   (d) Congenital heart defects

5. Commonest method used for prenatal diagnosis is
   (a) Ultrasonography
   (b) Maternal serum screening
   (c) Amniocentesis
   (d) Chorionic villus sampling

Answers

1, *c*; 2, *b*; 3. *d*; 4, *c*; 5, *a*.

CHAPTER 10

1. Placenta develops from
   (a) Decidua capsularis and chorion
   (b) Decidua capsularis and amnion
   (c) Decidua basalis and chorion
   (d) Decidua parietalis and trophoblast

2. Placental membrane in later stages of pregnancy mainly consists of
   (a) Cytotrophoblast and syncytiotrophoblast
   (b) Syncytiotrophoblast and fetal endothelium
   (c) Mesoderm and fetal endothelium
   (d) Syncytiotrophoblast only

3. All of the following are main functions of placenta, *except*
   (a) Transport of nutrients
   (b) Excretion of waste products
   (c) Growth of embryo and fetus
   (d) Exchange of gases O_2 and CO_2

4. Normal amount of amniotic fluid at full term is
   (a) 200 mL
   (b) 250 mL
   (c) 400 mL
   (d) 600 mL

5. Intervillous spaces of placenta contain
   (a) Fetal blood
   (b) Amniotic fluid
   (c) Maternal blood
   (d) Both fetal and maternal blood

6. Type of human placenta is
   (a) Epitheliochorial
   (b) Hemochorial
   (c) Endotheliochorial
   (d) Endothelioendothelial

7. In early pregnancy (i.e., up to 2 weeks), the *placental barrier* consists of all the structures, *except*
   (a) Syncytiotrophoblast
   (b) Cytotrophoblast
   (c) Extraembryonic mesoderm
   (d) Endothelium of fetal blood vessels

8. Pregnancy is maintained till term by
   (a) Follicle-stimulating hormone
   (b) Luteinizing hormone
   (c) Progesterone
   (d) Prostaglandins

Answers

1, *c*; 2, *b*; 3, *c*; 4, *c*; 5, *c*; 6, *b*; 7, *c*; 8, *c*.

CHAPTER 11

1. Skin develops from
   (a) Mesoderm and endoderm
   (b) Ectoderm and mesoderm
   (c) Ectoderm and endoderm
   (d) Surface ectoderm and neuroectoderm

2. Dendritic cells (melanoblasts) of skin are derived from
   (a) Ectoderm
   (b) Bone marrow
   (c) Endoderm
   (d) Neural crest

3. All of the following develop from ectoderm, *except*
   (a) Sweat glands
   (b) Dermis
   (c) Nail
   (d) Hair

4. Select *incorrect statement* about development of skin.
   (a) Epidermis is derived from ectoderm
   (b) Melanocytes are derived from neural crest cells
   (c) Langerhans cells are derived from endoderm
   (d) Dermis is derived from mesoderm

5. Three-layered epidermis in early development of skin does not consist of
   (a) Stratum basale
   (b) Intermediate layer
   (c) Periderm
   (d) Horny layer

6. Select *incorrect statement* about vernix caseosa.
   (a) It forms from exfoliated peridermal cells
   (b) It contains sebum
   (c) It protects fetal skin from toxic effects of amniotic fluid
   (d) It hinders the birth of fetus

7. All of the following are absent in the thick skin, *except*
   (a) Hair follicles
   (b) Arrector pili muscles
   (c) Sweat glands
   (d) Sebaceous glands

8. Select incorrect statement about melanocytes of the skin.
   (a) These develop from neural crest cells
   (b) These produce increased amount of melanin in response to ultraviolet light
   (c) In white races, their cell bodies are usually confined to basal layers
   (d) These begin producing melanin after birth

Answers

1, *b*; 2, *d*; 3, *b*; 4, *c*; 5, *d*; 6, *d*; 7, *c*; 8, *d*.

CHAPTER 12

1. All of the following develop by intramembranous ossification, *except*
   (a) Frontal bone
   (b) Parietal bone
   (c) Body of sphenoid bone
   (d) Tympanic part of temporal bone

2. All of the following bones develop by endochondral ossification, *except*
   (a) Ethmoid bone
   (b) Pterygoid processes of sphenoid
   (c) Petromastoid part of temporal bone
   (d) Occipital bone below superior nuchal line

3. All of the following are intersegmental in origin, *except*
   (a) Bodies of vertebrae
   (b) Intervertebral disks
   (c) Muscles of vertebral column
   (d) Spinal nerves supplying muscles of vertebral column

4. The mesodermal cells of sclerotomes
   (a) Around notochord form centrum of bodies of vertebrae
   (b) Around neural tube form vertebral arches
   (c) In body wall form trunk muscles
   (d) In between centrums of adjacent vertebrae form intervertebral disk

5. The costal element in the typical vertebra is a part of
   (a) Superior articular process
   (b) Inferior articular process
   (c) Transverse process
   (d) Spinous process

6. Structure responsible for growth in the length of bone is
   (a) Epiphysis
   (b) Diaphysis
   (c) Metaphysis
   (d) Epiphyseal cartilage

7. Fusion of two or more fingers or toes is called
   (a) Brachydactyly
   (b) Syndactyly
   (c) Polydactyly
   (d) Ectrodactyly

8. Secondary ossification center present at or just before birth (9th month of IUL) is present
   (a) At the distal end of femur
   (b) At the lower end of tibia
   (c) At the medial end of clavicle
   (d) At the lower end of radius

Answers
1, *c*; 2, *b*; 3, *b*; 4, *c*; 5, *c*; 6, *d*; 7, *b*; 8, *a*.

CHAPTER 13

1. Limb muscles develop from
   (a) Paraxial mesoderm
   (b) Lateral plate mesoderm
   (c) Splanchnic mesoderm
   (d) Neural crest cells

2. Muscles of tongue develop from
   (a) Preotic myotomes
   (b) Preoccipital myotomes
   (c) Occipital myotomes
   (d) Cervical myotomes

3. All of the following are preaxial muscles, *except*
   (a) Scalenes
   (b) Geniohyoid
   (c) Infrahyoid
   (d) Prevertebral

4. The hypomeric musculature of the body does not include
   (a) Extensor muscles of the vertebral column
   (b) Scalene muscles
   (c) Quadratus lumborum
   (d) Pelvic diaphragm

5. Select the *incorrect statement* about the development of muscles.
   (a) Epimeres form extensor muscle of spine
   (b) Hypomeres form prevertebral, intercostals, and abdominal muscles
   (c) Muscles derived from epimeres are supplied by ventral rami of spinal nerves
   (d) Cardiac muscle develops from splanchnic mesoderm

6. Muscle not derived from hypomeres in the cervical region is
   (a) Prevertebral
   (b) Infrahyoid
   (c) Laryngeal
   (d) Pharyngeal

7. All of the following are responsible for molecular regulation of muscle development, *except*
   (a) *BMP4*
   (b) *MyoD* genes
   (c) *MRFs*
   (d) Homeobox genes

8. Select the *incorrect statement.*
   (a) Most of the muscles of head and neck region are derived from somatomeres
   (b) Cardiac muscle and most of the smooth muscles are derived from splanchnic mesoderm
   (c) Extraocular muscles develop from preotic myotome
   (d) Muscles of iris develop from surface ectoderm

9. Preotic myotomes are arranged around
   (a) Otic capsule
   (b) Optic vesicle
   (c) Nasal capsule
   (d) None of the above

Answers
1, *a*; 2, *c*; 3, *c*; 4, *a*; 5, *c*; 6, *d*; 7, *d*; 8, *d*; 9, *b*.

CHAPTER 14

1. Pharyngeal arch supplied by two cranial nerves is
   (a) First pharyngeal arch
   (b) Second pharyngeal arch
   (c) Fourth pharyngeal arch
   (d) Sixth pharyngeal arch

2. Nerve supplying the muscles of sixth arch is
   (a) External laryngeal
   (b) Internal laryngeal
   (c) Recurrent laryngeal
   (d) None of the above

3. Derivatives of first pharyngeal arch do not include
   (a) Maxilla
   (b) Mandible
   (c) Masseter muscle
   (d) Orbicularis oculi muscle

4. Endodermal lining of tonsil is derived from
   (a) First pharyngeal pouch
   (b) Second pharyngeal pouch
   (c) Third pharyngeal pouch
   (d) Fourth pharyngeal pouch

5. First pharyngeal pouch forms
   (a) External auditory meatus
   (b) Middle ear and pharyngotympanic tube
   (c) Internal ear
   (d) Both middle and internal ears

6. First pharyngeal cleft forms
   (a) Internal auditory meatus
   (b) External auditory meatus
   (c) Tympanic cavity
   (d) Epitympanic recess

7. Parafollicular cells or C cells of thyroid gland develop from
   (a) First pharyngeal pouch
   (b) Second pharyngeal pouch
   (c) Third pharyngeal pouch
   (d) Caudal pharyngeal complex

8. Cartilage of the larynx which does not develop from fourth and sixth arch cartilages is
   (a) Epiglottis
   (b) Thyroid
   (c) Cricoid
   (d) Arytenoid

Answers
1, *a*; 2, *c*; 3, *d*; 4, *b*; 5, *b*; 6, *b*; 7, *d*; 8, *a*.

CHAPTER 15

1. The tongue develops from all the pharyngeal arches, *except*
   (a) First
   (b) Third
   (c) Fourth
   (d) Sixth

2. The parafollicular cells or C cells of thyroid gland develop from
   (a) First pharyngeal pouch
   (b) Second pharyngeal pouch
   (c) Third pharyngeal pouch
   (d) Fourth pharyngeal pouch

3. Select the *incorrect statement* about the development of tongue.
   (a) Development of tongue begins in the 4th week of IUL
   (b) Anterior two-third of tongue develops from two lingual swellings
   (c) Muscles of the tongue develop from occipital myotomes
   (d) Posterior-most part of tongue develops from third pharyngeal arch

4. Select the *incorrect statement* about the development of tongue.
   (a) Mucous membrane of the tongue is derived from the endoderm of the primitive foregut
   (b) Muscles of tongue develop from the mesoderm of the pharyngeal arches
   (c) Fibroareolar septa binding the muscles of tongue develop from mesenchyme of the pharyngeal arches
   (d) Muscles of tongue develop from occipital myotomes

5. All of the following provide general sensory innervation to the tongue, *except*
   (a) Lingual nerve
   (b) Chorda tympani nerve
   (c) Glossopharyngeal nerve
   (d) Superior laryngeal nerve

6. All of the following are true about development of lingual papillae and taste buds, *except*
   (a) Lingual papillae appear toward the end of the 8th week of IUL
   (b) Fungiform and filiform papillae appear late
   (c) Vallate and foliate papillae appear first
   (d) Taste buds develop by the inductive interaction between the epithelial cells of tongue and terminal branches of gustatory nerves innervating them

7. Select the *incorrect statement* about the development of thyroid.
   (a) First endocrine gland to develop
   (b) Begins to develop about 24 days after fertilization
   (c) Pyramidal lobe develops from the distal end of the thyroglossal duct
   (d) Starts functioning by the end of the 6th month

8. Thyroid gland starts functioning by the end of
   (a) 3rd month
   (b) 4th month
   (c) 5th month
   (d) 6th month

Answers

1, *d*; 2, *d*; 3, *d*; 4, *b*; 5, *b*; 6, *b*; 7, *d*; 8, *a*.

CHAPTER 16

1. Upper lip develops from all processes, *except*
   (a) Frontonasal process
   (b) Medial nasal processes
   (c) Lateral nasal processes
   (d) Maxillary processes

2. Nasolacrimal groove lies in the line of fusion of maxillary process and
   (a) Lateral nasal process
   (b) Medial nasal process
   (c) Mandibular process
   (d) Frontonasal process

3. Which of the following is the most common congenital anomaly of face?
   (a) Median cleft of upper lip
   (b) Unilateral cleft of upper lip
   (c) Unilateral cleft of upper lip with cleft palate
   (d) Unilateral cleft palate

4. Select *incorrect statement* about the development of nose.
   (a) Dorsum is formed by frontonasal process
   (b) Nasal cavities are formed by nasal pits
   (c) Choanae are formed by rupture of oronasal membranes
   (d) Apex is formed by lateral nasal process

5. All the paranasal air sinuses develop before birth, *except*
   (a) Maxillary
   (b) Ethmoidal
   (c) Frontal
   (d) Sphenoidal

6. Primary palate develops from
   (a) Frontonasal process
   (b) Maxillary processes
   (c) Mandibular processes
   (d) Lateral nasal processes

7. Secondary palate develops from
   (a) Frontonasal process
   (b) Median nasal process
   (c) Maxillary processes
   (d) Lateral nasal processes

8. Nasal septum develops from
   (a) Lateral nasal process
   (b) Frontonasal process
   (c) Nasobuccal membrane
   (d) Maxillary processes

Answers

1, *c*; 2, *a*; 3, *b*; 4, *d*; 5, *c*; 6, *a*; 7, *c*; 8, *b*.

CHAPTER 17

1. All of the following arteries supply primitive gut, *except*
   (a) Celiac artery
   (b) Superior mesenteric artery
   (c) Inferior mesenteric artery
   (d) Median sacral artery

2. During which week of IUL the buccopharyngeal membrane ruptures?
   (a) 4th
   (b) 6th
   (c) 8th
   (d) 10th

3. During which week of intrauterine life (IUL) the cloacal membrane ruptures?
   (a) 5th
   (b) 7th
   (c) 9th
   (d) 11th

4. All parts of the gastrointestinal tract (GIT) are solely derived from foregut, *except*
   (a) Pharynx
   (b) Esophagus
   (c) Stomach
   (d) Duodenum

5. All of the following are derivatives of the midgut, *except*
   (a) Duodenum distal to the entrance of common bile duct
   (b) Cecum
   (c) Left one-third of transverse colon
   (d) Appendix

6. All of the following statements are true for physiological hernia of midgut loop, *except*
   (a) It occurs because abdominal cavity fails to accommodate enlarging midgut loop
   (b) It occurs at the 6th week of IUL
   (c) It is reduced at the 10th week of IUL
   (d) It occurs only in female fetus

7. All of the following statements are correct about Meckel's diverticulum, *except*
   (a) It arises from antimesenteric border of ileum
   (b) It is persistence of vitellointestinal duct
   (c) It is about 2 cm in length
   (d) It is present about 2 feet proximal to ileocecal junction

8. All of the following statements are true about midgut rotation, *except*
   (a) Total anticlockwise rotation is 270°
   (b) First 90° anticlockwise rotation occurs within the umbilicus
   (c) Remaining 180° anticlockwise rotation occurs within the abdominal cavity
   (d) Nonrotation may cause gastroschisis

9. Select the *incorrect statement* about congenital megacolon.
   (a) It occurs due to the absence of parasympathetic ganglion in the colonic wall
   (b) It is produced due to failure of migration of neural crest cells in the wall of colon
   (c) It commonly affects sigmoid colon and rectum
   (d) It occurs due to the absence of sympathetic ganglia in the wall of colon

Answers

1, *d*; 2, *a*; 3, *b*; 4, *d*; 5, *c*; 6, *d*; 7, *c*; 8, *d*; 9, *d*.

CHAPTER 18

1. Liver develops from all of the following, *except*
   (a) Endoderm
   (b) Ectoderm
   (c) Septum transversum
   (d) Breaking of vitelline and umbilical veins

2. All of the following are derivatives of foregut, *except*
   (a) Stomach
   (b) Liver
   (c) Spleen
   (d) Pancreas

3. Dorsal pancreatic bud forms all parts of the pancreas, *except*
   (a) Upper part of head
   (b) Body
   (c) Tail
   (d) Uncinate process

4. Proximal part of main pancreatic duct (duct of Wirsung) develops from
   (a) Hepatic duct
   (b) Cystic duct
   (c) Ventral pancreatic duct
   (d) Dorsal pancreatic duct

5. Mesoderm of septum transversum forms all the elements of liver, *except*
   (a) Glisson's capsule
   (b) Peritoneal coverings
   (c) Blood vessels
   (d) Epithelial lining of bile ductules

6. Ectopic splenic tissue may be found at all sites, *except*
   (a) Gastrosplenic ligament
   (b) Hepatogastric ligament
   (c) Greater omentum
   (d) Left spermatic cord

7. The most fatal congenital anomaly of the liver is
   (a) Riedel lobe
   (b) Appendix of liver
   (c) Intrahepatic biliary atresia
   (d) Polycystic liver

8. The most common variation of pancreatic duct system is
   (a) Occlusion of accessory pancreatic duct
   (b) Discontinuation between dorsal and ventral pancreatic ducts
   (c) Inversion of pancreatic ducts
   (d) Absence of duodenal end of accessory pancreatic duct

Answers

1, *b*; 2, *c*; 3, *d*; 4, *c*; 5, *d*; 6, *b*; 7, *c*; 8, *a*.

CHAPTER 19

1. All of the following are involved in the development of mouth, *except*
   (a) Stomodeum
   (b) Oronasal membrane
   (c) Foregut
   (d) Buccopharyngeal membrane

2. Epithelium of all the following structures is ectodermal in origin, *except*
   (a) Hard palate
   (b) Sides of mouth
   (c) Lips
   (d) Tongue

3. Epithelial lining of all the following structures is endodermal in origin, *except*
   (a) Tongue
   (b) Floor of mouth
   (c) Soft palate
   (d) Hard palate

4. Select the *incorrect* statement about development of major salivary glands.
   (a) All develop from epithelial lining of primitive oral cavity
   (b) Epithelial buds of parotid glands arise from the angles of stomodeum
   (c) Epithelial buds of submandibular glands arise from the floor of linguogingival sulcus
   (d) Epithelial buds of sublingual gland arise from the floor of labiogingival sulcus

5. All of the following are the stages of development of tooth, *except*
   (a) Bud stage
   (b) Cap stage
   (c) Balloon stage
   (d) Bell stage

6. Which of the following provides the bulk and general form of the tooth?
   (a) Enamel
   (b) Dentin
   (c) Pulp
   (d) Cementum

7. All of the following are involved in the development of teeth (dentition), *except*
   (a) Ameloblasts
   (b) Odontoblasts
   (c) Osteoclasts
   (d) Osteocytes

8. Second hardest tissue in the body is
   (a) Enamel
   (b) Dentin
   (c) Bone
   (d) Hyaline cartilage

Answers

1, *b*; 2, *d*; 3, *d*; 4, *d*; 5, *c*; 6, *b*; 7, *d*; 8, *b*.

CHAPTER 20

1. First sign of development of the respiratory system is development of
   (a) Laryngotracheal groove
   (b) Primitive foregut
   (c) Respiratory diverticulum
   (d) Hypobranchial eminence

2. All of the following statements are true about surfactant, *except*
   (a) It is produced at the end of the 6th month of IUL
   (b) It forms a thin lining of alveoli
   (c) It reduces surface tension at the air–alveolar surface
   (d) It is produced by type I alveolar epithelial cells (type I pneumocytes)

3. *Blood–air barrier* in the lung consists of
   (a) Endoderm only
   (b) Mesoderm only
   (c) Mesoderm and endoderm
   (d) Mesoderm and ectoderm

4. All of the following statements are correct regarding respiratory diverticulum, *except*
   (a) It is an outgrowth of the ventral wall of foregut
   (b) It appears when embryo is about 4 weeks old
   (c) It is mesodermal in origin
   (d) It first appears as a midline laryngotracheal groove

5. Select the *incorrect statement* about the development of lung.
   (a) Right principal bronchus divides into three lobar bronchi
   (b) Left principal bronchus divides into two lobar bronchi

(c) By the end of 6th month, seven generations of subdivision of bronchi are formed
(d) Respiratory bronchioles are formed during canalicular stage of lung maturation

6. The stage of maturation of the lung that extends from 16 to 26 weeks is called
(a) Pseudoglandular stage
(b) Canalicular stage
(c) Terminal sac stage
(d) Alveolar stage

7. All laryngeal cartilages develop from neural crest mesenchyme of fourth and sixth pharyngeal arches, *except*
(a) Epiglottis
(b) Thyroid cartilage
(c) Cricoid cartilage
(d) Arytenoid cartilages

8. All of the following are features of alveolar stage of lung maturation, *except*
(a) Number of alveolar sac increases
(b) Blood capillaries come in intimate contact with the alveolar sacs
(c) Alveolar sac is lined by *type I* and *type II* pneumocytes
(d) *Type I pneumocytes* secrete surfactant

Answers

1, *a*; 2, *d*; 3, *c*; 4, *c*; 5, *c*; 6, *b*; 7, *a*; 8, *d*.

CHAPTER 21

1. The embryonic structure that does not contribute to the formation of diaphragm is
(a) Septum transversum
(b) Pleuroperitoneal membranes
(c) Dorsal mesogastrium
(d) Mesoderm of the body wall

2. Pericardial cavity is separated from the pleural cavity by
(a) Pleuroperitoneal membrane
(b) Pleuropericardial fold
(c) Pleuropericardial membrane
(d) Septum transversum

3. All of the following embryological events are involved in the development of the lesser sac, *except*
(a) Development of pneumoenteric recesses in the dorsal mesogastrium
(b) Regression of right pneumoenteric recess
(c) Rotation of stomach
(d) Formation of the greater omentum

4. Select the *incorrect statement* about intraembryonic coelom.
(a) It begins to develop near the end of the 3rd week
(b) It becomes horseshoe shaped by the 4th week
(c) Cranially, it communicates with extraembryonic coelom
(d) It divides lateral plate mesoderm into two layers

5. Select *incorrect statement* about pericardial cavity.
(a) It develops from the part of intraembryonic coelom that develops first
(b) It develops in the region of pericardial bar
(c) It communicates with the peritoneal cavity until the 3rd week
(d) It is separated from the pleural cavity by the pleuropericardial membrane

6. All of the following are correct about esophageal *hiatal hernia, except*
(a) Herniation of stomach through esophageal opening into the diaphragm
(b) It makes esophageal hiatus incompetent
(c) It causes projectile vomiting when infant is laid on its back after feeding
(d) It causes respiratory distress when infant is laid on the either side after feeding

7. All of the following statements are correct about CDH, *except*
(a) It occurs about once in 2200 births
(b) It occurs through foramen of Bochdalek
(c) About 99% newborns die
(d) Cause of death is respiratory distress

8. Which of the following is an *incorrect statement* about congenital diaphragmatic hernia?
   (a) Occurs through a defect in the posterolateral aspect of the diaphragm
   (b) Causes hypoplasia of the lungs
   (c) Can be detected prenatally in about 50% cases
   (d) Occurs mostly on the right side

Answers
1, *c*; 2, *c*; 3, *b*; 4, *c*; 5, *c*; 6, *d*; 7, *c*; 8, *d*.

CHAPTER 22

1. Heart starts beating on day
   (a) 16
   (b) 22
   (c) 28
   (d) 34

2. U-shaped loop of the heart tube
   (a) Has cranial arterial end
   (b) Has caudal venous end
   (c) Invaginates pericardial cavity from the dorsal side
   (d) Is initially suspended from ventral wall of the pericardial cavity by ventral mesogastrium

3. All of the following are dilatations of primary heart tube, *except*
   (a) Bulbus cordis
   (b) Primitive ventricle
   (c) Right atrium
   (d) Sinus venosus

4. All of the following contribute to the formation of interatrial septum, *except*
   (a) Septum primum
   (b) Septum secundum
   (c) Spiral septum
   (d) Septum spurium

5. Right valve of sinoatrial orifice forms all, *except*
   (a) Crista terminalis
   (b) Valve of inferior vena cava
   (c) Valve of coronary sinus
   (d) Septum spurium

6. All of the following are features of Fallot tetralogy, *except*
   (a) Interventricular septal defect
   (b) Overriding of aorta
   (c) Aortic stenosis
   (d) Hypertrophy of the right ventricle

7. All of the following form interventricular septum, *except*
   (a) Right bulbar ridge
   (b) Left bulbar ridge
   (c) Atrioventricular cushions
   (d) Spiral septum

8. Ventricles develop from
   (a) Distal part of bulbus cordis
   (b) Proximal part of bulbus cordis
   (c) Atrioventricular canals
   (d) Primitive ventricular chamber

Answers
1, *b*; 2, *d*; 3, *c*; 4, *c*; 5, *d*; 6, *c*; 7, *d*; 8, *d*.

CHAPTER 23

1. All of the following statements are true about aortic arch arteries, *except*
   (a) These are five in number
   (b) These are numbered I, II, III, IV, and V
   (c) These are numbered I, II, III, IV, and VI
   (d) These connect aortic sac horns with the dorsal aortae

2. Arch aorta does not develop from
   (a) Ventral part of aortic sac
   (b) Left horn of aortic sac
   (c) Left fourth aortic arch artery
   (d) Left seventh intersegmental artery

3. First aortic arch artery gives rise to
   (a) Maxillary artery
   (b) Hyoid artery
   (c) Stapedial artery
   (d) Facial artery

4. Select *incorrect statement* about ductus arteriosus.
   (a) It is derived from the distal part of the left sixth arch artery
   (b) It carries blood from the right ventricle to the dorsal aorta
   (c) The bradykinin secreted by lungs helps in its closure
   (d) It forms ligamentum venosum after birth

5. All arteries represent axis artery of upper limb, *except*
   (a) Axillary
   (b) Brachial
   (c) Posterior interosseous
   (d) Anterior interosseous

6. Axis artery of lower limb is represented by all, *except*
   (a) Inferior gluteal
   (b) Popliteal artery
   (c) Femoral artery
   (d) Plantar arch

7. All of the following contribute to the formation of the inferior vena cava, *except*
   (a) Posterior cardinal vein
   (b) Supracardinal vein
   (c) Intersubcardinal veins
   (d) Supracardinal–subcardinal anastomosis

8. Left renal vein is derived from all, *except*
   (a) Mesonephric vein
   (b) Subcardinal vein
   (c) Anastomosis between subcardinal veins
   (d) Supracardinal vein

9. Superior mesenteric vein is formed by
   (a) Vitelline vein
   (b) Umbilical vein
   (c) Anterior cardinal vein
   (d) Posterior cardinal vein

10. Left gonadal vein is formed by
   (a) Left supracardinal vein
   (b) Left sacrocardinal vein
   (c) Left posterior cardinal vein
   (d) Anastomosis between subcardinal veins

Answers

1, *b*; 2, *d*; 3, *a*; 4, *d*; 5, *c*; 6, *c*; 7, *c*; 8, *d*; 9, *b*; 10, *b*.

CHAPTER 24

1. Select the *incorrect statement* about the development of kidney.
   (a) Three successive kidneys develop in craniocaudal direction
   (b) The one which persists in the lumbar region to form a permanent kidney
   (c) The collecting system of kidney develops from ureteric bud
   (d) The development of the excretory system is induced by ureteric bud

2. Mesonephros
   (a) It forms in thoracolumbar region
   (b) It gives rise to excretory tubules
   (c) It appears at the beginning of the 3rd month
   (d) It functions only till the 10th week of IUL

3. All of the following are adult derivatives of ureteric bud, *except*
   (a) Renal pelvis
   (b) Minor calyces
   (c) Collecting tubules
   (d) Distal convoluted tubule

4. Ureteric bud arises from
   (a) Mesonephric duct
   (b) Paramesonephric duct
   (c) Vesicourethral canal
   (d) Urogenital sinus

5. Metanephric blastema gives rise to all, *except*
   (a) Bowman's capsule
   (b) Loop of Henle
   (c) Distal convoluted tubule
   (d) Collecting tubules

6. Definitive kidney develops from
   (a) Metanephros
   (b) Pronephros
   (c) Mesonephros
   (d) Wolffian duct

7. All of the following statements are true regarding horseshoe kidney, *except*
   (a) It occurs due to fusion of lower poles of two kidney
   (b) Inferior mesenteric artery lies ventral to isthmus
   (c) It lies at L1 vertebra level
   (d) Ureters pass anterior to the isthmus

8. Polycystic kidney
   (a) May be inherited as an autosomal recessive disorder
   (b) May be inherited as an autosomal dominant disorder
   (c) May occur due to splitting of ureteric bud
   (d) May occur due to dilatations in loops of Henle

9. Persistent lumen in urachus along its entire extent leads to a clinical condition called
   (a) Urachal sinus
   (b) Urachal cyst
   (c) Urachal fistula
   (d) Vitelline fistula

10. Absorption of mesonephric ducts in the urogenital sinus
   (a) Forms epithelial lining of trigone of urinary bladder
   (b) Makes mesonephric ducts and ureters to open separately in the urogenital sinus
   (c) Forms ejaculatory ducts in males
   (d) Forms ducts of Bartholin glands in females

Answers

1, *b*; 2, *c*; 3, *d*; 4, *a*; 5, *d*; 6, *a*; 7, *c*; 8, *d*; 9, *c*; 10, *a*.

CHAPTER 25

1. All of the following statements are correct regarding the development of testis, *except*
   (a) Primordial germ cells migrate from wall of yolk sac to the developing testis
   (b) Seminiferous tubules develop from second generation of sex cords
   (c) Rete testis is formed by first generation of sex cords
   (d) Leydig cells develop from mesoderm

2. All of the following statements are correct regarding the development of ovary, *except*
   (a) It develops from genital ridge in the upper lumbar region of posterior abdominal wall
   (b) Its primordial follicles are formed from primordial germ cells and coelomic epithelial cells
   (c) Two generations of sex cords form during its development
   (d) Its first generation of sex cords forms primordial follicles

3. In females, the paramesonephric duct (Mullerian duct) gives rise to all, *except*
   (a) Fallopian tubes
   (b) Cervix
   (c) Upper part of vagina
   (d) Vestibule of vagina

4. Genital swellings in females give rise to
   (a) Clitoris
   (b) Labia majora
   (c) Labia minora
   (d) Vagina

5. In males, mesonephric (Wolffian) duct gives rise to all, *except*
   (a) Rete testis
   (b) Efferent ductules
   (c) Duct of epididymis
   (d) Seminal vesicle

6. Genital swellings in males give rise to
   (a) Penis
   (b) Scrotal sac
   (c) Penile urethra
   (d) Prostate

7. Seminal vesicle develops from
   (a) Mullerian duct
   (b) Wolffian duct
   (c) Prostatic urethra
   (d) Membranous urethra

8. Congenital inguinal hernia in females may occur due to
   (a) Indecent of ovary
   (b) Presence of canal of Nuck
   (c) Shortening of gubernaculum of ovary
   (d) Absence of urogenital mesentery

9. Sinovaginal bulbs fuse to form
   (a) Clitoris
   (b) Vestibule of vagina
   (c) Vaginal plate
   (d) Uterovaginal canal

10. The phenotypic sexual differentiation of external genitalia begins at
   (a) 5th week of IUL
   (b) 7th week of IUL
   (c) 9th week of IUL
   (d) 11th week of IUL

11. Embryologically, the labia minora arise from
   (a) Paramesonephric ducts
   (b) Urethral folds
   (c) Sinovaginal bulbs
   (d) Genital swellings

Answers

1, *b*; 2, *d*; 3, *d*; 4, *b*; 5, *a*; 6, *b*; 7, *b*; 8, *b*; 9, *c*; 10, *b*; 11, *b*.

CHAPTER 26

1. All of the following are derivatives of neural crest, *except*
   (a) Neurons of dorsal root ganglia
   (b) Schwann cells
   (c) Melanoblasts of skin
   (d) Microglia

2. Lower end of the spinal cord of a 24-week-old embryo ends at the level of lower border of
   (a) First coccygeal vertebra
   (b) First sacral vertebra
   (c) Third lumbar vertebra
   (d) First lumbar vertebra

3. In adults, at which lumbar vertebral level the lower end of spinal cord ends?
   (a) Lower border of L3
   (b) Lower border of L2
   (c) Upper border of L1
   (d) Lower border of L1

4. All of the following are primary brain vesicles, *except*
   (a) Prosencephalon
   (b) Diencephalon
   (c) Mesencephalon
   (d) Rhombencephalon

5. Cerebellum develops from
   (a) Basal plate of metencephalon
   (b) Alar plate of metencephalon
   (c) Basal plate of myelencephalon
   (d) Alar plate of myelencephalon

6. During histogenesis of neural tube, the neuroepithelial cells lining neural canal form all, *except*
   (a) Ependymal cells
   (b) Neurons of ventral horns
   (c) Neurons of dorsal horns
   (d) Neurons of dorsal root ganglia

7. Fourth ventricle represents cavity of
   (a) Prosencephalon
   (b) Diencephalon
   (c) Mesencephalon
   (d) Rhombencephalon

8. All of the following statements are true regarding Arnold–Chiari malformation, *except*
   (a) It is not a congenital anomaly
   (b) Tonsils of cerebellum herniate through foramen magnum
   (c) Increase in CSF pressure
   (d) Stretching of IX, X, XI, and XII cranial nerves

9. All functional columns are present in the basal plate of hindbrain, *except*
   (a) General somatic efferent
   (b) General visceral efferent
   (c) Special somatic afferent
   (d) Special visceral efferent

10. All of the following statements are true regarding hydrocephalus, *except*
    (a) It occurs due to excessive production of CSF
    (b) It occurs due to blockage of passage of CSF circulation
    (c) It causes decreased intracranial pressure
    (d) It occurs due to microcephaly

Answers
1, *d*; 2, *b*; 3, *d*; 4, *b*; 5, *b*; 6, *d*; 7, *d*; 8, *a*; 9, *c*; 10, *c*.

CHAPTER 27

1. Which of the following components in the adrenal gland is formed by neural crest cells?
   (a) Zona glomerulosa
   (b) Zona fasciculata
   (c) Zona reticulata
   (d) Medulla

2. Rathke's pouch forms all, *except*
   (a) Pars anterior
   (b) Pars nervosa
   (c) Pars intermedia
   (d) Pars tuberalis

3. Infundibulum that grows from the floor of the third ventricle forms part of
   (a) Adenohypophysis
   (b) Neurohypophysis
   (c) Pars intermedia
   (d) Pars tuberalis

4. All of the following statements are correct regarding the development of adrenal gland, *except*
   (a) Its cortex forms from two episodes of proliferation of mesodermal cells of coelomic epithelium
   (b) Its medulla forms from neural crest
   (c) Its fetal cortex is absent at birth
   (d) The zona reticularis in its cortex is not formed until 3 years of age

Answers

1, *d*; 2, *b*; 3, *b*; 4, *c*.

CHAPTER 28

1. Select *incorrect statement* regarding the development of various components of the eye.
   (a) Retina develops from neuroectoderm
   (b) Lens develops from surface ectoderm
   (c) Vitreous body develops from endoderm
   (d) Sclera develops from mesoderm

2. Dilator and sphincter pupillae muscles of the iris develop from
   (a) Surface ectoderm
   (b) Neuroectoderm
   (c) Mesoderm
   (d) Neural crest cells

3. All of the following are derivatives of the dorsal part of otic vesicle, *except*
   (a) Saccule
   (b) Utricle
   (c) Semicircular canals
   (d) Endolymphatic duct

4. Auricular hillocks develop around the dorsal end/ends of
   (a) First pharyngeal arch
   (b) First and second pharyngeal arches
   (c) Second pharyngeal arch
   (d) Second and third pharyngeal arches

5. All of the following develop from hyoid arch, *except*
   (a) Helix
   (b) Antihelix
   (c) Tragus
   (d) Antitragus

6. All of the following develop from mesoderm, *except*
   (a) Substantia propria of the cornea
   (b) Ciliary muscle
   (c) Sphincter pupillae
   (d) Vitreous body

7. All of the following develop from first pharyngeal arch, *except*
   (a) Tensor tympani muscle
   (b) Stapedius muscle
   (c) Malleus
   (d) Incus

8. Select the *incorrect statement* regarding development of ear.
   (a) External auditory meatus develops from first pharyngeal cleft
   (b) Tubotympanic cavity develops from first pharyngeal pouch
   (c) Outer layer of tympanic membrane is ectodermal in origin
   (d) Antitragus develops from mandibular arch

Answers

1, *c*; 2, *b*; 3, *a*; 4, *b*; 5, *c*; 6, *c*; 7, *b*; 8, *d*.

CHAPTER 29

1. Each nucleotide consists of all of the following subunits, *except*
   (a) A molecule of deoxyribose sugar
   (b) A molecule of ribose sugar
   (c) A molecule of nitrogenous base
   (d) A molecule of phosphate

2. All of the following nitrogenous bases are present in a DNA molecule, *except*
   (a) Adenine
   (b) Thymine
   (c) Uracil
   (d) Guanine

3. Select the *incorrect statement* about the chromosomes.
   (a) Each chromosome presents a primary constriction called centromere
   (b) Number of chromosomes is not constant in a species
   (c) Each somatic cell contains 23 pairs of chromosomes
   (d) Females have two X chromosomes (XX) in each somatic cell

4. Select the *incorrect statement* about the Barr body.
   (a) Structurally, it represents an X chromosome that is genetically inactive

(b) Generally, it is located on the outer surface of nuclear membrane
(c) The number of Barr bodies in a cell is equal to the total number of X chromosomes minus one
(d) In neurons, it appears as a small dark body opposite the nucleolus

5. Select the *correct statement* about karyotyping.
   (a) Chromosomes are arranged in seven groups, referred to by letters A–G
   (b) Chromosomes of group A and group F are submetacentric
   (c) Chromosomes of group D and group G are metacentric
   (d) X chromosome belongs to group G and Y chromosome belongs to group C

6. Clinical conditions caused by trisomy include all of the following, *except*
   (a) Patau syndrome
   (b) Down syndrome
   (c) Klinefelter syndrome
   (d) Cri-du-chat syndrome

7. Clinical features of Down syndrome include all of the following, except
   (a) Oblique palpebral fissures with epicanthic folds
   (b) Presence of simian crease
   (c) Long protruding tongue
   (d) Long legs and arms

8. Select the *incorrect statement* about Klinefelter syndrome.
   (a) It is a trisomic condition found only in females
   (b) The affected individual is sex chromatin–positive
   (c) The affected individual has increased level of gonadotrophin
   (d) Lengths of legs and arms are usually longer than normal

9. Which of the following clinical condition is caused by monosomy?
   (a) Klinefelter syndrome
   (b) Turner syndrome
   (c) Down syndrome
   (d) Cri-du-chat syndrome

10. Select the *incorrect statement* about X-linked recessive inheritance.
   (a) It usually affects males
   (b) It usually affects females
   (c) It may affect females rarely
   (d) Females act as carriers

Answers

1, *b*; 2, *c*; 3, *b*; 4, *b*; 5, *a*; 6, *d*; 7, *d*; 8, *a*; 9, *b*; 10, *b*.

CHAPTER 30

1. Most susceptible period of pregnancy to teratogenesis is
   (a) 0–2 weeks
   (b) 3–8 weeks
   (c) 9–14 weeks
   (d) 15–38 weeks

2. Common cause of congenital birth defects is
   (a) Infection
   (b) Radiation
   (c) Genetic
   (d) Trauma

3. Amniocentesis is usually done between weeks
   (a) 8 and 10
   (b) 10 and 12
   (c) 12 and 14
   (d) 14 and 16

4. All of the following parameters are used during ultrasonography to determine the gestational age of fetus, *except*
   (a) Biparietal diameter (BPD)
   (b) Head circumference
   (c) Abdominal circumference
   (d) Crown-rump length

Answers

1, *b*; 2, *c*; 3, *d*; 4, *d*.

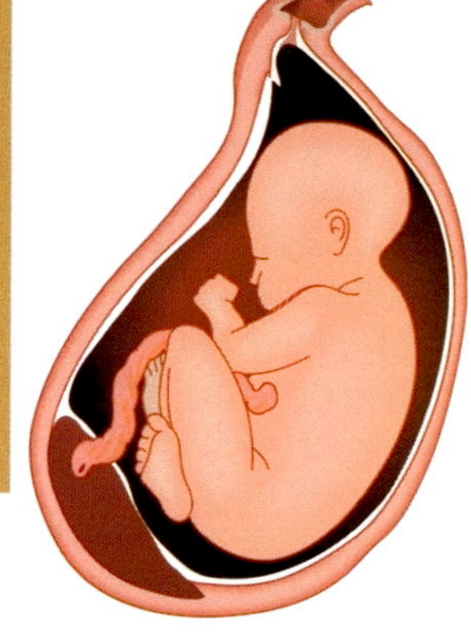

Index

D